Pain 2010—An Updated Review:
Refresher Course Syllabus

IASP Refresher Courses on Pain Management
held in conjunction with the 13th World Congress on Pain

August 29–September 2, 2010
Montreal, Quebec, Canada

IASP Scientific Program Committee

Jeffrey S. Mogil, PhD, Canada, *Chair*

Nadine Attal, MD, PhD, France

Rafael Benoliel, BDS, Israel

Phyllis Berger, BSc, South Africa

Mary Cardosa, MB BS, Malaysia

José Castro-Lopes, MD, PhD, Portugal, *ex officio*

Michael Caterina, MD, PhD, USA

Jun Chen, MD, PhD, China

Joyce De Leo, PhD, USA

Fernando de Queiróz Cunha, PhD, Brazil

Gerald Gebhart, PhD, USA, *ex officio*

Kathy Kreiter, USA, *ex officio*

Lance McCracken, PhD, United Kingdom

Karin Petersen, MD, USA

Srinivasa Raja, MD, USA

Martin Schmelz, MD, Germany

Michele Sterling, PhD, Australia

Bonnie Stevens, RN, PhD, Canada

Audun Stubhaug, MD, Norway

Victor Tortorici, PhD, Venezuela

Irene Tracey, PhD, United Kingdom

Hiroshi Ueda, PhD, Japan

Johannes Vlaeyen, PhD, Belgium

IASP PRESS® • SEATTLE

Preface

The chapters in this volume were written by the contributors to the Refresher Courses offered in conjunction with the 13th World Congress on Pain, held on August 29–September 2, 2010, in Montreal, Quebec, Canada.

Refresher Courses are among the most popular components of World Congresses, and this year saw the addition of several new courses and many new speakers. The courses, and by extension this book, truly cover the gamut of modern pain research and treatment, with topics ranging from state-of-the-art techniques (e.g., brain imaging, genetics, and animal and volunteer models) and treatments (e.g., interventional therapies, psychological therapies, and pharmacotherapies) to the state of the art in our understanding of pain disorders (e.g., cancer pain, neuropathic pain, musculoskeletal pain, complex regional pain syndrome, orofacial pain and headache, persistent postoperative pain, abdominal/pelvic pain, low back pain, and pediatric pain) and comorbidities (pain and addiction). I draw your attention especially to a few completely new courses, on pediatric pain, orofacial pain, and challenges in drug development. Whether you are new to pain research or a clinician looking to brush up your skills or thinking of delving into a new technique or treatment strategy, you'll find this book a valuable resource—a snapshot in time of the field of pain.

I wish to thank the speakers, both the many returning speakers and the "new blood," for their hard work and talents in writing these excellent chapters and preparing what are sure to be dynamic and effective presentations at the meeting. It has been genuinely useful and enjoyable for me personally to have read these contributions at the editing stage.

I also wish to express my deep gratitude to the Scientific Program Committee (especially Drs. Irene Tracey, Srinivasa Raja, and Johannes Vlaeyen, the Refresher Course Subcommittee), Dr. Jerry Gebhart (IASP President), Kathy Kreiter (IASP Executive Director), Terry Onustack (Meetings and Education Manager), and Elizabeth Endres and Irena Zlatanovic for their highly effective editorial assistance.

Jeffrey S. Mogil, PhD
Chair, Scientific Program Committee
13th World Congress on Pain

Acknowledgments

IASP wishes to thank the Ministère de la Santé et des Services sociaux du Québec for its financial support of the 13th World Congress on Pain's Refresher Course program.

IASP souhaite remercier le ministère de la Santé et des Services sociaux du Québec pour l'appui financier apporté au programme des cours de mise à niveau du 13ᵉ World Congress on Pain.

IASP thanks the following organizations that have expressed their commitment to pain education, research, and treatment throughout the world by becoming official sponsors of the 13th World Congress on Pain:

Diamond Level
Astellas Pharma Europe
Eli Lilly & Company
Grünenthal GmbH
MERCK
Mundipharma International Ltd.
Pfizer Inc.
Purdue Pharma LP USA
St. Jude Medical

Platinum Level
Purdue Pharma Canada

Gold Level
Archimedes Pharma Ltd.
Boston Scientific
Cephalon, Inc.
King Pharmaceuticals, Inc.
Mundipharma PTE Ltd.
Pfizer Canada
ProStrakan Group PLC
SonoSite International Ltd.

Silver Level
Endo Pharmaceuticals
Journal of Opioid Management
Medtronic Inc.
Nycomed Canada
QRxPharma

Bronze Level
Allergan, Inc.
IITC Life Sciences
Paladin Labs Inc.
Valeant Canada Limited
Wiley-Blackwell John Wiley & Sons Inc.

In addition, IASP thanks the following organizations that supported the Congress with local sponsorship funds:

Canada Level
Canadian Pain Society
Ministère de la Santé et des Services sociaux (MSSS)
Paladin Labs Inc.
Sanofi-Aventis Canada Inc.

Québec Level
Association québécoise de la douleur chronique (AQDC)
Charles River Laboratories Canada
IITC Inc./Life Sciences
Janssen-Ortho Inc.
Société québécoise de la douleur (SQD)
Stoelting Co.
Valeant Canada limitée/Limited

Montréal Level
Allergan Inc.
Bayer Inc.
Biovail Pharmaceuticals
CHUM - Hôtel Dieu/Centre de recherche du CHUM
MERCK Frosst Canada Ltée
Réseau québécois de recherche sur la douleur
Université de Montréal - Faculté de médecine
Université de Montréal - Faculté de médecine vétérinaire
University of Toronto - Center for the Study of Pain

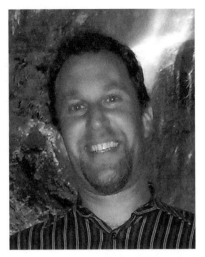

Jeffrey S. Mogil, PhD, was born in Toronto, Ontario, Canada, in 1966. He received a BSc (Honours) in Psychology from the University of Toronto in 1988, and a PhD in Neuroscience from UCLA in 1993. After a post-doctoral fellowship in Portland, Oregon, from 1993 to 1996, he joined the faculty of the Department of Psychology at the University of Illinois at Urbana-Champaign. He moved to McGill University in 2001, and is currently the E.P. Taylor Professor of Pain Studies (a Chair previously occupied by Dr. Ronald Melzack) and the Canada Research Chair in the Genetics of Pain (Tier I).

Dr. Mogil has made seminal contributions to the field of pain genetics and is the author of most major reviews of the subject, and the editor of the book, *The Genetics of Pain* (IASP Press, 2004). He is also a recognized authority in sex differences in pain and analgesia, and pain-testing methods in the laboratory mouse. Dr. Mogil is the author of over 150 journal articles and book chapters since 1992, and has given over 190 invited lectures in that same period. He holds or has held funding from the U.S. National Institutes of Health, the Canadian Institutes for Health Research, the Canada Foundation for Innovation, Genome Canada, Neuroscience Canada, the Louise and Alan Edwards Foundation, the Krembil Foundation, and the pharmaceutical and biotechnology industry. He is the recipient of numerous awards, including the Neal E. Miller New Investigator Award from the Academy of Behavioral Medicine Research (1998), the John C. Liebeskind Early Career Scholar Award from the American Pain Society (1998), the Patrick D. Wall Young Investigator Award from the International Association for the Study of Pain (2002), the Early Career Award from the Canadian Pain Society (2004), and a Neuropathic Pain Award from Pfizer Canada (2010). He currently serves as a Section Editor (Neurobiology) at the journal *PAIN* and is Chair of the Scientific Program Committee of the 13th World Congress on Pain.

Part 1
Neurobiology of Acute and Persistent Pain

Nociceptors, the Spinal Dorsal Horn, and Descending Modulation

Frank Porreca

Department of Pharmacology, University of Arizona Health Sciences Center, Tucson, Arizona, USA

Pain is defined by the International Association for the Study of Pain (IASP) as "an unpleasant sensory and emotional experience which we primarily associate with tissue damage or describe in terms of tissue damage, or both [52]." Whereas pain is considered to be an experience with sensory and cognitive and emotional components, nociception refers to the neural process by which stimuli that can elicit pain are detected by the nervous system. Specialized primary afferent sensory neurons, termed "nociceptors," are normally activated by high-threshold stimuli and transmit excitatory signals to the dorsal spinal cord. Sensory neurons have their cell bodies in the dorsal root ganglion (DRG) or the trigeminal ganglion. The peripheral sensory neurons are pseudounipolar, with an axonal stalk that bifurcates and sends projections to peripheral sites and to the dorsal horn of the spinal cord. Consequently, excitation of these sensory fibers can result in release of transmitters at both central and peripheral sites, the latter eliciting "neurogenic inflammation." High-intensity heat or mechanical stimuli or chemicals that can produce damage to tissues are termed "noxious" and are selectively detected by specific transducers localized at the peripheral terminals of nociceptors. Nociceptors are capable of encoding noxious stimuli, and critically, stimulation of nociceptors reliably elicits sensations that humans detect as pain. While most sensations are affectively neutral, pain is

unpleasant at threshold. It is this unpleasantness that serves as the teaching signal that allows avoidance of stimuli that can damage tissues [23,24]. Thus, pain is an important physiological mechanism that increases chances of survival.

Anatomical Characterization of Nociceptors

Primary afferent sensory neurons have been classified according to anatomical and electrophysiological characteristics. The Aβ fibers are large-diameter myelinated fibers with fast conduction. These neurons transmit almost exclusively non-nociceptive information. The medium-to-small diameter, thinly myelinated fibers are termed Aδ fibers, whereas nonmyelinated, slowly conducting fibers are designated as C-fibers. The Type I Aδ nociceptors, or high-threshold mechanoreceptors (HTM), respond to mechanical and chemical stimuli, but are also sensitive to high (>50°C) temperatures. Like other classes of nociceptors, these cells "sensitize" (see below) to both mechanical and thermal stimuli in the presence of tissue injury or inflammation. The Type II Aδ nociceptors respond to noxious thermal stimuli preferentially to mechanical stimuli [3,41,53].

As a class, the C-fiber nociceptors are polymodal, with populations of neurons responding to either heat, mechanical, or cold nociceptive stimuli.

Some C-fiber nociceptors are sensitive to heat and mechanical stimuli (CMH nociceptors), where others are referred to as "silent" or "sleeping" nociceptors; these nociceptors develop sensitivity to heat and chemical stimuli in the presence of injury or inflammation [53,88]. C fibers innervating the viscera are notable in that they respond to noninjurious stimuli such as stretching of hollow organs, while those fibers innervating teeth are responsive to nearly any intensity stimulus to elicit sensations of pain. Because Aδ nociceptors are myelinated and thus conduct at a faster rate than the unmyelinated C fibers, these nociceptors transmit what is called "first pain," which is the initial, sharp pain felt in response to pinch, pinprick, or noxious heat. The unmyelinated nociceptors transmit "second pain," comprising the more diffuse, dull, throbbing, and/or burning sensations that follow the first pain [3,41,53], and activity of these fibers is often the source of clinically relevant persistent pain.

C-fiber nociceptors have been categorized based on their dependence on trophic factors. The C fibers dependent on nerve growth factor (NGF) express the tyrosine kinase A (TrkA) neurotrophin receptor as well as the low-affinity p75 neurotrophin receptor. These nociceptors are peptidergic, expressing neurotransmitters including substance P and calcitonin gene-related peptide (CGRP) [71,72]. During development, NGF secreted by target tissue guides the development and differentiation of these sensory neurons. A second class of unmyelinated C-fiber nociceptors are deficient in the peptidic neurotransmitters, and they express the c-Ret and the GFR family of receptors that are the targets for glial-derived neurotrophic factors including GDNF, artemin, and neurturin [58]. The IB4 isolectin binds to this family of C-fiber nociceptors, which expresses the purinergic P2X3 receptor and the Mrg family of G-protein-coupled receptors. It is important to realize that these phenotypes are likely not "hard-wired," because the characteristics of these cells change dramatically in the presence of inflammation or nerve injury [3,88]. An important feature of nociceptors is their remarkable plasticity that can produce amplification of tissue signaling. One important mechanism of amplification is peripheral sensitization, in which thresholds for activation of the cells are diminished, resulting in enhanced excitability. Allodynia is present when normally non-noxious stimuli can now elicit sensations of pain, and hyperalgesia refers to exaggerated pain in response to normally painful stimuli [52,88].

Transduction Mechanisms of Pain

Although the observations that nociceptors respond to specific, high-threshold stimuli has been known for several decades, the specific process through which these stimuli are "transduced" into biological signals has only recently come to light. One important discovery contributing to our understanding of this process is the cloning of the transient receptor potential (TRP) family of ion channels. The TRP channels allow the influx of Na^+ and Ca^{2+} ions, resulting in depolarization and ultimately the possible generation of an action potential [67]. The first pain transducer to be elucidated was the TRPV1 ion channel. The TRPV1 ion channel was characterized by its activation by capsaicin, the ingredient in hot peppers that produces a burning sensation, by heat in excess of >43°C, and by low pH. The TRPV1 channel is present on most heat-sensitive nociceptors, including both Aδ and C fibers [10,11]. Mice with deletion of genes coding for the TRPV1 channel show diminished responses to noxious heat and an absence of thermal hyperalgesia after tissue injury. Conversely, proinflammatory agents, such as bradykinin and neurotrophins, that enhance responses to noxious heat also enhance the activation of the TRPV1 receptor [10,11]. Recent evidence has identified a family of oxidized linoleic acid metabolites, including 9- and 13-hydroxyoctadecadienoic acid (HODE), that are produced in response to noxious heat and may serve as endogenous activators of TRPV1 under normal and pathological pain conditions [61,62]. Subsequently, TRPV2, TRPV3, and TRPV4 channels have been identified and found to modulate thermal responses over a wide range of temperatures. The TRPV2 receptor, expressed on some Aδ fibers, also transduces noxious heat and is activated by temperatures >52°C. TRPV3 and TRPV4 are activated by temperatures between 25°C and 35°C, and detect warmth [3,67,88].

Menthol elicits a cool sensation and has been found to activate the TRPM8 channel. This channel is found on neurons that are sensitive to low temperatures (i.e., <25°C). Mice deficient in the expression of the TRPM8 channel show reduced behavioral responses to cool temperatures, but they still show avoidance of cold surfaces (<10°C). Moreover, approximately 4% of cold-sensitive afferent fibers show activation at low temperatures, suggesting the existence of another channel that is sensitive to noxious cold. Importantly, the expression of TRPM8 occurs in different neuronal populations from those expressing TRPV1, indicating functional segregation of these sensory modalities [5].

The TRPA1 channel has been proposed to be a channel that detects noxious (<15°C) cold [19]. It is activated by menthol and by icilin. However, it is also activated by mustard and cinnamon oil and produces a burning sensation [4]. Whether this channel is indeed an endogenous detector of noxious cold is not settled. One study performed with genetically altered mice that do not express the TRPA1 channel showed normal responses to cold stimuli [4], whereas in another study, responses to noxious cold below 0°C were diminished in TRPA1-null mice [44]. Moreover, unlike TRPM8, the TRPA1 channel is found on neurons expressing TRPV1, which could either argue against a role in cold sensitivity or explain the sensation of "burning" cold [88]. It was recently discovered that a mutation of the gene coding for an altered form of TRPA1 is responsible for the development of a heritable episodic human pain syndrome (termed "familial episodic pain syndrome" or FEPS), which is triggered by fatigue, fasting, and exposure to cold [43]. Afflicted individuals experience intense ongoing pain along with tachycardia and breathing difficulties during an attack. Studies performed with tissue obtained from individuals with the disorder showed that the TRPA1 channel is directly activated by cold and functions as a sensor for pain elicited by noxious cold [43]. This study validates TRPA1 as a transducer mediating human pain states.

In contrast to temperature-sensitive ion channels, the transducers for mechanical stimuli have not been clearly identified. Mechanosensitive channels were identified in *C. elegans* that belong to the degenerin/epithelial Na+ channel family (DEG/ENaC), and the mammalian orthologs of these channels are the acid-sensing ion channels (ASICs). The ASICs are present on low-threshold and high-threshold mechanoreceptors. However, deletion of ASIC1, ASIC2, or ASIC3 by genetic manipulations has produced only modest changes in mechanical sensitivity, and there is doubt that these channels are relevant to mechanical pain. Although the TRPV2, TRPV4, and TRPA1 channels have been investigated as potential mechanotransducers, none of them have yet been shown to posses the necessary characteristics. Accordingly, identification of the mechanical transducers still awaits further investigation.

Role of Sodium Channels in Pain Transmission

Voltage-gated sodium channels (VGSCs) are responsible for changes in membrane potentials that can either contribute to sensitization of nerve fibers or generate action potentials. Although several sodium channels are essential for nerve conduction, three of these, $Na_V1.7$, $Na_V1.8$ and $Na_V1.9$, are highly expressed in nociceptors. The role of the tetrodotoxin (TTX)-sensitive channel $Na_V1.7$ in pain has been confirmed by identification of several genetic mutations with important implications for nociceptive processing. Individuals with erythromelalgia, characterized by paroxysmal burning pain and vasodilatation of the extremities, as well as individuals with other paroxysmal pain disorders (e.g., paroxysmal extreme pain disorder, PEPD), demonstrate mutations of $Na_V1.7$ associated with increased function of the channel [15]. In contrast, individuals with mutations of $Na_V1.7$ resulting in loss of function suffer from congenital insensitivity to pain (CIP). These individuals do not experience pain with noxious stimuli and suffer injuries as a result of the loss of this protective function of pain. The $Na_V1.7$ channel is found on most nociceptors and accumulates at nerve endings [87]. Whereas this channel is known to have a critical role in the sensation of acute pain, its role in persistent pain states is unknown.

$Na_V1.8$ is a TTX-resistant channel that is specifically expressed in primary sensory neurons and is found in most nociceptors [45,73]. This channel generates the majority of inward Na+ current during the upstroke of action potentials in nociceptors, and it can allow neurons to repetitively fire in response to stimulation. Animal studies in models of nerve injury suggest that there is a redistribution of the $Na_V1.8$ channel after peripheral nerve injury, resulting in a decreased expression in the injured fibers but an increased expression in adjacent uninjured nerves. Reduction in expression of $Na_V1.8$ or inhibition of its activity has been associated with decreased behavioral expression of neuropathic pain in animal models [45,65].

Like $Na_V1.8$, $Na_V1.9$ is resistant to TTX. It mediates a persistent current with activation potential at −70 mV, close to the resting membrane potential, and this channel is active at the resting membrane potential and therefore may set the resting potential of nociceptors and can modulate the membrane potential in response to subthreshold stimuli [36]. The expression of $Na_V1.9$ is markedly reduced in injured nerve fibers in animal models of neuropathic pain. However, unlike

Na$_V$1.8, knockdown of this channel does not alter behavioral signs of neuropathic pain in animal models [45,65].

Role of Calcium Channels in Pain Transmission

Voltage-gated calcium channels (VGCCs) are critical elements that modulate neuronal excitation and transmitter release from nerve terminals [76]. The N-type VGCC has been identified on sensory neurons and is predominant on their nerve terminals. Activation of N-type calcium currents is critical to depolarization-coupled release of neurotransmitters, including substance P, CGRP, and glutamate, from primary afferent terminals. In conditions of chronic pain, it is believed that the expression of N-type VGCC is either increased or shows increased frequency of opening. The use of ω-conotoxin-GVIA to block N-type channel activity abolished increased activity of neurons postsynaptic to the primary afferent nociceptors in the spinal cord as well as behavioral signs of enhanced abnormal pain in animal models of nerve injury, and led to the development of its analog, ω-conotoxin-MVIIA, as ziconotide (Prialt*) [55,76]. This peptide is administered spinally for the management of severe, refractory pain.

The T-type VGCC is present in primary afferent neurons as well as on the spinal cord neurons postsynaptic to the central terminals of these fibers. Activation of the T-type VGCCs acts synergistically with the neurokinin-1 (NK1) receptor expressed on postsynaptic dorsal horn neurons in the activation of the *N*-methyl-D-aspartate (NMDA)/calcium channel complex of these cells, resulting in sensitization of these neurons to afferent inputs [39]. Blockade of the T-type VGCC produced a dose-dependent decrease in behavioral signs of neuropathic pain as well as electrophysiological signs of postsynaptic sensitization in animal models of nerve injury [17,39]. Its role in pain modulation makes the T-type VGCC an attractive target for drug development, and several compounds are under preclinical investigation as T-type channel blockers.

Transmission of Nociceptive Signals into the Central Nervous System

The primary afferent sensory fibers enter the central nervous system through the spinal cord, or, in the case of trigeminal ganglia neurons, at the level of the nucleus caudalis. The spinal dorsal horn is organized in discrete laminae that receive inputs from different types of fibers and serve different functions. The outermost laminae, lamina I, and the outer part of lamina II, which together make up the substantia gelatinosa, receive inputs from myelinated Aδ nociceptors and the peptidergic unmyelinated C-fiber nociceptors. The nonpeptidergic unmyelinated C-fiber nociceptors terminate on interneurons of the inner lamina II. The deeper laminae, III through V, receive inputs from the large-diameter myelinated Aβ fibers, which normally transmit innocuous sensory inputs, and lamina V also receives inputs from Aδ nociceptors. Laminae I and V are the source of most projection neurons to supraspinal sites such as the thalamus, parabrachial nucleus, and amygdala that send nociceptive inputs to higher cortical centers.

The concept of spinal modulation of nociceptive inputs was first elucidated by what became known as the "gate control theory" of pain [51]. This important and influential theory posited that both innocuous sensory inputs, mediated through large-diameter myelinated fibers, and noxious afferent inputs, mediated through unmyelinated C-fibers, converged on a transmission "T" cell in the spinal dorsal horn, which would project sensory inputs to supraspinal sites. In addition, the theory stated that large-diameter inputs excited a substantia gelatinosa ("SG") interneuron, whereas noxious C-fiber inputs inhibited the SG interneuron. The SG cell, in turn, exerted an inhibitory tone on the transmission T cell. Thus, a complex interplay between noxious and innocuous inputs could result in either enhanced or diminished transmission through the gate (i.e., the T cell). This theory attempted to explain clinically important phenomena such as summation of noxious stimuli or how innocuous stimuli could attenuate pain. In short, it was the first attempt to produce a testable hypothesis to explain the variations in individual responses to pain [24a]. Although the T and SG cells were not specified, and the theory as presented is now known to be anatomically incorrect, it was an important development as it triggered the intense research efforts in understanding mechanisms of pain and endogenous pain modulation that continue to this day.

The putative receptor for the neurotransmitter substance P, which is released from peptidergic nociceptors, is NK1. Although the population of lamina I neurons that express the NK1 receptor constitutes less than 5% of lamina I neurons, these cells account for more than 77% of the nociceptive-responsive cells of lamina I that project through the spinothalamic tract (STT), and they are important targets for peptidergic primary afferent nociceptors [12,78]. The remainder project to deeper laminae of the spinal cord and are able to promote sensitization of the deeper wide-dynamic-range neurons in a chronic pain state [78].

Under normal conditions, only noxious stimuli elicit internalization of the NK1 receptor in lamina I neurons. However, under conditions of inflammation or nerve injury, NK1 internalization is evoked by normally non-noxious stimuli, such as light brush, and occurs in deeper laminae as well as the outer laminae of the spinal dorsal horn [49,57]. This increased pattern of NK1 internalization is consistent with sensitization of the spinal cord neurons, and with lowered thresholds to initiate nocifensive responses as well as increased receptive fields of dorsal horn neurons. Blockade of the NK1 receptor alone, however, is insufficient to abolish acute or chronic pain [37,70,74]. Selective ablation of lamina I neurons expressing the NK1 receptor, accomplished by the spinal administration of substance P conjugated to saporin (SP-SAP), did not change normal nociceptive responses to acute noxious stimuli, but diminished behavioral and electrophysiological signs of enhanced pain sensitivity in animal models of inflammation and nerve injury. It was found that preventing ascending nociceptive inputs through lesion of the NK1 neurons of the outer lamina resulted in a loss of descending pain facilitation, which reversed signs of enhanced pain, suggesting the importance of spinal-supraspinal neuronal circuits for the maintenance of chronic pain states [78,79].

Like substance P, CGRP is released from peptidergic primary afferent nociceptors into the spinal dorsal horn. However, the neuronal targets for CGRP have not been as thoroughly characterized as the NK1 neurons. Evoked release of CGRP is increased in spinal tissue in animal models of inflammation or nerve injury, and manipulations that inhibit enhanced pain also abolish increased evoked release of CGRP. Release of CGRP from trigeminal neurons has been proposed as an important factor in migraine pain. Indeed, CGRP antagonists are now confirmed as effective in the treatment of migraine pain [18,63].

Potential Mechanisms of Analgesic Activity

Given that activation of nociceptors produces sensations of pain in humans, it is reasonable to pursue the development of pain-relieving strategies by altering the activity of these neurons. Analgesia can be expected either by diminishing neuronal excitation or by enhancing inhibition of primary afferent neurons and/or their postsynaptic targets in the spinal cord or nucleus caudalis. Lidocaine and other local anesthetics, because of their nonselective blockade of sodium channels, are useful for surgical and dental procedures but do not selectively inhibit pain. Blockade of all sensory fibers is not satisfactory as a means of long-term pain management. A recent study has shown that selective blockade of nociceptors can be achieved without affecting non-nociceptive sensory fibers [7,8]. The quaternary derivative of lidocaine, QX-314, was injected along with capsaicin to open the TRPV1 channel, allowing for selective inhibition of TRPV1-positive nociceptors. This concept was recently extended through the co-application of lidocaine, which also activates TRPV1 channels, with QX-314. This technique also allowed introduction of QX-314 into the nociceptor, resulting in a long-lasting, predominantly nociceptor-selective block, and suggesting sustained regional analgesia that could be achieved without the initial noxious activity elicited by capsaicin [7,8].

The development of blockers selective for specific sodium channels appears to have great therapeutic promise. Recent studies have shown that the small molecule A-803467 selectively blocks the $Na_V 1.8$ channel [40]. Moreover, A-803467 was found to block evoked activity of second-order spinal cord neurons in normal rats, and both evoked and spontaneous activity in neurons of nerve-injured rats. A-803467 attenuated acute nociception and blocked behavioral signs of neuropathic pain in animal models, presumably by attenuating the enhanced firing of, and transmitter release from, injured primary afferent nociceptors. Blockade of the $Na_V 1.8$ channel may lead to clinically relevant management of neuropathic pain. Selective blockers have not yet been developed for $Na_V 1.7$ or $Na_V 1.9$.

Blockade of the VGCCs also presents possible targets for pain modulation, possibly by inhibition of transmitter release. Blockade of the N-type VGCC is clinically validated, as shown by the use of ziconotide for the management of persistent refractory pain. However, a disadvantage of nonselective blockade of T-type VGCCs is that these channels are present in other tissue, such as cardiac cells. Gabapentin, initially developed as an anticonvulsant, was found to bind to the $\alpha_2\delta_1$ subunit of VGCCs, which is expressed in nociceptors [47]. This subunit of the channel, which is thought to be critical for trafficking VGCCs to the membrane to increase function, is upregulated in conditions of neuropathic pain. Gabapentin, and related compounds, are used clinically for management of neuropathic pain [28].

Opioids exert their analgesic effect by inhibition of both the primary afferent nociceptors and the second-order targets of the primary afferent fiber. Activation of the μ-opioid receptor inhibits Ca^{2+} channels and opens K^+ channels, which results in hyperpolarization [48]. In the central terminal of the primary afferent nociceptor, the result is decreased release of excitatory neurotransmitter into the spinal dorsal horn. Activation of μ-opioid receptors on the postsynaptic cell and the resulting hyperpolarization result in decreased sensitivity to released transmitters and diminished nociceptive inputs to higher pain-processing centers. Activation of opioid receptors is a clinically validated strategy, as demonstrated by the use of opiates as the most important medications for the control of moderate-to-severe pain [20].

Activation of the $α_2$-adrenergic receptor results in similar inhibitory effects on nociceptive signaling. Numerous studies in animals and human volunteers have shown that activation of spinal $α_2$-adrenergic receptors exerts a strong antinociceptive effect [21]. As in the case of opioid receptors, activation of $α_2$-adrenergic receptors hyperpolarizes neurons, thus reducing transmitter release and excitability in response to excitatory neurotransmitters. This mechanism underlies the potent antinociceptive synergy that exists between opioids and $α_2$-adrenergic receptor agonists [59,60]. Moreover, the utility of tricyclic antidepressants and other noradrenergic reuptake inhibitors (i.e., SNRIs) in neuropathic pain is likely to be mediated at least in part through the increased availability of norepinephrine at spinal $α_2$-adrenergic receptors [42,75].

Cannabinoid CB1 receptors are also localized on primary afferent neurons. As in the case of the opioid receptors (see below), the existence of selective receptors predicted the existence of endogenous ligands for the cannabinoid receptors. Endogenous ligands have been discovered, and activation of the CB1 receptor produces analgesia. Anandamide, Sanskrit for "internal bliss," was the first endocannabinoid to be isolated from the brain [14]. Activation of the cannabinoid CB1 receptors have been shown to produce acute antinociception and to block enhanced pain in animal models of inflammation and nerve injury [69,83]. Clinical studies performed with formulations containing derivatives of $Δ^9$-tetrahydrocannabinol have demonstrated efficacy in patients with neuropathic pain states [66].

Inhibition of responses of postsynaptic dorsal horn neurons to noxious inputs can also be produced by inhibition of the NMDA receptor. Activation of NMDA receptors opens Ca^{2+} channels that cause sensitization of dorsal horn neurons to sensory inputs [16]. Numerous studies performed with animal models have shown that blockade of the NMDA receptor does not produce antinociception, but reduces enhanced neuronal activity [1]. Inhibition of NMDA receptors has blocked the enhanced pain that occurs in models of neuropathic pain [84,85]. However, the clinical feasibility of NMDA-receptor blockade has been hampered by the occurrence of adverse effects. Recent studies have shown that memantine produces substantial pain relief in patients with phantom limb pain [29]. Ketamine, memantine, or dextromethorphan, which block NMDA-receptor activity, are useful in multiple clinical settings [77].

Descending Pain Modulation

The existence of an endogenous pain modulatory system has been hypothesized for many decades, based on the ability of individuals to seemingly ignore pain during moments of intense stress or immediate physical danger. The existence of a pain-regulatory mechanism was shown by microinjection of morphine into the periaqueductal gray (PAG), which surrounds the aqueduct of Sylvius between the third and fourth ventricles [81]. Subsequent studies revealed that several sites in the midbrain and medulla, when either microinjected with morphine or excited electrically, produced strong antinociception [27,46,50,56]. Electrical stimulation of the PAG was demonstrated to be clinically effective in relieving intractable pain, but it was soon abandoned because of adverse effects, including intense migraine-like headaches [38,68]. These studies contributed to the discovery of an endogenous opioidergic pain-modulatory system acting from supraspinal sites and modulating nociception at the level of the spinal cord.

Electrophysiological studies and lesioning experiments have revealed that the rostral ventromedial medulla (RVM) receives neuronal inputs from the PAG and is likely to be the final common relay in descending inhibition of nociception from supraspinal sites

[25]. Electrical stimulation and morphine microinjection into this region have produced antinociception. The RVM was shown to have a role as a relay, however, because inhibition of its activity with lidocaine blocks antinociception arising from electrical stimulation of the PAG. Descending projections from the RVM course through the dorsolateral funiculus (DLF) to the spinal dorsal horn, where they form synaptic contacts with primary afferent terminals as well as second-order neurons and thus modulate nociceptive inputs into the spinal cord. Descending modulation may be either positive (i.e., enhancing nociception) or negative (i.e., inhibiting nociception) [25].

Characterization of Antinociceptive and Pronociceptive Rostroventral Medulla Neurons

An intriguing finding was the existence of bidirectional pain modulation arising from the RVM, showing that this region modulates not only pain inhibition, but can also mediate a facilitation of pain, thus contributing to the enhanced pain seen in conditions of inflammation and nerve injury. Studies performed in anesthetized rats subject to noxious radiant heat applied to the tail revealed the existence of different populations of RVM neurons [25,26]. RVM neurons that showed an increase in firing just prior to the initiation of the nociceptive tail-flick reflex were thus termed "on-cells," and those that paused their ongoing firing just prior to the tail-flick were termed "off-cells" [25,26]. The activity of the "neutral" cells of the RVM did not correlate with nociceptive stimuli. This dichotomy in neuronal function is consistent with behavioral and electrophysiological studies that indicate bidirectional pain modulation. Low intensities of electrical or chemical stimulation applied to the RVM inhibited nociceptive responses, whereas higher levels of stimulation enhanced the same [82].

Further investigation revealed that the electrophysiological characteristics of the on-cells are consistent with a pronociceptive function. For example, manipulations that produce enhanced nociception, such as naloxone-precipitated withdrawal or prolonged exposure to a noxious stimulus, also produced an increase in on-cell activity. Inhibition of on-cell activity by microinjection of lidocaine into the RVM abolished enhanced pain. Of the RVM neurons, the on-cells are the only ones that are directly inhibited by morphine,

suggesting that these cells probably express μ-opioid receptors [34,35]. Furthermore, the on-cells are directly activated by cholecystokinin (CCK) [34,35], and there is a high degree of colocalization of CCK2 receptors with μ-opioid receptors on RVM neurons [90]. Based on these characteristics, these neurons are presumed to correspond to the RVM on-cells. Selective ablation of these neurons by saporin conjugated either to CCK or to the μ-opioid agonist dermorphin resulted in a loss of enhanced abnormal pain in animals with nerve injury, indicating that these neurons are likely to promote the enhanced pain state [64,90]. In contrast to the on-cells, the off-cells show enhanced firing frequency in the presence of opioids, whether administered systemically, into the RVM, or into the PAG. The enhanced off-cell activity is correlated with antinociception, and it is now known that disinhibition of off-cells is "necessary and sufficient" for analgesia [22,25].

Descending Serotonergic Pathways and Pain Modulation

The RVM is rich in serotonergic neurons with spinopetal projections, and early studies showed that spinal administration of nonselective serotonergic antagonists blocked antinociception produced by RVM stimulation. Stimulation of either the PAG or RVM was found to cause release of serotonin (5-hydroxytryptamine, 5-HT) in the spinal cord, and this effect was mimicked by spinally administered 5-HT agonists [13,89]. Recent studies, performed with antagonists selective for 5-HT receptor subtypes, show a more complicated picture, where the effect of spinal serotonin can be either inhibitory or facilitatory, depending on the receptor subtype activated. It is now accepted that activation of spinal 5-HT_{1A}, 5-HT_{1B}, 5-HT_{1D}, and 5-HT_{7} receptors inhibits nociception, whereas activation of the 5-HT_{2A} and 5-HT_{3} receptors facilitates nociception [80]. For example, the spinal administration of a 5-HT_{7} antagonist blocked the antinociceptive effect of morphine microinjected into the RVM, whereas that of a 5-HT_{3} antagonist blocked hyperalgesia induced by CCK administered into the RVM [80]. However, in spite of this evidence for an important serotonergic role for pain modulation, it is unclear whether 5-HT is present in direct projections from the RVM, because many on-cells and off-cells are γ-aminobutyric acid (GABA)ergic, whereas serotonergic projections represent the RVM "neutral" cells that do not respond to nociception.

Noradrenergic Systems and Pain Modulation

Like 5-HT, norepinephrine was found to be released into cerebrospinal fluid during antinociception produced by stimulation of the PAG or RVM. Moreover, antinociception arising from PAG or RVM stimulation was blocked by spinal administration of adrenergic antagonists, thus indicating a strong contribution of norepinephrine in antinociception associated with descending inhibition [13,30,31]. Whereas neither the PAG nor the RVM contain noradrenergic neurons, they are in communication with several important noradrenergic sites including the A5 (locus ceruleus), A6, and A7 (Kölliker-Füse) nuclei, which appear to contribute to antinociception. The locus ceruleus and A7 are important sources of noradrenergic projections to the superficial laminae of the spinal dorsal horn, which can inhibit the response of pain transmission neurons of the spinal dorsal horn through activation of the α_2-adrenergic receptors residing on the nerve terminals and on second-order dorsal horn neurons [2,6,9,86]. Activation of these α_2-adrenergic receptors is believed to underlie the antinociceptive effects of α_2-adrenergic agonists, such as clonidine, and to mediate the antinociceptive synergy with opioids, as described above.

Tricyclic antidepressants (TCAs) and mixed serotonin/norepinephrine reuptake inhibitors (i.e., SNRIs) probably exert their effectiveness against neuropathic pain by inhibiting norepinephrine reuptake and thus increasing the availability of norepinephrine at the α_2-adrenergic receptors in the spinal cord. The SNRIs duloxetine and milnacipran have been approved by the U.S. Food and Drug Administration as analgesics for diabetic neuropathy [54,75] and fibromyalgia [42], respectively. Emerging preclinical evidence also indicates that gabapentin may also exert its efficacy against neuropathic pain conditions by activating descending noradrenergic projections from the locus ceruleus [33]. Gabapentin elevated norepinephrine in spinal cerebrospinal fluid of surgical patients and reduced the amount of morphine required for relief of postoperative pain [32].

Conclusions

Modulation of the function and pathological activity of nociceptors offers multiple opportunities for the development of therapies for the relief of pain. Increased understanding of descending modulatory circuits also offers important opportunities for therapies for the treatment of pain. While descending inhibition has been clinically validated through the actions of opiate drugs and of neurotransmitter reuptake blockers, the mechanisms underlying descending facilitation and their role in chronic pain states remain to be validated. Nevertheless, these mechanisms are likely to offer further important opportunities for the treatment of pain. Finally, the adaptive changes that occur throughout the pain transmission system are likely to underlie the transition from acute to chronic pain, and these processes also will be important in new mechanisms that can offer pain relief. Ultimately, these strategies may be targeted to mechanisms that mediate pain in individual patients to offer effective pain relief while maintaining quality of life.

References

[1]   Aanonsen LM, Lei S, Wilcox GL. Excitatory amino acid receptors and nociceptive neurotransmission in rat spinal cord. Pain 1990;41:309–21.

[2]   Bajic D, Proudfit HK, Van Bockstaele EJ. Periaqueductal gray neurons monosynaptically innervate extranuclear noradrenergic dendrites in the rat pericoerulear region. J Comp Neurol 2000;427:649–62.

[3]   Basbaum AI, Bautista DM, Scherrer G, Julius D. Cellular and molecular mechanisms of pain. Cell 2009;139:267–84.

[4]   Bautista DM, Jordt SE, Nikai T, Tsuruda PR, Read AJ, Poblete J, Yamoah EN, Basbaum AI, Julius D. TRPA1 mediates the inflammatory actions of environmental irritants and proalgesic agents. Cell 2006;124:1269–82.

[5]   Bautista DM, Siemens J, Glazer JM, Tsuruda PR, Basbaum AI, Stucky CL, Jordt SE, Julius D. The menthol receptor TRPM8 is the principal detector of environmental cold. Nature 2007;448:204–8.

[6]   Beitz AJ. The organization of afferent projections to the midbrain periaqueductal gray of the rat. Neuroscience 1982;7:133–59.

[7]   Binshtok AM, Bean BP, Woolf CJ. Inhibition of nociceptors by TRPV1-mediated entry of impermeant sodium channel blockers. Nature 2007;449:607–10.

[8]   Binshtok AM, Gerner P, Oh SB, Puopolo M, Suzuki S, Roberson DP, Herbert T, Wang CF, Kim D, Chung G, Mitani AA, Wang GK, Bean BP, Woolf CJ. Coapplication of lidocaine and the permanently charged sodium channel blocker QX-314 produces a long-lasting nociceptive blockade in rodents. Anesthesiology 2009;111:127–37.

[9]   Cameron AA, Khan IA, Westlund KN, Willis WD. The efferent projections of the periaqueductal gray in the rat: a *Phaseolus vulgaris*-leucoagglutinin study. II. Descending projections. J Comp Neurol 1995;351:585–601.

[10] Caterina MJ, Julius D. The vanilloid receptor: a molecular gateway to the pain pathway. Annu Rev Neurosci 2001;24:487–517.

[11] Caterina MJ, Leffler A, Malmberg AB, Martin WJ, Trafton J, Petersen-Zeitz KR, Koltzenburg M, Basbaum AI, Julius D. Impaired nociception and pain sensation in mice lacking the capsaicin receptor. Science 2000;288:306–13.

[12] Cheunsuang O, Morris R. Spinal lamina I neurons that express neurokinin 1 receptors: morphological analysis. Neuroscience 2000;97:335–45.

[13] Cui M, Feng Y, McAdoo DJ, Willis WD. Periaqueductal gray stimulation-induced inhibition of nociceptive dorsal horn neurons in rats is associated with the release of norepinephrine, serotonin, and amino acids. J Pharmacol Exp Ther 1999;289:868–76.

[14] Devane WA, Hanus L, Breuer A, Pertwee RG, Stevenson LA, Griffin G, Gibson D, Mandelbaum A, Etinger A, Mechoulam R. Isolation and structure of a brain constituent that binds to the cannabinoid receptor. Science 1992;258:1946–9.

[15] Dib-Hajj SD, Rush AM, Cummins TR, Hisama FM, Novella S, Tyrrell L, Marshall L, Waxman SG. Gain-of-function mutation in $Na_V1.7$ in familial erythromelalgia induces bursting of sensory neurons. Brain 2005;128:1847–54.

[16] Dickenson AH, Sullivan AF. Evidence for a role of the NMDA receptor in the frequency dependent potentiation of deep rat dorsal horn nociceptive neurones following C fibre stimulation. Neuropharmacology 1987;26:1235–8.

[17] Dogrul A, Gardell LR, Ossipov MH, Tulunay FC, Lai J, Porreca F. Reversal of experimental neuropathic pain by T-type calcium channel blockers. Pain 2003;105:159–68.

[18] Doods H, Arndt K, Rudolf K, Just S. CGRP antagonists: unravelling the role of CGRP in migraine. Trends Pharmacol Sci 2007;28:580–7.

[19] Dunham JP, Leith JL, Lumb BM, Donaldson LF. Transient receptor potential channel A1 and noxious cold responses in rat cutaneous nociceptors. Neuroscience 2010;165:1412–9.

[20] Dworkin RH, O'Connor AB, Backonja M, Farrar JT, Finnerup NB, Jensen TS, Kalso EA, Loeser JD, Miaskowski C, Nurmikko TJ, et al. Pharmacologic management of neuropathic pain: evidence-based recommendations. Pain 2007;132:237–51.

[21] Eisenach JC, Hood DD, Curry R. Intrathecal, but not intravenous, clonidine reduces experimental thermal or capsaicin-induced pain and hyperalgesia in normal volunteers. Anesth Analg 1998;87:591–6.

[22] Fang FG, Haws CM, Drasner K, Williamson A, Fields HL. Opioid peptides (DAGO-enkephalin, dynorphin A$_{1-13}$, BAM 22P) microinjected into the rat brainstem: comparison of their antinociceptive effect and their effect on neuronal firing in the rostral ventromedial medulla. Brain Res 1989;501:116–28.

[23] Fields HL. Pain: an unpleasant topic. Pain 1999;Suppl 6:61–69.

[24] Fields HL. Understanding how opioids contribute to reward and analgesia. Reg Anesth Pain Med 2007;32:242–6.

[24a] Fields HL. Neuropathic pain: a brief conceptual history. In: Simpson DM, McArthur JC, Dworkin RH, editors. Neuropathic pain: mechanisms and management. New York: Oxford University Press; in press.

[25] Fields HL, Basbaum AI, Heinricher MM. Central nervous system mechanisms of pain modulation. In: McMahon SB, Koltzenburg M, editors. Melzack and Wall's textbook of pain, 5th ed. Edinburgh: Churchill Livingstone; 2005. p. 125–42.

[26] Fields HL, Bry J, Hentall I, Zorman G. The activity of neurons in the rostral medulla of the rat during withdrawal from noxious heat. J Neurosci 1983;3:2545–52.

[27] Gebhart GF. Opiate and opioid peptide effects on brain stem neurons: relevance to nociception and antinociceptive mechanisms. Pain 1982;12:93–140.

[28] Gordh TE, Stubhaug A, Jensen TS, Arner S, Biber B, Boivie J, Mannheimer C, Kalliomaki J, Kalso E. Gabapentin in traumatic nerve injury pain: a randomized, double-blind, placebo-controlled, crossover, multi-center study. Pain 2008;138:255–66.

[29] Hackworth RJ, Tokarz KA, Fowler IM, Wallace SC, Stedje-Larsen ET. Profound pain reduction after induction of memantine treatment in two patients with severe phantom limb pain. Anesth Analg 2008;107:1377–9.

[30] Hammond DL, Tyce GM, Yaksh TL. Efflux of 5-hydroxytryptamine and noradrenaline into spinal cord superfusates during stimulation of the rat medulla. J Physiol 1985;359:151–62.

[31] Hammond DL, Yaksh TL. Antagonism of stimulation-produced antinociception by intrathecal administration of methysergide or phentolamine. Brain Res 1984;298:329–37.

[32] Hayashida K, DeGoes S, Curry R, Eisenach JC. Gabapentin activates spinal noradrenergic activity in rats and humans and reduces hypersensitivity after surgery. Anesthesiology 2007;106:557–62.

[33] Hayashida K, Obata H, Nakajima K, Eisenach JC. Gabapentin acts within the locus coeruleus to alleviate neuropathic pain. Anesthesiology 2008;109:1077–84.

[34] Heinricher MM, McGaraughty S, Tortorici V. Circuitry underlying antiopioid actions of cholecystokinin within the rostral ventromedial medulla. J Neurophysiol 2001;85:280–6.

[35] Heinricher MM, Morgan MM, Fields HL. Direct and indirect actions of morphine on medullary neurons that modulate nociception. Neuroscience 1992;48:533–43.

[36] Herzog RI, Cummins TR, Waxman SG. Persistent TTX-resistant Na$^+$ current affects resting potential and response to depolarization in simulated spinal sensory neurons. J Neurophysiol 2001;86:1351–64.

[37] Hill R. NK1 (substance P) receptor antagonists: why are they not analgesic in humans? Trends Pharmacol Sci 2000;21:244–6.

[38] Hosobuchi Y, Adams JE, Linchitz R. Pain relief by electrical stimulation of the central gray matter in humans and its reversal by naloxone. Science 1977;197:183–6.

[39] Ikeda H, Heinke B, Ruscheweyh R, Sandkuhler J. Synaptic plasticity in spinal lamina I projection neurons that mediate hyperalgesia. Science 2003;299:1237–40.

[40] Jarvis MF, Honore P, Shieh CC, Chapman M, Joshi S, Zhang XF, Kort M, Carroll W, Marron B, Atkinson R, et al. A-803467, a potent and selective Na$_v$1.8 sodium channel blocker, attenuates neuropathic and inflammatory pain in the rat. Proc Natl Acad Sci USA 2007;104:8520–5.

[41] Julius D, Basbaum AI. Molecular mechanisms of nociception. Nature 2001;413:203–10.

[42] Kranzler JD, Gendreau RM. Role and rationale for the use of milnacipran in the management of fibromyalgia. Neuropsychiatr Dis Treat 2010;6:197–208.

[43] Kremeyer B, Lopera F, Cox JJ, Momin A, Rugiero F, Marsh S, Woods CG, Jones NG, Paterson KJ, Fricker FR, et al. A gain-of-function mutation in TRPA1 causes familial episodic pain syndrome. Neuron 2010;66:671–80.

[44] Kwan KY, Allchorne AJ, Vollrath MA, Christensen AP, Zhang DS, Woolf CJ, Corey DP. TRPA1 contributes to cold, mechanical, and chemical nociception but is not essential for hair-cell transduction. Neuron 2006;50:277–89.

[45] Lai J, Hunter JC, Porreca F. The role of voltage-gated sodium channels in neuropathic pain. Curr Opin Neurobiol 2003;13:291–7.

[46] Lewis VA, Gebhart GF. Evaluation of the periaqueductal central gray (PAG) as a morphine-specific locus of action and examination of morphine-induced and stimulation-produced analgesia at coincident PAG loci. Brain Res 1977;124:283–303.

[47] Li CY, Zhang XL, Matthews EA, Li KW, Kurwa A, Boroujerdi A, Gross J, Gold MS, Dickenson AH, Feng G, Luo ZD. Calcium channel alpha-a2delta1 subunit mediates spinal hyperexcitability in pain modulation. Pain 2006;125:20–34.

[48] Loose MD, Kelly MJ. Opioids act at mu-receptors to hyperpolarize arcuate neurons via an inwardly rectifying potassium conductance. Brain Res 1990;513:15–23.

[49] Mantyh PW, Clohisy DR, Koltzenburg M, Hunt SP. Molecular mechanisms of cancer pain. Nat Rev Cancer 2002;2:201–9.

[50] Mayer DJ, Wolfle TL, Akil H, Carder B, Liebeskind JC. Analgesia from electrical stimulation in the brainstem of the rat. Science 1971;174:1351–4.

[51] Melzack R, Wall PD. Pain mechanisms: a new theory. Science 1965;150:971–9.

[52] Merskey H, Bogduk N. Classification of chronic pain: descriptions of chronic pain syndromes and definitions of pain terms. Seattle: IASP Press; 1994.

[53] Meyer RA, Ringkamp M, Campbell JN, Raja SN. Peripheral mechanisms of cutaneous nociception. In: McMahon S, Koltzenburg M, editors. Wall and Melzack's textbook of pain. Philadelphia: Elsevier; 2008. p. 3–34.

[54] Mico JA, Ardid D, Berrocoso E, Eschalier A. Antidepressants and pain. Trends Pharmacol Sci 2006;27:348–54.

[55] Miljanich GP. Ziconotide: neuronal calcium channel blocker for treating severe chronic pain. Curr Med Chem 2004;11:3029–40.

[56] Mohrland JS, Gebhart GF. Effects of focal electrical stimulation and morphine microinjection in the periaqueductal gray of the rat mesencephalon on neuronal activity in the medullary reticular formation. Brain Res 1980;201:23–37.

[57] Nichols ML, Allen BJ, Rogers SD, Ghilardi JR, Honore P, Luger NM, Finke MP, Li J, Lappi DA, Simone DA, Mantyh PW. Transmission of chronic nociception by spinal neurons expressing the substance P receptor. Science 1999;286:1558–61.

[58] Orozco OE, Walus L, Sah DW, Pepinsky RB, Sanicola M. GFRalpha3 is expressed predominantly in nociceptive sensory neurons. Eur J Neurosci 2001;13:2177–82.

[59] Ossipov MH, Harris S, Lloyd P, Messineo E. An isobolographic analysis of the antinociceptive effect of systemically and intrathecally administered combinations of clonidine and opiates. J Pharmacol Exp Ther 1990;255:1107–16.

[60] Ossipov MH, Harris S, Lloyd P, Messineo E, Lin BS, Bagley J. Antinociceptive interaction between opioids and medetomidine: systemic additivity and spinal synergy. Anesthesiology 1990;73:1227–35.

[61] Patwardhan AM, Akopian AN, Ruparel NB, Diogenes A, Weintraub ST, Uhlson C, Murphy RC, Hargreaves KM. Heat generates oxidized linoleic acid metabolites that activate TRPV1 and produce pain in rodents. J Clin Invest 2010;120:1617–26.

[62] Patwardhan AM, Scotland PE, Akopian AN, Hargreaves KM. Activation of TRPV1 in the spinal cord by oxidized linoleic acid metabolites contributes to inflammatory hyperalgesia. Proc Natl Acad Sci USA 2009;106:18820–4.

[63] Petersen KA, Lassen LH, Birk S, Lesko L, Olesen J. BIBN4096BS antagonizes human alpha-calcitonin gene related peptide-induced headache and extracerebral artery dilatation. Clin Pharmacol Ther 2005;77:202–13.

[64] Porreca F, Burgess SE, Gardell LR, Vanderah TW, Malan TP Jr, Ossipov MH, Lappi DA, Lai J. Inhibition of neuropathic pain by selective ablation of brainstem medullary cells expressing the mu-opioid receptor. J Neurosci 2001;21:5281–8.

[65] Porreca F, Lai J, Bian D, Wegert S, Ossipov MH, Eglen RM, Kassotakis L, Novakovic S, Rabert DK, Sangameswaran L, Hunter JC. A comparison of the potential role of the tetrodotoxin-insensitive sodium channels, PN3/SNS and NaN/SNS2, in rat models of chronic pain. Proc Natl Acad Sci USA 1999;96:7640–4.

[66] Rahn EJ, Hohmann AG. Cannabinoids as pharmacotherapies for neuropathic pain: from the bench to the bedside. Neurotherapeutics 2009;6:713–37.

[67] Ramsey IS, Delling M, Clapham DE. An introduction to TRP channels. Annu Rev Physiol 2006;68:619–47.

[68] Raskin NH, Hosobuchi Y, Lamb S. Headache may arise from perturbation of brain. Headache 1987;27:416–20.

[69] Rice AS. Cannabinoids and pain. Curr Opin Investig Drugs 2001;2:399–414.

[70] Rost K, Fleischer F, Nieber K. [Neurokinin 1 receptor antagonists: between hope and disappointment]. Med Monatsschr Pharm 2006;29:200–5.

[71] Sah DW, Ossipov MH, Porreca F. Neurotrophic factors as novel therapeutics for neuropathic pain. Nat Rev Drug Discov 2003;2:460–72.

[72] Sah DW, Ossipov MH, Rossomando A, Silvian L, Porreca F. New approaches for the treatment of pain: the GDNF family of neurotrophic growth factors. Curr Top Med Chem 2005;5:577–83.

[73] Sangameswaran L, Fish LM, Koch BD, Rabert DK, Delgado SG, Ilnicka M, Jakeman LB, Novakovic S, Wong K, Sze P, et al. A novel tetrodotoxin-insensitive, voltage-gated sodium channel expressed in rat and human dorsal root ganglia. J Biol Chem 1997;272:14805–9.

[74] Sindrup SH, Graf A, Sfikas N. The NK1-receptor antagonist TKA731 in painful diabetic neuropathy: a randomised, controlled trial. Eur J Pain 2006;10:567–71.

[75] Smith T, Nicholson RA. Review of duloxetine in the management of diabetic peripheral neuropathic pain. Vasc Health Risk Manag 2007;3:833–44.

[76] Snutch TP. Targeting chronic and neuropathic pain: the N-type calcium channel comes of age. NeuroRx 2005;2:662–70.

[77] Suzuki M. Role of N-methyl-D-aspartate receptor antagonists in postoperative pain management. Curr Opin Anaesthesiol 2009;22:618–22.

[78] Suzuki R, Morcuende S, Webber M, Hunt SP, Dickenson AH. Superficial NK1-expressing neurons control spinal excitability through activation of descending pathways. Nat Neurosci 2002;5:1319–26.

[79] Suzuki R, Rahman W, Hunt SP, Dickenson AH. Descending facilitatory control of mechanically evoked responses is enhanced in deep dorsal horn neurones following peripheral nerve injury. Brain Res 2004;1019:68–76.

[80] Suzuki R, Rygh LJ, Dickenson AH. Bad news from the brain: descending 5-HT pathways that control spinal pain processing. Trends Pharmacol Sci 2004;25:613–7.

[81] Tsou K, Jang CS. Studies on the site of analgesic action of morphine by intracerebral micro-injection. Sci Sin 1964;13:1099–109.

[82] Urban MO, Gebhart GF. Supraspinal contributions to hyperalgesia. Proc Natl Acad Sci USA 1999;96:7687–92.

[83] Walker JM, Strangman NM, Huang SM. Cannabinoids and pain. Pain Res Manag 2001;6:74–9.

[84] Wang Z, Gardell LR, Ossipov MH, Vanderah TW, Brennan MB, Hochgeschwender U, Hruby VJ, Malan TP Jr, Lai J, Porreca F. Pronociceptive actions of dynorphin maintain chronic neuropathic pain. J Neurosci 2001;21:1779–86.

[85] Wegert S, Ossipov MH, Nichols ML, Bian D, Vanderah TW, Malan TP Jr, Porreca F. Differential activities of intrathecal MK-801 or morphine to alter responses to thermal and mechanical stimuli in normal or nerve-injured rats. Pain 1997;71:57–64.

[86] Westlund KN, Bowker RM, Ziegler MG, Coulter JD. Noradrenergic projections to the spinal cord of the rat. Brain Res 1983;263:15–31.

[87] Wood JN, Boorman JP, Okuse K, Baker MD. Voltage-gated sodium channels and pain pathways. J Neurobiol 2004;61:55–71.

[88] Woolf CJ, Ma Q. Nociceptors: noxious stimulus detectors. Neuron 2007;55:353–64.

[89] Yaksh TL, Wilson PR. Spinal serotonin terminal system mediates antinociception. J Pharmacol Exp Ther 1979;208:446–53.

[90] Zhang W, Gardell S, Zhang D, Xie JY, Agnes RS, Badghisi H, Hruby VJ, Rance N, Ossipov MH, Vanderah TW, Porreca F, Lai J. Neuropathic pain is maintained by brainstem neurons co-expressing opioid and cholecystokinin receptors. Brain 2009;132:778–87.

Correspondence to: Frank Porreca, PhD, Department of Pharmacology, University of Arizona Health Sciences Center, Tucson, AZ 85724, USA. Email: frankp@u.arizona.edu.

Dorsal Horn Plasticity and Neuron-Microglia Interactions

Michael W. Salter, MD, PhD

Program in Neurosciences and Mental Health, the Hospital for Sick Children; Department of Physiology;
University of Toronto Centre for the Study of Pain; Toronto, Ontario, Canada

The ability to appropriately respond to environmental stimuli that damage or threaten to damage tissue—noxious stimuli—has great survival value. Noxious stimuli are detected through a specialized system of noxious stimuli-detecting (that is, nociceptive) neurons, and in higher organisms responses to noxious stimulation lead to acute nociceptive pain. Nociceptive pain is a crucial defensive mechanism that warns an individual of recent, ongoing, or imminent damage to the body, and it is produced as the physiological outcome of normal functioning of peripheral and central nervous systems. By contrast, chronic pain, which is inflammatory or neuropathic, is the result of aberrant functioning of peripheral or central nervous systems that have been pathologically modified [66,67]. Typically, chronic pain is not directly related to nociception, and it may persist long after any tissue damage that may have initiated the nociceptive pain has subsided. There are no known defensive, or other helpful, functions of chronic pain. Rather, chronic pain may be insidious and destructive to the life of the individual who is suffering from it. Pathological alterations that underlie and amplify chronic pain occur in the peripheral nervous system or in numerous sites within the central nervous system, leading to the concept that chronic pain is a group of mechanistically separable nervous system disorders produced by one or more abnormal cellular signaling mechanisms.

The somatosensory gateway in the central nervous system (CNS) is in the spinal cord dorsal horn, which is not a simple relay station. Rather, it is a complex nociceptive processing network through which inputs from the periphery are transduced and modulated by local, as well as descending, excitatory and inhibitory control mechanisms [66,67]. The output of this network is transmitted to areas of the CNS involved in sensory, emotional, autonomic, and motor processing. Normally, the output is balanced by excitatory and inhibitory processes. But in pathological pain states, the output of the dorsal horn nociceptive network is greatly increased. The major mechanisms for increased output of the nociceptive network are: (1) enhancing excitatory synaptic transmission, via the *N*-methyl-D-aspartate (NMDA) receptor subtype of glutamate receptor (NMDAR), or (2) suppressing inhibitory mechanisms mediated by γ-aminobutyric acid (GABA) and glycine receptors. Abundant evidence indicates that the increased activity of the nociceptive network involves substantial interactions between neurons and non-neuronal cells, in particular microglia, in the dorsal horn [20,56].

Synaptic Transmission and Short-Lasting Plasticity

Synaptic Transmission from Primary Afferents to Dorsal Horn Neurons Is Excitatory

Synaptic input from all primary sensory afferents onto second-order neurons in the dorsal horn is excitatory. Like the vast majority of synapses in the CNS, this excitation is mediated by glutamate released from the presynaptic terminals, which produces an excitatory postsynaptic potential (EPSP) in the dorsal horn neurons. EPSPs evoked by low-frequency action potential discharge of the primary afferents are mediated principally by activation of the α-amino-3-hydroxyl-5-methyl-4-isoxazole-propionate (AMPA) [21] and kainate [27] subtypes of glutamate receptor. Unlike most regions of the CNS, a large portion of synaptic transmission at primary afferent synapses is mediated by calcium-permeable AMPA receptors [53], providing the opportunity for these receptors to participate in synaptic plasticity. Under basal conditions, the NMDA subtype of glutamate receptor, which is also localized at excitatory primary afferent synapses and is a key to pain neuroplasticity (see below), contributes little to the postsynaptic responses to low-frequency presynaptic action potentials. The lack of NMDAR contribution arises as a consequence of tonic inhibition of current flow by pore blockade by extracellular Mg^{2+} at the resting membrane potential current flow, and because the activity per se of NMDARs is tonically downregulated by biasing of kinase/phosphatase regulatory systems toward dephosphorylation. It is important to appreciate that even with primary afferents that may be considered "slow," from the perspective of axonal conduction velocity, the synaptic transmission to second-order neurons is the means of this fast glutamatergic transmission [34,66].

Inhibitory Synaptic Transmission in the Dorsal Horn

Although action potential discharge by dorsal horn neurons is driven by glutamatergic EPSPs, the activity of these neurons is powerfully suppressed by inhibitory inputs that act pre- or postsynaptically [11,31,66]. The predominant inhibition is that produced postsynaptically by GABA and/or glycine, released from dorsal horn inhibitory interneurons, which themselves are excited by primary afferent inputs, as well as by inputs from descending neurons. These neurons evoke fast inhibitory postsynaptic potentials (IPSPs) mediated by $GABA_A$ and glycine receptors, respectively. As is well known, these receptors are ligand-gated Cl^- channels, the opening of which normally suppresses generation of action potentials by hyperpolarizing the membrane and by "shunting" the postsynaptic cell [40]. Postsynaptic inhibition may also be produced by activation of metabotropic receptors, i.e., G-protein-coupled receptors, such

as $GABA_B$, adenosine and opioid receptors, which typically produce postsynaptic hyperpolarization by means of activating K^+ channels. Discharge of dorsal horn neurons is also inhibited presynaptically by suppression of the release of glutamate from primary afferent terminals. This presynaptic inhibition involves many of the same chemical mediators that cause postsynaptic inhibition, with receptors localized on the presynaptic terminals of primary afferents [67].

Control of Nociceptive Output from the Dorsal Horn by Integration of Excitation and Inhibition

The efficacy of excitatory synaptic transmission and of the coupling between EPSPs and action potential generation are fundamentally important for controlling the activity of neurons in the nociceptive network within the dorsal horn. There are various cellular and molecular mechanisms for increasing, or decreasing, the strength of glutamatergic synapses and the efficiency by which this synaptic input produces action potentials. It is the increase in action potential discharge in dorsal horn nociceptive neurons that is key to pain hypersensitivity. These mechanisms range from those that are very rapid in onset, and typically also rapidly reversible, to those that are more slowly developing and persistent. The integration of these various mechanisms, based on the short- and long-term past electrical and biochemical history of the dorsal horn neurons, is a major means for controlling the output of the nociceptive dorsal horn network.

Windup: Rapid-Onset and Reversible Enhancement of Excitatory Transmission

At low rates of discharge, primary afferent nociceptors primarily release glutamate. However, noxious peripheral stimulation that is more intense or sustained induces primary afferent nociceptors to discharge at higher frequencies, resulting in release of peptide neuromodulators such as substance P and calcitonin gene-related peptide (CGRP), together with glutamate, from central nociceptor terminals. These peptides act on their cognate G-protein-coupled receptors to produce depolarizing synaptic potentials lasting up to tens of seconds [8]. These slow EPSPs can greatly facilitate temporal summation of fast EPSPs, with cumulative depolarization of the dorsal horn neurons that is accentuated by feedforward recruitment of NMDAR current through relief of the Mg^{2+} blockade of the channels [46]. The current flow through NMDARs leads to a rise in intracellular Ca^{2+} levels. Moreover, the sustained depolarization may also recruit voltage-gated Ca^{2+} channels, causing a further boost in the level of intracellular Ca^{2+} and triggering plateau potentials mediated by Ca^{2+}-activated nonselective cation channels [36]. The end result of these processes is a progressive increase in the action potential discharge in dorsal horn nociceptive neurons during a train of nociceptive peripheral stimuli [66] that is commonly referred to as "windup" [33]. The summation leading to windup is reversed within seconds when the initiating input from primary afferent nociceptors ends, and there appear to be no long-term consequences to windup. Nevertheless, in conjunction with persisting forms of plasticity, windup can greatly enhance the nociceptive output of the dorsal horn.

Persistent Synaptic Plasticity in the Dorsal Nociceptive Network

Nociceptive neurons in the dorsal horn neurons exhibit mechanistically distinct forms of activity-dependent persistent enhancement of responsiveness to nociceptive inputs that are often referred to together as "central sensitization" [65]. One form of plasticity is a heterosynaptic plasticity that outlasts the initiating stimulus for tens of minutes (classic central sensitization) [51,52], and a second is a homosynaptic long-term potentiation elicited by brief high-frequency inputs [41,43]. In addition, there are pre- and postsynaptic transcription-dependent changes in synaptic function that take longer to manifest (hours), but which last for prolonged periods (days) [70]. Finally, a reduction in the level of tonic and phasic inhibition also facilitates the output of the nociceptive network [5,35].

The processes that produce central sensitization are initiated by inputs of peripheral nociceptors, whereas central sensitization is not evoked by inputs from primary afferents that are non-nociceptive. These nociceptive inputs initiate intracellular signaling cascades, leading to an orchestrated series of modifications of neuronal network behavior consisting of enhancement of excitatory postsynaptic responses. One consequence of this signaling is an increase in the gain of nociceptive output neurons, resulting in increased responses to the same input from primary afferents. A second consequence of sensitization of dorsal horn neurons is unmasking of subthreshold inputs, such that neurons are recruited to discharge in response to stimuli that

were previously subliminal [67]. Thus, when the dorsal horn nociceptive processing system is sensitized, a given noxious peripheral stimulus will evoke increased responses of individual nociceptive dorsal neurons and, as well, there is an increase in the overall number of nociceptive output neurons activated.

Heterosynaptic Potentiation in Dorsal Horn Nociceptive Neurons

The most prominent form of persistent plasticity in the dorsal horn is a rapid-onset, activity-dependent increase in the excitability of nociceptive dorsal horn neurons as a result of a barrage of nociceptor afferent input as short as 10–20 seconds [3,68]. Activity-dependent heterosynaptic central potentiation may manifest within seconds of an appropriate nociceptive conditioning stimulus, and if the stimulus is maintained, even at low levels, the central sensitization persists up to several hours or even longer. After this sensitization by nociceptor-conditioning stimuli, normally subliminal inputs become sufficient to activate dorsal horn neurons, and responses of synapses not activated by the conditioning/initiating stimulus are enhanced, which is clear evidence that the potentiation is heterosynaptic [45].

As a result of heterosynaptic potentiation, low-threshold sensory fibers activated by innocuous stimuli such as light touch can, after the induction of the heterosynaptic sensitization, activate normally high-threshold nociceptive neurons, providing a neural substrate for the clinical phenomenon of allodynia. Thus, although evoked by a non-noxious stimulus in the periphery, allodynia may arise as a result of changes in sensory processing within the CNS. This phenomenon is prominent in the neurons in the most superficial layer of the dorsal horn, lamina I, where the phenotype of neurons may switch from purely nociceptive to nociceptive/non-nociceptive [26].

Heterosynaptic potentiation in nociceptive dorsal horn neurons is realized as a decrease in discharge threshold due to the recruitment of previously subthreshold non-nociceptive afferent inputs, as an increase in the responsiveness of dorsal horn neurons (i.e., an increase in the number of action potentials elicited by a suprathreshold input), and as an expansion of the excitatory cutaneous or deep receptive fields. The unmasking of subthreshold inputs causes nociceptive dorsal horn neurons to discharge in response to stimuli in surrounding regions of the periphery, producing a spread of sensitivity beyond the site of the tissue damage that may be a neural substrate for secondary hyperalgesia, whereby stimuli outside an area of injury are experienced as painful.

Heterosynaptic potentiation is produced as a consequence of the engagement of multiple intracellular signaling cascades in dorsal horn neurons, cascades that were effectively dormant before activation by fast neurotransmitters such as glutamate or modulators such as substance P, brain-derived neurotrophic factor (BDNF), or Eph-B. This process leads to enhanced excitatory postsynaptic responses and depressed inhibition [22,66]. Two major classes of mechanisms contribute to the resultant increased synaptic efficacy: (1) post-translational processing of ion channel/receptors or associated regulatory proteins altering intrinsic functional properties, and (2) cell-surface expression and trafficking of channels in primary sensory and dorsal horn neurons due to the trafficking of receptors to the membrane [30]. Additionally, regulation of K^+ channels may contribute to heterosynaptic potentiation: the coupling between synaptic inputs and action potential generation in dorsal horn neurons can be enhanced through downregulating $K_v4.2$ channels, the major contributor to A-type K^+ currents [17], and the balance between metabotropic glutamate receptor (mGluR) and $GABA_B$-receptor activation can switch the intrinsic firing properties of deep dorsal horn neurons from a tonic to a plateau or even an endogenous bursting pattern, through modulation of the inwardly rectifying K^+ channel, Kir3 [10].

Long-Term Potentiation in Dorsal Horn Nociceptive Neurons

A conceptually simple means to sensitize central pain transmission neurons is to homosynaptically increase the efficacy of the excitatory primary afferent inputs onto these neurons. Brief, high-frequency primary afferent stimulation does induce a potentiation of AMPA-receptor-mediated responses at synapses onto second-order neurons [22,43]. The potentiation is prevented by pharmacological blockade of NMDA receptors, and it persists for as long as experimentally observable, up to many hours. The lasting enhancement of monosynaptic excitatory synaptic responses at primary afferent-second order synapses in pain pathways shares common signaling cascades with the NMDA-receptor-dependent form of long-term potentiation (LTP) of excitatory synaptic transmission observed in many regions of the CNS, which resemble many aspects

of the signaling responsible for heterosynaptic sensitization described above.

Nociceptive neurons in the dorsal horn exhibit a distinct form of homosynaptic potentiation. This synaptic enhancement persists for hours or days after nociceptive synaptic stimulation and is thus a form of LTP [43,66]. LTP is observed in neurokinin-1 (NK1)-expressing neurons in spinal lamina I, and it can be evoked by brief periods of either high-frequency electrical stimulation (~100 Hz) [41] or low-frequency electrical stimulation (i.e. 2 Hz) at C-fiber strength [19]. Activation of NMDARs [18] and group I mGluRs [2] is involved in the induction of LTP. Homosynaptic plasticity is bidirectional, and under certain circumstances, glutamatergic synapses in the dorsal horn may show long-term depression (LTD) [44].

Homosynaptic potentiation of AMPA-receptor responses at synapses on dorsal horn neurons can occur experimentally in response to brief, high-frequency nociceptor stimulation [41]. The potentiation is restricted to the activated synapse and is persistent. Nociceptors do not usually fire at high frequencies, and therefore homosynaptic potentiation was thought to be limited to very intense stimuli producing a spatially and modality-constrained, if long-lasting, facilitation. However, recently it has been demonstrated that homosynaptic LTP may occur at primary afferent firing rates that match those produced by peripheral noxious stimulation [43]. Nevertheless, homosynaptic LTP alone cannot account for the spatial spread of pain hypersensitivity, nor for the facilitation of non-nociceptive inputs in nociceptive dorsal horn neurons; these common features of clinical chronic pain can only be accounted for by heterosynaptic potentiation.

Phosphorylation of NMDARs in Nociceptive Sensitization in the Dorsal Horn

The function of NMDARs is regulated by the balance of activity of protein kinases and phosphoprotein phosphatases acting at serine/threonine or tyrosine residues. Tyrosine phosphorylation of NMDARs appears critical for triggering and maintaining pain hypersensitivity induced by inflammation or peripheral nerve injury [15,29,30], with the non-receptor tyrosine kinase, Src, and the phosphatase, striatal-enriched tyrosine phosphatase (STEP), having major roles [42]. Src and STEP are themselves subject to regulation, and they provide a point of convergence through which sustained enhancement of NMDARs may facilitate excitatory synaptic transmission in nociceptive neurons (see Fig. 1). The facilitation may occur through the enhanced NMDAR currents per se (Fig. 1, middle) or through triggering enhancement of AMPA receptor currents (Fig. 1, right). Importantly, the basal sensory thresholds and acute nociceptive behavior are not dependent upon Src phosphorylation-mediated upregulation of NMDAR function (Fig. 1, left), indicating that the kinase is not essential for acute pain but rather is important in chronic pain hypersensitivity [29].

Src-dependent phosphorylation of NMDARs is involved in both inflammatory pain and neuropathic pain, as inferred from the effects of a 10-amino-acid peptide derived from Src unique domain fused with the protein transduction domain of HIV Tat protein (Src40-49Tat), rendering the peptide membrane permeant [29]. Src40-49Tat uncouples Src from the NMDAR complex, thereby inhibiting Src-mediated upregulation of NMDARs [14]. Administering Src40-49Tat reverses mechanical, thermal, and cold pain hypersensitivity induced by inflammation and peripheral nerve injury (PNI), without changing basal sensory thresholds and

acute nociception. Furthermore, no confounding sedation, motor deficit, or learning and memory impairment was observed at doses that suppress pain hypersensitivity. Thus, uncoupling Src from the NMDAR complex prevents phosphorylation-mediated enhancement of these receptors and thereby inhibits pain hypersensitivity while avoiding the deleterious consequence of directly blocking NMDARs [24].

Microglia-Neuron Signaling Mediates Enhanced Transmission after Peripheral Nerve Injury

The dominant theme in research on pain, as in all of neurobiology, for most of the past 100 years has been to understand the role of neurons. Until recently, glial cells were generally considered to serve primarily housekeeping roles in the nervous system. However, this view has changed radically in the last half-decade, in particular for the role of microglia in pain resulting from PNI. In the healthy CNS microglia are not dormant [7,37] as thought until recently, but instead engage in continuous

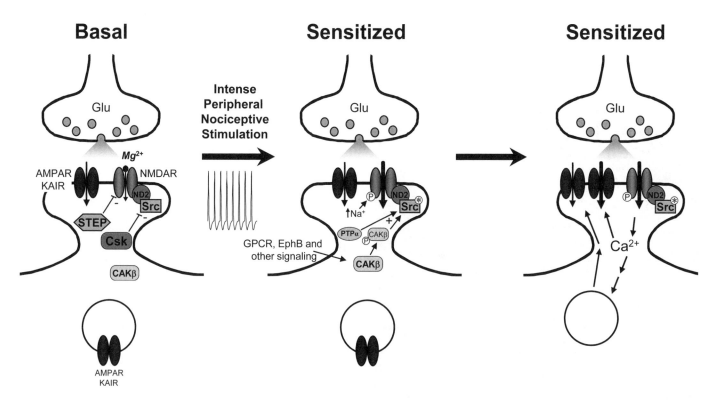

Fig. 1. A model for the role of sensitization of nociceptive dorsal horn neuron in pain hypersensitivity. Left: under basal conditions, NMDA-receptor (NMDAR) activity is suppressed by partial blockade of the channel by Mg^{2+} and by the activity of the protein tyrosine phosphatase, STEP, and the kinase, Csk. AMPAR, AMPA receptor; KAIR, kainate receptor. Middle: nociceptive input increases NMDAR-mediated currents (1) by relief of Mg^{2+} inhibition; (2) by activation of Src (Src*) via the actions of PTPα and activated CAKβ (CAKβ-P), which overcomes the suppression by STEP; and (3) by sensitizing the NMDARs to raised intracellular [Na^+]. GPCR, G-protein-coupled receptor. Right: upregulation of NMDAR function allows a large boost in entry of Ca^{2+}, which binds to calmodulin (CaM), causing activation of CaMKII (not illustrated). The enhancement of glutamatergic transmission is ultimately expressed through increased number of AMPARs/KAIRs in the postsynaptic membrane and/or through enhanced AMPA/KAIR activity.

surveillance of the local environment and respond to various stimuli that threaten physiological homeostasis. Responsive microglia undergo a diversity of types of changes, including proliferation; alterations in morphology, gene expression, and function [39]; and recruitment of bone-marrow-derived cells from the blood [70]. Responses of microglia in the dorsal horn (e.g., see Fig. 2) are concomitant with the development of neuropathic pain behaviors in all PNI models tested in rodents: spinal nerve ligation, chronic constriction injury, and dorsal rhizotomy [9,58,64].

Following PNI a series of changes occur in microglia within the spinal dorsal horn [6,12,28,50]. Within hours, the microglia start to respond, as evidenced by the small soma becoming hypertrophic and the long and thin processes withdrawing [12]. Subsequently, microglia proliferate, with the proliferation peaking about 3 days after nerve injury [13]. The microglia show an increased level of a number of "marker" proteins including CD11b [6,12,28,58], toll-like receptor 4 (TLR4) [50], cluster determinant 14 (CD14) [50], CD4 [49], and major histocompatibility complex (MHC) class II protein [48,49]. Many reports have demonstrated a correlation between signs of microglial response and PNI-induced pain hypersensitivity. But the fact that microglia have a causal role in these nerve-injury-evoked pain behaviors

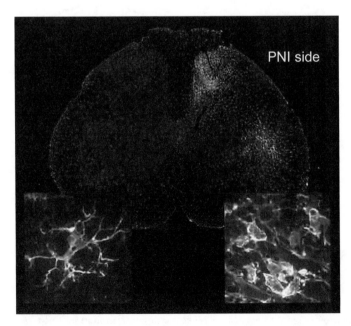

Fig. 2. Microglia in the spinal cord respond to injury to a peripheral nerve. Immunofluorescence for the microglia-specific protein, iba1, is shown in the photomicrographs of transverse section through lumbar spinal cord of a rat 14 days after sciatic nerve injury. The entire section is shown in the background, and the insets show enlargements of regions of superficial dorsal horn on the non-injured (left) or injured side (right).

was demonstrated in studies implicating $P2X_4$ receptors ($P2X_4Rs$) [58] and p38 mitogen-activated protein (MAP) kinase [23].

Microglia-Neuron Signaling: $P2X_4$ Receptors, BDNF, and KCC2

Mechanical hypersensitivity following spinal nerve ligation is reversed by pharmacological $P2X_4R$ blockade by means of an intrathecally administered antagonist [58]. $P2X_4Rs$ were found to be expressed neither in neurons nor in astrocytes, but in microglia. $P2X_4R$ expression, normally low in the naive spinal cord, progressively increases in the days following nerve injury, with a time course that parallels that of the development of mechanical hypersensitivity. In addition, suppressing the rise in $P2X_4R$ level by intrathecally administered antisense RNA prevents the development of mechanical hypersensitivity, and PNI does not cause a change in mechanical threshold in $P2X_4R$ null mutant mice [62]. Thus, microglial $P2X_4Rs$ in the spinal cord are necessary for mechanical hypersensitivity after nerve injury. Sufficiency of $P2X_4R$ stimulation in microglia for development of mechanical hypersensitivity was demonstrated by "microglia transfer experiments" in which microglia in primary culture are administered intrathecally in animals that were otherwise naive. When the microglia are stimulated in vitro by adenosine triphosphate (ATP), to activate $P2X_4Rs$, the animals develop mechanical hypersensitivity progressively over the course of the 3–5 hours following the administration. In contrast, transferring unstimulated microglia does not alter tactile sensitivity, nor does administering vehicle or ATP-only controls.

A key step for producing mechanical hypersensitivity is the increase in expression of $P2X_4Rs$ [58] that is initiated by PNI. The signals that cause upregulation of $P2X_4R$ expression are most likely produced by action potential discharge in primary afferents in the injured nerve [47]. Within the spinal cord, key intermediaries are fibronectin/integrin [59,60], interferon γ and its receptor, the interferon γ receptor [57], and the tyrosine kinase, Lyn [61]. On the other hand, $P2X_4Rs$ themselves are not required for microglia to proliferate, change morphology, and upregulate "markers" such as CD11b, because all of these changes occur in mice lacking $P2X_4Rs$ [62]. Because $P2X_4R$-null mice do not develop mechanical hypersensitivity after PNI, the changes in morphology, proliferation, and marker increase cannot per se be necessary for the hypersensitivity. Rather, these changes may be upstream in pathways leading to $P2X_4R$ upregulation, or in pathways that are not directly causative for PNI-induced mechanical hypersensitivity.

Ultimately, the signaling initiated by $P2X_4R$ activation in the microglia must be transmitted to the nociceptive neurons in the dorsal horn, and must cause increased discharge activity in the nociceptive processing network. While this enhanced responsiveness could potentially arise from alteration of intrinsic passive or active membrane conductances, increased excitatory drive, or suppressed inhibition, it is known that after PNI there is a prominent suppression of inhibition in dorsal horn neurons that is critical for producing mechanical hypersensitivity [5,35]. In particular, mechanical hypersensitivity in neurons of spinal lamina I following peripheral nerve injury involves reduction in the expression of the K^+-Cl^- cotransporter, KCC2, normally responsible for the extrusion of Cl^- from the cell [5]. As a consequence, after peripheral nerve injury there is a rise in intracellular Cl^- in lamina I dorsal horn neurons, resulting in a depolarizing shift in the anion reversal potential (E_{anion}) and hyperexcitability by means of dramatically reducing GABA$_A$-ergic and glycinergic inhibition. In about one-third of lamina I neurons, GABA produces frank excitation rather than inhibition. Local blockade or knockdown of spinal KCC2 in naive rats markedly reduces nociceptive threshold, confirming that disruption of anion homeostasis in lamina I neurons is sufficient to produce neuropathic pain behaviors. Although sensitization after PNI is displayed by many cells in both the superficial and deep laminae of the dorsal horn, the impact in terms of pain hypersensitivity may be most important for lamina I spinothalamic or spinoparabrachial projection neurons, particularly those expressing the NK1 receptor [1,16].

That stimulating $P2X_4Rs$ on microglia acts via this mechanism was shown by intrathecal injection of $P2X_4R$-stimulated microglia, which causes a rise in intracellular Cl^- in lamina I neurons, reducing inhibition and converting GABA$_A$-ergic responses to excitation [4]. Moreover, pharmacological blockade of $P2X_4R$ acutely reverses the rise in intracellular Cl^- in lamina I neurons after PNI. Thus, the issue of how microglia signal to neurons reduces to the issue of how microglia signal to lamina I neurons to effect the shift in E_{anion} that contributes to enhancing neuronal responses. This signaling might potentially occur through the release of one or more diffusible chemical messengers

from microglia upon stimulation of $P2X_4Rs$. Indeed, activated microglia are known to secrete a number of diffusible chemical messengers, including interleukin-1β, interleukin-6, and tumor necrosis factor-α. Release of these factors in the spinal cord has been hypothesized to contribute to nerve-injury-induced pain hypersensitivity [32,56,63].

Microglia also express and release neurotrophic factors such as BDNF, and in hippocampal neurons BDNF mediates anion gradient shifts, leading to increased Cl^- [38]. In addition, it has been reported that BDNF heterozygous knockout mice show attenuated pain hypersensitivity following nerve injury as compared to wild-type mice [69]. Thus, these lines of evidence point to BDNF as a primary candidate signaling molecule between microglia and neurons. Consistent with this reasoning, intrathecal application of BDNF mimics the mechanical hypersensitivity and alteration in E_{anion} caused by PNI or by administering $P2X_4R$-stimulated microglia, demonstrating that BDNF is sufficient to cause tactile hypersensitivity and to raise intracellular Cl^- in lamina I neurons. The mechanical hypersensitivity produced by PNI is reversed by a function-blocking antibody against TrkB, the cognate receptor for BDNF, and by a BDNF-sequestering fusion protein (TrkB-Fc), implying that BDNF-TrkB signaling is necessary for neuropathic pain hypersensitivity.

The intracellular biochemical pathway by which $P2X_4R$-stimulation causes release of BDNF has been found to be mediated by Ca^{2+} influx, leading to activation of p38 MAP kinase, which causes release of premade BDNF and also increases transcription and translation of BDNF [55]. Demonstrating that p38 MAP kinase is a cellular intermediary in the release of BDNF evoked by stimulating microglial P2X4Rs provides a unifying mechanism for observations that the ongoing expression of neuropathic pain behaviors requires both the activation of $P2X_4Rs$ and p38 MAP kinases (see above). The results unify previous seemingly disparate findings and point to signaling of $P2X_4Rs$ and p38 MAP kinase in microglia as being critical for the involvement of BDNF in neuropathic pain after PNI.

Microglia-Induced Disinhibition and NMDAR Synaptic Transmission

GABAergic and glycinergic inhibition within the dorsal horn strongly suppresses polysynaptic inputs from primary afferents to lamina I neurons, such that these neurons mainly discharge only in response to inputs from primary afferent nociceptors. Pharmacological blockade of GABA$_A$ and glycine receptors, or of KCC2, unmasks polysynaptic excitatory synaptic transmission [54] from inputs that largely arise from non-nociceptive primary afferents, switching the functional phenotype of lamina I neurons from nociceptive only to nociceptive/non-nociceptive [25]. Applying P2X$_4$R-stimulated microglia to the spinal cord in vivo similarly unmasks excitatory non-nociceptive synaptic inputs to lamina I neurons, phenocopying the change in response characteristics of these cells after PNI (see Fig. 3). Thus, disinhibition is manifested as

an increase in the output of the dorsal horn nociceptive network. In vitro, the unmasking of polysynaptic inputs by blocking GABA$_A$ and glycine receptors depends upon NMDARs [54]. Thus, by causing disinhibition in the dorsal horn, microglia-neuron signaling following peripheral nerve injury may facilitate NMDAR-dependent polysynaptic transmission. Collectively, the results provide the basis for a conceptual model whereby P2X$_4$-receptor stimulation of microglia causes release of BDNF, which then acts on dorsal horn neurons to raise intracellular Cl$^-$ and produce the resultant enhancement of neuronal responsiveness (see Fig. 4).

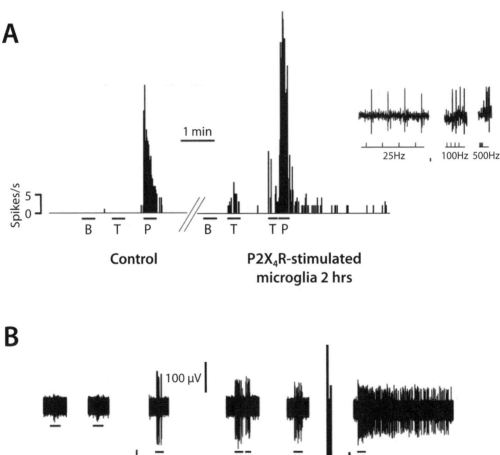

Fig. 3. Administering P2X$_4$-receptor (P2X$_4$R)-stimulated microglia recapitulates the changes in responses of lamina I projection neurons seen after peripheral nerve injury. (A) Responses of a lamina I projection neuron to innocuous brush (B) or touch (T) or noxious pinch (P) under basal conditions (left) or 2 hours after administering P2X$_4$R-stimulated microglia (right). (B) Responses of a lamina I projection neuron in a naïve animal (left) or in a different animal after peripheral neuron injury (PNI). The inset shows the extracellularly recorded discharge activity from each neuron.

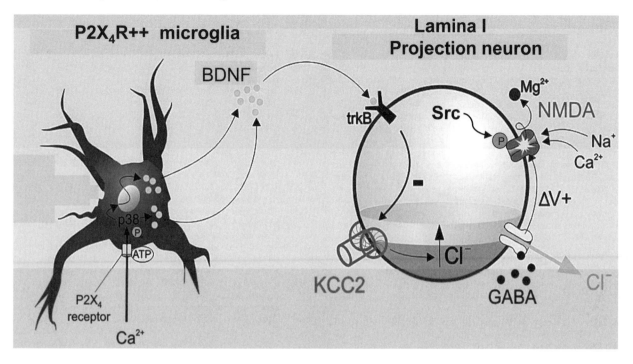

Fig. 4. A model for pain hypersensitivity induced by peripheral nerve injury. After peripheral nerve injury microglia in the dorsal horn increase expression of $P2X_4$ receptors ($P2X_4Rs$), stimulation of which causes the microglia to release brain-derived neurotrophic factor (BDNF). BDNF, acting on TrkB receptors, causes downregulation of KCC2, causing intracellular Cl^- concentration to increase and thereby decreasing inhibition of the neurons. Depolarizing $GABA_A$ responses facilitate NMDA-receptor (NMDAR) currents by reducing Mg^{2+} blockade of the receptor. Concomitantly, Src kinase upregulates NMDAR function.

Conclusions

Enhancement of excitatory synaptic responses of projection neurons within the dorsal horn nociceptive network, directly or through suppression of inhibition, is a key process that increases the gain of nociceptive transmission and leads to pain hypersensitivity. In recent years, it has become apparent that the key molecular mechanisms in the dorsal horn are not restricted to neurons but also involve glial cells. Understanding how microglia-neuron signaling impacts synaptic transmission and plasticity is anticipated to lead to strategies for the diagnosis and management of chronic pain that were not previously anticipated by a view of pain plasticity solely focused on neurons.

Acknowledgments

The author is supported by grants from the Canadian Institutes of Health Research, the Krembil Foundation, and the Ontario Neurotrauma Foundation. He holds a Canada Research Chair (Tier I), in Neuroplasticity and Pain, and is an International Scholar of the Howard Hughes Medical Institute.

References

[1] Allen BJ, Rogers SD, Ghilardi JR, Menning PM, Kuskowski MA, Basbaum AI, Simone DA, Mantyh PW. Noxious cutaneous thermal stimuli induce a graded release of endogenous substance P in the spinal cord: imaging peptide action in vivo. J Neurosci 1997;17:5921–7.

[2] Azkue JJ, Liu XG, Zimmermann M, Sandkuhler J. Induction of long-term potentiation of C fibre-evoked spinal field potentials requires recruitment of group I, but not group II/III metabotropic glutamate receptors. Pain 2003;106:373–9.

[3] Cook AJ, Woolf CJ, Wall PD, McMahon SB. Dynamic receptive field plasticity in rat spinal cord dorsal horn following C-primary afferent input. Nature 1987;325:151–3.

[4] Coull JA, Beggs S, Boudreau D, Boivin D, Tsuda M, Inoue K, Gravel C, Salter MW, De Koninck Y. BDNF from microglia causes the shift in neuronal anion gradient underlying neuropathic pain. Nature 2005;438:1017–21.

[5] Coull JA, Boudreau D, Bachand K, Prescott SA, Nault F, Sik A, De Koninck P, De Koninck Y. Trans-synaptic shift in anion gradient in spinal lamina I neurons as a mechanism of neuropathic pain. Nature 2003;424:938–42.

[6] Coyle DE. Partial peripheral nerve injury leads to activation of astroglia and microglia which parallels the development of allodynic behavior. Glia 1998;23:75–83.

[7] Davalos D, Grutzendler J, Yang G, Kim JV, Zuo Y, Jung S, Littman DR, Dustin ML, Gan WB. ATP mediates rapid microglial response to local brain injury in vivo. Nat Neurosci 2005;8:752–8.

[8] De Koninck Y, Henry JL. Substance P-mediated slow excitatory postsynaptic potential elicited in dorsal horn neurons in vivo by noxious stimulation. Proc Natl Acad Sci USA 1991;88:11344–8.

[9] DeLeo JA, Yezierski RP. The role of neuroinflammation and neuroimmune activation in persistent pain. Pain 2001;90:1–6.

[10] Derjean D, Bertrand S, Le MG, Landry M, Morisset V, Nagy F. Dynamic balance of metabotropic inputs causes dorsal horn neurons to switch functional states. Nat Neurosci 2003;6:274–81.

[11] Dickenson AH, Chapman V, Green GM. The pharmacology of excitatory and inhibitory amino acid-mediated events in the transmission and modulation of pain in the spinal cord. Gen Pharmacol 1997;28:633–8.

[12] Eriksson NP, Persson JK, Svensson M, Arvidsson J, Molander C, Aldskogius H. A quantitative analysis of the microglial cell reaction in central primary sensory projection territories following peripheral nerve injury in the adult rat. Exp Brain Res 1993;96:19–27.

[13] Gehrmann J, Banati RB. Microglial turnover in the injured CNS: activated microglia undergo delayed DNA fragmentation following peripheral nerve injury. J Neuropathol Exp Neurol 1995;54:680–8.

[14] Gingrich JR, Pelkey KA, Fam SR, Huang Y, Petralia RS, Wenthold RJ, Salter MW. Unique domain anchoring of Src to synaptic NMDA receptors via the mitochondrial protein NADH dehydrogenase subunit 2. Proc Natl Acad Sci USA 2004;101:6237–42.

[15] Guo W, Zou S, Guan Y, Ikeda T, Tal M, Dubner R, Ren K. Tyrosine Phosphorylation of the NR2B subunit of the NMDA receptor in the spinal cord during the development and maintenance of inflammatory hyperalgesia. J Neurosci 2002;22:6208–17.

[16] Honor P, Menning PM, Rogers SD, Nichols ML, Basbaum AI, Besson JM, Mantyh PW. Spinal substance P receptor expression and internalization in acute, short-term, and long-term inflammatory pain states. J Neurosci 1999;19:7670–8.

[17] Hu HJ, Carrasquillo Y, Karim F, Jung WE, Nerbonne JM, Schwarz TL, Gereau RW. The kv4.2 potassium channel subunit is required for pain plasticity. Neuron 2006;50:89–100.

[18] Ikeda H, Heinke B, Ruscheweyh R, Sandkuhler J. Synaptic plasticity in spinal lamina I projection neurons that mediate hyperalgesia. Science 2003;299:1237–40.

[19] Ikeda H, Stark J, Fischer H, Wagner M, Drdla R, Jager T, Sandkuhler J. Synaptic amplifier of inflammatory pain in the spinal dorsal horn. Science 2006;312:1659–62.

[20] Inoue K, Tsuda M. Microglia and neuropathic pain. Glia 2009;57:1469–79.

[21] Jessell TM, Jahr CE. Fast and slow excitatory transmitters at primary afferent synapses in the dorsal horn of the spinal-cord. Advances in pain research and therapy. New York: Raven Press; 1985. p. 31–9.

[22] Ji RR, Kohno T, Moore KA, Woolf CJ. Central sensitization and LTP: do pain and memory share similar mechanisms? Trends Neurosci 2003;26:696–705.

[23] Jin SX, Zhuang ZY, Woolf CJ, Ji RR. p38 mitogen-activated protein kinase is activated after a spinal nerve ligation in spinal cord microglia and dorsal root ganglion neurons and contributes to the generation of neuropathic pain. J Neurosci 2003;23:4017–22.

[24] Kalia LV, Kalia SK, Salter MW. NMDA receptors in clinical neurology: excitatory times ahead. Lancet Neurol 2008;7:742–55.

[25] Keller AF, Beggs S, Salter MW, De Koninck Y. Disrupting anion homeostasis in the spinal dorsal horn replicates the enhanced excitability of Lamina I projection neurons observed following peripheral nerve injury. Soc Neurosci Abstracts 2005;31.

[26] Keller AF, Beggs S, Salter MW, De Koninck Y. Transformation of the output of spinal lamina I neurons after nerve injury and microglia stimulation underlying neuropathic pain. Mol Pain 2007;3:27.

[27] Li P, Wilding TJ, Kim SJ, Calejesan AA, Huettner JE, Zhuo M. Kainate-receptor-mediated sensory synaptic transmission in mammalian spinal cord. Nature 1999;397:161–4.

[28] Liu L, Tornqvist E, Mattsson P, Eriksson NP, Persson JK, Morgan BP, Aldskogius H, Svensson M. Complement and clusterin in the spinal cord dorsal horn and gracile nucleus following sciatic nerve injury in the adult rat. Neuroscience 1995;68:167–79.

[29] Liu XJ, Gingrich JR, Vargas-Caballero M, Dong YN, Sengar A, Beggs S, Wang SH, Ding HK, Frankland PW, Salter MW. Treatment of inflammatory and neuropathic pain by uncoupling Src from the NMDA receptor complex. Nat Med 2008;14:1325–32.

[30] Liu XJ, Salter MW. Glutamate receptor phosphorylation and trafficking in pain plasticity in spinal cord dorsal horn. Eur J Neurosci 2010; in press.

[31] Malcangio M, Bowery NG. GABA and its receptors in the spinal cord. Trends Pharmacol Sci 1996;17:457–62.

[32] Marchand F, Perretti M, McMahon SB. Role of the immune system in chronic pain. Nat Rev Neurosci 2005;6:521–32.

[33] Mendell LM. Modifiability of spinal synapses. Physiol Rev 1984;64:260–324.

[34] Moore KA, Baba H, Woolf CJ. Synaptic transmission and plasticity in the superficial dorsal horn. Prog Brain Res 2000;129:63–80.

[35] Moore KA, Kohno T, Karchewski LA, Scholz J, Baba H, Woolf CJ. Partial peripheral nerve injury promotes a selective loss of GABAergic inhibition in the superficial dorsal horn of the spinal cord. J Neurosci 2002;22:6724–31.

[36] Morisset V, Nagy F. Ionic basis for plateau potentials in deep dorsal horn neurons of the rat spinal cord. J Neurosci 1999;19:7309–16.

[37] Nimmerjahn A, Kirchhoff F, Helmchen F. Resting microglial cells are highly dynamic surveillants of brain parenchyma in vivo. Science 2005;308:1314–8.

[38] Payne JA, Rivera C, Voipio J, Kaila K. Cation-chloride co-transporters in neuronal communication, development and trauma. Trends Neurosci 2003;26:199–206.

[39] Perry VH. Modulation of microglia phenotype. Neuropathol Appl Neurobiol 1994;20:177.

[40] Prescott SA, De Koninck Y. Gain control of firing rate by shunting inhibition: roles of synaptic noise and dendritic saturation. Proc Natl Acad Sci USA 2003;100:2076–81.

[41] Randic M, Jiang MC, Cerne R. Long-term potentiation and long-term depression of primary afferent neurotransmission in the rat spinal cord. J Neurosci 1993;13:5228–41.

[42] Salter MW, Kalia LV. Src kinases: a hub for NMDA receptor regulation. Nat Rev Neurosci 2004;5:317–28.

[43] Sandkuhler J. Understanding LTP in pain pathways. Mol Pain 2007;3:9.

[44] Sandkuhler J. Models and mechanisms of hyperalgesia and allodynia. Physiol Rev 2009;89:707–58.

[45] Simone DA, Baumann TK, Collins JG, LaMotte RH. Sensitization of cat dorsal horn neurons to innocuous mechanical stimulation after intradermal injection of capsaicin. Brain Res 1989;486:185–9.

[46] Sivilotti LG, Thompson SW, Woolf CJ. Rate of rise of the cumulative depolarization evoked by repetitive stimulation of small-caliber afferents is a predictor of action potential windup in rat spinal neurons in vitro. J Neurophysiol 1993;69:1621–31.

[47] Suter MR, Berta T, Gao YJ, Decosterd I, Ji RR. Large A-fiber activity is required for microglial proliferation and p38 MAPK activation in the spinal cord: different effects of resiniferatoxin and bupivacaine on spinal microglial changes after spared nerve injury. Mol Pain 2009;5:53.

[48] Sweitzer SM, DeLeo JA. The active metabolite of leflunomide, an immunosuppressive agent, reduces mechanical sensitivity in a rat mononeuropathy model. J Pain 2002;3:360–8.

[49] Sweitzer SM, White KA, Dutta C, DeLeo JA. The differential role of spinal MHC class II and cellular adhesion molecules in peripheral inflammatory versus neuropathic pain in rodents. J Neuroimmunol 2002;125:82–93.

[50] Tanga FY, Raghavendra V, DeLeo JA. Quantitative real-time RT-PCR assessment of spinal microglial and astrocytic activation markers in a rat model of neuropathic pain. Neurochem Int 2004;45:397–407.

[51] Thompson SW, Woolf CJ, Sivilotti LG. Small-caliber afferent inputs produce a heterosynaptic facilitation of the synaptic responses evoked by primary afferent A-fibers in the neonatal rat spinal cord in vitro. J Neurophysiol 1993;69:2116–28.

[52] Thompson SWN, King AE, Woolf CJ. Activity-dependent changes in rat ventral horn neurones in vitro; summation of prolonged afferent evoked postsynaptic depolarizations produce a d-APV sensitive windup. Eur J Neurosci 1990;2:638–49.

[53] Tong CK, MacDermott AB. Both Ca²⁺-permeable and -impermeable AMPA receptors contribute to primary synaptic drive onto rat dorsal horn neurons. J Physiol 2006;575:133–44.

[54] Torsney C, MacDermott AB. Disinhibition opens the gate to pathological pain signaling in superficial neurokinin 1 receptor-expressing neurons in rat spinal cord. J Neurosci 2006;26:1833–43.

[55] Trang T, Beggs S, Wan X, Salter MW. P2X4-receptor-mediated synthesis and release of brain-derived neurotrophic factor in microglia is dependent on calcium and p38-mitogen-activated protein kinase activation. J Neurosci 2009;29:3518–28.

[56] Tsuda M, Inoue K, Salter MW. Neuropathic pain and spinal microglia: a big problem from molecules in 'small' glia. Trends Neurosci 2005;28:101–7.

[57] Tsuda M, Masuda T, Kitano J, Shimoyama H, Tozaki-Saitoh H, Inoue K. IFN-gamma receptor signaling mediates spinal microglia activation driving neuropathic pain. Proc Natl Acad Sci USA 2009;106:8032–7.

[58] Tsuda M, Shigemoto-Mogami Y, Koizumi S, Mizokoshi A, Kohsaka S, Salter MW, Inoue K. P2X4 receptors induced in spinal microglia gate tactile allodynia after nerve injury. Nature 2003;424:778–83.

[59] Tsuda M, Toyomitsu E, Komatsu T, Masuda T, Kunifusa E, Nasu-Tada K, Koizumi S, Yamamoto K, Ando J, Inoue K. Fibronectin/integrin system is involved in P2X₄ receptor upregulation in the spinal cord and neuropathic pain after nerve injury. Glia 2008;56:579–85.

[60] Tsuda M, Toyomitsu E, Kometani M, Tozaki-Saitoh H, Inoue K. Mechanisms underlying fibronectin-induced upregulation of P2X₄R expression in microglia: distinct roles of PI3K-Akt and MEK-ERK signaling pathways. J Cell Mol Med 2009;13:3251–9.

[61] Tsuda M, Tozaki-Saitoh H, Masuda T, Toyomitsu E, Tezuka T, Yamamoto T, Inoue K. Lyn tyrosine kinase is required for P2X₄ receptor upregulation and neuropathic pain after peripheral nerve injury. Glia 2008;56:50–8.

[62] Ulmann L, Hatcher JP, Hughes JP, Chaumont S, Green PJ, Conquet F, Buell GN, Reeve AJ, Chessell IP, Rassendren F. Up-regulation of P2X4 receptors in spinal microglia after peripheral nerve injury mediates BDNF release and neuropathic pain. J Neurosci 2008;28:11263–8.

[63] Watkins LR, Maier SF. Glia: a novel drug discovery target for clinical pain. Nat Rev Drug Discov 2003;2:973–85.

[64] Watkins LR, Milligan ED, Maier SF. Glial proinflammatory cytokines mediate exaggerated pain states: implications for clinical pain. Adv Exp Med Biol 2003;521:1–21.

[65] Woolf CJ. Evidence for a central component of post-injury pain hypersensitivity. Nature 1983;306:686–8.

[66] Woolf CJ, Salter MW. Neuronal plasticity: increasing the gain in pain. Science 2000;288:1765–9.

[67] Woolf CJ, Salter MW. Plasticity and pain: role of the dorsal horn. In: McMahon SB, Koltzenburg M, editors. Melzack and Wall's textbook of pain, 5th ed. Elsevier; 2006. p. 91–106.

[68] Woolf CJ, Wall PD. Relative effectiveness of C primary afferent fibers of different origins in evoking a prolonged facilitation of the flexor reflex in the rat. J Neurosci 1986;6:1433–42.

[69] Yajima Y, Narita M, Usui A, Kaneko C, Miyatake M, Narita M, Yamaguchi T, Tamaki H, Wachi H, Seyama Y, Suzuki T. Direct evidence for the involvement of brain-derived neurotrophic factor in the development of a neuropathic pain-like state in mice. J Neurochem 2005;93:584–94.

[70] Zhang J, Shi XQ, Echeverry S, Mogil JS, De KY, Rivest S. Expression of CCR2 in both resident and bone marrow-derived microglia plays a critical role in neuropathic pain. J Neurosci 2007;27:12396–406.

Correspondence to: Dr. Michael W. Salter, The Hospital for Sick Children, 555 University Avenue, Toronto, Ontario M5G 1X8, Canada. Email: mike.salter@utoronto.ca.

Part 2
Cancer Pain: From Mechanisms to Treatment

Mechanisms of Cancer Pain: Experimental Data

3

Sital Patel, BSc, and Anthony H. Dickenson, PhD, FmedSci

Department of Neuropharmacology, University College London, London, United Kingdom

Improvements in the detection and treatment of cancers have resulted in patients surviving longer, but at a high cost of decreased quality of life, and severe pain is often a major contributor [36]. Bone metastases are frequently predictive of pain, and bone cancer pain is in fact the most common cancer-related pain; approximately 90% of cancer patients experience bone pain, and only about half of these have even temporary relief from conventional therapies [31].

Patients experience a triad of pain states consisting of background pain, spontaneous pain, or incident pain. The intermittent nature of spontaneous and incident pains makes them hard to treat, and it is very difficult for patients with bone metastases to attain freedom from pain on movement [30].

Currently, treatment of bone cancer involves a number of approaches including radiotherapy, chemotherapy, surgical intervention, pharmacotherapy, or a combination of these treatments. However, several novel compounds are currently under investigation, including denosumab, osteoprotegerin analogues, and anti-angiogenic agents [35]. In terms of pharmacotherapy for the pain associated with bone metastases, the main classes of drugs used are bisphosphonates, nonsteroidal anti-inflammatory drugs (NSAIDs), and opioids. Nonpharmacological treatments for the palliation of bone cancer include radiopharmaceuticals, of which the newer beta-emitting isotopes display better pharmacokinetic and decay properties [33].

Animal models of human diseases represent an area with a proven track record for value to translational research, particularly in the field of chronic pain; we have greater knowledge of nociceptive processing at the peripheral, spinal, and supraspinal level thanks to investigation in animal models of inflammatory and neuropathic pain. Until recently, cancer pain has been studied much less than other pains, but things are starting to change. Understanding the mechanisms of cancer pain was revolutionized by the development of animal models by Patrick Mantyh and colleagues [44]. Cancer-induced bone pain (CIBP) is a unique pain state but with some mechanisms overlapping those of chronic inflammatory and neuropathic pain. This chapter is an overview of current preclinical knowledge of mechanisms and treatments of cancer pain.

Cancer pain can be considered to be a mixed-mechanism pain, and not a single neuropathic, visceral, or somatic pain state. It is a complex syndrome where inflammatory, neuropathic, and ischemic mechanisms are often involved, and at more than a single site. Inflammation-induced changes will be caused by direct tissue damage resulting from tumor growth as well as by the release of pain mediators by the cancer cells themselves. The neuropathic pain component can be due to pre-existing cancer-induced damage to sensory nerves such as infiltration or compression, as well as subsequent interventions such as chemotherapy and surgery that in turn may cause neuropathy. Although the effectiveness of drugs used to treat neuropathic pain (such as gabapentin or carbamazepine) in attenuating both behavioral and neuronal measures in certain animal models of CIBP may suggest neuropathic mechanisms, the actions of these drugs are not exclusive to neuropathic pain, and thus drug efficacy cannot be used as a diagnosis.

Clinically, patients could present with a combination of positive and negative signs such as sensory loss (numbness), spontaneous pain, allodynia, hyperalgesia, and paresthesia [39], which indicate neuropathy, together with descriptors such as burning, tingling, shooting, "pins-and-needles-like," and electric-shock-like pains. However, some of the positive symptoms will also occur when the pain is inflammatory. Research so far has revealed CIBP to be a unique pain state, and therefore it will be interesting to apply the questionnaires that aid the diagnosis of neuropathic pain to cancer patients.

Peripheral Sensitization after Inflammation

Many inflammatory mediators are released by tissue injury, and these can directly activate and sensitize nociceptor terminals to subsequent thermal, mechanical, and chemical stimuli, and also stimulate the antidromic release of transmitters from collateral branches of sensory nerves (neurogenic inflammation). A myriad of events and interactions produce a sensitizing "soup" of mediators in the vicinity of the nociceptor terminal, which go on to produce peripheral inflammation. In particular, some intracellular second messengers, such as adenosine triphosphate (ATP), cyclic adenosine monophosphate (cAMP), and protein kinase C-ε (PKCε), and molecular sensors, such as the capsaicin receptor, transient potential receptor vanilloid 1 (TRPV1), and the sensory-nerve-specific or selective families of sodium channels, are emerging as important molecules in integrating signals and generating peripheral sensitization [2,10].

Pharmacotherapy of Cancer-Induced Bone Pain

The treatment algorithm for CIBP in terms of pharmacotherapy currently consists of anticonvulsants, antidepressants, antiarrhythmics, steroids, N-methyl-D-aspartate (NMDA) receptor antagonists, sympatholytic agents, and topical agents such as lidocaine creams and patches. However, the World Health Organization's three-step pain relief ladder recommends nonopioids such as NSAIDs as the first drug to try, followed by the addition of mild opioids and adjuvants such as anticonvulsants, steroids, and bisphosphonates in Step 2, and finally stronger opioids with or without adjuvants in Step 3. Nonpharmacological strategies include psychological and physical treatments such as hypnotherapy, cognitive-behavioral therapy, and transcutaneous electrical nerve stimulation (TENS).

Nonsteroidal Anti-Inflammatory Drugs

In terms of pharmacotherapy, NSAIDs are the first step on the analgesic ladder for CIBP relief, and even where the severity of pain requires progression to other analgesics, administration of NSAIDs may continue to be advantageous due to possible additive effects [30]. NSAIDs inhibit the cyclooxygenase (COX) pathway of arachidonic acid breakdown, thus reducing the formation of prostaglandins. The rationale for their use in CIBP is based on preventing activation and sensitization of primary afferents by prostaglandins. However, trials of NSAIDs in cancer pain that include bone metastases do not specify effects on incident pain, and there is a general lack of clinical evidence to support a significant analgesic effect of NSAIDs in CIBP [51]. Side effects associated with NSAIDs include bleeding, gastrointestinal ulceration, and renal toxicity. The new class of COX-2-selective antagonists have been reported to inhibit cancer cell growth [47].

It has been demonstrated in murine and rat models that chronic bisphosphonate treatment reduces destruction of bone and sensory nerves innervating the bone, as well as movement-evoked bone pain [57,46]. Selective inhibition of COX-2 (by NS-398) in the murine model has been shown to reduce spontaneous pain, bone destruction, and tumor growth [40] supporting, the previously reported evidence for antitumorigenic properties of this class of drug [47] and the involvement of prostaglandin sensitization of primary afferents in this pain state. However, a different study in the murine model [43] showed that whereas nonselective inhibition of COX (with indomethacin) significantly reduced mechanically evoked pain, inhibition of COX-1 (with SC560) or COX-2 (with celecoxib) was ineffective. The discrepancy between the investigations may be due to differences in effects on spontaneous and evoked pain, or differing selectivity for COX-2. There are similar discrepancies in rat models of CIBP, where acute dosing with the COX-2 antagonist celecoxib has been shown to be ineffective [28], whereas another investigation in the same model showed chronic administration of the COX-2 antagonists lumiracoxib and valdecoxib to significantly reduce pain behavior [14]. Here the different findings could be due to acute versus chronic administration regimes or, again, differing selectivity for COX-2. Currently underway is a Phase 2 trial investigating the anticancer activity of a novel COX-2-specific inhibitor, apricoxib, in combination with either docetaxel or pemetrexed, in patients with lung cancer. The primary measure is time to disease progression, and the study is due to be completed in June, 2010. Previous Phase 2a data from a trial investigating the analgesic affects of apricoxib found that it had a favorable safety profile in addition to being a potent analgesic in postoperative dental pain [38]. It is clear that further investigation is necessary to evaluate the use of this class of drug in CIBP.

Bisphosphonates

Bisphosphonates inhibit osteoclastic bone resorption and therefore reduce pain in patients by decreasing the osteolytic effect of the tumor. Bisphosphonates have been reported to potentiate the effects of analgesics in treating CIBP, although the effect is modest and does not allow for reduction of the dose of analgesic [30]. Side effects associated with bisphosphonates include gastrointestinal tract toxicity, fever, and electrolyte abnormalities.

A paucity of knowledge surrounding the mechanisms driving CIBP has hindered the development of better treatments for this type of chronic pain. Based on knowledge of the sensory innervation of bone and factors released by tumor cells and inflammatory infiltrate, we can infer some of the processes driving this type of chronic pain. There is a rich supply of sensory nerves to the periosteum, bone marrow, and mineralized bone [26]. Therefore, destruction of bone architecture in regions with sensory innervation will result in direct mechanical damage of these afferent fibers and lead to pain. Furthermore, stretching of the periosteum due to growth of tumor within the bone, or nerve entrapment after pathological fracture or by the invading tumor itself, may also result in pain [30].

Other Agents

As well as resulting from mechanical damage or distension of primary afferents by tumors invading the bone, pain may arise due to stimulation of nociceptors by factors released by tumor cells and the accompanying inflammatory infiltrate. In addition to cancer cells, tumors are made up of a number of cell types including macrophages, neutrophils, and T-cells, and they release a plethora of growth factors, cytokines, interleukins, chemokines, prostanoids, and endothelins [42,48], resulting in activation of primary afferents that express receptors for many of these factors. Furthermore, the local environment of the tumor is made more acidic [16], and this decrease in pH can activate acid-sensing ion channels (ASICs) expressed by primary afferents.

The vanilloid receptor, TRPV1, a cation channel activated by noxious heat and capsaicin and expressed by nociceptors, is also activated by decreases in pH, and protons decrease the temperature threshold for TRPV1 activation. The local acidosis induced by cancers not only causes activation of primary afferents, but in addition facilitates osteoclastic bone destruction. Osteoclast formation and activation are reliant on macrophage colony-stimulating factor (M-CSF) and on the interaction between the receptor activator for nuclear factor κB (RANK; expressed on osteoclast precursors) with the RANK ligand (RANK-L; expressed on various cell types including osteoblasts) in an acidic environment. The natural balance of bone remodeling is controlled by both osteoblast and osteoclast activity; however, this process is interrupted by tumor-induced overexpression of the RANK receptor and increased RANK-L signaling.

Potential novel targets for attenuating CIBP identified by investigation in these models include: the bradykinin B_1 receptor, as pharmacological blockade of B_1 has been shown to block pain in early and advanced stages of CIBP [45]; the TRPV1 receptor, as chronic administration of a TRPV1 antagonist or disruption of the TRPV1 gene will significantly attenuate ongoing and movement-evoked pain [15]; and endothelin receptors, as pharmacological blockade of ET_A reduced ongoing and movement-evoked pain and, with chronic administration, reduced neurochemical indices of peripheral and central sensitization [34]. One of the first targets identified in the murine model was RANK-L. As mentioned previously, osteoprotegerin acts as a decoy receptor for RANK-L, preventing RANK-L-driven stimulation of osteoclast activity [21], and was demonstrated to reduce skeletal destruction, pain and the spinal neurochemical alterations in the model [19]. Following

Phase 3 clinical trials and currently under U.S. Federal Drug Administration (FDA) review is denosumab, a fully human monoclonal antibody, which specifically targets RANK-L.

Other novel agents under investigation include radiopharmaceuticals such as Alpharadin, which is an alpha-particle emitting treatment of bone metastases in patients with cancer. Early clinical trial data have been favorable in comparison to placebo, showing a decrease in bone-alkaline phosphatase levels. High levels of alkaline phosphatase in the blood are indicative of osteoblastic bone tumors. Phase 3 trials for Alpharadin are currently underway [24].

Hypertrophy of astrocytes, increased expression of dynorphin and c-Fos, and internalization of substance P receptors have all been reported in models of neuropathic and inflammatory pain [1,32]. Conversely, whereas substance P levels in primary afferent neurons are elevated in models of inflammation and decreased in models of neuropathy, they are not altered in the murine bone cancer model [44]. Thus, the neurochemical alterations occurring in this model are unique, reflecting a pain state that differs in some aspects but shares some features of neuropathy and inflammation. These findings alone start to give indications as to why current pharmacotherapy is not very effective, even though neuropathy and inflammation are clearly contributors to CIBP, as discussed in the previous sections. Thus, these different underlying mechanisms may interact and will probably require distinct drug treatments. Interesting to note is the fact that breast cancer metastases are either mixed or predominantly osteolytic in comparison to prostate cancer metastases, which form predominantly osteoblastic lesions [59]. Therefore, the primary cancer may affect the usefulness of newer more targeted therapies.

Animal Studies of Cancer-Induced Bone Pain

The original Mantyh model has been further developed to involve different bones such as the calcaneus [55], humerus [56], and tibia [29], as well as different cell lines, including fibrosarcoma [56], melanoma, and adenocarcinoma [41]. The latter study showed that the different cell lines caused distinct localization and extent of bone destruction, type of pain behavior, and neurochemical reorganization of the spinal cord, demonstrating that multiple mechanisms

are involved in generating and maintaining CIBP. A study in 2005 used a more mixed lytic/blastic tumor in mice [17]. Injection of prostate carcinoma cells into the femora of mice resulted in a similar temporal development of allodynic behavior as in the other models. Anti-nerve growth factor (NGF) therapy in these mice almost eliminated pain behavior without affecting tumor growth or bone destruction, thus showing an important role for NGF in driving CIBP, at least in osteoblastic disease, and highlighting NGF receptors (or anti-NGF therapy) as an important new target for pharmacotherapy.

Effects of Carbamazepine in the Animal Model

In recent unpublished studies we observed that systemic carbamazepine reduced pain-like ipsilateral hypersensitivity to mechanical and cooling stimuli in a mammary cell line (MRMT-1) model of CIBP and also reduced mechanical and thermal suprathreshold neuronal excitability in the dorsal horn, seen at time of peak behavior after injection of MRMT-1 cells into the tibia. The drug had no effect on the same measures in control animals, highlighting a role of abnormal sodium channel activity in the generation and maintenance of neuronal excitability in CIBP.

One useful property of carbamazepine is that it shows properties of state-dependency—that is, it preferentially acts on sodium channels that are repetitively firing rather than those that are less active. Ectopic firing of neurons in damaged neurons is thought to be a driving factor in the development of neuropathic pain. The peripheral changes that accompany CIBP could be hypothesized to also induce abnormal firing of sodium channels.

The clustering of sodium channels and/or the change in channel kinetics may lead to increased neuronal firing, providing a biochemical substrate through which carbamazepine may act to modulate the peripheral nociceptive drive [8]. Moreover, carbamazepine has been shown to modulate the activity of $Na_v1.8$, a sodium channel that is found predominantly in unmyelinated C fibers [7]. This channel has a limited nerve distribution and is found predominantly in fine sensory fibers, which means that it could be a highly selective pain target.

Role of $\alpha_2\delta$ Calcium Channel Subunits

Neuropathic pain results from nerve damage, which among a wide range of etiologies and different origins can include trauma, diabetes, herpes infection, and cancer. There are several well-established animal models of neuropathic pain, in which many genes change their expression in the cell bodies of damaged nerves. In particular, calcium channels, responsible for converting peripheral activity into transmitter release and thus allowing peripheral messages to activate spinal neurons, are altered by nerve injury. Importantly, there is a huge upregulation of the calcium channel accessory subunit $\alpha_2\delta_1$, for both mRNA and protein, in both the dorsal root ganglia (DRG) corresponding to the nerve damage and the spinal cord dorsal horn. This increase of $\alpha_2\delta_1$ coincides with the onset of tactile allodynia [22]. Voltage-gated calcium channels of the Ca_V1 and Ca_V2 classes consist of an α_1 subunit, associated with a β-subunit and an $\alpha_2\delta$-subunit. The principal effect of calcium channel $\alpha_2\delta_1$ subunits is to increase the functional expression of the channels. The $\alpha_2\delta_1$ subunit role in development of neuropathic pain is evidenced by mice globally overexpressing $\alpha_2\delta_1$ having allodynia in the absence of nerve damage [23]. The antiallodynic and antihyperalgesic gabapentinoid drugs, pregabalin and gabapentin, are $\alpha_2\delta$ ligands. Finally, mice with a mutant $\alpha_2\delta_1$ subunit that fails to bind gabapentinoids develop neuropathic pain but do not respond to these drugs [13]. However, the molecular mechanism that explains the ability of these drugs to alleviate neuropathic pain in vivo has been lacking. Gabapentin produces a substantial inhibition of calcium currents when applied chronically but not acutely in vitro, by reducing the proportion of Ca_V1 and $\alpha_2\delta$ subunits at their functional site of action, the cell membrane [18]. Gabapentin therefore is an inhibitor of movement of the channel; that is, it modulates calcium channel trafficking.

Recently we used a rat model of neuropathic pain to investigate whether gabapentinoid drugs inhibit the trafficking of $\alpha_2\delta_1$ from DRG cell bodies to their presynaptic terminals in the dorsal horn of the spinal cord in vivo, and under conditions that resemble therapeutic use. We analyzed the distribution of $\alpha_2\delta_1$ in DRGs, axons, and spinal cord in the ligated region, and we determined the effect of chronic pregabalin treatment on $\alpha_2\delta_1$ distribution. Our findings indicate that pregabalin does inhibit the trafficking of $\alpha_2\delta_1$ subunits in vivo [4].

Due to its proven effects in these chronic pain conditions and their contribution to CIBP, we have tested gabapentin in our rat model of CIBP. We found that chronic (but not acute) treatment with systemic gabapentin significantly reduced pain behavior and, moreover, normalized the hyperexcitable dorsal horn response *and* reset the neuronal populations [11]. Cessation of gabapentin treatment resulted in a return to the uninhibited pain state, showing that permanent changes, such as anatomical reorganization, are unlikely to account for CIBP, and that neuronal physiology probably has a more prominent role.

The antihyperalgesic effects of gabapentin have also been confirmed in the murine model of CIBP, where chronic systemic treatment attenuated ongoing and movement-evoked pains [34]. These findings along with our own imply that for more adequate pain control in CIBP, combination therapy of an opioid with gabapentin for example may be useful, particularly if (as has been shown to be the case in neuropathic pain) there is a synergistic action between morphine and gabapentin [27]. Furthermore, a spino-bulbo-spinal pathway with a facilitatory action at spinal 5-HT$_3$ receptors, which we found to be activated in CIBP, has been shown to be a determinant not only of abnormal behavioral and neuronal activity in neuropathic pain, but also of the efficacy of gabapentin [50].

Enhanced Neuronal Responses in the Animal Model

In the model of CIBP, not only do neurons show enhanced responses, indicative of hyperexcitability, but we reported the alteration of the ratio between nociceptive-specific (i.e., pain-only) cells and wide-dynamic-range (WDR) neurons (responding to innocuous and noxious inputs) in the superficial dorsal horn. Compared to sham-operated rats, animals with CIBP had an increased proportion of WDR neurons, which also showed hyperexcitable responses to mechanical, thermal, and electrical stimuli. As some of these superficial cells will be NK1-expressing projection neurons, this could translate to increased transmission of signals to the brain areas involved in the affective component of pain, as well as access of lower threshold inputs. This does in fact fit with the clinical condition of bone cancer and neuropathy correlating with increased anxiety and depression [30], and the hyperresponsivity to low-threshold stimuli may be important in terms of the mechanical allodynia seen behaviorally in the animal models.

This shift in populations was a change that had not been reported previously in any chronic pain model, but the hyperexcitability of WDR neurons we reported was confirmed in a murine model [20], thus demonstrating again the high probability of translational validity of these models. Subsequently, we showed a temporal correlation between the development of pain behavior and the neuronal alterations in the superficial dorsal horn [11]. Correlates between behavioral and neuronal alterations have not yet been widely studied in chronic pain states, a void that is also present in other areas of neuroscience. Our investigations showing a relationship between behavioral alterations and neuronal responses indicate the latter as the most suitable substrate for pharmacological study, being suprathreshold responses more clinically relevant than the threshold-level behavioral responses. In addition, these investigations contribute to evidence for a major role of superficial dorsal horn neurons in the regulation and behavioral expression of pain sensitivity [58].

Increased excitability may be generated in both spinal and supraspinal pathways. Superficial dorsal horn NK1-expressing neurons have been shown to form the origin of a spino-bulbo-spinal loop which, with ascending information relaying to the rostroventral medulla (RVM) and then descending to return to the spinal cord, produces a facilitatory action at spinal $5-HT_3$ receptors. This loop modulates mechanical and thermal nociceptive transmission and is necessary for full coding of inputs by spinal neurons [49]. Furthermore, this circuit will receive input from centers such as the parabrachial area and amygdala, involved in the affective component of pain, and so may amplify and prolong the sensation to a painful stimulus so that emotional state may alter the perception of pain. Pain and mood share neurological pathways in the central nervous system (CNS) and have similar neurochemical bases, in particular their modulation by monoamine systems. This provides the substrate through which pain can influence mood, giving rise to comorbidities or secondary symptoms such as anxiety and depression, and by the same pathways, may permit mood to exacerbate pain; indeed, patients with depression often present with symptoms that include medically unexplained pain, with the mean prevalence of such pain cited as 65% [3]. Thus, at any given time and for any given nociceptive stimulus, the overall pain experience can be influenced by emotional state (the psychological context in which the stimulus is received), emotional traits (the psychological characteristics of the recipient), and cognitive set (e.g., attention and vigilance).

Descending Facilitation and Serotonin

In order to assess the role of the descending serotonergic facilitatory pathway in CIBP, we measured the effects of spinally administered ondansetron, a selective $5-HT_3$-receptor antagonist, on electrical, mechanical, and thermally evoked dorsal horn neuronal responses in animals with CIBP compared to sham-operated rats [12]. We found that spinal ondansetron reduced mechanical- and thermal-evoked dorsal horn neuronal responses in all animals, suggesting that the pathway is normally active, but the effects of ondansetron were significantly greater in animals injected with MRMT-1 (compared to sham-operated rats), suggesting that there is increased activation of this excitatory serotonergic pathway in CIBP.

Opioids

The translational studies mentioned so far based on behavioral, neurochemical, and neuronal characterizations have already shed some light on the pathophysiological mechanisms underlying CIBP, but what have we learned from pharmacological investigations? As mentioned previously, opioids, although with side effects, remain the mainstay for treatment of severe pain from malignancy in the bone, and at present represent the most widely studied class of drug in CIBP models. The first studies with morphine added to the growing body of evidence suggesting CIBP to be a unique pain state, as efficacy of acute systemic administration was far lower than in inflammatory models [25,56]. These and subsequent investigations have also shown that with acute opioid administration, high doses are necessary to significantly reduce pain behavior [53]. This finding is consistent with the clinical problem of high doses of opioids being necessary to combat incident pain, as discussed previously.

We used a chronic dosing schedule in order to monitor the efficacy of morphine over time against CIBP [52]. We found that from the first dose, morphine effectively reduced pain behavior, but pre- versus post-morphine testing revealed that the analgesic effects were wearing off between doses. We also found that acute, systemic injection of morphine on postoperative day 15 (equivalent to the last day of treatment in the chronic morphine group) significantly reduced pain behavior, although not to the same extent as in the chronically treated animals at this time point. These data support the use of a chronic opioid treatment regime in CIBP, although moderate affects of acute administration were also observed during this investigation. This may explain the necessity to use higher systemic doses to attenuate pain in other studies, where investigations were carried out at later postoperative days when the pain has become more severe.

Electrophysiological characterization in our chronically treated animals revealed that the hyperexcitability of superficial dorsal horn neurons is attenuated, although not reversed, and furthermore that the abnormally high ratio of WDR cells remains. This finding, suggesting that even with chronic morphine treatment there is still greater access of low-threshold stimuli to brain regions involved in pain processing, may relate to the problems of controlling incident pain with opioids in the clinic.

Purines

Purines such as ATP have been implicated in a variety of pathological conditions. ATP is released by damaged tissues and causes pain in human volunteers. Eight ATP receptors have been identified so far, and of these $P2X_3$ is of particular interest because it is expressed selectively and predominantly on small-diameter nociceptive sensory neurons [9]. In the periphery, ATP can act to sensitize sensory nerve endings, and centrally $P2X_3$ receptors can be found expressed on the DRGs and central terminals of sensory fibers, where they can presynaptically modulate the release of glutamate and γ-aminobutyric acid (GABA) onto dorsal horn neurons. These neurons are also sensitive to capsaicin since the TRPV1 receptor is found coexpressed with the $P2X_3$ receptor, suggesting a role in the transmission of nociceptive information [9,6]. Moreover, the $P2X_3$-expressing sensory neurons terminate in the superficial lamina, further implicating the role of this receptor subtype in modulating pain. However, there is a subset of $P2X_3$-expressing receptors on DRG neurons, which are insensitive to capsaicin and terminate onto deeper laminae in the dorsal horn.

More recently we have investigated the affects of a dual $P2X_3$- and $P2X_{2/3}$-selective antagonist on deep dorsal horn WDR neurons in the CIBP model (unpublished data). In keeping with our previous work, these animals also displayed neuronal hypersensitivity to both mechanical and thermal stimuli. The spinal application of a novel dual $P2X_3$ and $P2X_{2/3}$ antagonist, AF-353, dose-dependently reduced responses of electrically evoked Aδ and C fibers, and postdischarge, with

no affect on Aβ fibers. Dose-dependent reductions of neuronal responses were observed following application of mechanical and thermal stimuli. Previous work has shown that primary afferents from the bone, periosteum, and joint capsule of mice are predominantly peptidergic [26]. However, $P2X_3$ receptors—the predominant subtype in DRG—terminate in inner lamina II; that is, they associate with IB-4-binding nonpeptidergic neurons [5,54]. Therefore, the ability of a $P2X_3$- and $P2X_{2/3}$-receptor-specific antagonist to attenuate neuronal hypersensitivity in the CIBP model following spinal application is an unexpected finding. A study mentioned earlier [17] revealed that treatment with an antibody to NGF in a model of metastatic prostate cancer tumor to bone significantly reduced pain behaviors. NGF has been known to play a significant role in the generation and modulation of pain in bone cancer and neuropathic pain models. Additionally, NGF induces de novo expression of $P2X_3$ in axons projecting to lamina I and outer lamina II, where DRG neurons expressing the peptidergic neuromodulators, substance P and calcitonin gene-related peptide (CGRP), terminate [37]. Since it is primarily the peptidergic afferents that arise from bone tissue, it is therefore reasonable to infer that NGF-induced de novo expression of $P2X_3$ on sensory neurons of peptidergic afferents may have a role in driving CIBP. Thus the spinal application of AF-353 could affect neuronal hypersensitivity in our MRMT-1-cell-induced CIBP model.

Conclusion

Cancer-induced bone pain is a unique pain state, incorporating somatic, visceral, and ischemic mechanisms. Damage by the tumor itself and the release of mediators in its vicinity provide the peripheral drive of signaling to the spinal cord. Spinally, the flow of signaling up from the periphery and down from higher brain centers alters the processing of this information, resulting in the enhanced perception of pain.

Animal models have facilitated the understanding of the events that take place in the periphery, spinally, and supraspinally, to create and maintain the pain, in addition to revealing novel, druggable targets. However, given the structural and chemical changes that contribute to this pain state, it is difficult to target a single mechanism. We believe that polytherapy is the way forward, incorporating new drugs when they become available.

References

[1] Abbadie C, Brown JL, Mantyh PW, Basbaum AI. Spinal cord substance P receptor immunoreactivity increases in both inflammatory and nerve injury models of persistent pain. Neuroscience 1996;70:201–9.

[2] Akopian AN, Sivilotti L, Wood JN. A tetrodotoxin-resistant voltage-gated sodium channel expressed by sensory neurons. Nature 1996;379:257–62.

[3] Bair MJ, Robinson RL, Katon W, Kroenke K. Depression and pain comorbidity: a literature review. Arch Intern Med 2003;163:2433–45.

[4] Bauer CS, Nieto-Rostro M, Rahman W, Tran-Van-Minh A, Ferron L, Douglas L, Kadurin I, Sri Ranjan Y, Fernandez-Alacid L, Millar NS, et al. The increased trafficking of the calcium channel subunit $\alpha_2\delta_1$ to presynaptic terminals in neuropathic pain is inhibited by the $\alpha_2\delta$ ligand pregabalin. J Neurosci 2009;29:4076–88.

[5] Bradbury EJ, Burnstock G, McMahon SB. The expression of P2X$_3$ purinoreceptors in sensory neurons: effects of axotomy and glial-derived neurotrophic factor. Mol Cell Neurosci 1998;12:256–68.

[6] Burnstock G, Wood JN. Purinergic receptors: their role in nociception and primary afferent neurotransmission. Curr Opin Neurobiol 1996;6:526–32.

[7] Cardenas CA, Cardenas CG, de Armendi AJ, Scroggs RS. Carbamazepine interacts with a slow inactivation state of Na$_V$1.8-like sodium channels. Neurosci Lett 2006;408:129–34.

[8] Chapman V, Suzuki R, Chamarette HL, Rygh LJ, Dickenson AH. Effects of systemic carbamazepine and gabapentin on spinal neuronal responses in spinal nerve ligated rats. Pain 1998;75:261–72.

[9] Chen CC, Akopian AN, Sivilotti L, Colquhoun D, Burnstock G, Wood JN. A P2X purinoceptor expressed by a subset of sensory neurons. Nature 1995;377:428–31.

[10] Dib-Hajj SD, Tyrrell L, Black JA, Waxman SG. NaN, a novel voltage-gated Na channel, is expressed preferentially in peripheral sensory neurons and down-regulated after axotomy. Proc Natl Acad Sci USA 1998;95:8963–8.

[11] Donovan-Rodriguez T, Dickenson AH, Urch CE. Gabapentin normalizes spinal neuronal responses that correlate with behavior in a rat model of cancer-induced bone pain. Anesthesiology 2005;102:132–40.

[12] Donovan-Rodriguez T, Urch CE, Dickenson AH. Evidence of a role for descending serotonergic facilitation in a rat model of cancer-induced bone pain. Neurosci Lett 2006;393:237–42.

[13] Field MJ, Cox PJ, Stott E, Melrose H, Offord J, Su TZ, Bramwell S, Corradini L, England S, Winks J, et al. Identification of the $\alpha_2\delta_1$ subunit of voltage-dependent calcium channels as a molecular target for pain mediating the analgesic actions of pregabalin. Proc Natl Acad Sci USA 2006;103:17537–42.

[14] Fox A, Medhurst S, Courade JP, Glatt M, Dawson J, Urban L, Bevan S, Gonzalez I. Anti-hyperalgesic activity of the cox-2 inhibitor lumiracoxib in a model of bone cancer pain in the rat. Pain 2004;107:33–40.

[15] Ghilardi JR, Rohrich H, Lindsay TH, Sevcik MA, Schwei MJ, Kubota K, Halvorson KG, Poblete J, Chaplan SR, Dubin AE, et al. Selective blockade of the capsaicin receptor TRPV1 attenuates bone cancer pain. J Neurosci 2005;25:3126–31.

[16] Griffiths JR. Are cancer cells acidic? Br J Cancer 1991;64:425–7.

[17] Halvorson KG, Kubota K, Sevcik MA, Lindsay TH, Sotillo JE, Ghilardi JR, Rosol TJ, Boustany L, Shelton DL, Mantyh PW. A blocking antibody to nerve growth factor attenuates skeletal pain induced by prostate tumor cells growing in bone. Cancer Res 2005;65:9426–35.

[18] Hendrich J, Van Minh AT, Heblich F, Nieto-Rostro M, Watschinger K, Striessnig J, Wratten J, Davies A, Dolphin AC. Pharmacological disruption of calcium channel trafficking by the $\alpha_2\delta$ ligand gabapentin. Proc Natl Acad Sci USA 2008;105:3628–33.

[19] Honore P, Luger NM, Sabino MA, Schwei MJ, Rogers SD, Mach DB, O'Keefe PF, Ramnaraine ML, Clohisy DR, Mantyh PW. Osteoprotegerin blocks bone cancer-induced skeletal destruction, skeletal pain and pain-related neurochemical reorganization of the spinal cord. Nat Med 2000;6:521–8.

[20] Khasabov SG, Ghilardi JR, Mantyh PW, Simone DA. Spinal neurons that express NK-1 receptors modulate descending controls that project through the dorsolateral funiculus. J Neurophysiol 2005;93:998–1006.

[21] Lacey DL, Timms E, Tan HL, Kelley MJ, Dunstan CR, Burgess T, Elliott R, Colombero A, Elliott G, Scully S, et al. Osteoprotegerin ligand is a cytokine that regulates osteoclast differentiation and activation. Cell 1998;93:165–76.

[22] Li CY, Song YH, Higuera ES, Luo ZD. Spinal dorsal horn calcium channel $\alpha_2\delta_1$ subunit upregulation contributes to peripheral nerve injury-induced tactile allodynia. J Neurosci 2004;24:8494–9.

[23] Li CY, Zhang XL, Matthews EA, Li KW, Kurwa A, Boroujerdi A, Gross J, Gold MS, Dickenson AH, Feng G, Luo ZD. Calcium channel $\alpha_2\delta_1$ subunit mediates spinal hyperexcitability in pain modulation. Pain 2006;125:20–34.

[24] Liepe K. Alpharadin, a 223Ra-based alpha-particle-emitting pharmaceutical for the treatment of bone metastases in patients with cancer. Curr Opin Investig Drugs 2009;10:1346–58.

[25] Luger NM, Sabino MA, Schwei MJ, Mach DB, Pomonis JD, Keyser CP, Rathbun M, Clohisy DR, Honore P, Yaksh TL, Mantyh PW. Efficacy of systemic morphine suggests a fundamental difference in the mechanisms that generate bone cancer vs. inflammatory pain. Pain 2002;99:397–406.

[26] Mach DB, Rogers SD, Sabino MC, Luger NM, Schwei MJ, Pomonis JD, Keyser CP, Clohisy DR, Adams DJ, O'Leary P, Mantyh PW. Origins of skeletal pain: sensory and sympathetic innervation of the mouse femur. Neuroscience 2002;113:155–66.

[27] Matthews EA, Dickenson AH. A combination of gabapentin and morphine mediates enhanced inhibitory effects on dorsal horn neuronal responses in a rat model of neuropathy. Anesthesiology 2002;96:633–40.

[28] Medhurst SJ, Walker K, Bowes M, Kidd BL, Glatt M, Muller M, Hattenberger M, Vaxelaire J, O'Reilly T, Wotherspoon G, et al. A rat model of bone cancer pain. Pain 2002;96:129–40.

[29] Menendez L, Lastra A, Fresno MF, Llames S, Meana A, Hidalgo A, Baamonde A. Initial thermal heat hypoalgesia and delayed hyperalgesia in a murine model of bone cancer pain. Brain Res 2003;969:102–9.

[30] Mercadante S. Malignant bone pain: pathophysiology and treatment. Pain 1997;69:1–18.

[31] Meuser T, Pietruck C, Radbruch L, Stute P, Lehmann KA, Grond S. Symptoms during cancer pain treatment following WHO guidelines: a longitudinal follow-up study of symptom prevalence, severity and etiology. Pain 2001;93:247–57.

[32] Nichols ML, Lopez Y, Ossipov MH, Bian D, Porreca F. Enhancement of the antiallodynic and antinociceptive efficacy of spinal morphine by antisera to dynorphin A (1–13) or MK-801 in a nerve-ligation model of peripheral neuropathy. Pain 1997;69:317–22.

[33] Paes FM, Serafini AN. Systemic metabolic radiopharmaceutical therapy in the treatment of metastatic bone pain. Semin Nucl Med 2010;40:89–104.

[34] Peters CM, Lindsay TH, Pomonis JD, Luger NM, Ghilardi JR, Sevcik MA, Mantyh PW. Endothelin and the tumorigenic component of bone cancer pain. Neuroscience 2004;126:1043–52.

[35] Petrut B, Simmons C, Broom R, Trinkaus M, Clemons M. Pharmacotherapy of bone metastases in breast cancer patients. Expert Opin Pharmacother 2008;9:937–45.

[36] Portenoy RK. Managing cancer pain poorly responsive to systemic opioid therapy. Oncology (Williston Park) 1999;13(5 Suppl 2):25–9.

[37] Ramer MS, Bradbury EJ, McMahon SB. Nerve growth factor induces P2X$_3$ expression in sensory neurons. J Neurochem 2001;77:864–75.

[38] Rao PP, Grover RK. Apricoxib, a COX-2 inhibitor for the potential treatment of pain and cancer. IDrugs 2009;12:711–22.

[39] Rasmussen PV, Sindrup SH, Jensen TS, Bach FW. Symptoms and signs in patients with suspected neuropathic pain. Pain 2004;110:461–9.

[40] Sabino MA, Ghilardi JR, Jongen JL, Keyser CP, Luger NM, Mach DB, Peters CM, Rogers SD, Schwei MJ, de Felipe C, Mantyh PW. Simultaneous reduction in cancer pain, bone destruction, and tumor growth by selective inhibition of cyclooxygenase-2. Cancer Res 2002;62:7343–9.

[41] Sabino MA, Luger NM, Mach DB, Rogers SD, Schwei MJ, Mantyh PW. Different tumors in bone each give rise to a distinct pattern of skeletal destruction, bone cancer-related pain behaviors and neurochemical changes in the central nervous system. Int J Cancer 2003;104:550–8.

[42] Safieh-Garabedian B, Poole S, Allchorne A, Winter J, Woolf CJ. Contribution of interleukin-1 beta to the inflammation-induced increase in nerve growth factor levels and inflammatory hyperalgesia. Br J Pharmacol 1995;115:1265–75.

[43] Saito O, Aoe T, Yamamoto T. Analgesic effects of nonsteroidal antiinflammatory drugs, acetaminophen, and morphine in a mouse model of bone cancer pain. J Anesth 2005;19:218–24.

[44] Schwei MJ, Honore P, Rogers SD, Salak-Johnson JL, Finke MP, Ramnaraine ML, Clohisy DR, Mantyh PW. Neurochemical and cellular reorganization of the spinal cord in a murine model of bone cancer pain. J Neurosci 1999;19:10886–97.

[45] Sevcik MA, Ghilardi JR, Halvorson KG, Lindsay TH, Kubota K, Mantyh PW. Analgesic efficacy of bradykinin B1 antagonists in a murine bone cancer pain model. J Pain 2005;6:771–5.

[46] Sevcik MA, Luger NM, Mach DB, Sabino MA, Peters CM, Ghilardi JR, Schwei MJ, Rohrich H, De Felipe C, Kuskowski MA, Mantyh PW. Bone cancer pain: the effects of the bisphosphonate alendronate on pain, skeletal remodeling, tumor growth and tumor necrosis. Pain 2004;111:169–80.

[47] Sheng H, Shao J, Kirkland SC, Isakson P, Coffey RJ, Morrow J, Beauchamp RD, DuBois RN. Inhibition of human colon cancer cell growth by selective inhibition of cyclooxygenase-2. J Clin Invest 1997;99:2254–9.

[48] Sorkin LS, Xiao WH, Wagner R, Myers RR. Tumour necrosis factor-alpha induces ectopic activity in nociceptive primary afferent fibres. Neuroscience 1997;81:255–62.

[49] Suzuki R, Morcuende S, Webber M, Hunt SP, Dickenson AH. Superficial NK1-expressing neurons control spinal excitability through activation of descending pathways. Nat Neurosci 2002;5:1319–26.

[50] Suzuki R, Rahman W, Rygh LJ, Webber M, Hunt SP, Dickenson AH. Spinal-supraspinal serotonergic circuits regulating neuropathic pain and its treatment with gabapentin. Pain 2005;117:292–303.

[51] Urch C. The pathophysiology of cancer-induced bone pain: current understanding. Palliat Med 2004;18:267–74.

[52] Urch CE, Donovan-Rodriguez T, Gordon-Williams R, Bee LA, Dickenson AH. Efficacy of chronic morphine in a rat model of cancer-induced bone pain: behavior and in dorsal horn pathophysiology. J Pain 2005;6:837–45.

[53] Vermeirsch H, Nuydens RM, Salmon PL, Meert TF. Bone cancer pain model in mice: evaluation of pain behavior, bone destruction and morphine sensitivity. Pharmacol Biochem Behav 2004;79:243–51.

[54] Vulchanova L, Riedl MS, Shuster SJ, Stone LS, Hargreaves KM, Buell G, Surprenant A, North RA, Elde R. P2X$_3$ is expressed by DRG neurons that terminate in inner lamina II. Eur J Neurosci 1998;10:3470–8.

[55] Wacnik PW, Eikmeier LJ, Ruggles TR, Ramnaraine ML, Walcheck BK, Beitz AJ, Wilcox GL. Functional interactions between tumor and peripheral nerve: morphology, algogen identification, and behavioral characterization of a new murine model of cancer pain. J Neurosci 2001;21:9355–66.

[56] Wacnik PW, Kehl LJ, Trempe TM, Ramnaraine ML, Beitz AJ, Wilcox GL. Tumor implantation in mouse humerus evokes movement-related hyperalgesia exceeding that evoked by intramuscular carrageenan. Pain 2003;101:175–86.

[57] Walker K, Medhurst SJ, Kidd BL, Glatt M, Bowes M, Patel S, McNair K, Kesingland A, Green J, Chan O, Fox AJ, Urban LA. Disease modifying and anti-nociceptive effects of the bisphosphonate, zoledronic acid in a model of bone cancer pain. Pain 2002;100:219–29.

[58] Yezierski RP, Yu CG, Mantyh PW, Vierck CJ, Lappi DA. Spinal neurons involved in the generation of at-level pain following spinal injury in the rat. Neurosci Lett 2004;361:232–6.

[59] Yin JJ, Pollock CB, Kelly K. Mechanisms of cancer metastasis to the bone. Cell Res 2005;15:57–62.

Correspondence to: Prof. Anthony H. Dickenson, PhD, FmedSci, Department of Neuropharmacology, University College London, Gower Street, London WC1E 6BT, United Kingdom. Email: anthony.dickenson@ucl.ac.uk.

Pharmacological Management of Cancer Pain

Sebastiano Mercadante, MD

Anesthesia and Intensive Care Unit and Pain Relief and Palliative Care Unit, La Maddalena Cancer Center, Palermo, Italy

Pain is a prevalent symptom experienced by at least 30% of patients undergoing oncological treatment for metastatic disease and by more than 70% of advanced cancer patients [5]. In 1986, the World Health Organization (WHO) published a set of guidelines for cancer pain management based on the three-step analgesic ladder [29]. The main aim of WHO guidelines was to legitimize the prescribing of strong opioids, arising from evidence of poor management of cancer pain due to reluctance of health care professionals, institutions, and government to use opioids because of fears of addition, tolerance, and illegal abuse.

The application of the WHO analgesic ladder is reported to achieve satisfactory pain relief in up to 90% of patients with cancer pain. Despite considerable experience proving its feasibility and efficacy [14,27,30], in the era of evidence-based medicine the three-step ladder has been criticized for the lack of robust data supporting this approach.

Studies validating the WHO analgesic ladder have been shown to have methodological limitations, including the circumstances during which assessments were made, small sample sizes, retrospective analyses, high rates of exclusions and dropout, inadequate follow-up, and a lack of comparison with levels of pain before the introduction of the analgesic ladder approach [11].

Thus, many problems are unresolved due a lack of controlled studies on this subject. Needing attention are a better definition of the role of nonsteroidal anti-inflammatory drugs (NSAIDs), issues surrounding the prolonged use of NSAIDs in cancer pain, and the utility of Step 2 of the WHO ladder (see below). Moreover, the indications for using different strong opioids and alternate routes of administration to improve pain relief in difficult pain situations are not well established. The proportion of patients who do not benefit from these treatments remains unclear, and how the opioid response may be improved with the use of adjuvants is also uncertain. Finally, different countries apply the WHO ladder approach differently depending on the availability of drugs.

Steps of the Analgesic Ladder

Step 1

The first step in the WHO analgesic ladder involves the use of a nonopioid drug with or without an adjuvant analgesic. Studies of various nonopioid analgesics have been performed, either alone or combined with opioids, but heterogeneity of study designs and outcomes and short study lengths have precluded meta-analyses. From the data available, nonopioid analgesics appear more effective than placebo. No superior safety or efficacy was demonstrated for any of the drugs within this class, and slight advantages were found in trials of combinations of an nonopioid analgesic with an opioid, compared with either type of drug used alone [13]. Some studies suggest a different role for nonopioid analgesics, administered in patients already on opioids, to reinforce analgesia in patients with difficult pain control or who tend to develop adverse effects with increasing doses of opioids [20]. The conclusions of this study are intriguing, because the reluctance of North American physicians to use NSAIDs and conversely their extensive, and sometimes exaggerated, use in European countries may find a compromise based on these data. Patients could be started on opioids alone and then have nonopioid analgesics added, for example in conditions where pain is particularly sensitive to this class of drugs, or to reduce opioid escalation when adverse effects develop.

Although adverse effects occurred infrequently in previous large studies, those side effects were not appropriately assessed. The development of ulcer or renal toxicity might not be apparent with short-term dosing [13], and the specific long-term safety profile of NSAIDs has never been established in randomized studies.

Step 2

The role of "weak opioids" in the treatment of moderate cancer pain has been questioned, and it has been speculated that this step could be bypassed entirely. A meta-analysis conducted by Eisenberg et al. [7] reported that no significant differences in pain relief were noted when the use of nonopioids alone was compared to nonopioids plus opioids for moderate pain. However, these results were based on single-dose studies or studies involving a small number of patients, and it is likely that their regular clinical use would be more effective than would be predicted by single-dose administration data. Previous studies underlined the role of opioids for moderate pain (namely dextropropoxyphene and codeine), in comparison to morphine in terms of efficacy and adverse effects. In opioid-naive-patients, a more favorable balance between side effects and analgesia occurred when Step 2 opioids were administered compared to low doses of morphine used to bypass Step 2 [9,23].

On the other hand, other studies assessed the use of strong opioids in opioid-naive patients (bypassing Step 2). Doses of 25 µg/h of fentanyl have been used successfully [24,25], although this is the equivalent of 60 mg/day of oral morphine, which is a considerable dosage for opioid-naive patients, with a high risk of producing adverse effects and reducing patient

compliance. This observation was confirmed in a study where transdermal fentanyl used at doses of 25 µg/h was better tolerated in codeine-using patients compared to opioid-naive patients [28].

In a more recent study the sequential treatment proposed by WHO was compared with a direct administration of strong opioid as the first step [12]. Treatments provided good analgesia, although the group treated with opioids first had better pain relief, greater patient satisfaction, and fewer therapeutic interventions. However, nausea was more frequently reported in the strong opioid group. Only 50% of patients in the control (WHO ladder) group needed strong opioids in doses similar to those used in patients who received strong opioids first [12]. Unfortunately, the initial doses of strong opioids were not mentioned in the text, making evaluation of data difficult, because initial doses have large effects on compliance, efficacy, and tolerability.

Morphine used at very low doses in opioid-naive patients may offer different advantages, including greater tolerability while providing analgesia. The rationale is to replace opioids for moderate pain with morphine used in doses equivalent to the range commonly prescribed in clinical practice [16,21,]. A subsequent study confirmed that 30 mg/day of oral morphine provides excellent analgesia in opioid-naive patients [6]. Of course, patients with severe pain are already candidates to receive strong opioids at consistent doses of the equivalent of about 60 mg/day of oral morphine, according to the WHO guidelines, so this approach should be reserved for patients with moderate pain, potentially requiring Step 3 drugs.

Step 3

Morphine is the most frequently used opioid in cancer pain management. Although morphine remains a cornerstone for the management of cancer pain, due to its track record of clinical experience and its wide availability in a variety of formulations, no clear data exist about the superiority of any opioid over another [10,16].

A substantial minority of patients treated with oral morphine (10–30%) do not have a successful outcome because of excessive adverse effects, inadequate analgesia, or a combination [4]. Individualization of therapy has been emphasized to minimize side effects and improve the analgesic response. It is now recognized that individual patients vary greatly in their response to different opioids [18]. Patients who obtain poor analgesic efficacy or tolerability with one opioid will frequently tolerate another opioid better. A shift from one opioid to another is recommended when the adverse effect/analgesic equation is skewed toward the side-effect component, despite an aggressive adjuvant treatment. Opioid rotation has been shown to be useful in opening the therapeutic window and establishing a more advantageous analgesia/toxicity relationship. By substituting opioids and using lower doses than expected (according to equivalency conversion tables), it is possible in most cases not only to reduce or relieve the symptoms of opioid toxicity and manage patients who are highly tolerant to previously used opioids, but also to improve analgesia. This strategy uses much lower doses of alternative opioids in patients who are unresponsive to high doses of morphine [18]. The biological basis for the individual variability in sensitivity to opioids is multifactorial, and many aspects remain unclear [14]. Although the conversion ratio between opioids in such circumstances remains unpredictable, morphine, oxycodone, and hydromorphone seem to be more manageable in the clinical context. Methadone, which is chemically distinct from morphine, oxycodone, or hydromorphone, shows some peculiarities that make it unique. Individual response varies remarkably from opioid to opioid, due to asymmetric tolerance, different efficacies, pharmacokinetic profiles, and nonopioid effects, such as an anti-N-methyl-D-aspartate (anti-NMDA) effect. The correct conversion ratio from morphine to methadone is quite complex and is particularly debated in the literature. It appears that the previous dose of morphine is the determinant in the choice of the dose of methadone in a proportional manner. However, many factors may affect the conversion ratio [1,19]. The concepts of equianalgesia are hard to apply in the clinical setting, where patients suffer adverse effects from opioids with poor analgesia in most circumstances, a critical condition that requires immediate intervention. Highly tolerant patients who are receiving high doses of opioids unsuccessfully should be carefully monitored.

Alternative Routes of Administration

Many patients will develop tolerance to most of the undesirable side effects of opioids (such as nausea/vomiting or sedation) over a period of several days. However, certain patients may not be able to tolerate oral medications because of esophageal motility problems or gastrointestinal obstruction (e.g., head and neck or esophageal cancer, or bowel obstruction), or they may have nausea and vomiting, limiting the utility of the oral route. Finally, some patients are unable to swallow due to the site of their cancer or because they are neurologically impaired. In these cases, an alternative form of analgesia must be used. Alternative routes of administration, including the intravenous and subcutaneous, as well as the transdermal routes, are advocated in such circumstances [3].

The intravenous route of administration is indicated for those patients whose pain cannot be controlled by a less invasive route or for those who already have central venous access. The major disadvantage of this route is that it requires some expertise and is more complex to manage, especially at home. On the other hand, this route is more rapid, allowing for an immediate effect in emergency conditions. Different opioids are available as an intravenous solution in most countries, including morphine, hydromorphone, fentanyl, alfentanil, sufentanil, and methadone. For patients requiring parenteral opioids who do not have indwelling intravenous access, the subcutaneous route can be used. This simple method of parenteral administration involves inserting a small plastic cannula on an area of the chest, abdomen, upper arms, or thighs and attaching the tubing to an infusion pump. The limiting factor is the volume of fluid that can be injected per hour, often requiring more concentrated solutions. Most drugs used by the intravenous route can also be used by subcutaneous infusion, except methadone, which can induce local toxicity. The oral-parenteral ratio for morphine is 2:1 or 3:1 [10]. Intravenous or subcutaneous opioid infusions can be given as continuous infusions or can be administered via a patient-controlled analgesia (PCA) device, which provides continuous infusion plus on-demand boluses. Confused or uncooperative patients may not be the best candidates for PCA use.

The transdermal route is a very comfortable route of administration. For patients who are unable to take oral medications, the transdermal route is a priority option for maintaining continuous plasma concentrations of opioids. Two drugs are available, fentanyl and buprenorphine, due to their potency and lipophilicity. A transdermal fentanyl-oral morphine conversion ratio of 1:70 to 1:100 has been suggested. For buprenorphine, the buprenorphine-oral morphine conversion ratio ranges from 1:60 to 1:80.

The sublingual administration of opioids is particularly beneficial in the patient with cancer who is unable to tolerate oral administration because of nausea/vomiting or dysphagia. It may also be attractive in patients who cannot receive parenteral opioids because of lack of venous access or contraindications for subcutaneous drug administration. Because sublingual venous drainage is systemic rather than portal, hepatic first-pass elimination can be avoided. On the other hand, the transmucosal or sublingual route also offers the potential for more rapid absorption and onset of action relative to the oral route. This route is thus particularly useful for treating breakthrough pain, which requires a fast opioid effect. Lipophilic drugs are better absorbed than are hydrophilic drugs, and thus fentanyl and buprenorphine are mostly used by this route.

Treatment of Breakthrough Pain

Breakthrough pain has been defined as a transitory increase in pain intensity over a baseline pain of moderate intensity in patients receiving a regularly administered analgesic treatment. However, transitory pain may occur in patients with no baseline pain at all. Moreover, pain exacerbations may also occur in patients with severe baseline pain in uncontrolled situations. The intermittent pain may be induced by movement, defined as incident pain, or may be unrelated to activity and thus less predictable [26].

A rescue dose of opioid can provide a means to treat breakthrough pain in patients already stabilized on a baseline opioid regimen. The use of a short half-life opioid, such as immediate-release morphine, is suggested. The most effective doses remain unknown, although clinicians suggest a dose roughly equivalent to about 15% of the total daily opioid dose, administered as needed every 2–3 hours. Titration of the rescue dose according to the characteristics of breakthrough pain should be attempted in an individualized manner to identify the most appropriate dose, as the approach to opioid supplemental dosing has been based solely on anecdotal experience. However, the onset of action of an oral dose may be too slow (more than 30 minutes), and better results may be obtained with a parenteral rescue dose. Although the intravenous route is the fastest, subcutaneous administration is associated with an acceptable onset of effect and should be considered equivalent in terms of efficacy. PCA is an interesting modality to deliver drugs as needed. It appears that the demand dose is important to the success of PCA, and the initial set-up of the PCA system will influence the therapeutic outcome. However, there are limitations in the use of such pumps.

Oral transmucosal dosing is a recent noninvasive approach to the rapid onset of analgesia. Highly lipophilic agents may pass rapidly through the oral mucosa, avoiding first-pass metabolism and achieving active plasma concentrations within minutes. Fentanyl, incorporated in a hard matrix on a handle, is rapidly absorbed. It has been shown to have an onset of pain relief similar to that of intravenous morphine, within 10–15 minutes. When the fentanyl matrix dissolves, approximately 25% of the total fentanyl concentration crosses the buccal mucosa and enters the bloodstream. The remaining amount is swallowed, and about one-third of this part is absorbed, thus achieving a total bioavailability of 50%. However, this approach requires the active participation and collaboration of patients, who are often unable to use the stick. New formulations, such as effervescent, intranasal, or sublingual fentanyl, provide rapid analgesia and seem to be more acceptable to patients [8].

Adjuvants

Adjuvants comprise a wide range of drugs commonly prescribed to improve opioid analgesia. Antidepressants and anti-epileptics are most frequently administered as coanalgesics in the presence of neuropathic pain, in combination with opioids. Despite the relative efficacy demonstrated by this class of drugs in chronic noncancer conditions, evidence of the benefit of such a combination in cancer pain management is weak. Gabapentin was effective in reducing the mean global score and dysesthesia, but not allodynia, compared to placebo in patients with neuropathic cancer pain that was not adequately controlled by systemic opioids [2]. However, the magnitude and duration of benefit for patients remains questionable in clinical practice. Similarly, amitriptyline added to opioids was able to reduce the worst pain only, while producing greater central adverse effects, in comparison to patients receiving opioids alone [17].

Thus, the role of adjuvants remains poorly defined, at least in advanced cancer patients receiving opioids, and further data from well-designed and robust studies are needed. In particular, information is required regarding the timing of starting these drugs.

Conclusion

The WHO method remains of paramount importance and should continue to be encouraged when treating advanced cancer patients with pain, considering the high chances of success, ranging between 70% and 90%. Despite the lack of strong evidence to produce unbiased estimates of the proportion of patients in whom the ladder produces satisfactory results, and the fact that no controlled studies with other methods have been conducted to assess its validity, we should not underestimate the educational value of this simple approach. The correct use of the WHO method can lead to adequate long-term pain control in most patients with advanced cancer disease. Wider dissemination of the WHO guidelines among health care workers is still necessary to raise the standard of treatment before introducing other unvalidated treatments, as many cancer patients still suffer from unrelieved pain due to inappropriate pain management, insufficient knowledge and education, the physician's limited experience regarding the management of cancer pain, and legal and political issues surrounding opioid prescription and use.

It seems clear, however, that individualization will provide optimal treatment. Thus, a profound knowledge of drug characteristics and good experience in evaluating patients' response, together with recognition of possible alternative treatments, still remain the keys to success.

References

[1] Benitez-Rosario M, Salinas-Martin A, Aguirre-Jaime A, Perez-Mendez L, Feria M. Morphine-methadone opioid rotation in cancer patients: analysis of dose predicting factors. J Pain Symptom Manage 2009;37:1061–8.

[2] Caraceni A, Zecca E, Bonezzi C, Arcuri E, Tur RY, Maltoni M, Visentin M, Gorni G, Martini C, Tirelli W, Barbieri M, De Conno F. Gabapentin for neuropathic cancer pain: a randomized controlled trial from the Gabapentin Cancer Pain Study Group. J Clin Oncol 2004;22:2909–17.

[3] Cherny NJ, Chang V, Frager G, Ingham JM, Tiseo PJ, Popp B, Portenoy RK, Foley KM. Opioid pharmacotherapy in the management of cancer pain. Cancer 1995;76:1288–93.

[4] Cherny N, Ripamonti C, Pereira J, Davis C, Fallon M, McQuay H, Mercadante S, Pasternak G, Ventafridda V; Expert Working Group of the European Association of Palliative Care Network. Strategies to manage the adverse effects of oral morphine: an evidence-based report. J Clin Oncol 2001;19:2542–54.

[5] Cleeland CS, Gonin R, Hatfield AK, Edmonson JH, Blum RH, Stewart JA, Pandya KJ. Pain and its treatment in outpatients with metastatic cancer. N Engl J Med 1994;330:592–6.

[6] De Conno F, Ripamonti C, Fagnoni E, Brunelli C, Luzzani M, Maltoni M, Arcuri E, Bertetto O; MERITO Study Group. The MERITO Study: a multicentre trial of the analgesic effect and tolerability of normal-release oral morphine during "titration phase" in patients with cancer pain. Palliat Med 2008;22:214–21.

[7] Eisenberg E, Berkey C, Carr DB, Mosteller F, Chalmers C. Efficacy and safety of non steroidal anti-inflammatory drugs for cancer pain: a meta-analysis. J Clin Oncol 1994;12:2756–65.

[8] Grape S, Schug SA, Lauer S, Schug BS. Formulations of fentanyl for the management of pain. Drugs 2010;70:57–72.

[9] Grond S, Radbruch L, Meuser T, Loick G, Sabatowski R, Lehmann K. High-dose tramadol in comparison to low-dose morphine for cancer pain relief. J Pain Symptom Manage 1999;18:174–9.

[10] Hanks GW, Conno F, Cherny N, Hanna M, Kalso E, McQuay HJ, Mercadante S, Meynadier J, Poulain P, Ripamonti C, et al.; Expert Working Group of the Research Network of the European Association for Palliative Care. Morphine and alternative opioids in cancer pain: the EAPC recommendations. Br J Cancer 2001;84:587–93.

[11] Jadad AR, Browman GP. The WHO analgesic ladder for cancer pain management. JAMA 1995;274:1870–3.

[12] Marinangeli F, Ciccozzi A, Leonardis M, Aloisio L, Mazzei A, Paladini A, Porzio G, Marchetti P, Varrassi G. Use of strong opioids in advanced cancer pain: a randomized trial. J Pain Symptom Manage 2004;27:409–16.

[13] McNicol E, Strassels S, Goudas L, Lau J, Carr D. Nonsteroidal anti-inflammatory drugs, alone or combined with opioids, for cancer pain: a systematic review. J Clin Oncol 2004;22:1975–92.

[14] Mercadante S. Pain treatment and outcome in advanced cancer patients followed at home. Cancer 1999;85:1849–58.

[15] Mercadante S. Opioid rotation in cancer pain. rationale and clinical aspects. Cancer 1999;86:1856–66.

[16] Mercadante S. Opioid titration in cancer pain: a critical review. Eur J Pain 2007;11:823–30.

[17] Mercadante S, Arcuri E, Tirelli W, Villari P, Casuccio A. Amitriptyline in neuropathic cancer pain in patients on morphine therapy: a randomized placebo-controlled, double-blind crossover study. Tumori 2002;88:239–42.

[18] Mercadante S, Bruera E. Opioid switching: a systematic and critical review. Cancer Treat Rev 2006;32:304–15.

[19] Mercadante S, Ferrera P, Villari P, Casuccio A, Intravaia G, Mangione S. Frequency, indications, outcomes, and predictive factors of opioid switching in an acute palliative care unit. J Pain Symptom Manage 2009;37:632–41.

[20] Mercadante S, Fulfaro F, Casuccio A. A randomised controlled study on the use of anti-inflammatory drugs in patients with cancer on morphine therapy: effect on dose-escalation and pharmacoeconomic analysis. Eur J Cancer 2002;38:1358–63.

[21] Mercadante S, Porzio G, Ferrera P, Fulfaro F, Aielli F, Ficorella C, Verna L, Tirelli W, Villari P, Arcuri E. Low morphine dose in opioid-naive cancer patients with pain. J Pain Symptom Manage 2006;31:242–7.

[22] Mercadante S, Porzio G, Ferrera P, Fulfaro F, Aielli F, Verna L, Villari P, Ficorella C, Gebbia V, Riina S, Casuccio A, Mangione S. Sustained-release oral morphine versus transdermal fentanyl and oral methadone in cancer pain management. Eur J Pain 2008;12:1040–6.

[23] Mercadante S, Salvaggio L, Dardanoni G, Agnello A, Garofalo S. Dextropropoxyphene versus morphine in opioid-naive cancer patients with pain. J Pain Symptom Manage 1998;15:76–81.

[24] Mystakidou K. Pain management of cancer patients with transdermal fentanyl: a study of 1828 step I, II & III transfers. J Pain 2004;5:119–32.

[25] Mystakidou K, Tsilika E, Kouloulias V, Kouvaris I, Georgaki S, Vlahos L. Long-term cancer pain management in morphine pre-treated and opioid naive patients with transdermal fentanyl. Int J Cancer 2003;107:486–92.

[26] Portenoy RK, Hagen NA. Breakthrough pain: definition, prevalence, and characteristics. Pain 1990;41:273–81.

[27] Ventafridda V, Tamburini M, Caraceni A, De Conno F, Naldi F. A validation study of the WHO method for cancer pain relief. Cancer 1987;59:850–6.

[28] Vielvoye-Kerlmeer A, Mattern C, Uitendaal M. Transdermal fentanyl in opioid-naive cancer patients: an open trial using transdermal fentanyl for the treatment of chronic cancer pain in opioid-naive patients and a group using codeine. J Pain Symptom Manage 2000;19:185–92.

[29] World Health Organization. Cancer pain relief and palliative care. Geneva: World Health Organization; 1990.

[30] Zech DFJ, Grond S, Lynch J, Hertel D, Lehmann KA. Validation of World Health Organization guidelines for cancer pain relief: a 10-year prospective study. Pain 1995;63:65–76.

Correspondence to: Dr. Sebastiano Mercadante, Anesthesia and Intensive Care Unit and Pain Relief and Palliative Care Unit, La Maddalena Cancer Center, Palermo, Via san Lorenzo 312, 90146 Palermo, Italy. Email: terapiadeldolore@ lamaddalenanet.it.

Interventional Procedures in the Treatment of Refractory Cancer Pain

Allen W. Burton

Department of Pain Medicine, MD Anderson Cancer Center, Houston, Texas, USA

"We don't beat the Reaper by living longer. We beat the Reaper by living well." Professor Randy Pausch uttered this statement during his famous last lecture at Carnegie Mellon University prior to his death from pancreatic cancer in 2008 [28]. As opposed to the widely-used World Health Organization (WHO) approach of utilizing opioids first, many now advocate a mechanism-based approach to cancer pain treatment [1]. According to the old dogma, cancer pain was as a problem mainly toward the end of life in the context of metastatic, progressive disease, whereas new data show pain to be problematic throughout the cancer care cycle [1]. The effective management of acutely painful surgeries and related treatments may limit the development of chronic pain states in long-term survivors [7]. Effective treatment strategies include multidisciplinary, multimodal care, incorporating (1) combinations of long-acting opioids for constant pain with short-acting opioids for incidental pain; (2) "adjuvant" coanalgesics including nonsteroidal anti-inflammatory drugs, anticonvulsants, antidepressants, and topical agents to optimize analgesia and minimize opioid doses, thereby reducing opioid-related side effects; (3) prophylactic treatment of constipation, nausea, and other common troublesome symptoms; and (4) interventional options for pain control, including nerve blocks, spinal infusions, vertebral augmentation, and other procedures. Lastly (5), psychological evaluation and support must not be overlooked. This chapter will focus on the role of procedures as part of the overall cancer treatment and in the overall context of palliative care. I will discuss traditional analgesic procedures in addition to briefly highlighting neurodestructive procedures, vertebroplasty and kyphoplasty, fracture stabilization, tumor ablation, and other procedures. Finally, the decision-making relating to the role, timing, and special risks of procedures in the cancer patient will be highlighted. This monograph is devoted to the science and decision-making aspects of interventional cancer pain techniques; for a "how-to" approach, the interested reader is directed to Rathmell or Brown's excellent atlases of interventional pain procedures [5,32].

Decision Making

In traditional pain management teachings, several arbitrary distinctions are usually created. Cancer pain, chronic pain (often called "nonmalignant" pain), and acute pain are viewed as distinct clinical entities with unique treatment strategies. In fact, these distinct clinical entities represent slightly different aspects of common pathophysiological states that blend together in a disease continuum. Therefore, there is much overlap in appropriate therapeutic approaches to "cancer pain." For example, optimal acute pain management for cancer surgery may be important to the patient's overall

Pain 2010—An Updated Review: Refresher Course Syllabus
edited by Jeffrey S. Mogil
IASP Press, Seattle, © 2010

43

outcome in the avoidance of chronic pain and perhaps even improved survival [42].

When considering the need for procedural intervention in the patient with progressive cancer, the clinician faces a complex decision-making algorithm that generally reduces to two decisive criteria: failure to achieve adequate pain relief through pharmacological means and pain anatomically amenable to an intervention [40]. These issues usually generate a referral to an interventionalist, often—but not necessarily—an anesthesiologist. Often, the patient's pharmacological options have been exhausted, and the referral for an intervention occurs very far along in the disease process—essentially at the very end stages of life. However, this traditional approach (that is, the WHO ladder), placing interventions on the fourth step, is not always in the patient's best interest [1,8]. In many cases of localized, severe pain, the risk and benefit ratio swings in favor of an interventional pain-relieving procedure well before the pharmacological approaches are exhausted. Typically, the procedure will not substitute for the ongoing use of other pain control modalities, but it can improve pain relief and allow for a reduction in systemic medications and their side effects. The interventional specialist must determine if a procedure is likely to provide tangible benefit and make sure there is no contraindication to the procedure (pancytopenia, hemodynamic instability, etc.). Finally, especially in terms of spinal infusions, advanced planning for home care and appropriate follow-up care are critical [23].

Spinal Infusions

Two broad groups of patients—those with poor pain relief despite numerous analgesic trials and those with unacceptable side effects from analgesics—may benefit from neuraxial analgesic infusions [9,13,38,39]. There have been many reports of successful analgesia with epidural and intrathecal infusion [9]. In our center, we have moved almost exclusively to the intrathecal route (except in the immediate postoperative period) [9]. The reason for favoring the intrathecal route is economic; we have seen similar analgesia with much lower infusion rates and volumes. Whereas the epidural infusion regularly uses 10 cc's or more per hour, intrathecal administration usually runs at 0.5 cc's per hour, saving numerous resources in addition to reducing the frequency of changing external bags. The clinical equivalence of the intrathecal and epidural routes has been confirmed

by other groups [24]. Neuraxial infusions can be implemented in a variety of ways and with various medications and equipment, as outlined below.

In patients with progressive disease and a short survival time, a percutaneous catheter, porta-cath, "Du Pens" percutaneous catheter, or tunneled "epidural" catheter (usually placed in the intrathecal space) with an external pump may be most cost-effective, and most easily adjustable in the home care setting [13]. Recent meta-analysis of complications related to home use of external intrathecal catheters reveals a low rate of serious complications. The rate of superficial infection was 2.3% and that of deep infection was 1.4%, with the authors calculating that every 71st patient had a deep infection after 54 days of therapy, with the risk of bleeding and neurological injury estimated at 0.9% and 0.4%, respectively [2]. Therefore, in cancer pain patients with a short life expectancy, with adequate home resources, an external intrathecal catheter can be considered an effective and low-cost option. One decision-making algorithm published by our group is shown in Fig. 1 [29].

Patients being considered for an implanted pain pump will need a trial infusion that is similar in many ways to the external infusion described above. Issues around pump implantation and management are covered in a nice "how we do it" article by Smith and Coyne [37]. These patients will generally have a longer life expectancy, or in some cases they have chronic cancer pain in a nonterminal setting. The optimal medication for infusion is a subject for a longer monograph, but expert recommendations for polyanalgesia exist and have been recently updated [15]. In terms of chronic noncancer versus cancer pain, the main difference is a more rapid, aggressive dose and drug titration in cancer patients. In our center, the preferred first-line analgesic is often hydromorphone, alone or in combination with bupivacaine. In refractory cases, ziconotide may be added or substituted as a potent non-opioid neuraxial analgesic [33].

Other Cancer Analgesic Procedures

Vertebroplasty is the injection of a painful, fractured vertebral body with bone cement, generally polymethylmethacrylate. Kyphoplasty adds the placement of balloons into the vertebral body with an inflation/deflation sequence to create a cavity and perhaps restore height prior to the cement injection.

These procedures are performed in a percutaneous fashion on an outpatient (or short stay) basis, usually with monitored anesthesia care or heavy sedation. The mechanism of action is unknown, but is postulated that stabilization of the fracture leads to analgesia. The procedure is indicated for painful vertebral compression fractures due to osteoporosis or malignancy. The ideal candidate has severe axial (nonradiating) pain due to a fractured vertebrae. Patients who receive no benefit from a short course of conservative therapy, including analgesics and bracing, are generally considered good candidates for one of these procedures. Patients with painful fractures more than 1 year old are not likely to obtain substantial benefit from vertebroplasty or kyphoplasty, unless there is evidence of a fracture non-union (such as edema on an MRI or a positive bone scan). Pain relief is seen in around two-thirds of patients, and even those with advanced disease may find significant improvement in quality of life [10,19,21]. In patients with advanced metastatic disease, these procedures can be combined with local tumor ablation, or sequenced with spinal radiation therapy as needed [20]. Finally, patients with painful spinal metastasis and neurological compromise may be candidates for spinal surgery up to and including vertebrectomy, which in many cases provides significant improvement in quality of life and may increase lifespan as well [12].

Tumor Ablation (Radiofrequency/Cryoablation) and Cementoplasty

Local tumor ablation with or without addition of bone cement is a recent addition to the cancer pain treatment armamentarium. Several studies show favorable local pain relief following tumor ablation. Studies are underway to determine which technique is optimal [11]. When a fracture is impending due to extensive lytic involvement, bone cement may be injected into the void created by the tumor ablation. This procedure is often done in the hip, femur, and pelvis [27].

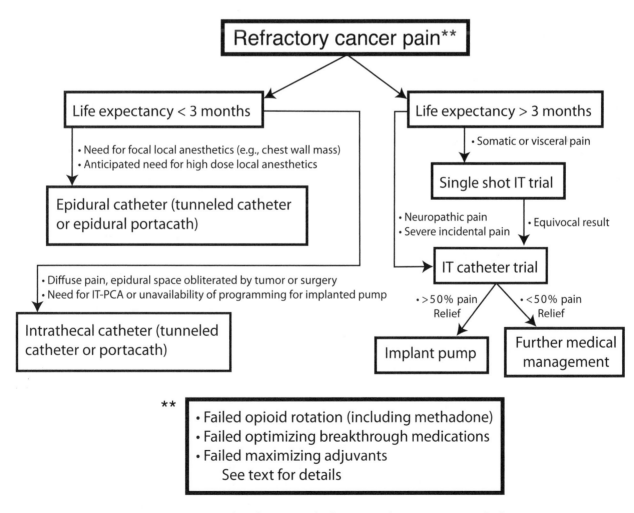

Fig. 1. Decision making for neuraxial infusions in refractory cancer pain [29].

Neurosurgical Ablative Techniques

In some cases of pain refractory to the aforementioned techniques, including spinal analgesic infusion, ablative neurosurgical techniques may be useful. Overall, the use of these techniques has dropped precipitously over the years, presumably as other effective pain control therapies have been implemented. In many centers, it can be difficult to find the local neurosurgical expertise to perform some of these procedures. The most commonly used procedures include anterolateral cordotomy for lateralized pain, midline myelotomy for pelvic pain, rhizotomy and/or dorsal root entry zone lesioning for plexopathic pain, and finally various ablative procedures used in the past including pituitary ablation for bone pain. Many authors and centers, particularly outside the United States, view cordotomy as a valuable technique in managing refractory cancer pain [31]. Techniques mainly used experimentally or in chronic pain states include deep brain stimulation or cortical stimulation [18].

Surgical Techniques

In many pathological cancer pain states, surgical techniques may be highly effective as palliative techniques. These include vertebrectomy for metastatic disease in selected cases and fixation of pathologically fractured long bones [12]. Placement of venting gastrostomy and feeding jejunostomy tubes, or diverting ostomies, may provide effective palliation of visceral symptoms associated with gastric outlet obstruction [16]. Other shunting procedures may be helpful with malignant pleural effusions or ascites. More recently, a variety of less invasive stenting procedures have been developed for the bronchus, esophagus, and many hollow viscera [35].

Neurolytic Blocks

Neurolytic blocks are often extremely helpful in patients with advanced cancer, debilitation, and severe, refractory pain syndromes. In many cases, clinicians may wish to, where feasible, perform a "test block" with local anesthetic to ensure that the patient obtains analgesia from the block and does not find the sensory changes uncomfortable [22]. Unfortunately, the amount of pain relief obtained with the neurolytic block may fall short of that achieved with the local anesthetic block.

With head and neck cancers, the pain is often diffuse and crosses tissue planes/nerve distributions, making the role of neurolytic blocks limited. Some patients will have focal pains that are amenable to the following blocks: peripheral trigeminal (i.e., supraorbital, mental), trigeminal, sphenopalatine, glossopharyngeal, occipital, and superficial cervical plexus [41].

Visceral pain has a discrete innervation that makes it amenable to neurolytic blockade. For upper abdominal pain associated with pancreatic, liver, or gastric tumor, the celiac plexus block has been advocated. Numerous approaches and medications have been tried and compared in the literature, with good support for favorable clinical outcomes in more than two-thirds of patients undergoing the block [17]. In our center, we use a posterior approach guided by fluoroscopy, with two needles placed in the retrocrural space. We inject local anesthetic followed by 50–100% alcohol or 8–10% phenol solution up to a volume of 20 cc's. Other approaches that have been advocated include transgastric (via an endoscope) and anterior (with ultrasound guidance) [6,26]. The anterior approach with ultrasound is very exciting for potential application at the bedside in a hospice setting [3]. The majority of patients undergoing celiac block will experience orthostatic hypotension due to visceral vasodilatation and diarrhea due to the unopposed parasympathetic effect. Neurologically, there is a small risk of paraplegia [14].

For pain in the pelvic viscera, the superior hypogastric block, more recently the inferior hypogastric plexus block, and the ganglion impar block have been described and used, although not as widely as the celiac block [30,34]. The superior hypogastric block should reduce pain coming from the bladder, uterus, vagina, prostate, urethra, testes, descending colon, and rectum. An anterior approach has also been described for patients who cannot lie prone [25]. Blocking the inferior hypogastric plexus, which lies anterior to the sacrum at approximately the S2 level, may provide pain relief for rectal pain according to recent case reports. The ganglion of impar lies just anterior to the sacrococcygeal junction and is easily blocked with an injection just anterior to the sacrum. This procedure often provides pain relief for perineal pain without risk of incontinence [30].

Risks of neurolytic blocks nearly always include deafferentation pain, which is the main reason neurolytic blockade is not used in the chronic pain setting. Further, with the celiac plexus block there is a risk of paralysis, probably due to anterior spinal artery vasospasm and infarct. With the hypogastric plexus block, we have seen several cases of lower extremity hip flexor weakness due to inadvertent spread of neurolytic agent to the psoas muscle with a partial denervation of the lumbar plexus (unpublished data). We have modified our technique to ensure medial needle placement and medial dye spread prior to neurolytic injection. As neurolytic blocks are relatively rare, the incidence of complication is difficult to determine, but weakness or paralysis are estimated to occur with less than 5% incidence and perhaps less than 1%. Such blocks are clearly reserved for the patient with progressive cancer and refractory pain.

Other special circumstances include neurolysis of peripheral nerves, including the intercostals or other peripheral branches. Intercostal neurolysis can produce short-term relief, with one group finding a median duration of effect to be 3 weeks, although in their series of 25 patients, one-third experienced analgesia until the end of life [43]. These authors found optimal outcomes using a diagnostic block, followed by a 10% phenol injection in those obtaining relief with the diagnostic block.

Subarachnoid or epidural neurolysis has been conducted in highly refractory cases where bladder and bowel function are already compromised. Slatkin and Rhiner reported four cases of phenol saddle blocks with reasonably good outcomes, with the use of 0.6–1.0 mL of 6% phenol in glycerin injected via subarachnoid injection in cases of highly refractory pelvic cancer pain [36]. This report also nicely reviews the literature.

Conclusions

As opposed to the automatic WHO approach of utilizing opioids first, many experts now advocate a mechanism-based approach to cancer pain treatment [1]. Old dogma relegated cancer pain to the end-of-life situation with metastatic, progressive disease, whereas new data show pain to be problematic throughout the cancer care cycle. The effective management of acutely painful surgeries and related treatments may limit the development of chronic pain states in long-term survivors. The best treatment strategies include a careful multidisciplinary assessment with an approach individualized to the patient's needs [1]. Finally, in cases of indolent cancer or remission, cancer pain syndromes effectively become chronic pain states in nearly all aspects. Thus, in these situations, optimal success will be seen through the use of chronic pain multidisciplinary

assessment and treatment strategies. The goals of treatment in chronic postcancer pain or "success" are slightly altered from the "Freedom from cancer pain" label above the WHO ladder to the more realistic: "Optimal functioning, optimal analgesia, and effective coping with ongoing pain."

In my view, the WHO ladder concept is outdated and vastly oversimplified in 2010, and I advocate a mechanism-based use of all the above therapies in the context of the patient's pain syndrome. More resource commitment to support ongoing research into unrelieved cancer pain is essential [4].

References

[1] Ahmedzai SH, Boland J. The total challenge of cancer pain in supportive and palliative care. Curr Opin Support Palliat Care 2007;1:3–5.
[2] Aprili D, Bandschapp O, Rochlitz C, Urwyler A, Ruppen W. Serious complications associated with external intrathecal catheters used in cancer pain patients. A systematic review and meta-analysis. Anesthesiology 2009;111:1346–55.
[3] Bhatnagar S, Gupta D, Mishra S, Thulkar S, Chauhan H. Bedside ultrasound-guided celiac plexus neurolysis with bilateral paramedian needle entry technique can be an effective pain control technique in advanced upper abdominal cancer pain. J Palliat Med 2008;11:1195–9.
[4] Brawley OW, Smith DE, Kirch RA. Taking action to ease suffering: advancing cancer pain control as a health care priority. CA Cancer J Clin 2009;59:285–89.
[5] Brown DL. Atlas of regional anesthesia, 3rd edition. Philadelphia: Elsevier Saunders; 2006.
[6] Burton AW. Celiac plexus blocks: wider application warranted for treating pancreatic cancer pain. J Support Oncol 2009;7:88–9.
[7] Burton AW, Fanciullo GJ, Beasley RD, Fisch MJ. Chronic pain in the cancer survivor: a new frontier. Pain Med 2007;8:189–98.
[8] Burton AW, Hamid B. Current challenges in cancer pain management: does the WHO ladder approach still have relevance? Expert Rev Anticancer Ther 2007;7:1501–2.
[9] Burton AW, Rajagopal A, Shah HN, Mendoza T, Cleeland CS, Hassenbusch SJ, Arens JF. Epidural and intrathecal analgesia is effective in treating refractory cancer pain. Pain Med 2004;5;239–47.
[10] Burton AW, Reddy SK, Shah HN, Tremont-Lukats I, Mendel E. Percutaneous vertebroplasty—a technique to treat refractory spinal pain in the setting of advanced metastatic disease: a case series. J Pain Symptom Manage 2005;30:87–95.
[11] Callstrom MR, Charboneau JW, Goetz MP, Rubin J, Wong GY, Sloan JA, Novotny PJ, Lewis BD, Welch TJ, Farrell MA, et al. Painful metastases involving bone: feasibility of percutaneous CT- and US-guided radio-frequency ablation. Radiology 2002;224:87–97.
[12] Choi D, Crockard A, Bunger C, Harms J, Kawahara N, Mazel C, Melcher R, Tomita K. Review of metastatic spine tumour classification and indications for surgery: the consensus statement of the Global Spine Tumour Study Group. Eur Spine J 2010;19:215–22.
[13] Crul BJ, Delhaas EM. Technical complications during long-term subarachnoid or epidural administration of morphine in terminally ill cancer patients: a review of 140 cases. Reg Anesth 1991;16:209–13.
[14] Davies DD. Incidence of major complications of neurolytic celiac plexus block. J Roy Soc Med 1993;86:264–6.
[15] Deer T, Krames ES, Hassenbusch SJ, Burton AW, Caraway D, Du Pen S, Eisenach J, Erdek M, Grigsby E, Kim P, Levy R, et al. Polyanalgesic Consensus Conference 2007: Recommendations for the management of pain by intraspinal (intrathecal) drug delivery: report of an expert interdisciplinary panel. Neuromodulation 2007;10:300–28.
[16] Easson AM and Pisters PWT. The role of palliative surgery. In: Fisch MJ, Burton AW, editors. Cancer pain management New York: McGraw Hill; 2007. p. 263–70.
[17] Eisenberg E, Carr DB, Chalmers TC. Neurolytic celiac plexus block for treatment of cancer pain: a meta-analysis. Anesth Analg 1995;80:290–5.
[18] Fenstermaker RA. Neurosurgical invasive techniques for cancer pain: a pain specialist's view. Curr Rev Pain 1999;3:190–7.

[19] Fourney DR, Schomer DF, Nader R, Chlan-Fourney J, Suki D, Ahrar K, Rhines LD, Gokaslan ZL. Percutaneous vertebroplasty and kyphoplasty for painful vertebral body fractures in cancer patients. J Neurosurg 2003;98:21–30.

[20] Georgy BA. Bone cement deposition patterns with plasma-mediated radio-frequency ablation and cement augmentation for advanced metastatic spine lesions. Am J Neuroradiol 2009;30:1197–202.

[21] Hentschel SJ, Burton AW, Fourney DR, Rhines LD, Mendel E. Percutaneous vertebroplasty and kyphoplasty performed at a cancer center: refuting proposed contraindications. J Neurosurg Spine 2005;2:436–40.

[22] Lamacraft G, Cousins MJ. Neural blockade in chronic and cancer pain. Int Anesthesiol Clin 1997;35:131–53.

[23] Mercadante S. Intrathecal morphine and bupivacaine in advanced cancer pain patients implanted at home. J Pain Symptom Manage 1994;9:201–7.

[24] Mercadante S, Villari P, Cascuccio A, Marrazzo A. A randomized-controlled study of intrathecal versus epidural thoracic analgesia in patients undergoing abdominal cancer surgery. J Clin Monit Comput 2008;22:293–8.

[25] Mishra S, Bhatnagar S, Gupta D, Thulkar S. Anterior ultrasound-guided superior hypogastric plexus neurolysis in pelvic cancer pain. Anaesth Intensive Care 2008; 36:732–5.

[26] Moore JC, Adler DG. Celiac plexus neurolysis for pain relief in pancreatic cancer. J Support Oncol 2009;783–7.

[27] Munk PL, Rashid F, Heran MK, Papirny M, Liu DM, Malfair D, Badii M, Clarkson PW. Combined cementoplasty and radiofrequency ablation in the treatment of painful neoplastic lesions of bone. J Vasc Interv Radiol 2009;20:903–11.

[28] Pausch R, Zaslow J. The last lecture. New York: Hyperion; 2008.

[29] Phan PC, Are M, Burton AW. Neuraxial infusions. Tech Reg Anesth Pain Manag 2005;9:152–60.

[30] Plancarte R, deLeon-Casasola OA, El-Helaly M, Allende S, Lema MJ. Neurolytic superior hypogastric plexus block for chronic pelvic pain associated with cancer. Reg Anesth 1997;22:562–8.

[31] Raslan AM. Percutaneous computed tomography-guided radiofrequency ablation of upper spinal cord pain pathways for cancer-related pain. Neurosurgery 2008;62(Suppl 1):226–33.

[32] Rathmell JP. Atlas of image guided intervention in regional anesthesia and pain medicine. Philadelphia: Lippincott Williams & Wilkins; 2006.

[33] Rauck RL, Wallace MS, Burton AW, Kapural L, North JM. Intrathecal ziconotide for neuropathic pain: a review. Pain Pract 2009;9:327–37.

[34] Schultz DM. Inferior hypogastric plexus blockade: a transsacral approach. Pain Physician 2007;10:757–63.

[35] Sharma P, Kozarek R. Role of esophageal stents in benign and malignant disease. Am J Gastroenterol 2010;105:258–73.

[36] Slatkin NE, Rhiner M. Phenol saddle blocks for intractable pain at the end of life: report of four cases and literature review. Am J Hosp Palliat Care 2003;20:62–6.

[37] Smith TJ, Coyne PJ. How to use implantable intrathecal drug delivery systems for refractory cancer pain. J Support Oncol 2003;1:73–6.

[38] Smith TJ, Coyne PJ, Staats PS, Deer T, Stearns LJ, Rauck RL, Boortz-Marx RL, Buchser E, Català E, Bryce DA, Cousins M, Pool GE. An implantable drug delivery system for refractory cancer pain provides sustained pain control, less drug related toxicity and possibly better survival compared to comprehensive medical management. J Clin Oncol 2005;16:825–33.

[39] Smith TJ, Staats PS, Deer T, Stearns LJ, Rauck RL, Boortz-Marx RL, Buchser E, Català E, Bryce DA, Coyne PJ, Pool GE; Implantable Drug Delivery Systems Study Group. Randomised clinical trial of an implantable drug delivery system compared with comprehensive medical management for refractory cancer pain; impact on pain, drug-related toxicity and survival. J Clin Oncol 2002;20:4040–9.

[40] Swarm R, Anghelescu DL, Benedetti C, Boston B, Cleeland C, Coyle N, Deleon-Casasola OA, Eidelman A, Eilers JG, Ferrell B, et al.; National Comprehensive Cancer Network (NCCN). Adult cancer pain. J Natl Compr Canc Netw 2007;5:726–51.

[41] Varghese BT, Koshy RC, Sebastian P, Joseph E. Combined sphenopalatine ganglion and mandibular nerve, neurolytic block for pain due to advanced head and neck cancer. Palliat Med 2002;16:447–8.

[42] Vila H, Liu J, Kavasmaneck D. Paravertebral block: new benefits from an old procedure. Curr Opin Anaesthesiol 2007;20:316–8.

[43] Wong FCS, Lee TW, Yuen KK, Lo SH, Sze WK, Tung SY. Intercostal nerve block for cancer pain: effectiveness and selection of patients. Hong Kong Med J 2007;13:266–70.

Correspondence to: Prof. Allen W. Burton, MD, Department of Pain Medicine, MD Anderson Cancer Center, 1400 Holcombe-409, Houston, TX 77030, USA. Email: awburton@mdanderson.org.

Part 3
The Basics of Brain Imaging

Functional MRI Studies of Pain Processing

6

Irene Tracey, PhD

Oxford Centre for Functional Magnetic Resonance Imaging of the Brain, Department of Clinical Neurology, and Nuffield Department of Anaesthetics, University of Oxford, John Radcliffe Hospital, Oxford, United Kingdom

This chapter will focus on how functional magnetic resonance imaging (fMRI) can be used to dissect physiological and psychological characteristics of the pain experience. I will discuss how other magnetic resonance (MR)-related measures can be used, such as quantitative cerebral blood flow (for measuring tonic pain), morphometry, tractography, and spectroscopic measures (for measuring potential neurodegeneration and maladaptive plasticity), to improve our understanding of pain processing within the human central nervous system (CNS) from a structural, functional, and metabolic perspective.

Basic Principles of Imaging Techniques: Pros and Cons

To appreciate the utility of these new methodologies, it is important to understand what they measure, and by implication what their limitations are with regard to providing information about neural activity within the human brain or spinal cord.

Functional neuroimaging refers to the measurement and localization of neural activity that results from the performance of a task, whether sensory, motor, or cognitive. Fig. 1 illustrates the main imaging modalities in use today and shows what physiological correlate of brain activity they measure. There is a "cost" or balance between the spatial and temporal information achievable and the "invasiveness" required

if high resolution is desired in both domains, as illustrated in Fig. 2. It is clear from these diagrams that human brain activity can be measured and imaged using several techniques, but that two basic classes of mapping technique have evolved: (1) those that map or localize the underlying electrical activity of the brain and (2) those that map local physiological or metabolic consequences of altered brain electrical activity. Among the former are the noninvasive neural electromagnetic techniques of electroencephalography (EEG) and magnetoencephalography (MEG). These methods allow exquisite temporal resolution of neural processes (typically over a 10–100-ms time scale), but they suffer from relatively poor spatial resolution (between one and several centimeters). The benefits of EEG and MEG will be discussed in the chapter by Iannetti in this volume. Positron emission tomography (PET) and functional magnetic resonance imaging (fMRI) methods (Table I) are in the second category. They can be made sensitive to the changes in regional blood perfusion, blood volume (for example, using injected magnetic resonance contrast agents), or blood oxygenation that accompanies neuronal activity. Blood-oxygenation-level-dependent (BOLD) fMRI, which is sensitive primarily to the last of these variables, allows an image spatial resolution that is of the order of a few millimeters, with a temporal resolution of several seconds (limited by the hemodynamic response itself, which lags behind neuronal activity).

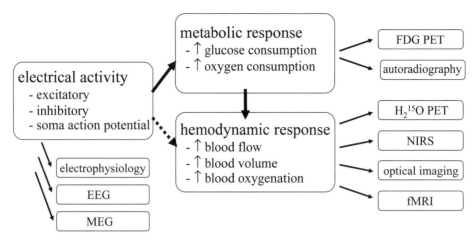

Fig. 1. The main imaging modalities in use today and the physiological correlate of brain activity they measure. EEG, electroencephalography; FDG, fluorodeoxyglucose; fMRI, functional magnetic resonance imaging; MEG, magnetoencephalography; NIRS, near-infrared spectroscopy; PET, positron emission tomography.

PET and fMRI thus measure brain activity indirectly, by imaging changes in blood flow, blood oxygenation, or local metabolic changes. Currently, PET and fMRI are the most extensively used tools in neuroimaging research in humans. The temporal resolution of PET is on the order of tens of seconds, while for fMRI it is shorter, which has significant advantages, as discussed later. Furthermore, fMRI is a completely noninvasive tool, unlike PET, which requires injection of a radioligand, and this feature provides added flexibility in terms of paradigm designs and patient studies. However, as discussed more extensively in the chapter by Schweinhardt in this volume, PET provides the additional opportunity for examining specific neurotransmitters or receptors and therefore, unlike fMRI,

has increased biological specificity. PET and MRI can therefore be employed to provide information on the anatomical structure and the neurochemical composition of the central nervous system (CNS), which along with functional information, yields a systems view of pain processing within the CNS. Advances in our ability to "label" receptors, neurotransmitters, or even intracellular substrates allow techniques based on PET (and to lesser extent MRI) to image their function and distribution within the CNS. These "labels" provide a "visual report" from the scene of cellular events. Molecular imaging has thus been defined as the measurement and imaging of biological processes in vivo at the molecular and cellular level.

Table I
Comparison of fMRI and PET imaging techniques

Modality	BOLD fMRI	^{15}O-Water PET
Working principle	Detects changes in the magnetic field due to variations in the oxyhemoglobin : deoxyhemoglobin ratio	Detects the radioactive isotopes that are tagged onto the molecule of interest
Availability	Most tertiary medical centers	Isotopes are short-lived and must be generated by a nearby cyclotron
Invasiveness	Completely noninvasive	Employs radioisotopes; requires intravenous access as minimum
Spatial resolution	1–2 mm	5 mm at best
Temporal resolution	Hundreds of milliseconds	Minutes
Experimental design	Flexible; limited mainly by noise and magnetic environment	Limited by tracer half-life and radiation dose
Derived data	Unable to quantify the physiological baseline	Able to quantify the physiological baseline

Abbreviations: BOLD fMRI, blood-oxygenation-level-dependent functional magnetic resonance imaging; PET, positron emission tomography.

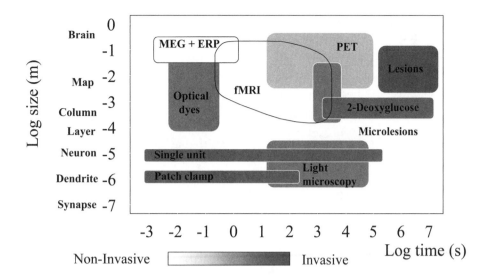

Fig. 2. Relative invasiveness of imaging modalities. ERP, event-related potential; MEG, magnetoencephalography.

The Basis for Blood-Oxygen-Level-Dependent Functional MRI

The most common form of fMRI used is BOLD fMRI. The signal from BOLD imaging depends on the relative concentrations of oxyhemoglobin and deoxyhemoglobin in the local vasculature. The disproportionate increase in cerebral blood flow that accompanies neural activity results in a relative decrease in the concentration of deoxygenated hemoglobin. Deoxygenated hemoglobin is a paramagnetic molecule. It distorts the local magnetic field and causes a loss of signal. Thus, the decrease of deoxygenated hemoglobin leads to higher signal intensities that contrast against surrounding tissue. During image analysis, the BOLD signal that is expected to result from the stimulus is modeled mathematically. The model is compared to the signal that is measured during the experiment itself. Statistical maps are constructed and superimposed on a structural brain image to indicate where the measured signal best fits the model. Further details regarding data analysis and background information on fMRI can be found at www.fmrib.ox.ac.uk/fsl.

The Cerebral Signature for Pain Perception

Over the last decade, FMRI and PET functional imaging studies have revealed the large distributed brain network that is accessed during processing of noxious inputs. Several cortical and subcortical brain regions are commonly activated by noxious stimulation, including the anterior cingulate cortex (ACC), insular cortex, frontal and prefrontal cortices (PFC), primary and secondary somatosensory cortices (S1 and S2, respectively), thalamus, basal ganglia, cerebellum, amygdala, hippocampus, and regions within the parietal and temporal cortices. This network is though to reflect the complexity of pain as an experience and is often called the "pain matrix."

The matrix can be simplistically thought of as having lateral components (sensory-discriminatory, involving areas such as the primary and secondary somatosensory cortices, thalamus, and posterior parts of the insula) and medial components (affective-cognitive-evaluative, involving areas such as the anterior parts of the insula, ACC, and PFC) [1]. However, because different brain regions play a more- or less-active role depending upon the precise interplay of the factors involved in influencing pain perception (e.g., cognition, mood, and injury), the "pain matrix" is not a defined entity.

A recent meta-analysis of human data from different imaging studies provides clarity regarding the regions most commonly found active during an acute pain experience as measured by PET and fMRI [3]. These areas include the primary and secondary somatosensory cortices, insular cortex, ACC, and PFC, as well as the thalamus. This is not to say that these areas are the fundamental core network of human nociceptive processing (and if they were ablated it would cure all pain), although studies investigating acute pharmacologically induced analgesia do show predominant effects in this core network that suggest their overall importance in influencing pain perception [18]. Other regions such as the basal ganglia, cerebellum, amygdala, hippocampus, and areas within the parietal and temporal cortices can also be active depending upon the particular set of circumstances for a given individual.

A "cerebral signature" for pain is perhaps how we should define the network; it is necessarily unique for each individual [15]. This unique signature is particularly relevant, given the very recent awareness of how great a role our genes play in the perception of pain related to a noxious stimulus or due to injury. For example, individuals homozygous for the met158 allele of the catechol-O-methyltransferase gene (*COMT*) polymorphism (val158met) showed diminished regional mu-opioid system responses to pain (measured using PET) and higher sensory and affective ratings for experimentally induced pain compared with heterozygotes [19]. The link between our genes and pain perception during acute and chronic pain experiences is one of the most exciting areas of pain research at present; the field is being led primarily by animal studies, but with fast translation to human studies [10]. Functional imaging is poised to provide phenotypic information that is based on objective mechanistic data in conjunction with reported pain symptomatology. As such, it has the potential to provide the intermediary between genetics and behavior.

For brevity, it is not possible to provide a full account of what is currently known regarding how various factors such as cognition, context, mood, and injury alter the CNS to modulate the experience of pain. Other reviews provide this information [2,5,12,15,16,17]. Instead, I will give a brief introduction to other methods that are currently being used to understand pain processing in the human CNS.

Other Magnetic Resonance-Based Measures of Neuronal Function and Systems Pain Processing

Techniques such as magnetic resonance spectroscopy (MRS), diffusion tractography imaging, pharmacological MRI, quantitative cerebral blood flow mapping, and volumetric imaging are currently being applied to the study of human disease, including pain. These methods enable us to examine different aspects of structure and function within the human CNS in chronic pain states. Combined with advances in how we analyze the data, as well as integration of fMRI with other techniques, these methods provide us with unprecedented opportunities to unravel this complex and heterogeneous medical problem noninvasively in humans.

Structural Imaging

Magnetic Resonance Volumetry

MR volumetry involves the use of automated analysis techniques that allow the segmentation and measurement of gray and white matter volumes of a structural brain image. Application of this technique for the sensitive assessment of cerebral atrophy in Alzheimer's disease and its progression is well established. Apkarian and colleagues [4] first reported the application of this technique to chronic pain research. They found significant cerebral atrophy in chronic pain patients, even after accounting for age-related brain volume decreases. Patients with chronic back pain showed a loss of gray matter volume equivalent to that seen in 10–20 years of normal aging. The loss was localized to the bilateral dorsolateral prefrontal cortex and right thalamus [4]. Thereafter, studies involving a range of chronic pain conditions have revealed gray matter losses in several other areas implicated in nociceptive processing [13].

The dramatic extent of neurodegeneration in chronic pain states evidenced by these studies has compelled the shift in our approach to chronic pain from symptom to disease. There is now a pressing need to perform more advanced structural imaging measures and analyses to better quantify these effects. The challenge is in determining the possible causal factors that produce such neurodegeneration in patients. Candidate factors include the chronic pain condition itself (i.e., excitotoxic events due to barrage of nociceptive inputs), the pharmacological agents prescribed, or perhaps the physical lifestyle change subsequent to becoming a chronic pain patient. Carefully controlled longitudinal studies are required, as this area rapidly becomes an active topic of research: a recent review assesses these data and how they affect our current definition of chronic pain as a possible disease in its own right [13].

Diffusion Tensor Imaging

Diffusion of water in white matter tracts is directionally dependent (anisotropic) on the orientation of axon bundles. Diffusion tensor imaging (DTI) is an MRI-based technique that measures the anisotropic motion of water in different regions of the brain, and after subsequent processing, calculates a principal direction of diffusion for water in each imaging voxel. Using DTI, Hadjipavlou and colleagues [8] defined connections between the periaqueductal gray and separately for the nucleus cuneiformis (part of the brainstem reticular formation implicated in central sensitization), to the

PFC, amygdala, thalamus, hypothalamus, and rostro-ventral medial medulla bilaterally. Such data show the existence of the anatomical circuitry that mediates the top-down influences on pain processing in humans. Characterization of anatomical connectivity by DTI, in concert with neuroimaging techniques that identify areas of functional or structural alterations in chronic pain patients, is now being performed [6], and such research will more fully inform the neurobiology that instantiates the chronic pain state.

Neurochemical Imaging

Proton Magnetic Resonance Spectroscopy

Proton magnetic resonance spectroscopy (MRS) produces signals that are reported as frequencies that may be assigned to molecules of biological interest. An example is *N*-acetyl aspartate (NAA), an amino acid derivative located in neurons. Apkarian and colleagues [7] have demonstrated reductions in NAA concentrations (implying neuronal loss) in the dorsolateral PFC of patients with chronic lower back pain. The study adds to the current hypothesis that neurodegeneration might be occurring in the chronic pain state. More recent studies aiming to examine the role of glutamate in chronic pain states show promising results [9].

Quantitative Perfusion Imaging

It is possible to detect functional activation caused by painful stimuli using an alternative MRI-based non-invasive technique called arterial spin labeling. This technique measures cerebral blood flow directly and quantitatively, and therefore it is capable of measuring ongoing activity rather than evoked, brief stimuli as normally measured using BOLD-based fMRI. It is therefore ideally suited to examine the neural activity underpinning the ongoing, tonic pain that is often reported by patients. Studies are now beginning to use this technique, with very promising early findings [11,14].

Conclusions

Neuroimaging techniques that noninvasively provide functional or structural information regarding the CNS have unequivocally shown that the brains of patients with chronic pain are significantly more affected than was previously anticipated.

Neuroimaging data acquisition and analytical techniques are improving rapidly. These advances when applied to pain research will allow us to further examine how mechanisms of chronic pain gleaned from animal studies map to human neurobiology. This field is of considerable interest to all, from the laboratory-based animal researcher to the chronic pain clinician. We envisage that data obtained from such techniques will not reside solely within the laboratory but will progressively move into clinical practice to aid decisions on diagnosis and treatment choices.

References

[1] Albe-Fessard D, Berkley KJ, Kruger L, et al. Diencephalic mechanisms of pain sensation. Brain Res 1985;356:217–96.

[2] Apkarian AV, Baliki MN, Geha PY. Towards a theory of chronic pain. Prog Neurobiol 2009;87:81–97.

[3] Apkarian AV, Bushnell MC, Treede RD, Zubieta JK. Human brain mechanisms of pain perception and regulation in health and disease. Eur J Pain 2005;9:463–84.

[4] Apkarian AV, Sosa Y, Sonty S, et al. Chronic back pain is associated with decreased prefrontal and thalamic gray matter density. J Neurosci 2004;24:10410–5.

[5] Craig AD. Interoception: the sense of the physiological condition of the body. Curr Opin Neurobiol 2003;13:500–5.

[6] Geha PY, Baliki MN, Harden RN, Bauer WR, Parrish TB, Apkarian AV. The brain in chronic CRPS pain: abnormal gray-white matter interactions in emotional and autonomic regions. Neuron 2008;60:570–81.

[7] Grachev ID, Fredrickson BE, Apkarian AV. Abnormal brain chemistry in chronic back pain: an in vivo proton magnetic resonance spectroscopy study. Pain 2000;89:7–18.

[8] Hadjipavlou G, Dunckley P, Behrens TE, Tracey I. Determining anatomical connectivities between cortical and brainstem pain processing regions in humans: a diffusion tensor imaging study in healthy controls. Pain 2006;123:169–78.

[9] Harris RE, Sundgren PC, Craig AD, Kirshenbaum E, Sen A, Napadow V, Clauw DJ. Elevated insular glutamate in fibromyalgia is associated with experimental pain. Arthritis Rheum 2009;60:3146–52.

[10] LaCroix-Fralish ML, Mogil JS. Progress in genetic studies of pain and analgesia. Annu Rev Pharmacol Toxicol 2009;49:97–121.

[11] Owen DG, Clarke CF, Ganapathy S, Prato FS, St Lawrence KS. Using perfusion MRI to measure the dynamic changes in neural activation associated with tonic muscular pain. Pain 2010;148:375–86.

[12] Schweinhardt P, Lee M, Tracey I. Imaging pain in patients: is it meaningful? Curr Opin Neurol 2006;19:392–400.

[13] Tracey I, Bushnell MC. How neuroimaging studies have challenged us to rethink: is chronic pain a disease? J Pain 2009;10:1113–20.

[14] Tracey I, Johns E. The pain matrix: reloaded or reborn as we image tonic pain using arterial spin labelling. Pain 2010 148:359–60.

[15] Tracey I, Mantyh PW. The cerebral signature for pain perception and its modulation. Neuron 2007;55:377–91.

[16] Wiech K, Ploner M, Tracey I. Neurocognitive aspects of pain perception. Trends Cogn Sci 2008;12:306–13.

[17] Wiech K, Tracey I. The influence of negative emotions on pain: behavioral effects and neural mechanisms. Neuroimage 2009;47:987–94.

[18] Wise RG, Rogers R, Painter D, et al. Combining fMRI with a pharmacokinetic model to determine which brain areas activated by painful stimulation are specifically modulated by remifentanil. Neuroimage 2002;16:999–1014.

[19] Zubieta JK, Heitzeg MM, Smith YR, et al. COMT val158met genotype affects mu-opioid neurotransmitter responses to a pain stressor. Science 2003;299:1240–3.

Correspondence to: Professor Irene Tracey, PhD, FMRIB Centre, Department of Clinical Neurology and Nuffield Department of Anaesthetics, University of Oxford, John Radcliffe Hospital, Headington, OX3 9DU, England, United Kingdom. Email: irene@fmrib.ox.ac.uk.

The Basics of Positron Emission Tomography

Petra Schweinhardt, MD, PhD

Department of Neurology and Neurosurgery and Faculty of Dentistry, McGill University, Montreal, Quebec, Canada

Overview of PET Imaging

Basic Principles

Positron emission tomography (PET) imaging relies on the detection of the distribution of radioactivity emitted by radionuclides. Radionuclides used for PET are radioactive isotopes that emit positrons when they decay. Since positrons are the anti-particles to electrons, they possess the same mass (511 keV/c^2, where keV = kiloelectronvolt and c = the speed of light), but the opposite charge. For PET, molecules of biological interest are labeled with positron-emitting isotopes. Molecules that are commonly labeled include receptor ligands or molecules of metabolic pathways, such as glucose. In theory, any molecule of interest could be labeled and used for PET imaging. Tracer amounts of the labeled molecule (i.e., amounts too small to exhibit any pharmacological or biological effect) are administered to the subject (usually intravenously, but other routes of administration—such as inhalation—are possible, depending on the molecule). The labeled molecule becomes concentrated in its respective location (e.g., a dopamine receptor antagonist accumulates at dopamine receptors), and positrons are emitted as the isotope decays.

When positrons encounter an electron, both particles are annihilated, and a pair of annihilation (gamma) photons of 511 keV, which move in opposite directions, are emitted. The 511-keV photons are either absorbed (by photoelectric absorption) or attenuated (by Compton scattering) by the scintillation detectors in the scanner. The scintillators reemit the absorbed energy in the form of a visible light, which is then multiplied by the photomultiplier tubes. Detection of the two opposite 511-keV photons *in coincidence* by two detectors is the basis of PET imaging. Photons that do not arrive in temporal pairs (i.e., within a timing window of a few nanoseconds) are ignored.

Connecting the two points of the detector ring where the two photons of a temporal pair were detected with a straight line creates a "line of response" (LOR) along which the annihilation event is known to have occurred. Many annihilation events are associated with positron emission of the tracer that has accumulated in a given location. This is exploited to determine the location of the tracer, because it allows the determination of intersecting LORs. However, localization is imprecise for several reasons, which affects spatial resolution. First, positrons travel some distance in the surrounding tissue before being annihilated and emitting gamma rays (up to a few millimeters, depending on the tissue and the positron emitter). Second, the two photons of a temporal pair are not emitted at exactly 180° but at an angle that is slightly smaller (noncollinearity). Drawing a straight LOR therefore introduces some error. At zero kelvins, the angle between the two gamma photons would be exactly 180°. At higher temperatures, there is some residual momentum associated with the positron, and therefore, the two annihilation photons are not emitted exactly at 180°. The maximum deviation between the observed LOR and the original annihilation line is ±0.25°.

Spatial Resolution

The spatial resolution—that is, the minimum distance between two points that can be detected—of a PET image depends on several factors. One important factor is the intrinsic resolution of the scintillation detectors, which is related to their size. Inherent in PET imaging and degrading spatial resolution is the fact that the annihilation site is not identical to the site of positron emission. Obviously, it is the location of positron emission we are interested in, but the photons that are detected by the scintillators originate at the site of annihilation. The distance (or range) a positron travels before being annihilated decreases with tissue density but increases with its energy. As a result, tracers labeled with different isotopes provide different spatial resolutions. For example, positrons emitted by fluorine-18 have a lower energy than positrons emitted by carbon-11, and therefore, ^{18}F-tracers provide better spatial resolution. The noncollinearity described above further decreases spatial resolution. Additional factors that influence spatial resolution include scatter coincidences and the image reconstruction method used. The typical effective spatial resolution of human PET experiments is in the order of 4–6 mm.

Temporal Aspects of Image Acquisition

There are two fundamental approaches to PET data acquisition: static and dynamic imaging. For static imaging, counts of activity detected by the scintillators are summed over a predetermined time period. This image does not contain any temporal information; it indicates solely the magnitude and the spatial distribution of radioactivity. However, when static imaging is combined with radioisotopes that have very short half-lives, temporal information can be obtained. Oxygen-15 has a half-life of about 2 minutes, and consequently, multiple injections can be performed in a session, with each injection providing a single image of brain activity over about 1 minute. After a 10-minute interval, another injection can be performed because the radioactivity from the previous injection is virtually nonexistent. Dynamic PET imaging involves a sequence of continuous

acquisitions ("frames"), which range in duration from a few seconds to over 20 minutes (the longer frame length towards the end is necessary to compensate for the loss of signal due to radioactive decay). Data from each frame are independently reconstructed to form a set of images, which can be visualized and used to estimate physiological parameters. Acquisition time depends on the isotope: scans using carbon-11 tracers are typically 40–60 minutes in length, whereas dynamic acquisition for fluorine-18 tracers usually lasts 60–90 minutes.

Radiotracers

In theory, PET technology can be used to trace any substance in vivo in humans, provided it can be labeled with a radionuclide. Suitable radionuclides are isotopes with relatively short half-lives, in order to keep the effective biological radiation dose relatively low. Carbon-11 (^{11}C, half-life ~ 20 minutes), fluorine-18 (^{18}F, half-life ~ 110 minutes), or oxygen-15 (^{15}O, half-life ~ 2 minutes) are commonly used radionuclides. To label a molecule of interest, different pathways depending on the nuclide can be used. For ^{11}C reactions, ^{11}C-labeled methyliodide is often used to introduce a methyl group into a molecule. For many ^{18}F-labeling reactions, nucleophilic substitution reactions are used, although there are other ways to introduce the ^{18}F into a biomolecule. (In organic and inorganic chemistry, nucleophilic substitution is a fundamental class of substitution reaction in which an "electron-rich" nucleophile selectively bonds with or attacks the positive charge of an atom attached to a group or atom called the "leaving group"; the positive atom is referred to as an "electrophile.") The radioactively labeled molecule is called a "hot tracer," whereas any molecule with the original, stable isotope is called a "cold tracer." In any radiotracer production process, the stable isotope is present in some of the compound molecules due to a "dilution" with the stable isotope during the labeling reaction, and this plays an important role with regard to the specific activity of the compound administered.

Due to the short half-lives of the PET radionuclides, many tracers have to be produced on site, which requires a cyclotron and a radiochemistry laboratory. A cyclotron suitable for this type of work is available for approximately US$1–3 million; additional significant costs stem from the electronic control of the system, the extensive shielding required, and the disposal of nuclear waste. Tracers containing ^{18}F, which has a half-life of approximately 110 minutes, can be produced off site and transported to imaging facilities within 2–4 hours. This convenience certainly contributes to the success of the only commonly used radiotracer, ^{18}F-fluorodeoxyglucose (FDG), which is widely used in clinical oncology. Several tracers have been developed to study brain function and structure. For example, radioactively labeled water (labeled using ^{15}O) can be used to measure blood flow, very much according to the same principles employed in magnetic resonance (MR)-based techniques, such as blood-oxygen-level-dependent (BOLD)-sensitive imaging or arterial spin labeling (ASL). There are distinct advantages of each technique; a strength of PET activation studies is measuring tonic activation over several minutes. Several radiotracers have been developed for PET that are ligands or substrates for specific neuroreceptor subtypes (e.g., ^{11}C-raclopride and ^{18}F-fallypride for dopamine D_2/D_3 receptors), transporters (e.g., ^{11}C-McN 5652 and ^{11}C-DASB for serotonin transporters), or enzymes (e.g., ^{18}F-L-6-fluorodopa [^{18}F–FDOPA] for aromatic amino acid decarboxylase, involved in the synthesis of monoamines). Imaging of dopamine and opioid receptors is discussed in more detail below.

Specific Activity

Specific activity is defined as the amount of radioactivity per mol of compound. Or, differently put, the ratio between the radioactively labeled compound and the total amount of compound (labeled and unlabeled). It follows that the more tracer that was not successfully labeled with the radionuclides, the lower the specific activity. It also follows that as time elapses between production of the tracer and tracer administration, specific activity decreases because the radionuclides decay. There are two important implications. First, saturation effects might occur due to receptor occupancy by the cold tracer in receptor systems that have small numbers of available binding sites, and consequently, the signal would be decreased. Second, with a low specific activity, there is a safety risk of injecting higher than tracer amounts; that is, amounts with a pharmacological effect. This risk occurs because the amount of tracer to be injected is measured in radioactivity units and therefore, is based only on hot tracer; with a low specific activity, more unlabeled tracer is present for a given dose of radioactivity. There can be unwanted side effects when substances are injected that have a narrow "therapeutic" range; that is, when the dose needed for imaging is not much lower than the dose leading to side effects.[1] Generally speaking, the higher the specific activity, the better. For tracers with moderately high affinity, a specific activity of 10 GBq/μmol is considered standard, and for high-affinity receptor ligands, 100 GBq/μmol or higher is recommended [6]. (The SI unit of radioactivity is becquerel (Bq); 1 Bq is defined as one decay per second.)

Safety Considerations

Only one commonly used radiotracer, ^{18}F-FDG, holds approval by the U.S. Food and Drug Administration (FDA) for use in humans. However, non-approved radiotracers can be used, in the U.S., Canada, and Europe, for research purposes under certain conditions. In Europe, for example, a process called "in-house production" is permitted, which means that non-approved tracers can be used on approval of a clinical trial application (CTA) or with local ethics committee approval. In Canada, the governmental department with responsibility for national public health, Health Canada, permits the use of other radiotracers with "established safety profiles" for human research, because Health Canada recognizes that "application of CTA requirements to positron emitting radiopharmaceuticals research studies is thought to place an undue regulatory burden on the researchers in this field and impede basic research involving positron emitting radiopharmaceuticals in Canada." The Canadian exposure limits are enforced by Health Canada and the Canadian Nuclear Safety Commission, but they are based on the guidelines published by the International Atomic Energy Agency based in Vienna. Exposure limits as specified by Health Canada are a whole-body single dose of 20 mSv and an annual

---

[1] Consider the following example. In an experiment, 370 mBq of the μ-opioid-receptor agonist ^{11}C-carfentanil is to be injected into a subject. Directly after production, the specific activity was determined to be 24 GBq/μmol. If the tracer is administered immediately, the amount of carfentanil injected is 24 GBq/μmol = 370 mBq/x, i.e., x = 0.154 μmol. Since the molar mass of carfentanil is 394.5 g/mol, this corresponds to 6.1 μg. Considering that not more than 0.1 μg/kg body weight should be injected, this amount would be acceptable for a person weighing at least 60 kg. If, however, there is a 10-minute delay between production and administration (e.g., because the subject is not yet positioned on the scanner bed), specific activity decreases to 18 GBq/μmol, and consequently, 9 μg of carfentanil is injected. This procedure is potentially dangerous for a subject weighing less than 90 kg because it might result in side effects associated with μ-opioid-receptor activation such as respiratory depression.

dose of 20 mSv. (The physical aspects of radiation are measured in gray [Gy], referring to how much energy has been absorbed. Sievert [Sv] is the unit of dose equivalent and attempts to reflect the biological effects of the radiation absorbed by the tissues.) A typical dynamic scan using a ^{11}C-tracer exposes the subject to between 5 and 10 mSv, which means that repeated scanning within one year is feasible in research studies.

Imaging the Dopaminergic System in the Context of Pain

Several radiotracers are available that can be used to study different aspects of the brain's dopaminergic system. Dopaminergic neurons are present mainly in the ventral tegmental area (VTA) of the midbrain, the substantia nigra pars compacta (SNc), and the arcuate nucleus of the hypothalamus. Pathways that might be of particular importance for pain processing are the nigrostriatal system, which originates in the SNc and projects to the dorsal striatum, and the mesocorticolimbic system, which starts in the VTA and projects to the frontal cortex and to limbic areas including the amygdala and the nucleus accumbens (NAc). At present, there is conclusive evidence for five different types of dopamine receptors that are categorized as D_1-like receptors (D_1 and D_5) and D_2-like receptors (D_2, D_3, and D_4). In the dorsal striatum, D_2 receptors are dominant, whereas in the mesolimbic and mesocortical projections, D_1 and D_3 receptors also play an important role. Several PET tracers have been used to study presynaptic (dopamine synthesis, transport, and storage) and postsynaptic (receptor) function. ^{18}F-FDOPA accumulates in dopaminergic neurons, more precisely in presynaptic vesicles, after decarboxylation to ^{18}F-dopamine by the aromatic amino acid decarboxylase (AAAD). FDOPA PET reflects DOPA transport into the neurons, DOPA decarboxylation, and dopamine storage capacity. FDOPA is, however, not strictly specific for dopaminergic cells because it also accumulates in regions with high concentrations of serotonin or norepinephrine. Healthy subjects injected with ^{18}F-FDOPA show high uptake in areas with high AAAD activity—that is, the caudate and putamen as well as the midbrain [4]. AAAD activity is reduced in diseases with degeneration of dopaminergic neurons, mainly Parkinson's disease and related disorders. Interestingly, one small study in fibromyalgia patients has reported decreased ^{18}F-FDOPA uptake compared to control sub-

jects in several brain regions, including the midbrain, medial thalamus, hippocampus, anterior cingulate cortex, and insular cortex [16].

Dopamine uptake from the synaptic cleft is mediated via the dopamine transporter (DAT). DAT is essential for recycling dopamine back into the presynaptic neuron. Its blockage, for example by psychostimulants such as cocaine and methylphenidate, leads to a massive rise in synaptic dopamine levels. Several PET tracers that allow measuring DAT levels are available and have chiefly been employed in investigations of drug abuse and Parkinson's disease. No published reports on the application of this method to the study of pain can be retrieved using the key words "DAT" and "PET" and "pain" in PubMed as of February 2010.

Several radioligands are available to study dopamine receptors in humans. In general, two types of studies can be conducted with radioligands: baseline or challenge studies. Studies performed without a challenge inform about the receptor's binding capacity at rest, which is influenced by several factors, including endogenous tonic neurotransmitter levels, receptor density, and receptor affinity. Challenge studies investigate to which degree the radioligand is displaced by competitive binding of the neurotransmitter released by the challenge (e.g., administration of painful stimulation). Displacement is conveniently described by a change in binding potential (BP). The BP of a receptor ligand is the number of maximally available receptors (B_{max}) relative to the equilibrium dissociation constant, K_d (BP = B_{max}/K_d). K_d is the rate with which the ligand binds to the receptor relative to the rate with which the ligand dissociates from the receptor.[2]

In the context of pain, the D_1-receptor tracer ^{11}C-NNC 756 has been used to compare baseline striatal binding potentials in patients with burning mouth syndrome and healthy control subjects [5]. In contrast to striatal D_2 binding potentials, which were investigated in the same study using the tracer ^{11}C-raclopride, no difference was observed. D_2-binding potential was

---

[2] The equilibrium dissociation constant, K_d, is a specific type of an equilibrium constant that quantifies the tendency of a compound to dissociate into its components. In the case of a receptor and its ligand, the ligand bound to the receptor corresponds to the compound; the unbound ligand and the unoccupied receptor correspond to the components. The concentration of the two components (unbound ligand and unoccupied receptor) multiplied divided by the concentration of the compound (receptors occupied by the ligand) corresponds to the dissociation constant (K_d = ([A] × [B])/[AB]). It follows that a low value for K_d corresponds to a high concentration of receptors occupied by the ligand, and hence to high affinity of the ligand for the receptor.

increased in the putamen of the patient group, which might signify a decline in endogenous tonic dopamine levels. Alternatively, increased binding potential could be caused by increased receptor density or affinity. It is important to point out that these alternative explanations cannot be differentiated with PET receptor studies in which binding potentials are measured. Although it is possible to determine B_{max} and K_d in human PET experiments, binding potentials are much more widely used because measurement of B_{max} and K_d often require multiple measurements with different specific activities to obtain reliable results.

The D_2-receptor antagonist ^{11}C-raclopride has been the most commonly used PET tracer to study the dopaminergic system in the context of pain. A challenge study using ^{11}C-raclopride found that whereas healthy subjects displayed decreased binding potentials in response to an experimental pain stimulus (indicative of dopamine release), binding potentials in fibromyalgia patients remained unchanged compared to the control condition [17]. An elegant series of experiments by Scott and colleagues demonstrated decreased striatal ^{11}C-raclopride binding potentials both during the anticipation and during the pain administration phase of placebo analgesia [12,13]. It is important to emphasize that due to the relatively low receptor affinity of ^{11}C-raclopride (K_d = 8 nM), only binding potentials in the striatum (which has the highest density of D_2 receptors) can be reliably measured. High-affinity tracers such as ^{11}C-FLB 457, ^{11}C-fallypride, or ^{18}F-fallypride are available to investigate extrastriatal areas with lower densities of D_2 receptors. For completeness, it should be noted that all D_2 radioligands discussed above have some affinity to D_3 receptors.

Opioid Receptor Imaging and Pain

Carfentanil is an extremely potent (8 to 10 thousand times the potency of morphine) [10] and high-affinity (K_d = 0.05 nM) [3] mu-opioid receptor agonist. After intravenous administration of ^{11}C-carfentanil, the highest concentrations are seen in the thalamus and amygdala, with intermediate levels in the frontal, temporal, and parietal cortices, anterior cingulate cortex, caudate nucleus, and hippocampus [11]. As discussed above, the "therapeutic" window between the dose that is necessary for receptor imaging and the dose that produces respiratory side effects is relatively small. The amount administered must be kept under 0.1 μg/kg body weight. Importantly for

the study of pain, analgesia might be induced if too much carfentanil is administered. ^{11}C-carfentanil has been used to study opioid release during acute pain challenges in healthy subjects [1,19]. It has been suggested that the degree of opioid release is inversely related to the individual's pain sensitivity in several regions, including the thalamus, amygdala and cingulate cortex [19]. Well-designed studies of placebo analgesia showed further increases of opioid release during placebo analgesia compared to control conditions with the identical pain challenge [14,18].

Diprenorphine, which is a close derivative of naloxone, is another high-affinity ligand (K_d = 0.2 nM) that is used to study the opioidergic system. Diprenorphine binds with the same affinity to mu, delta, and kappa receptors. Diprenorphine has been labeled with both ^{11}C and ^{18}F; the majorities of studies thus far have used ^{11}C-diprenorphine. If the distribution of ^{11}C-diprenorphine is normalized to the thalamus, it becomes apparent that the specific binding[3] of diprenorphine is higher in the temporal cortex, anterior cingulate cortex, and caudate nucleus compared to ^{11}C-carfenatil, which is in accordance with the high density of all three opioid receptors in these regions. ^{11}C-diprenorphine was used early on to compare baseline binding potentials in chronic pain patients with rheumatoid arthritis to those of healthy participants [7]. Patients showed reduced binding potentials, compatible with either tonic opioid release or reduced receptor density. In fact, both explanations might apply because tonically increased opioid levels can lead to receptor internalization [2]. More recent studies specifically compared ^{11}C-diprenorphine binding in neuropathic pain of central and peripheral origin [8]. Whereas the observation of reduced opioid receptor binding in patients with peripheral neuropathic pain is reminiscent of the early study in rheumatoid arthritis patients, patients with central neuropathic pain showed more pronounced decreases of ^{11}C-diprenorphine binding *contralateral* to the pain. Interestingly, opioid-binding decreases were

---

[3] Specific binding describes binding to the structure of interest, such as opioid receptors. Unspecific binding refers to all other binding, including to membranes due to lipophilicity or receptors of no interest. Unspecific binding is usually proportional to the concentration of radioligand because membrane binding, which does not saturate in this range, is the most important source of unspecific binding. For quantification, binding in a region of interest, where specific binding is hypothesized or known to occur, is often compared to a reference region that is known to be devoid of specific binding (e.g., due to the lack of the receptor of interest) and that should therefore control for unspecific binding. The underlying assumption is that unspecific binding is the same across different brain regions.

more extensive than brain anatomical lesions, suggesting metabolic depression and/or degeneration of opioid-receptor-bearing neurons secondary to central lesions [8]. ^{11}C-diprenorphine PET has also been used to demonstrate that motor cortex stimulation in pain patients is related to the release of endogenous opioids [9]. In addition to frequently being labeled with ^{11}C, diprenorphine has also been labeled with [18]F (e.g., ref. [15]). To date, only a few pain studies have been performed using ^{18}F-diprenorphine, which has the same advantages as any ^{18}F tracer compared to an ^{11}C tracer, including better spatial resolution and potentially greater sensitivity due to a longer half-life.

References

[1] Bencherif B, Fuchs PN, Sheth R, Dannals RF, Campbell JN, Frost JJ. Pain activation of human supraspinal opioid pathways as demonstrated by [11C]-carfentanil and positron emission tomography (PET). Pain 2002;99:589–98.

[2] Christie MJ. Cellular neuroadaptations to chronic opioids: tolerance, withdrawal and addiction. Br J Pharmacol 2008;154:384–96.

[3] Frost JJ, Wagner HN Jr, Dannals RF, Ravert HT, Links JM, Wilson AA, Burns HD, Wong DF, McPherson RW, Rosenbaum AE, et al. Imaging opiate receptors in the human brain by positron tomography. J Comput Assist Tomogr 1985;9:231–6.

[4] Garnett ES, Firnau G, Nahmias C. Dopamine visualized in the basal ganglia of living man. Nature 1983;305:137–8.

[5] Hagelberg N, Forssell H, Rinne JO, Scheinin H, Taiminen T, Aalto S, Luutonen S, Nagren K, Jaaskelainen S. Striatal dopamine D1 and D2 receptors in burning mouth syndrome. Pain 2003;101:149–54.

[6] Herholz K, Herscovitch P, Heiss W-D. Positron emitters and tracers. In: Herholz K, Herscovitch P, Heiss WD, editors. NeuroPet. Berlin: Springer; 2004. p. 187–8.

[7] Jones AK, Cunningham VJ, Ha-Kawa S, Fujiwara T, Luthra SK, Silva S, Derbyshire S, Jones T. Changes in central opioid receptor binding in relation to inflammation and pain in patients with rheumatoid arthritis. Br J Rheumatol 1994;33:909–16.

[8] Maarrawi J, Peyron R, Mertens P, Costes N, Magnin M, Sindou M, Laurent B, Garcia-Larrea L. Differential brain opioid receptor availability in central and peripheral neuropathic pain. Pain 2007;127:183–94.

[9] Maarrawi J, Peyron R, Mertens P, Costes N, Magnin M, Sindou M, Laurent B, Garcia-Larrea L. Motor cortex stimulation for pain control induces changes in the endogenous opioid system. Neurology 2007;69:827–34.

[10] Mather LE. Clinical pharmacokinetics of fentanyl and its newer derivatives. Clin Pharmacokinet 1983;8:422–46.

[11] Sadzot B, Frost JJ. Pain and opiate receptors: considerations for the design of positron emission tomography studies. Anesth Prog 1990;37:113–20.

[12] Scott DJ, Stohler CS, Egnatuk CM, Wang H, Koeppe RA, Zubieta JK. Individual differences in reward responding explain placebo-induced expectations and effects. Neuron 2007;55:325–36.

[13] Scott DJ, Stohler CS, Egnatuk CM, Wang H, Koeppe RA, Zubieta JK. Placebo and nocebo effects are defined by opposite opioid and dopaminergic responses. Arch Gen Psychiatry 2008;65:220–31.

[14] Wager TD, Scott DJ, Zubieta JK. Placebo effects on human mu-opioid activity during pain. Proc Natl Acad Sci USA 2007;104:11056–61.

[15] Wester HJ, Willoch F, Tolle TR, Munz F, Herz M, Oye I, Schadrack J, Schwaiger M, Bartenstein P. 6-O-(2-[18F]fluoroethyl)-6-O-desmethyl-diprenorphine ([18F]DPN): synthesis, biologic evaluation, and comparison with [11C]DPN in humans. J Nucl Med 2000;41:1279–86.

[16] Wood PB, Patterson JC 2nd, Sunderland JJ, Tainter KH, Glabus MF, Lilien DL. Reduced presynaptic dopamine activity in fibromyalgia syndrome demonstrated with positron emission tomography: a pilot study. J Pain 2007;8:51–8.

[17] Wood PB, Schweinhardt P, Jaeger E, Dagher A, Hakyemez H, Rabiner EA, Bushnell MC, Chizh BA. Fibromyalgia patients show an abnormal dopamine response to pain. Eur J Neurosci 2007;25:3576–82.

[18] Zubieta JK, Bueller JA, Jackson LR, Scott DJ, Xu Y, Koeppe RA, Nichols TE, Stohler CS. Placebo effects mediated by endogenous opioid activity on mu-opioid receptors. J Neurosci 2005;25:7754–62.

[19] Zubieta JK, Smith YR, Bueller JA, Xu Y, Kilbourn MR, Jewett DM, Meyer CR, Koeppe RA, Stohler CS. Regional mu opioid receptor regulation of sensory and affective dimensions of pain. Science 2001;293:311–5.

Correspondence to: Petra Schweinhardt, MD, PhD, Strathcona Building, Room 2/38F, 3640 University Street, McGill University, Montreal, QC, Canada H3A 2B2. Email: petra.schweinhardt@mcgill.ca.

Electrocortical Responses to Nociceptive Stimulation in Humans

Giandomenico Iannetti, MD, PhD

Department of Neuroscience, Physiology and Pharmacology, University College London, United Kingdom

EEG and MEG: What Do They Measure?

The ongoing electrical activity of the human brain can be directly sampled through the skull, using one or an array of electrodes placed on the scalp. The recording of electrical activity (the electroencephalogram, EEG), or its magnetic counterpart (the magnetoencephalogram, MEG), reflects summated and synchronized postsynaptic potentials in populations of cortical neurons [49], thus providing a direct measure of spontaneous or stimulus-evoked underlying neuronal activity on a millisecond time scale [42]. In contrast to their high temporal resolution, EEG and MEG scalp signals have a rather low spatial resolution, because each scalp electrode/sensor records a spatially blurred mixture of neural activities. In particular, the skull and meningeal structures surrounding the brain exert a spatial low-pass filtering on electrical currents detected by EEG, thus preventing discrimination between distinct but proximal neural sources.

It is important to note that just a fraction of total brain activity is measured in EEG/MEG recordings. Indeed, only low-frequency neuronal activities (i.e., slow postsynaptic potentials, and not action potentials) that happen *synchronously* in *large populations* of neurons located in open-field cortical structures are measurable using scalp EEG/MEG.

The distribution of the electrical potential or of the magnetic field at a given time across the scalp can be used to infer the location of the underlying neural sources (the so-called "inverse problem"), using models of how neural activity translates into scalp potentials. However, because an infinite number of source configurations can explain any given distribution of scalp potentials, additional assumptions must be made (e.g., the number and configuration of contributing sources, as well as anatomical constraints on their locations), thus limiting the trustworthiness of these approaches.

Event-Related EEG and MEG Responses

Fast-rising sensory, motor, or cognitive events (such as a high-power laser pulse delivered to the skin) elicit transient changes in the ongoing EEG (called event-related potentials, ERPs) and MEG (called event-related fields, ERFs). These changes can be either phase-locked or non-phase-locked to the sensory event, and they are often, using a somewhat misleading but widely used nomenclature, referred to as "evoked" (when phase-locked) and "induced" (when non-phase-locked). The detection of phase-locked responses relies on across-trial averaging in the time domain. The waveform obtained expresses the average scalp potential as a function of time relative to the onset of the sensory event. Across-trial averaging has been used for a long time in both basic and clinical pain research. Because across-trial averaging in the time domain cancels out non-phase-locked responses, these responses must first be transformed in the time-frequency domain in each single trial (using a windowed Fourier or a continuous wavelet transform), and then averaged. The detection of non-phase-locked responses is a much newer field, which has only recently been applied to basic pain research [34].

Because of their small magnitude, the identification of these brain responses relies on signal processing methods to enhance their signal-to-noise ratio (SNR). The most widely used approach is across-trial averaging (both in the time domain and in the time-frequency domain). The basic assumption underlying this procedure is that elicited responses are stationary (i.e., their latency and morphology do not vary across trials) and will therefore be unaffected by the averaging procedure, while the ongoing electrical brain activity behaves as noise unrelated to the event, and will therefore be largely canceled out by the averaging procedure, thus enhancing the SNR. Across-trial averaging has a crucial cost, in that all the information concerning across-trial variability of response latency and amplitude is lost. However, this variability, which is particularly high in nociceptive responses, reflects important, physiologically relevant factors such as differences in stimulus parameters (duration, intensity, and location) and fluctuations in vigilance, expectation, attentional focus, or task strategy.

To prevent the loss of this meaningful information contained in the trial-to-trial variability of event-related EEG and MEG response, a significant effort is being devoted to develop analytical approaches that, using wavelet filtering and multiple linear regression, estimate latency and amplitude of nociceptive-evoked responses in each single trial [17,32]. These estimates facilitate the utility of EEG and MEG in studying sensory systems, by exploring the single-trial dynamics between different features of these responses, behavioral variables (e.g., intensity of perception, reaction time), and also measurements of brain activity obtained using different neuroimaging modalities (e.g., functional magnetic resonance imaging) [19,31]. These methods, which explore response dynamics at the level of single-trials, can provide new insights into the functional significance of the different brain processes elicited by nociceptive stimulation in humans (for a review, see [37]).

Stimulation of Nociceptive Afferents in EEG and MEG Studies of Pain

The study of any sensory system requires the availability of a quantifiable stimulus that selectively activates the sensory system under investigation. The issue of the selectivity of sensory stimuli is especially relevant in the study of nociception, which is a submodality of the somatosensory system. Until recently, in contrast with other sensory systems (e.g., auditory, visual), specific nociceptive stimulators had not been available. Transcutaneous electrical stimuli are easy to control, and they activate the peripheral afferents in a highly synchronous manner. However, the large diameter of Aβ non-nociceptive afferents results in an activation threshold that is lower than that of Aδ- and C-fiber nociceptive afferents. Thus, when the intensity of electrical stimulation is above the threshold of nociceptive afferents, the coactivation of mechanoreceptors is unavoidable. For this reason, the use of noxious heat stimuli, which activate a molecular transduction mechanism that is specific for nociception [23], has received great attention.

The introduction of high-power radiant heat stimulators (lasers) in sensory physiology in the 1970s [33] revolutionized the study of the nociceptive system. Indeed, nociceptive free nerve endings belonging to Aδ and C fibers are mostly located in the epidermis, whereas non-nociceptive fibers terminate more deeply, in the dermis. Laser pulses produce a transient heating of the most superficial skin layers. Thus, laser pulses are nociceptive-specific both from a physical perspective (i.e., they use a nociceptive-specific transduction mechanism) and from a spatial perspective (i.e., they heat only the most superficial skin layers, where nociceptors are located), and they activate Aδ or C skin nociceptors selectively, without coactivating deeper, tactile mechanoreceptors [46]. In addition, due to their physical properties (their monochromatic nature, high spectral density, and fast energy transfer), laser pulses activate peripheral afferents in a synchronous fashion, making this technique optimal to elicit time-locked responses in the ongoing EEG.

For all these reasons, laser stimulators are now recognized as the most accurate way to elicit pain in human experiments [12]. Radiant heat has limitations as well: long interstimulus intervals (usually >5 s) must separate two stimuli applied at the same location, to avoid skin overheating; nociceptor habituation and/or sensitization may occur; and baseline skin temperature has to be carefully monitored throughout data collection, as its variations affect the target skin temperature and can lead to misinterpretations. Fast-rising contact heat stimulators have recently been proposed as an alternative, but the application of the thermode on the skin unavoidably results in the concomitant stimulation of low-threshold mechanoreceptors, which represents a potentially serious confounding factor. Furthermore, the profile of temperature increase, which is known at the surface of the thermode, is delayed and attenuated by thermal conduction between the skin surface and nociceptive nerve terminals [2].

To overcome the problems related to noxious heat stimulation, intra-epidermal electrical stimulation has been suggested as an alternative method to produce a selective activation of skin nociceptors [4,22,24]. This method relies on the idea that small, concentric electrodes can generate electric currents spatially restricted to the epidermal layers and activate nociceptors selectively. Converging evidence indicates that, provided that low intensities of stimulation are used, intra-epidermal electrical stimulation can selectively activate skin nociceptors (Fig. 1). [40].

Nociceptive Evoked Responses: Functional Significance

Brief laser pulses selectively excite Aδ- and C-fiber free nerve endings located in the superficial layers of the skin [5]. They elicit a number of brain responses that can be detected in the EEG and MEG both in the time domain (e.g., laser-evoked potentials, LEPs) [9] and in the time-frequency domain [34]. LEPs comprise a number of waves that are time-locked to the onset of the stimulus.

The largest wave is a negative–positive complex (called N2–P2, peaking at 200–350 ms when stimulating the hand dorsum), which is maximal at the scalp vertex and is similar in shape, scalp topography, and sensitivity to various experimental factors affecting vertex potentials elicited by virtually any kind of transient

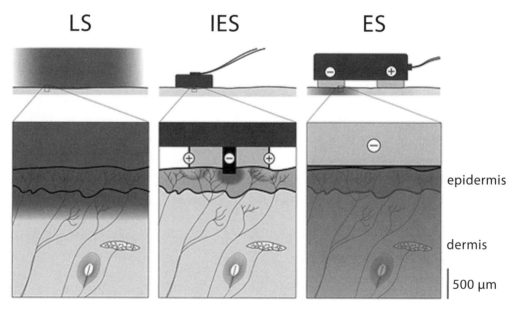

Fig. 1. Schematic representation of nociceptive laser stimulation (LS), nociceptive intra-epidermal electrical stimulation (IES), and non-nociceptive transcutaneous electrical stimulation (ES) of the hairy skin. Only Aδ and C nociceptive free nerve endings are located in the epidermis. Non-nociceptive myelinated endings (e.g., Ruffini and Pacini corpuscles) are located deeper in the dermis. Left panel: the increase in skin temperature generated by LS activates selectively heat-sensitive nociceptive afferents located in the epidermis. Middle panel: because the electric current generated by IES is spatially restricted to the epidermis, when applied at twice the perceptive threshold, it selectively activates the nociceptive free nerve endings located in the epidermis. Right panel: the electric current generated by ES activates preferentially deeper large-diameter non-nociceptive myelinated nerve fibers, because these fibers have a lower electrical activation threshold than small-diameter nociceptive afferents. Modified from Mouraux et al. [40].

sensory stimulus. This N2–P2 complex is preceded by a smaller negative wave (N1) that overlaps in time and space with the larger subsequent N2 wave and has a maximal distribution over the temporocentral region contralateral to the stimulated side [17]. Several studies have shown that the N1, N2, and P2 waves reflect a combination of cortical activities originating from the primary and secondary somatosensory cortices, the insula, and the anterior cingulate cortex [15].

Nociceptive laser pulses also elicit non-phase-locked brain responses related to the activation of Aδ fibers [34,44,47]. These responses consist of a short-lasting event-related synchronization (ERS), starting about 160 ms after onset of stimulation of the hand dorsum, followed by a long-lasting event-related desynchronization (ERD), starting about 500 ms after stimulus onset. The frequency of both responses is centered around 10 Hz. The neural generators and the functional significance of these two responses remain largely unknown.

Both EEG and MEG studies have shown that the magnitude of nociceptive-evoked responses may correlate extremely well with the energy of the applied stimulus and, even better, with the perceived intensity of pain [1,3,8,14,16,20,35,43,45,50]. However, recent studies have shown that, in a number of circumstances, the magnitude of the elicited brain responses (both in the time domain and in the time-frequency domain) can be clearly dissociated from both the intensity of the nociceptive stimulus and the intensity of perceived pain [10,11,13,18,25,36,41], indicating that the magnitude of ERPs elicited by noxious stimuli is largely determined by the saliency of the eliciting stimulus, rather than by pain perception per se.

When a nociceptive stimulus is repeated at a short and constant interstimulus interval, it elicits an ERP of smaller magnitude (e.g., [38]). This effect of stimulus repetition is largely determined by the duration of the interstimulus interval: the shorter the interval, the more pronounced the response decrement [6,48,53,55]. Previous studies have shown that the effect of stimulus repetition on the magnitude of nociceptive ERPs cannot be attributed to refractoriness of the afferent neural pathways or of the underlying cortical generators. Indeed, stimulus repetition affects the magnitude of nociceptive ERPs only if the interstimulus interval remains constant from trial to trial, but it does not have such an effect if the interstimulus interval is varied randomly from trial to trial [36]. In other words,

the effect of stimulus repetition appears to be strongly conditioned by the *context* within which the repetition occurs. The response reduction observed when the interstimulus interval is constant across trials could thus be the result of both bottom-up and top-down modulations, related to the fact that the repeated stimulus is both less novel and less unpredictable.

Importantly, a large number of studies have shown that the magnitude of vertex potentials elicited by non-nociceptive somatosensory, and even nonsomatosensory stimuli (e.g., auditory or visual stimuli), is similarly modulated by stimulus repetition. Indeed, the amplitude of these vertex potentials is strongly reduced only when stimuli are repeated using a constant interstimulus interval, but not when stimuli are repeated using a varying interstimulus interval [7,30,56]. This finding suggests that nociceptive ERPs and vertex potentials reflect similar brain processes, which are largely multimodal (i.e., independent of the activated sensory channel) and are strongly dependent on the context in which the stimuli are presented.

The influence of attentional context on the magnitude of nociceptive-evoked responses has been also investigated in experiments examining the effect of novelty (i.e., the difference in one or more physical dimensions in relation to previously occurring stimuli). In a series of elegant studies, Legrain et al. [e.g., 27–29] have shown that when a long, regular, and monotonous sequence of nociceptive laser stimuli are presented, and a small number of novel stimuli (<20%) are randomly interspersed within this sequence, novel nociceptive stimuli elicit ERPs of increased magnitude, regardless of the physical property defining the novel stimulus from the standard stimulus (e.g., an increase in stimulus energy or a change in location).

These findings suggest that the observed effect of novelty is related not to the processing of a particular physical feature of the stimulus, but to novelty per se. Given that the magnitude of the EEG responses elicited by nociceptive stimuli seems largely determined by factors that are known to modulate stimulus saliency (e.g., novelty and uncertainty), it is reasonable to hypothesize that this multimodal network is mainly devoted to the detection of and reaction to salient sensory input [18].

When the EEG responses elicited by nociceptive stimuli perceived as painful are quantitatively compared with the brain responses elicited by non-nociceptive somatosensory stimuli, as well as by auditory and visual stimuli, it seems that the ERPs elicited by nociceptive stimuli can be entirely explained by a combination of multimodal neural activity (i.e., neural activity that is elicited by any sensory stimulus, independently of sensory modality) and somatosensory-specific, but not nociceptive-specific, neural activity (i.e., neural activity that is elicited by both nociceptive and non-nociceptive somatosensory stimuli) (Fig. 2) [39]. Interestingly, the source analysis of the multimodal neural activity underlying nociceptive ERPs showed that it was optimally modeled by generators located in bilateral operculoinsular areas and in the anterior cingulate cortex—that is, all the areas commonly thought to generate the nociceptive-evoked EEG and MEG responses. Whereas the multimodal activity explains almost entirely the N2–P2 complex, the somatosensory-specific activity explains approximately half of the N1 wave. This and other findings provide converging evidence that whereas the N1 wave represents an early stage of sensory processing related to the ascending nociceptive input, the N2–P2 complex represents a later stage of processing that, albeit largely multimodal, is more related to the perceptual outcome of the nociceptive input [26].

Nociceptive Evoked Responses: Clinical Usefulness

Laser-evoked potentials have been convincingly demonstrated to be related to the activation of type II A-mechano-heat nociceptors and spinothalamic neurons located in the anterolateral quadrant of the spinal cord [51,52]. Because of this specificity in the afferent somatosensory pathways, LEPs are useful to document dysfunctions of small-fiber primary sensory afferents; to investigate the function of spinothalamic tract, brainstem, and thalamocortical projections conveying thermonociceptive signals; or to explore the effect of a given experimental factor on the transmission and processing of nociceptive input. Their clinical usefulness is increased by the ability of laser pulses to elicit cortical responses when applied to virtually all skin territories, including glabrous skin [21,54]. For these reasons, LEPs have been recommended as the easiest and most reliable neurophysiological method of assessing the function of nociceptive pathways and diagnosing clinical pain of neuropathic origin [12]. Indeed, even if LEPs reflect cortical activities that are not entirely specific for the nociceptive system, their generation still relies on the functional state of that system, both at peripheral and central levels.

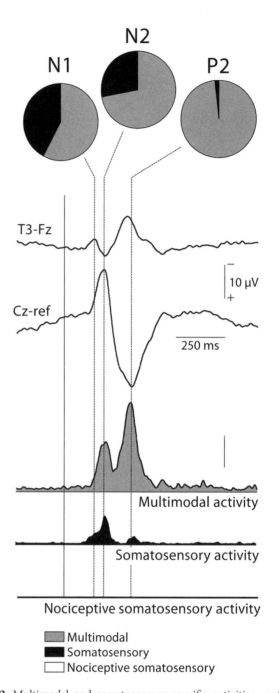

Fig. 2. Multimodal and somatosensory-specific activities contributing to the laser-evoked potential (LEP) waveform. LEPs appear as a large negative-positive biphasic wave (N2–P2), maximal at the scalp vertex (shown here at Cz vs. nose reference). An earlier negative wave (N1) precedes the N2–P2 complex. The N1 (shown here at T3 vs. Fz) is maximal over the temporocentral area contralateral to the stimulated side. The greater part of the LEP waveform is explained by multimodal brain activity (i.e., activity that is also elicited by stimulation of other sensory modalities). The time course of this multimodal activity, expressed as global field power (μV^2), is shown in gray. Note how multimodal activity explains the greater part of the N1 and N2 waves and almost all of the P2 wave. Somatosensory-specific brain activity (i.e., activity elicited by both nociceptive and non-nociceptive somatosensory stimuli) also contributes to the LEP waveform. The time course of somatosensory-specific activity is shown in black. Note how its contribution is largely confined to the time interval corresponding to the N1 and N2 waves. Also note the lack of nociceptive-specific somatosensory activity contributing to the LEP. Modified from Mouraux and Iannetti [39].

References

[1] Arendt-Nielsen L. Characteristics, detection, and modulation of laser-evoked vertex potentials. Acta Anaesthesiol Scand Suppl 1994;101:7–44.

[2] Baumgartner U, Cruccu G, Iannetti GD, Treede RD. Laser guns and hot plates. Pain 2005;116:1–3.

[3] Beydoun A, Morrow TJ, Shen JF, Casey KL. Variability of laser-evoked potentials: attention, arousal and lateralized differences. Electroencephalogr Clin Neurophysiol 1993;88(3):173–81.

[4] Bromm B, Meier W. The intracutaneous stimulus: a new pain model for algesimetric studies. Methods Find Exp Clin Pharmacol 1984;6:405–10.

[5] Bromm B, Treede RD. Nerve fibre discharges, cerebral potentials and sensations induced by CO_2 laser stimulation. Hum Neurobiol 1984;3:33–40.

[6] Bromm B, Treede RD. Human cerebral potentials evoked by CO2 laser stimuli causing pain. Exp Brain Res 1987;67:153–62.

[7] Budd TW, Michie PT. Facilitation of the N1 peak of the auditory ERP at short stimulus intervals. Neuroreport 1994;5:2513–6.

[8] Carmon A, Dotan Y, Sarne Y. Correlation of subjective pain experience with cerebral evoked responses to noxious thermal stimulations. Exp Brain Res 1978;33:445–53.

[9] Carmon A, Mor J, Goldberg J. Evoked cerebral responses to noxious thermal stimuli in humans. Exp Brain Res 1976;25:103–7.

[10] Chapman CR, Chen AC, Colpitts YM, Martin RW. Sensory decision theory describes evoked potentials in pain discrimination. Psychophysiology 1981;18:114–20.

[11] Clark JA, Brown CA, Jones AK, El-Deredy W. Dissociating nociceptive modulation by the duration of pain anticipation from unpredictability in the timing of pain. Clin Neurophysiol 2008;119:2870–8.

[12] Cruccu G, Anand P, Attal N, Garcia-Larrea L, Haanpaa M, Jorum E, Serra J, Jensen TS. EFNS guidelines on neuropathic pain assessment. Eur J Neurol 2004;11:153–62.

[13] Dillmann J, Miltner WH, Weiss T. The influence of semantic priming on event-related potentials to painful laser-heat stimuli in humans. Neurosci Lett 2000;284:53–6.

[14] Frot M, Magnin M, Mauguiere F, Garcia-Larrea L. Human SII and posterior insula differently encode thermal laser stimuli. Cereb Cortex 2007;17:610–20.

[15] Garcia-Larrea L, Frot M, Valeriani M. Brain generators of laser-evoked potentials: from dipoles to functional significance. Neurophysiol Clin 2003;33:279–92.

[16] Garcia-Larrea L, Peyron R, Laurent B, Mauguiere F. Association and dissociation between laser-evoked potentials and pain perception. Neuroreport 1997;8:3785–9.

[17] Hu L, Mouraux A, Hu Y, Iannetti GD. A novel approach for enhancing the signal-to-noise ratio and detecting automatically event-related potentials (ERPs) in single trials. Neuroimage 2010;50:99–111.

[18] Iannetti GD, Hughes NP, Lee MC, Mouraux A. Determinants of laser-evoked EEG responses: pain perception or stimulus saliency? J Neurophysiol 2008;100:815–28.

[19] Iannetti GD, Mouraux A. Combining EEG and fMRI in pain research. In: Lemieux L, Mulert C, editors. EEG-fMRI: physiological basis, technique, and applications. London: Springer; 2009. p. 365–84

[20] Iannetti GD, Zambreanu L, Cruccu G, Tracey I. Operculoinsular cortex encodes pain intensity at the earliest stages of cortical processing as indicated by amplitude of laser-evoked potentials in humans. Neuroscience 2005;131:199–208.

[21] Iannetti GD, Zambreanu L, Tracey I. Similar nociceptive afferents mediate psychophysical and electrophysiological responses to heat stimulation of glabrous and hairy skin in humans. J Physiol 2006;577:235–48.

[22] Inui K, Tran TD, Hoshiyama M, Kakigi R. Preferential stimulation of Aδ fibers by intra-epidermal needle electrode in humans. Pain 2002;96:247–52.

[23] Julius D, Basbaum AI. Molecular mechanisms of nociception. Nature 2001;413:203–10.

[24] Kaube H, Katsarava Z, Kaufer T, Diener H, Ellrich J. A new method to increase nociception specificity of the human blink reflex. Clin Neurophysiol 2000;111:413–6.

[25] Lee MC, Mouraux A, Iannetti GD. Characterizing the cortical activity through which pain emerges from nociception. J Neurosci 2009;29:7909–16.

[26] Lee MC, Mouraux A, Iannetti GD. Characterizing the cortical activity through which pain emerges from nociception. J Neurosci 2009;29:7909–16.

[27] Legrain V, Guerit JM, Bruyer R, Plaghki L. Attentional modulation of the nociceptive processing into the human brain: selective spatial attention, probability of stimulus occurrence, and target detection effects on laser evoked potentials. Pain 2002;99:21–39.

[28] Legrain V, Guerit JM, Bruyer R, Plaghki L. Electrophysiological correlates of attentional orientation in humans to strong intensity deviant nociceptive stimuli, inside and outside the focus of spatial attention. Neurosci Lett 2003;339:107–10.

[29] Legrain V, Perchet C, Garcia-Larrea L. Involuntary orienting of attention to nociceptive events: neural and behavioral signatures. J Neurophysiol 2009;102:2423–34.

[30] Loveless N, Hari R, Hamalainen M, Tiihonen J. Evoked responses of human auditory cortex may be enhanced by preceding stimuli. Electroencephalogr Clin Neurophysiol 1989;74:217–27.

[31] Mayhew SD, Dirckx SG, Niazy RK, Iannetti GD, Wise RG. EEG signatures of auditory activity correlate with simultaneously recorded fMRI responses in humans. Neuroimage 2010;49:849–64.

[32] Mayhew SD, Iannetti GD, Woolrich MW, Wise RG. Automated single-trial measurement of amplitude and latency of laser-evoked potentials (LEPs) using multiple linear regression. Clin Neurophysiol 2006;117:1331–44.

[33] Mor J, Carmon A. Laser emitted radiant heat for pain research. Pain 1975;1:233–7.

[34] Mouraux A, Guerit JM, Plaghki L. Non-phase locked electroencephalogram (EEG) responses to CO_2 laser skin stimulations may reflect central interactions between A partial partial differential- and C-fibre afferent volleys. Clin Neurophysiol 2003;114:710–22.

[35] Mouraux A, Guerit JM, Plaghki L. Non-phase locked electroencephalogram (EEG) responses to CO_2 laser skin stimulations may reflect central interactions between Aδ- and C-fibre afferent volleys. Clin Neurophysiol 2003;114:710–22.

[36] Mouraux A, Guerit JM, Plaghki L. Refractoriness cannot explain why C-fiber laser-evoked brain potentials are recorded only if concomitant Aδ-fiber activation is avoided. Pain 2004;112:16–26.

[37] Mouraux A, Iannetti GD. Across-trial averaging of event-related EEG responses and beyond. Magn Reson Imaging 2008;26:1041–54.

[38] Mouraux A, Iannetti GD. A review of the evidence against the "first come first served" hypothesis. Comment on Truini et al. [Pain 2007;131:43–7]. Pain 2008;136:219–21.

[39] Mouraux A, Iannetti GD. Nociceptive laser-evoked brain potentials do not reflect nociceptive-specific neural activity. J Neurophysiol 2009;101:3258–69.

[40] Mouraux A, Iannetti GD, Plaghki L. Low intensity intra-epidermal electrical stimulation can activate Adelta-nociceptors selectively. Pain 2010; Epub May 24.

[41] Mouraux A, Plaghki L. Cortical interactions and integration of nociceptive and non-nociceptive somatosensory inputs in humans. Neuroscience 2007;150:72–81.

[42] Nunez PL, Srinivasan R. Electric fields of the brain: the neurophysics of EEG. New York: Oxford University Press; 2006.

[43] Ohara S, Crone NE, Weiss N, Treede RD, Lenz FA. Amplitudes of laser evoked potential recorded from primary somatosensory, parasylvian and medial frontal cortex are graded with stimulus intensity. Pain 2004;110:318–28.

[44] Ohara S, Crone NE, Weiss N, Treede RD, Lenz FA. Cutaneous painful laser stimuli evoke responses recorded directly from primary somatosensory cortex in awake humans. J Neurophysiol 2004;91:2734–46.

[45] Plaghki L, Delisle D, Godfraind JM. Heterotopic nociceptive conditioning stimuli and mental task modulate differently the perception and physiological correlates of short CO_2 laser stimuli. Pain 1994;57:181–92.

[46] Plaghki L, Mouraux A. How do we selectively activate skin nociceptors with a high power infrared laser? Physiology and biophysics of laser stimulation. Neurophysiol Clin 2003;33:269–77.

[47] Ploner M, Gross J, Timmermann L, Pollok B, Schnitzler A. Pain suppresses spontaneous brain rhythms. Cereb Cortex 2006;16:537–40.

[48] Raij TT, Vartiainen NV, Jousmaki V, Hari R. Effects of interstimulus interval on cortical responses to painful laser stimulation. J Clin Neurophysiol 2003;20:73–9.

[49] Speckmann E, Elger C. Introduction to the neurophysiological basis of the EEG and DC potentials. In: Niedermeyer E, Lopes Da Silva F, editors. Electroencephalography: basic principles, clinical applications, and related fields. Baltimore: Lippincott, Williams and Wilkins; 1999. p. 15–27.

[50] Timmermann L, Ploner M, Haucke K, Schmitz F, Baltissen R, Schnitzler A. Differential coding of pain intensity in the human primary and secondary somatosensory cortex. J Neurophysiol 2001;86:1499–503.

[51] Treede RD, Lankers J, Frieling A, Zangemeister WH, Kunze K, Bromm B. Cerebral potentials evoked by painful, laser stimuli in patients with syringomyelia. Brain 1991;114:1595–1607.

[52] Treede RD, Meyer RA, Campbell JN. Myelinated mechanically insensitive afferents from monkey hairy skin: heat-response properties. J Neurophysiol 1998;80:1082–93.

[53] Truini A, Galeotti F, Cruccu G, Garcia-Larrea L. Inhibition of cortical responses to Adelta inputs by a preceding C-related response: testing the "first come, first served" hypothesis of cortical laser evoked potentials. Pain 2007;131:341–7.

[54] Truini A, Haanpaa M, Zucchi R, Galeotti F, Iannetti GD, Romaniello A, Cruccu G. Laser-evoked potentials in post-herpetic neuralgia. Clin Neurophysiol 2003;114:702–9.

[55] Truini A, Rossi P, Galeotti F, Romaniello A, Virtuoso M, De Lena C, Leandri M, Cruccu G. Excitability of the Adelta nociceptive pathways as assessed by the recovery cycle of laser evoked potentials in humans. Exp Brain Res 2004;155:120–3.

[56] Wang AL, Mouraux A, Liang M, Iannetti GD. The enhancement of the N1 wave elicited by sensory stimuli presented at very short inter-stimulus intervals is a general feature across sensory systems. PLoS ONE 2008;3:e3929.

Correspondence to: Giandomenico Iannetti, MD, PhD, Department of Neuroscience, Physiology and Pharmacology, Medical Sciences Building, University College London, Gower Street, London WC1E 6BT, United Kingdom. Email: g.iannetti@ucl.ac.uk.

Part 4

From Basic Science to Management of Chronic Musculoskeletal Pain

9

From Basic Science to Management of Chronic Musculoskeletal Pain

Lars Arendt-Nielsen, PhD,[a] Thomas Graven-Nielsen, PhD,[a] Bruce L. Kidd, DM, FRCP,[b]
and César Fernández-de-las-Peñas, PT, PhD[c]

[a]Center for Sensory-Motor Interaction, Department of Health Science and Technology, Aalborg University, Aalborg, Denmark; [b]William Harvey Research Institute, Barts and The London, Queen Mary School of Medicine and Dentistry, London, United Kingdom; [c]Department of Physical Therapy, Occupational Therapy, Rehabilitation and Physical Medicine, University of Rey Juan Carlos, Madrid, Spain

Peripheral and central sensitization are important mechanisms for musculoskeletal pain conditions. Musculoskeletal pain is a major clinical problem, and further research into the peripheral and central neurobiological mechanisms is required to improve understanding, diagnosis, and therapy. This chapter will focus on the clinical manifestations of localized and widespread musculoskeletal pain, and on methods to assess the underlying mechanisms involved. Experimental techniques to assess the mechanisms underlying deep-tissue hyperalgesia, temporal summation, descending control, and referred pain are available, and these techniques reflect different mechanisms and act as proxies for the symptoms seen in patients (e.g., spreading of pain, tenderness, and widespread hyperalgesia) and offer additional information about the mechanisms involved that could lead to revised treatment strategies (Fig. 1). Furthermore, central sensitization is a potential mechanism involved in the transition from acute to chronic widespread pain.

This chapter will apply a translational musculoskeletal pain research approach in which basic animal science is translated into human experimental pain models for investigating fundamental pain mechanisms in healthy volunteers. As healthy volunteers do not behave as a surrogate for a sensitized chronic pain patient, pain models are needed where healthy volunteers can transiently be transformed into a patient.

These models would act as a proxy for clinical symptoms where mechanisms such as peripheral or central sensitization can be mimicked. Finally, the mechanisms discovered can be further investigated and possibly modulated in patients with musculoskeletal pain problems (Fig. 2).

Basic Aspects of Musculoskeletal Pain

Fundamental aspects of nociception from musculoskeletal structures are covered in the following sections.

Basic Aspects of Muscle Pain

Muscle pain presents as localized, regional, or widespread pain (Fig. 1). As one clinical pain condition transitions to another, more and more sensory abnormalities occur [28], with widespread hyperalgesia in chronic conditions. Evidence from the literature indicates that the intensity of ongoing pain [75] as well as the duration of pain [59] determines the degree of generalized muscle hyperalgesia (Fig. 3). This point is fundamental because it underpins the importance of ongoing nociception for the chronification process.

Myofascial pain syndrome is an example of a regional muscle pain condition characterized by localized tenderness and pain caused by active trigger points. The affected muscles often display increased fatigability,

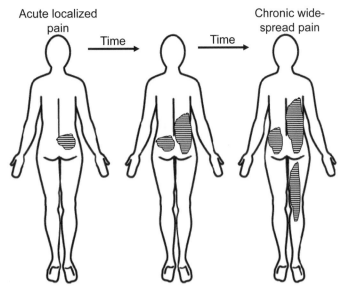

Fig. 1. A sketch of what is often seen when pain develops from a localized acute pain problem into a chronic widespread pain condition. The spreading of where the pain is perceived (hatched areas) and the associated generalized sensitization develop over time, and the patient experiences aggravated pain over time. It is assumed that intervention at an early stage may reduce this generalization or even prevent it from occurring.

stiffness, subjective weakness, pain on movement, and slightly restricted range of motion that is unrelated to joint restrictions.

The sensation of acute deep-tissue pain is the result of activation of group III (Aδ-fiber) and group IV (C-fiber) polymodal muscle nociceptors [105]. The nociceptors can be sensitized by release of neuropeptides from the nerve endings. This process may eventually lead to hyperalgesia and central sensitization of dorsal horn neurons, manifesting as prolonged neuronal discharges, increased responses to defined noxious stimuli, responses to non-noxious stimuli, and expansion of the receptive field [105,111,126]. In humans, little information is available on the peripheral neuronal correlate of muscle nociceptor activation, and few microneurographic studies have been published [100,129] due to difficulties in recording and directly activating the muscle nociceptors. Other quantitative techniques are needed, therefore, and quantitative sensory testing may help to assess muscle pain, muscle hyperalgesia, and referred pain.

Basic Aspects of Tendon/Ligament Pain

Within the mixed group of musculoskeletal pain complaints are the tendinopathies. Rotator cuff, lateral elbow, and Achilles tendinopathy are well-recognized examples. The wide range of treatments and lack of consensus among clinicians might reflect a lack of knowledge

regarding not only etiology, but also basic sensitivity and nociceptive properties of tendon tissues. Alfredson and Lorentzon [1] found high microdialysate glutamate levels in painful Achilles tendinopathy subjects.

Cat tendon tissue was found to have a dense innervation of group III and IV afferent fibers [107]. Mense and Simons [108] highlighted the increased innervation density of neuropeptide-containing fibers in rat calcaneal tendon peritendineum tissue compared to the associated muscle. Substance P and calcitonin-gene related peptide (CGRP) immunoreactivity has been demonstrated in human tendon tissue [22,37] indicating a thin-fiber sensory innervation (most likely serving a nociceptive function). The nerve endings are mostly found around small arterioles and blood vessels in the tissue [22,37].

The nociceptive characteristics of tendinous tissue have been described experimentally by tendon tissue injections of hypertonic saline to study pain reactions and the pattern of referred pain [68]. The tendon tissue was more sensitive to the experimental pain stimulus compared with similar injections in the muscle tissue. Furthermore, *N*-methyl-D-aspartate (NMDA) and transient receptor potential vanilloid 1 (TRPV1) receptors were shown to be functionally relevant in tendon tissue

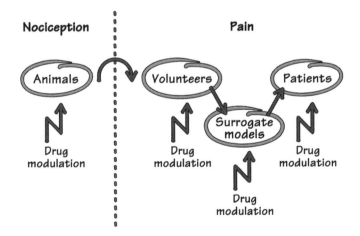

Fig. 2. A sketch of the translational research approach in the study of musculoskeletal pain. The information from animal models is translated into human volunteer studies attempting to discover and assess fundamental mechanisms. This process can be further elaborated using surrogate models for inducing conditions in healthy volunteers (e.g., peripheral sensitization, central sensitization, or spreading sensitization) that mimic the symptoms seen in patients. This research provides the basis for translating this fundamental knowledge into better understanding of the mechanisms involved and symptoms observed in patients with musculoskeletal pain. At the different levels in this translational process, new or existing compounds can be evaluated and targeted for the management of the mechanisms involved in musculoskeletal pain.

as peritendinous injections of glutamate and capsaicin, respectively, effectively induced tendon pain [69].

Basic Aspects of Bone-Related Pain

Bone-associated pain is very frequent in the clinic and is difficult to treat [39]. Osteoarthritis is one of the most common diseases worldwide, and the major source of osteoarthritis-associated pain derives from nociceptive receptors in the superficial bone and joint structures. Another common bone disorder is osteoporosis, which leads to decreased density and bone fragility and thereby bone-associated pain [44]. Cancer patients with bone metastases suffer from bone-associated pain, and animal models have been developed to delineate the underlying pain mechanisms and to help in the development of new and better treatment regimens [98].

The underlying origin of bone-associated pain is still not fully understood in either animals or humans. Kellgren [84] investigated the pain sensitivity of bone by drilling holes in human bone and found that this procedure did not cause any pain when the periosteum was carefully anesthetized. The periosteum is innervated by unmyelinated nociceptive afferents, and pressure stimulation seems capable of activating these fibers [74]. Animal studies indicate that δ-opioid receptors located on those peripheral endings play an important role in controlling bone-associated nociception [24]. This information could lead to design of better management regimens for bone-related pains—a significant clinical problem. Periosteum pain sensitivity has not been thoroughly investigated, although injection of hypertonic saline around the periosteum caused more pain than did intramuscular injections [72].

Basic Aspects of Joint Pain

Joint pain is a major clinical problem [25]. Inflammatory joint diseases, such as rheumatoid arthritis (RA), are the prominent reason for joint pain at younger ages, whereas osteoarthritis (OA) is more prevalent in the elderly. OA pain is normally localized, but it can be referred, for example, from an arthritic hip to the knee.

Most of the basic information on the neurobiology of joint pain comes from inflammatory models. Direct animal models exist for OA, but they do not translate very well into humans. Continuous and intense nociceptive input from the OA-damaged knee joint may in addition drive central sensitization in animals [101]. Impairment of descending inhibition lowers

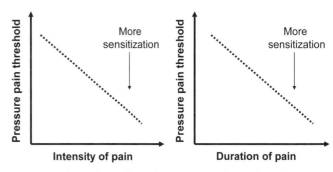

Fig. 3. Ample evidence from the literature shows that the intensity as well as the duration of the nociceptive input is important for driving the process of generalized muscle hyperalgesia. The sketch summarizes the findings on how increased intensity, ongoing clinical pain, and increased duration of the pain condition result in increased muscle hyperalgesia as assessed by pressure pain thresholds.

the excitation threshold of spinal cord neurons to joint nociceptive input, increases the receptive fields of neurons, and increases ongoing discharges [120].

Disease hallmarks in OA are articular cartilage degeneration and joint space narrowing, but generally, pain etiology is unclear. Peripheral nociceptors may be sensitized by, for example, inflamed synovium and damaged subchondral bone, but most often there is a discrepancy between physical damage of joint and pain symptoms [49]. The joint nerves contain Aβ, Aδ, and C fibers [121]. Corpuscular endings of Aβ fibers are identified in ligaments and in the fibrous capsule. C fibers are identified in all structures of the joint except the normal cartilage. A particular group of C fibers (silent nociceptors) do not respond to noxious mechanical stimuli under normal conditions but only with ongoing inflammation [122].

Muscle and joint tissues in rats show differing sensory responses to experimental pain, with prolonged allodynia in joint compared to muscle tissue [131]. It would appear prudent to assume that human muscle and other deep tissue (joint, tendon, and tendon–bone junction) would similarly display differing sensory manifestations to experimental pain. From all human joint structures including ligaments, fibrous capsule, adipose tissue, meniscus, periosteum, and synovial layer, but not cartilage, pain can be evoked by mechanical, thermal, and chemical stimuli [45,85].

We have recently been working on a new joint-pain-mapping technology where pressure pain thresholds are assessed from many locations over the joint. By mapping the threshold levels onto the MRI-extracted three-dimensional joint surface, it is now possible to get an impression of the regions of the joint (e.g., the knee) that are sensitized the most [11].

This sensitization can later (1) be related to the radiological findings or (2) be modulated by analgesic or anti-inflammatory compounds.

General Central Mechanisms in Musculoskeletal Pain

Referred Pain

Many musculoskeletal conditions are accompanied by local and/or referred pain, as has been known for many years [84]. Referred pain is a true central phenomenon. Pain located at the source of pain is termed "local pain" or "primary pain," whereas pain felt in a different region, away from the source of pain, is termed "referred pain." A clear distinction between spread of pain and referred pain is not possible at the moment, and these phenomena may also share common pathophysiological mechanisms. Central sensitization may be reflected by the size and location of the area of referred pain. Animal studies show expansion and development of new receptive fields by noxious muscle stimuli [76]. In the context of referred pain, the unmasking of new receptive fields due to central sensitization could mediate this phenomenon [71,106]. The frequency of referred pain from prolonged mechanical stimulation on the anterior tibial muscle is significantly higher than for brief stimulation, indicating the time-dependency of referred pain [68]. Moreover, saline-induced referred pain occurred less frequently in healthy subjects treated with ketamine compared with a placebo treatment [124], indicating the involvement of central sensitization.

Referred pain has been used extensively as a diagnostic tool in the clinic. In clinical practice, it is very common to see that pain in one region (e.g., the neck, shoulder, or hip) spreads to another (e.g., the arm, hand, or knee). Pain from muscles and joints is usually described as deep and diffuse and difficult to locate precisely [8]. In patients with musculoskeletal pain, the symptoms may be the summation of referred pain from multiple tissues (e.g., ligaments and muscles at the same time), making it more difficult to establish the right diagnosis. Referred pain from muscle tissues may be similar to referred pain elicited by other tissues, such as joints [23].

Temporal Summation

The facilitated pain response to sequential stimuli of equal strength is defined as temporal summation, and it mimics the initial phase of the wind-up process measured in animal dorsal horn neurons [9]. To elicit temporal summation, a stimulus is repeated at constant intervals, for example, five times with a frequency of 1 Hz, at constant intensity. The intensity of the five constant stimuli is increased gradually until the subject feels an increase in pain perception during the repeated stimulation. Repeated tapping on a muscle by a pressure probe has recently been used to assess the efficacy of temporal summation, and temporal summation was found to be more potent for deep tissue stimulation compared with skin stimulation [112].

The facilitated degree of temporal summation indicates an enhanced central integrative mechanism (central sensitization). Therefore, facilitated temporal summation of pain in patients with chronic musculoskeletal pain might suggest the involvement of central sensitization [133,134,137]. The threshold for the withdrawal reflex during repeated stimulation is significantly lower in fibromyalgia and whiplash patients compared with healthy controls, indicating central sensitization in these patients [18].

Descending Modulation

The manifestation of central sensitization may also be due to an imbalance between descending inhibition and facilitation, which can also be assessed experimentally. Painful heterotopic conditioning stimuli (thermal, mechanical, electrical, or chemical) have been utilized to evoke diffuse noxious inhibitory control (DNIC), which is the decreased pain perception induced by phasic painful stimulation given elsewhere in the body than the heterotopic stimulus (i.e., counterirritation). It has been suggested that a dysfunction of DNIC mechanisms may be an important contributor to the clinical manifestations of chronic pain [13]. A recent study demonstrated reduced activation of the rostral anterior cingulate cortex in fibromyalgia patients compared with healthy control subjects; this brain area is probably essential in descending pain control [81].

Transition from Localized Acute Pain to Chronic Widespread Pain

Today there are no definitive models explaining the transition from localized to widespread musculoskeletal pain conditions. It is likely that that the initial excitation and sensitization of nociceptors due to tissue damage will cause sufficient nociceptive input to the central pain systems to cause central sensitization of dorsal horn neurons or higher brain centers. The mechanisms of central sensitization may involve an imbalance between descending inhibition and facilitation. Reorganization of higher brain centers may also take place in parallel or after the sensitization of second-order neurons.

New and advanced quantitative pain assessment technologies have been developed to obtain more detailed information about the spreading of musculoskeletal hyperalgesia. Measuring pressure pain thresholds from many locations makes it possible to assess and quantify localized hyperalgesia versus generalized muscle hyperalgesia [21] and provides new diagnostic possibilities.

Musculoskeletal Pain Management

This section will describe some typical conditions of musculoskeletal pain in detail, highlight potential mechanisms involved, and focus on potential strategies for relevant pain management.

Myofascial Pain Conditions

The myofascial pain syndrome represents the clinical manifestation of muscle referred pain and is characterized by muscle trigger points (TrPs). The referred pain patterns reported with injection of different algogenic substances commonly used in experimental pain models for eliciting both local and referred pain from muscle tissues, such as hypertonic saline [12,71], bradykinin and serotonin [15], capsaicin [143], substance P [16], glutamate [135], nerve growth factor (NGF) [136], or acidic saline [60], are similar to the referred pain patterns described in the *Trigger Point Manual* [130].

The most accepted definition of TrPs states that "a TrP is a hyperirritable spot within a taut band of a skeletal muscle that is painful on muscle stimulation (compression, stretch, overload or contraction) which responds with a referred pain that is perceived distantly from the spot" [130]. The duration of referred pain could be as short as a few seconds or as long as a few hours or days (sometimes indefinitely) and is described as deep, diffuse, burning, tightening, or pressing pain. Muscle referred pain can spread cranially/caudally or ventrally/dorsally, and the intensity and spreading area are positively correlated to the degree of TrP activity (i.e., the irritability of the nervous system).

From a clinical point of view, there are active and latent TrPs. Active TrPs are characterized by local and referred pain reproduction of the clinical symptomatology reported by the patient, and the pain is recognized by the patient as a "usual" pain [130]. Latent TrPs are identified as local and referred pain not reproducing any pain symptoms familiar or usual for a patient [130]. Both active and latent TrPs provoke motor dysfunctions—muscle weakness, inhibition, increased motor irritability (spasm), muscle imbalance, and altered motor recruitment [96,97]—in the affected muscle [130].

The generation of a TrP may result from a variety of factors including repetitive muscle overuse, muscle overload, psychological stress, and joint dysfunctions. Particular attention has been paid to injured or overloaded muscle fibers in the pathogenesis of TrPs [31,67,80,138]. Some authors have hypothesized that muscle trauma, repetitive low-intensity muscle overload, or intense eccentric contractions may create a vicious cycle of events, wherein damage to the sarcoplasmic reticulum or the cell membrane may lead to an increase in calcium concentration, an activation of actin and myosin filaments, a relative shortage of adenosine triphosphate (ATP), and an impaired calcium pump [67,130].

Two recent microdialysis studies showed that the concentrations of bradykinin, CGRP, substance P, tumor necrosis factor-α, interleukin-1β, serotonin, and norepinephrine were significantly higher in active muscle TrPs when compared to latent TrPs or non-TrP areas [127,128]. Other studies have recently shown the existence of both nociceptive (hyperalgesia) and non-nociceptive (allodynia) hypersensitivity [94] and that large-diameter muscle afferents may be involved in pain and mechanical hyperalgesia [142] at muscle TrPs. Additionally, there is indication of an association between muscle TrPs and the sympathetic nervous system [30,32,63,104].

The presence of multiple TrPs (spatial summation) or the presence of TrPs during prolonged periods of time (temporal summation) may potentially sensitize the dorsal spinal cord and supraspinal structures by prolonged nociceptive afferent barrage into the central nervous system [55].

Among the different interventions directed at inactivating TrPs, manual therapy is the first treatment option [43]. Different interventions have been suggested, including static compression [53,61,66,130], massage [130], stretching [130], muscle energy techniques [117], strain-counterstrain [77], neuromuscular approaches [77,115], and manipulative interventions

[52]. Several studies have demonstrated that active TrPs are related to different pain syndromes such as mechanical idiopathic neck pain [54], chronic tension-type headache [58,59], lateral epicondylalgia [51], migraine [26,53], shoulder pain [64], whiplash syndrome [47], fibromyalgia syndrome [65], cluster headache [27], and carpal tunnel syndrome [116]. All these studies found that the referred pain elicited by active TrPs reproduced the pain pattern in these pain conditions. In fact, the presence of active TrPs has been related to the development of central sensitization in headaches [57] and fibromyalgia syndrome [65].

In addition, several studies have reported that inactivation of active TrPs was associated with significant improvement in different chronic pain conditions, such as chronic pelvic pain [4,5], neck pain [66], migraine [27], or tension-type headache [56], supporting the relevance of including TrP management into multimodal approaches for chronic pain. The clinical acceptance and usefulness of trigger point evaluation across disciplines is still hampered by the lack of good inter- and intra-observer reliability studies.

Ligament and Tendon Pain Conditions

Rupture of a ligament results in joint instability, and in this case the first choice of treatment is surgery. However, data about ligament pain are scarce. The long dorsal sacroiliac ligament has been considered relevant in different pain syndromes such as low back pain [141] and peripartum pelvic pain [140]. A recent anatomical study has found that sacroiliac joint pain may be due to an entrapment neuropathy of the lateral branches of the dorsal sacral rami at the long posterior sacroiliac ligament [103]. These studies support a possible role of ligament pain in chronic pain conditions.

There is no consensus for the treatment of ligament pain. The injection of various compounds aimed at producing a sclerosing effect has been used to treat ligament pain injuries for more than 100 years [35]. Some authors promote the use of prolotherapy for the management of ligament pain; however, the Cochrane Review concluded that the evidence is conflicting regarding the efficacy of prolotherapy injections for patients with chronic low back pain [36]. When used alone, prolotherapy is not an effective treatment for chronic low back pain [36]. When combined with spinal manipulation, exercise, and other co-interventions, prolotherapy may improve chronic low back pain and disability [36]. Furthermore, a recent study has demonstrated that prolotherapy

injections created an inflammatory response, but this response was variable, and overall not uniformly different from that caused by saline injections or needle-stick procedures [82]. Therefore, the use of prolotherapy for the management of ligament pain should be conducted with caution at this moment.

The use of physical therapy, particularly manual therapy, to manage ligament pain has attracted some support, although evidence for efficacy is scarce. A recent case report has shown the effectiveness of a positional stretching technique of the coracohumeral ligament on a 51-year-old female diagnosed with phase I frozen shoulder [118]. However, a cause-and-effect relationship cannot be inferred from a case report. Nevertheless, the use of manual therapy in ligament sprains (e.g., ankle sprain) is supported by the literature [139].

Joint Pain Conditions

Osteoarthritis (OA) is a major cause of disability in the elderly and has a high prevalence in society. Among the joints associated with OA, the knee is the most commonly affected. Knee OA is a frequent cause of disability [41]. Although pain from deep tissue is difficult to assess precisely, pressure pain thresholds have been found to be useful in assessing pain reactions in OA patients [78].

Peripheral and central sensitization may be among the underlying mechanisms of pain in OA [78], and for chronic musculoskeletal pain in general [7]. Bajaj et al. [17] found that knee OA patients experienced stronger pain and larger referred pain areas to experimental muscle stimulation outside the affected joint, which is another reflection of central sensitization [7]. Chronic musculoskeletal pain patients in general have generalized deep-tissue hyperalgesia and increased responses to experimental painful stimulation [73,99,113,133]. Patients with chronic musculoskeletal pain such as OA [90], temporomandibular disorders [86], and widespread muscle pain such as fibromyalgia [40,89,93] have impaired diffuse noxious inhibitory control (DNIC) that may contribute significantly to the enhanced pain response and the spread of pain to larger body areas.

The management regimens for RA and OA have changed dramatically in recent years. Early referral for specialist opinion is recommended for any patient with RA or suspected synovitis of undetermined cause [2]. Effective communication and education are vital, together with ready access to a multidisciplinary team.

The early use of either conventional disease-modifying antirheumatic drug (DMARD) therapy or biological DMARD therapy offers the prospect of very significant disease control, and in the case of the biological therapy, disease remission [38].

Current opinion favors the use of a combination of conventional or biological DMARDs, ideally within the first 3 months of diagnosis; this should include methotrexate and at least one other DMARD, plus short-term glucocorticoids [70]. In some patients, the very rapid reduction in pain scores following introduction of anti-tumor necrosis factor agents suggests a direct analgesic effect over and above more general anti-inflammatory effects, although this possibility remains unproven [79].

The general principles for the use of analgesic agents in RA and other inflammatory arthropathies are the same as for other musculoskeletal disorders. Acetaminophen (paracetamol) plus codeine combinations are widely used, although objective evidence for efficacy is limited by the paucity of clinical trials. Adverse events limit widespread applicability, although titration of the dose to effect is useful in overcoming these problems [87]. The long-term use of stronger opioids in chronic musculoskeletal conditions remains controversial [83], but recent developments in oral and transdermal sustained-release formulations have increased both the safety and utility of these agents.

Nonsteroidal anti-inflammatory drugs (NSAIDs) continue to be used widely for symptomatic therapy of RA [46], although their long-term use has been reduced in consequence of increased awareness of significant toxicity issues. Gastrointestinal events, including perforation, ulceration, and bleeding, are well documented [91]. Other well-recognized problems include edema and renal insufficiency, with the development of coxibs (cyclooxygenase-2 inhibitors) serving to highlight the additional cardiovascular risks associated with these agents. Other clinically useful strategies include combining NSAIDs with tramadol or with weak opioids, although there are surprisingly few adequately designed randomized controlled trials to provide objective support for these approaches.

The role of antidepressants in relieving pain and depression in RA is not clear, although some studies suggest an effect on both pain and morning stiffness [14]. For the most part, these agents remain useful as adjuvant therapy and are not considered front-line analgesic agents in most musculoskeletal disorders.

As is the case for RA, clinical guidelines for the management of OA stress the importance of both pharmacological and nonpharmacological approaches [3,144]. Patient education and self-management programs reduce overall pain scores and improve general well-being [42]. Weight loss [50] and adherence to an exercise program also play a vital role in symptomatic knee OA [110]. Other interventions shown to be of benefit include knee taping in patients with patellofemoral OA [43], as well as wedged insoles and shoe orthoses [119]. Transcutaneous nerve stimulation may play a role in some individuals [29].

For many years, oral analgesics such as acetaminophen and NSAIDs have been the mainstay treatment for symptomatic OA. To an even greater extent than in RA, the increased awareness of NSAID toxicity has seen a move away from the long-term use of these agents in symptomatic OA. Combination therapies, as discussed above, are used widely. Stronger opioids such as transdermal fentanyl are effective in reducing pain scores and improving function in patients with knee and hip OA [92]. Overall, however, the relative lack of efficacy and the many safety issues surrounding both NSAIDs and opioids have led the pharmaceutical industry to invest massively in finding new compounds for managing OA pain, and promising results have been published using monoclonal NGF antibodies in OA pain [123].

Other pharmacological approaches include the use of topical therapies such as NSAID creams and gels, which have a much better safety record (adverse events <1.5%) compared with oral administration. Systemic reviews also support the use of topically applied capsaicin, with a limited number of trials reporting benefit in OA [102]. Approximately one-third of patients report local adverse events with topical capsaicin, usually burning discomfort at the site of application.

Intra-articular steroid injections are widely used to control symptoms in OA, although the duration of symptom relief may be relatively short, with effects lasting only a few weeks [20]. Intra-articular hyaluronic acid (hyluronan) is a high-molecular-weight polysaccharide that has symptomatic benefits similar to intra-articular steroids, although the onset of action is delayed, with effects lasting up to 12 months [95]. Glucosamine and chondroitin sulfate have enjoyed striking popularity for the treatment of OA and enjoyed favorable early reports. However, a more recent, large-scale trial failed to show benefit over placebo [33].

A large proportion of patients with arthritic pain seek help from complementary or alternative sources, with acupuncture being a popular choice. Recent individual randomized controlled trials have reported conflicting results in patients with arthritic pain, although a couple of systematic reviews provide generally favorable support, with symptomatic benefits over both sham acupuncture and placebo [48].

TENS (transcutaneous electrical nerve stimulation) has an established a general role in the treatment of chronic pain, although few studies have assessed the efficacy of the technique for arthritic pain. Underlying mechanisms of action remain unclear, but in studies of experimental joint inflammation TENS reduces spinal stimulatory neurotransmitters (glutamate, aspartate) and at the same time activates modulatory opioid, serotonin, and/or muscarinic receptors to reduce pain behaviors [132]. In clinical studies, TENS has been found to be as effective as exercise and better than placebo for controlling arthritic pain, although combination approaches produce the most favorable results [29].

Bone-Related Pain Conditions

Bone and joint pain may be difficult to separate because cartilage degradation in joint diseases eventually activates bone structures and related nociceptive endings. Skeletal involvement is a frequent and troublesome complication affecting many patients with neoplastic disease. Once cancer cells establish in the bone, the normal process of bone turnover is disturbed, and pain may occur normally as a mix of nociceptive and neuropathic pain. The inhibition of bone resorption and hypercalcemia can be reduced by the use of bisphosphonates, which in addition reduce the pain. A survey from a multidisciplinary cancer pain clinic showed that 32% of patients were referred with pain related to bone metastases [19]. Pain from bone metastases is manifested in a variety of ways, including referred pain, muscle spasms, or paroxysms of stabbing pain, particularly when bony lesions are accompanied by nerve compression. The pain mechanism is often correlated with the clinical features, but the intensity of pain experienced is often disproportional to the size or degree of bone involvement. Pain may be evoked during standing, walking, sitting, turning, lifting, and coughing. The pathophysiological mechanism of pain in patients with bone metastases in the absence of a fracture is poorly understood. The presence of pain is not correlated with the type of tumor, the location, number, and size of metastases, or the gender or age of patients [114].

The use of analgesics according to the World Health Organization (WHO) ladder is recommended. There is no clear evidence that NSAIDs have any specific efficacy in malignant bone pain. Because of its intermittent nature, bone pain is difficult to manage without causing unacceptable side effects such as sedation [109]. Breakthrough pain is a major challenge because rapid- and short-acting opioids may cause withdrawal hyperalgesia [6].

Vertebral collapse associated with osteoporosis is also a major cause of bone pain. In addition to traditional pain treatment, calcitonin has also proven to have analgesic effects in such conditions [10].

As the δ-opioid receptor seems to be expressed on nociceptors located in the periostium, interaction with this receptor may be beneficial for treating bone-related pain. The opioid drug buprenorphine (or its metabolites) seems to interact with the δ-receptor and at the same time has an antihyperalgesic effect [88], suggesting this opioid as an interesting possibility for the treatment of bone-related pain [125].

As the study of treatment options for bone-related pain is still in its infancy, the hope is that the knowledge from basic research will translate into development of new compounds for better and safer management of the many bone-related pain problems.

References

[1]   Alfredson H, Lorentzon R. Chronic tendon pain: no signs of chemical inflammation but high concentrations of the neurotransmitter glutamate. Implications for treatment? Curr Drug Targets 2002;3:43–54.

[2]   American College of Rheumatology. Ad hoc Committee on Clinical Guidelines: guidelines for the management of rheumatoid arthritis. Arthritis Rheum 2002;46:328–46.

[3]   American College of Rheumatology. Subcommittee on Osteoarthritis Guidelines: recommendations for the medical management of osteoarthritis of the hip and knee. Arthritis Rheum 2000;43:1905–15.

[4]   Anderson RU, Wise D, Sawyer T, Chan C. Sexual dysfunction in men with chronic protatitis/chornic pelvic pain syndrome: Improvement after trigger point release and paradoxical relaxation training. J Urol 2006;176:1534–9.

[5]   Anderson RU, Sawyer T, Wise D, Morey A, Nathanson B. Painful myofascial trigger points and pain sites in men with chronic prostatitis/chronic pelvic pain syndrome. J Urol 2009;182:2753–8.

[6]   Angst MS, Koppert W, Pahl I, Clark DJ, Schmelz M. Short-term infusion of the mu-opioid agonist remifentanil in humans causes hyperalgesia during withdrawal. Pain 2003;106:49–57.

[7]   Arendt-Nielsen L, Graven-Nielsen T. Central sensitization in fibromyalgia and other musculoskeletal disorders. Curr Pain Headache Rep 2003;7:355–61.

[8]   Arendt-Nielsen L, Graven-Nielsen T. Muscle pain: sensory implications and interaction with motor control. Clin J Pain 2008;24:291–8.

[9]   Arendt-Nielsen L, Graven-Nielsen T. Translational aspects of musculoskeletal pain: from animals to patients. In: Graven-Nielsen T, Arendt-Nielsen L, Mense S, editors. Fundamentals of musculoskeletal pain. Seattle: IASP Press; 2008. p. 347–66.

[10] Arendt-Nielsen L, Hoeck HC, Karsdal MA, Christiansen C. Role of calcitonin in management of musculoskeletal pain. Rheumatol Rep 2009;1:39–42.

[11] Arendt-Nielsen L, Nie H, Laursen MB, Laursen BS, Madeleine P, Simonsen OH, Graven-Nielsen T. Sensitization in patients with painful knee osteoarthritis. Pain 2010; in press.

[12] Arendt-Nielsen L, Svensson P. Referred muscle pain: basic and clinical findings. Clin J Pain 2001;17:11–9.

[13] Arendt-Nielsen L, Yarnitsky D. Experimental and clinical applications of quantitative sensory testing applied to skin, muscles and viscera. J Pain 2009;10:556–72.

[14] Ash G, Dickens CM, Creed FH, Jayson MI, Tomenson B. The effects of dothiopin on subjects with rheumatoid arthritis and depression. Rheumatology 1999;38:959–67.

[15] Babenko V, Graven-Nielsen T, Svensson P, Drewes AM, Jensen TS, Arendt-Nielsen L. Experimental human muscle pain and muscular hyperalgesia induced by combinations of serotonin and bradykinin. Pain 1999;82:1–8.

[16] Babenko V, Graven-Nielsen T, Svensson P, Drewes AM, Jensen TS, Arendt-Nielsen L. Experimental human muscle pain induced by intramuscular injections of bradykinin, serotonin, and substance P. Eur J Pain 1999;3:93–102.

[17] Bajaj P, Bajaj P, Graven-Nielsen T, Arendt-Nielsen L. Osteoarthritis and its association with muscle hyperalgesia: an experimental controlled study. Pain 2001;93:107–14.

[18] Banic B, Petersen-Felix S, Andersen OK, Radanov BP, Villiger PM, Arendt-Nielsen L, Curatolo M. Evidence for spinal cord hypersensitivity in chronic pain after whiplash injury and in fibromyalgia. Pain 2004;107:7–15.

[19] Banning A, Sjøgren P, Henriksen H. Pain causes in 200 patients referred to a multidisciplinary cancer pain clinic. Pain 1991;45:45–8.

[20] Bellamy N, Campbell J, Robinson V, Gee T, Bourne R, Wells G. Intraarticular corticosteroid for treatment of osteoarthritis. Cochrane Database Syst Rev 2005;(2):CD005328.

[21] Binderup AT, Arendt-Nielsen L, Madeleine P. Cluster analysis of pressure pain threshold maps from the trapezius muscle. Comput Methods Biomech Biomed Engin 2010; Epub Feb 8.

[22] Bjur D, Alfredson H, Forsgren S. The innervation pattern of the human Achilles tendon: studies of the normal and tendinosis tendon with markers for general and sensory innervation. Cell Tissue Res 2005;320:201–6.

[23] Bogduk N. The neck and headaches. Neurol Clin North Am 2004;22:151–71.

[24] Brainin-Mattos J, Smith ND, Malkmus S, Rew Y, Goodman M, Taulane J, Yaksh TL. Cancer-related bone pain is attenuated by a systemically available delta-opioid receptor agonist. Pain 2006;122:174–81.

[25] Breivik H, Beverly C, Ventafridda V, Cohen R, Gallacher D. Survey of chronic pain in Europe: prevalence, impact on daily life, and treatment. Eur J Pain 2006;10:287–333.

[26] Calandre EP, Hidalgo J, García-Leiva JM, Rico-Villademoros F. Trigger point evaluation in migraine patients: an indication of peripheral sensitization linked to migraine predisposition? Eur J Neurol 2006;13:244–9.

[27] Calandre EP, Hidalgo J, Garcia-Leiva JM, Rico-Villademoros F, Delgado-Rodriguez A. Myofascial trigger points in cluster headache patients: a case series. Head Face Med 2008;30:4–32.

[28] Carli G, Suman AL, Biasi G, Marcolongo R. Reactivity to superficial and deep stimuli in patients with chronic musculoskeletal pain. Pain 2002;100:259–69.

[29] Cheing GL, Hui-Chan CW. Would the addition of TENS to exercise training produce better physical performance outcomes in people with knee osteoarthritis that either intervention alone? Clin Rehabil 2004;18:487–97.

[30] Chen JT, Chen SM, Kuan TS, Chung KC, Hong CZ. Phentolamine effect on the spontaneous electrical activity of active loci in a myofascial trigger spot of rabbit skeletal muscle. Arch Phys Med Rehabil 1998;79:790–4.

[31] Chen SM, Chen JT, Kuan TS, Hong J, Hong CZ. Decrease in pressure pain thresholds of latent myofascial trigger points in the middle finger extensors immediately after continuous piano practice. J Musculoskel Pain 2000;8:83–92.

[32] Chung JW, Ohrbach R, McCall WDJr. Effect of increased sympathetic activity on electrical activity from myofascial painful areas. Am J Phys Med Rehabil 2004;83:842–50.

[33] Clegg DO, Reda DJ, Harris CL, Klein MA, O'Dell JR, Hooper MM, Bradley JD, Bingham CO 3rd, Weisman MH, Jackson CG, et al. Glucosamine, chondroitin sulfate, and the two in combination for painful knee osteoarthritis. N Engl J Med 2006;354:795–808.

[34] Cushnaghan J, McCarthy C, Dieppe P. Taping the patella medially: a new treatment for osteoarthritis of the knee joint. BMJ 1994;308:753–5.

[35] Dagenais S, Haldeman S, Wooley JR. Intraligamentous injection of sclerosing solutions (prolotherapy) for spinal pain: a critical review of the literature. Spine J 2005;5:310–28.

[36] Dagenais S, Yelland MJ, Del Mar C, Schoene ML. Prolotherapy injections for chronic low-back pain. Cochrane Database Syst Rev 2007;(2):CD004059.

[37] Danielson P, Alfredson H, Forsgren S. Immunohistochemical and histochemical findings favoring the occurrence of autocrine/paracrine as well as nerve-related cholinergic effects in chronic painful patellar tendon tendinosis. Microsc Res Tech 2006;69:808–19.

[38] Deighton C, O'Mahony R, Tosh J, Turner C, Rudolf M. Management of rheumatoid arthritis: summary of NICE guidance. BMJ 2009;338:710–2.

[39] Delaney A, Fleetwood-Walker SM, Colvin LA, Fallon M. Translational medicine: cancer pain mechanisms and management. Br J Anaesth 2008;101:87–94.

[40] de Souza JB, Potvin S, Goffaux P, Charest J, Marchand S. The deficit of pain inhibition in fibromyalgia is more pronounced in patients with comorbid depressive symptoms. Clin J Pain 2009;25:123–7.

[41] Dieppe PA. Relationship between symptoms and structural change in osteoarthritis: what are the important targets for therapy? J Rheumatol 2005;32:1147–9.

[42] Dieppe PA, Lohmander LS. Pathogenesis and management of pain in osteoarthritis. Lancet 2005;365:965–73.

[43] Dommerholt J, Bron C, Franssen JLM. Myofascial trigger points: an evidence informed review. J Man Manip Ther 2006;14:203–21.

[44] Downey PA, Siegel MI. Bone biology and the clinical implications for osteoporosis. Phys Ther 2006;86:77–91.

[45] Dye SF, Vaupel GL, Dye CC. Conscious neurosensory mapping of the internal structures of the human knee without intraarticular anesthesia. Am J Sports Med 1998;26:773–7.

[46] Emery P, Suarez-Almazor M. Rheumatoid arthritis. Clin Evid 2003;9:1349–71.

[47] Ettlin T, Schuster C, Stoffel R, Brüderlin A, Kischka U. A distinct pattern of myofascial findings in patients after whiplash injury. Arch Phys Med Rehabil 2008;89:1290–3.

[48] Ezzo J, Hadhazy V, Birch S, Lao L, Kaplan G, Hochberg M, Berman B. Acupuncture for osteoarthritis of the knee: a systematic review. Arthritis Rheum 2001;44:819–25.

[49] Felson DT. The sources of pain in knee osteoarthritis. Curr Opin Rheumatol 2005;17:624–8.

[50] Felson DT, Zhang Y, Anthony JM, Naimark A, Anderson JJ. Weight loss reduces the risk for symptomatic osteoarthritis in women. The Framingham Study. Ann Intern Med 1992;116:772–9.

[51] Fernández-Carnero J, Fernández-de-las-Peñas C, De-La-Llave-Rincón AI, Ge HY, Arendt-Nielsen L. Prevalence of and referred pain from myofascial trigger points in the forearm muscles in patients with lateral epicondylalgia. Clin J Pain 2007;23:353–60.

[52] Fernández-de-las-Peñas C. Interaction between trigger points and joint hypo-mobility: a clinical perspective. J Man Manip Ther 2009;17:74–7.

[53] Fernández-de-las-Peñas C, Alonso-Blanco C, Fernández J, Miangolarra-Page JC. The immediate effect of ischemic compression technique and transverse friction massage on tenderness of active and latent myofascial triggers points: a pilot study. J Bodyw Mov Ther 2006;10:3–9.

[54] Fernández-de-las-Peñas C, Alonso-Blanco C, Miangolarra JC. Myofascial trigger points in subjects presenting with mechanical neck pain: a blinded, controlled study. Man Ther 2007;12:29–33.

[55] Fernández-de-las-Peñas C, Caminero AB, Madeleine P, Guillem-Mesado A, Ge HY, Arendt-Nielsen L, Pareja JA. Multiple active myofascial trigger points and pressure pain sensitivity maps in the temporalis muscle are related in women with chronic tension type headache. Clin J Pain 2009;25:506–12.

[56] Fernández-de-las-Peñas C, Cleland JA, Cuadrado ML, Pareja JA. Predictor variables for identifying patients with chronic tension type headache who are likely to achieve short-term success with muscle trigger point therapy. Cephalalgia 2008;28:264–75.

[57] Fernández-de-las Peñas C, Cuadrado ML, Arendt-Nielsen L, Simons DG, Pareja JA. Myofascial trigger points and sensitisation: an updated pain model for tension type headache. Cephalalgia 2007;27:383–93.

[58] Fernández-de-las Peñas C, Ge HY, Arendt-Nielsen L, Cuadrado ML, Pareja JA. Referred pain from trapezius muscle trigger point shares similar characteristics with chronic tension type headache. Eur J Pain 2007;11:475–82.

[59] Fernández-de-las-Peñas C, Ge HY, Arendt-Nielsen L, Cuadrado ML, Pareja JA. The local and referred pain from myofascial trigger points in the temporalis muscle contributes to pain profile in chronic tension type headache. Clin J Pain 2007;23:786–92.

[60] Frey Law LA, Sluka KA, McMullen T, Lee J, Arendt-Nielsen L, Graven-Nielsen T. Acidic buffer induced muscle pain evokes referred pain and mechanical hyperalgesia in humans. Pain 2008;140:254–64.

[61] Fryer G, Hodgson L. The effect of manual pressure release on myofascial trigger points in the upper trapezius muscle. J Bodyw Mov Ther 2005;9:248–55.

[62] Fujiwara A, Tamai K, An HS, Shimizu K, Yoshida H, Saotome K. The interspinous ligament of the lumbar spine. Magnetic resonance images and their clinical significance. Spine 2000;25:358–63.

[63] Ge HY, Fernández-de-las-Penas C, Arendt-Nielsen L. Sympathetic facilitation of hyperalgesia evoked from myofascial tender and trigger points in patients with unilateral shoulder pain. Clin Neurophysiol 2006;117:1545–50.

[64] Ge HY, Fernández-de-las-Peñas C, Madeleine P, Arendt-Nielsen L. Topographical mapping and mechanical pain sensitivity of myofascial trigger points in the infraspinatus muscle. Eur J Pain 2008;12:859–65.

[65] Ge HY, Nie H, Madeleine P, Danneskiold-Samsøe B, Graven-Nielsen T, Arendt-Nielsen L. Contribution of the local and referred pain from active myofascial trigger points in fibromyalgia syndrome. Pain 2009;147:233–40.

[66] Gemmell H, Miller P, Nordstrom H. Immediate effect of ischaemic compression and trigger point pressure release on neck pain and upper trapezius trigger points: a randomized controlled trial. Clin Chiropract 2008;11:30–6.

[67] Gerwin RD, Dommerholt D, Shah JP. An expansion of Simons' integrated hypothesis of trigger point formation. Curr Pain Head Rep 2004;8:468–75.

[68] Gibson W, Arendt-Nielsen L, Graven-Nielsen T. Referred pain and hyperalgesia in human tendon and muscle belly tissue. Pain 2006;120:113–23.

[69] Gibson W, Arendt-Nielsen L, Sessle BJ, Graven-Nielsen T. Glutamate and capsaicin-induced pain, hyperalgesia and modulatory interactions in human tendon tissue. Exp Brain Res 2009;194:173–82.

[70] Goekoop-Ruiterman YP, de Vries-Bouwstra JK, Allaart CF, van Zeben D, Kerstens PJ, Hazes JM, Zwinderman AH, Ronday HK, Han KH, Westedt ML, et al. Clinical and radiographic outcomes of four different treatment strategies in patients with early rheumatoid arthritis (the BeSt study): a randomized, controlled trial. Arthritis Rheum 2005;52:3381–90.

[71] Graven-Nielsen T. Fundamentals of muscle pain, referred pain, and deep tissue hyperalgesia. Scand J Rheumatol 2006;122(Suppl):1–43.

[72] Graven-Nielsen T, Arendt-Nielsen L, Svensson P, Jensen TS. Experimental muscle pain: a quantitative study of local and referred pain in humans following injection of hypertonic saline. J Musculoskel Pain 1997;5:49–69.

[73] Graven-Nielsen T, Aspegren Kendall S, Henriksson KG, Bengtsson M, Sorensen J, Johnson A, Gerdle B, Arendt-Nielsen L. Ketamine reduces muscle pain, temporal summation, and referred pain in fibromyalgia patients. Pain 2000;85:483–91.

[74] Gronblad M, Liesi P, Korkala O, Karaharju E, Polak J. Innervation of human bone periosteum by peptidergic nerves. Anat Rec 1984;209:297–9.

[75] Herren-Gerber R, Weiss S, Arendt-Nielsen L, Petersen-Felix S, Di Stefano G, Radanov BP, Curatolo M. Modulation of central hypersensitivity by nociceptive input in chronic pain after whiplash injury. Pain Med 2004;5:366–76.

[76] Hoheisel U, Mense S, Simons DG, Yu X-M. Appearance of new receptive fields in rat dorsal horn neurons following noxious stimulation of skeletal muscle: a model for referral of muscle pain? Neurosci Lett 1993;153:9–12.

[77] Ibáñez-García J, Alburquerque-Sendín F, Rodríguez-Blanco C, Girao D, Atienza-Meseguer A, Planella-Abella S, Fernández-de-Las Peñas C. Changes in masseter muscle trigger points following strain-counter-strain or neuro-muscular technique. J Bodyw Mov Ther 2009;13:2–10.

[78] Imamura M, Imamura ST, Kaziyama HH, Targino RA, Hsing WT, de Souza LP, Cutait MM, Fregni F, Camanho GL. Impact of nervous system hyperalgesia on pain, disability, and quality of life in patients with knee osteoarthritis: a controlled analysis. Arthritis Rheum 2008;59:1424–31.

[79] Inglis JJ, Nissim A, Lees DM, Hunt SP, Chernajovsky Y, Kidd BL. The differential contribution of tumour necrosis factor to thermal and mechanical hyperalgesia during chronic inflammation. Arthritis Res Ther 2005;7:807–16.

[80] Itoh K, Okada K, Kawakita K. A proposed experimental model of myofascial triggers points in human muscle after slow eccentric exercise. Acupunct Med 2004;22:2–13.

[81] Jensen KB, Kosek E, Petzke F, Carville S, Fransson P, Marcus H, Williams SC, Choy E, Giesecke T, Mainguy Y, Gracely R, Ingvar M. Evidence of dysfunctional pain inhibition in fibromyalgia reflected in rACC during provoked pain. Pain 2009;144:95–100.

[82] Jensen KT, Rabago DP, Best TM, Patterson JJ, Vanderby R Jr. Early inflammatory response of knee ligaments to prolotherapy in a rat model. J Orthop Res 2008;26:816–23.

[83] Kalso E, Edwards JE, Moore RA, McQuay HJ. Opioids in chronic non-cancer pain: systematic review of efficacy and safety. Pain 2004;112:372–80.

[84] Kellgren JH. On the distribution of pain arising from deep somatic structures with charts of segmental pain areas. Clin Sci 1939;4:35–46.

[85] Kellgren JH, Samuel EP. The sensitivity and innervation of the articular capsule. J Bone Joint Surg 1950;4:193–205.

[86] King CD, Wong F, Currie T, Mauderli AP, Fillingim RB, Riley JL, 3rd. Deficiency in endogenous modulation of prolonged heat pain in patients with irritable bowel syndrome and temporomandibular disorder. Pain 2009;143:172–8.

[87] Kjaersgaard-Andersen P, Nafei A, Skov O, Madsen F, Andersen HM, Kroner K, Hvass I, Gjoderum O, Pedersen L, Branebjerg PE. Codeine plus paracetamol versus paracetamol in longer-term treatment of chronic pain due to osteoarthritis of the hip. A randomised, double-blind, multi-centre study. Pain 1990;43:309–18.

[88] Koppert W, Ihmsen H, Körber N, Wehrfritz A, Sittl R, Schmelz M, Schüttler J. Different profiles of buprenorphine-induced analgesia and antihyperalgesia in a human pain model. Pain 2005;118:15–22.

[89] Kosek E, Ekholm J, Hansson P. Increased pressure pain sensibility in fibromyalgia patients is located deep to the skin but not restricted to muscle tissue. Pain 1995;63:335–9.

[90] Kosek E, Ordeberg G. Lack of pressure pain modulation by heterotopic noxious conditioning stimulation in patients with painful osteoarthritis before, but not following, surgical pain relief. Pain 2000;88:69–78.

[91] Laine L. Gastrointestinal effects of NSAIDs and coxibs. J Pain Symptom Manage 2003;25:S32–40.

[92] Langford R, McKenna F, Ratcliffe S, Vojtassak J, Richarz U. Transdermal fentanyl for improvement of pain and functioning in osteoarthritis: a randomized, placebo-controlled trial. Arthritis Reum 2006;54:1829–37.

[93] Lautenbacher S, Rollman GB. Possible deficiencies of pain modulation in fibromyalgia. Clin J Pain 1997;13:189–96.

[94] Li LT, Ge HY, Yue SW, Arendt-Nielsen L. Nociceptive and non-nociceptive hypersensitivity at latent myofascial trigger points. Clin J Pain 2009;25:132–7.

[95] Lo GH, LaValley M, McAlindon T, Felson DT. Intra-articular hyaluronic acid in treatment of knee osteoarthritis: a meta-analysis. JAMA 2003;290:3115–21.

[96] Lucas KR. The impact of latent trigger points on regional muscle function. Curr Pain Headache Rep 2008;12:344–9.

[97] Lucas KR, Polus BI, Rich PA. Latent myofascial trigger points: their effects on muscle activation and movement efficiency. J Bodyw Mov Ther 2004;8:160–6.

[98] Luger NM, Mach DB, Sevcik MA, Mantyh PW. Bone cancer pain: from model to mechanism to therapy. J Pain Symptom Manage 2005;29:S32–46.

[99] Madeleine P, Lundager B, Voigt M, Arendt-Nielsen L. Sensory manifestations in experimental and work-related chronic neck-shoulder pain. Eur J Pain 1998;2:251–60.

[100] Marchettini P, Simone DA, Caputi G, Ochoa JL. Pain from excitation of identified muscle nociceptors in humans. Brain Res 1996;740:109–16.

[101] Martindale JC, Wilson AW, Reeve AJ, Chessell IP, Headley PM. Chronic secondary hypersensitivity of dorsal horn neurones following inflammation of the knee joint. Pain 2007;133:79–86.

[102] Mason L, Moore RA, Derry S, Edwards JE, McQuay HJ. Systematic review of topical capsaicin for the treatment of chronic pain. BMJ 2004;328:991.

[103] McGrath C, Nicholson H, Hurst P. The long posterior sacroiliac ligament: a histological study of morphological relations in the posterior sacroiliac region. Joint Bone Spine 2009;76:57–62.

[104] McNulty WH, Gevirtz R, Hubbard D, Berkoff G. Needle electromyographic evaluation of trigger point response to a psychological stressor. Psychophysiology 1994;31:313–6.

[105] Mense S. Nociception from skeletal muscle in relation to clinical muscle pain. Pain 1993;54:241–89.

[106] Mense S. Referral of muscle pain. New aspects. Am Pain Soc J 1994;3:1–9.

[107] Mense S, Meyer H. Different types of slowly conducting afferent units in cat skeletal muscle and tendon. J Physiol 1985;363:403–17.

[108] Mense S, Simons DG. Muscle pain: understanding its nature, diagnosis and treatment. Philadelphia: Lippincott Williams and Wilkins; 2001. p. 29.

[109] Mercadante S. Malignant bone pain: pathophysiology and treatment. Pain 1997;69:1–18.

[110] Messier SP, Loeser RF, Miller GD, Morgan TM, Rejeski WJ, Sevick MA, Ettinger WH, Pahor M, Williamson JD. Exercise and dietary weight loss in overweight and obese older adults with knee osteoarthritis: the Arthritis, Diet, and Activity Promotion Trial. Arthritis Rheum 2004;50:1501–10.

[111] Neugebauer V, Schaible HG. Evidence for a central component in the sensitization of spinal neurons with joint input during development of acute arthritis in cat's knee. Neurophysiology 1990;64:299–311.

[112] Nie H, Arendt-Nielsen L, Andersen H, Graven-Nielsen T. Temporal summation of pain evoked by mechanical stimulation in deep and superficial tissue. J Pain 2005;6:348–55.

[113] O'Neill S, Manniche C, Graven-Nielsen T, Arendt-Nielsen L. Generalized deep-tissue hyperalgesia in patients with chronic low-back pain. Eur J Pain 2007;11:415–20.

[114] Oster MW, Vizel M, Turgeon LR. Pain of terminal cancer patients. Arch Intern Med 1978;138:1801–2.

[115] Palomeque-del-Cerro L, Fernández-de-las-Peñas C. Neuromuscular approaches. In: Fernández-de-las-Peñas C, Arendt-Nielsen L, Gerwin R, editors. Tension type and cervicogenic headache: pathophysiology, diagnosis and treatment. Boston: Jones & Bartlett; 2009. p. 327–38.

[116] Qerama E, Kasch H, Fuglsang-Frederiksen A. Occurrence of myofascial pain in patients with possible carpal tunnel syndrome: a single-blinded study. Eur J Pain 2009;13:88–91.

[117] Rodríguez-Blanco C, Fernández-de-las-Peñas C, Hernández-Xumet JE, Algaba C, Rabadán M, de la Quintata M. Changes in active mouth opening following a single treatment of latent myofascial trigger points in the masseter muscle involving post-isometric relaxation or strain/counter-strain. J Bodyw Mov Ther 2006;10:197–206.

[118] Ruiz JO. Positional stretching of the coracohumeral ligament on a patient with adhesive capsulitis: a case report. J Man Manip Ther 2009;17:58–63.

[119] Sasaki T, Yasuda K. Clinical evaluation of the treatment of osteoarthritic knees using a newly designed wedge insole. Clin Orthop 1987;221:181–7.

[120] Schaible HG. Spinal mechanisms contributing to joint pain. Novartis Found Symp 2004;260:4–22.

[121] Schaible HG, Richter F, Ebersberger A, Boettger MK, Vanegas H, Natura G, Vazquez E, Segond von Banchet G. Joint pain. Exp Brain Res 2009;196:153–62.

[122] Schaible HG, Schmidt RF. Activation of groups III and IV sensory units in medial articular nerve by local mechanical stimulation of knee joint. J Neurophysiol 1983;49:35–44.

[123] Schnitzer TJ, Lane NE, Smith MD, Brown MT. Efficacy and safety of PF04383119 for moderate to severe pain due to osteoarthritis (OA) of the knee: a randomized trial. Abstracts of the 12th World Congress on Pain 2008; abstract PT214.

[124] Schulte H, Graven-Nielsen T, Sollevi A, Jansson Y, Arendt-Nielsen L, Segerdahl M. Pharmacological modulation of experimental phasic and tonic muscle pain by morphine, alfentanil and ketamine in healthy volunteers. Acta Anaesthesiol Scand 2003;47:1020–30.

[125] Schutter U, Ritzdorf I, Heckes B. [Treatment of chronic osteoarthritis pain: effectivity and safety of a 7 day matrix patch with a low dose buprenorphine.] MMW Fortschr Med 2008;150(Suppl 2):96–103.

[126] Sessle BJ, Hu JW, Yu X-M. Brainstem mechanisms of referred pain and hyperalgesia in the orofascial and temporomandibular region In: Vecchiet L, Albe-Fessard D, Lindblom U, Giamberardino MA, editors. New trends in referred pain and hyperalgesia. Amsterdam: Elsevier; 1993. p. 59–71.

[127] Shah JP, Danoff JV, Desai MJ, Parikh S, Nakamura LY, Phillips TM, Gerber LH. Biochemicals associated with pain and inflammation are elevated in sites near to and remote from active myofascial trigger points. Arch Phys Med Rehabil 2008;89:16–23.

[128] Shah JP, Phillips TM, Danoff JV, Gerber LH. An in vitro microanalytical technique for measuring the local biochemical milieu of human skeletal muscle. J Appl Physiol 2005;99:1977–84.

[129] Simone DA, Marchettini P, Caputi G, Ochoa JL. Identification of muscle afferents subserving sensation of deep pain in humans. J Neurophysiol 1994;72:883–9.

[130] Simons DG, Travell JG. Myofascial pain and dysfunction: the trigger point manual, 2nd ed, Vol. 1. Baltimore: Lippincott William & Wilkins, 1999. p. 278–307.

[131] Sluka KA. Stimulation of deep somatic tissue with capsaicin produces longlasting mechanical allodynia and heat hypoalgesia that depends on early activation of the cAMP pathway. J Neurosci 2002;22:5687–93.

[132] Sluka KA, Vance CG, Lisi TL. High-frequency, but not low-frequency transcutaneous electrical nerve stimulation reduces aspartate and glutamate release in the spinal cord dorsal horm. J Neurochem 2005;95:1794–801.

[133] Staud R, Cannon RC, Mauderli AP, Robinson ME, Price DD, Vierck CJ Jr. Temporal summation of pain from mechanical stimulation of muscle tissue in normal controls and subjects with fibromyalgia syndrome. Pain 2003;102:87–95.

[134] Staud R, Craggs JG, Perlstein WM, Robinson ME, Price DD. Brain activity associated with slow temporal summation of C-fiber evoked pain in fibromyalgia patients and healthy controls. Eur J Pain 2008;12:1078–89.

[135] Svensson P, Cairns BE, Wang K, Arendt-Nielsen L. Glutamate-evoked pain and mechanical allodynia in the human masseter muscle. Pain 2003;101:221–7.

[136] Svensson P, Cairns BE, Wang K, Arendt-Nielsen L. Injection of nerve growth factor into human masseter muscle evokes long-lasting mechanical allodynia and hyperalgesia. Pain 2003;104:241–7.

[137] Sörensen J, Graven-Nielsen T, Henriksson KG, Bengtsson M, Arendt-Nielsen L. Hyperexcitability in fibromyalgia. J Rheumatol 1998;25:152–5.

[138] Treaster D, Marras WS, Burr D, Sheedy JE, Hart D. Myofascial trigger point development from visual and postural stressors during computer work. J Electromyogr Kinesiol 2006;16:115–24.

[139] Van der Wees PJ, Lenssen AF, Hendriks EJ, Stomp DJ, Dekker J, de Bie RA. Effectiveness of exercise therapy and manual mobilisation in ankle sprain and functional instability: a systematic review. Aust J Physiother 2006;52:27–37.

[140] Vleeming A, de Vries HJ, Mens JM, van Wingerden JP. Possible role of the long dorsal sacroiliac ligament in women with peripartum pelvic pain. Acta Obstet Gynecol Scand 2002;81:430–6.

[141] Vleeming A, Pool-Goudzwaard AL, Hammudoghlu D, Stoeckart R, Snijders CJ, Mens JM. The function of the long dorsal sacroiliac ligament: its implication for understanding low back pain. Spine 1996;21:556–62.

[142] Wang YH, Ding XL, Zhang Y, Chen J, Ge HY, Arendt-Nielsen L, Yue SW. Ischemic compression block attenuates mechanical hyperalgesia evoked from latent myofascial trigger points. Exp Brain Res 2010;202:265–70.

[143] Witting N, Svensson P, Gottrup H, Arendt-Nielsen L, Jensen TS. Intramuscular and intradermal injection of capsaicin: a comparison of local and referred pain. Pain 2000;84:407–12.

[144] Zhang W, Doherty M, Arden N, Bannwarth B, Bijlsma J, Gunther KP, Hauselmann HJ, Herrero-Beaumont G, Jordan K, Kaklamanis P, et al. EULAR evidence based recommendations for the management of hip osteoarthritis: report of a task force of the EULAR Standing Committee for International Clinical Studies Including Therapeutics (ESCISIT). Ann Rheum Dis 2005;64:669–81.

Correspondence to: Lars Arendt-Nielsen, PhD, Center for Sensory-Motor Interaction (SMI), Department of Health Science and Technology, Aalborg University, Fredrik Bajers Vej 7, Bld. D3, DK-9220 Aalborg E, Denmark. Email: LAN@hst.aau.dk.

Part 5

Utility and Development of Pain Models:
Animals to Humans

Utility and Development of Pain Models: Animals to Humans

10

Martin Schmelz, MD,[a] **Gary J. Bennett, PhD,**[b] **and Karin L. Petersen, MD**[c]

[a]*Department of Anesthesiology and Intensive Care Medicine, Medical Faculty, University of Heidelberg, Mannheim, Germany;*
[b]*Department of Anesthesia and Faculty of Dentistry, McGill University, Montreal, Quebec, Canada;* [c]*Department of Neurology,
UCSF Pain Clinical Research Center, University of California, San Francisco, California, USA*

Pain models are commonly used to investigate pathophysiological mechanisms, potential therapeutic targets, and efficacy of new analgesic compounds. Theoretically, this approach appears straightforward. It is, in fact, an iterative process in which companies are asking for crucial targets in order to develop compounds, and basic researchers are asking for compounds in order to test crucial targets. Regardless of this procedural problem, experimental pain models represent the main tool to test for analgesic efficacy of new compounds. As far as the predictive value for the analgesic efficacy in chronic pain patients is concerned, the main challenge of the approach is determining to what degree mechanisms overlap between animal and human experimental pain models and clinical pain conditions. This challenge is even more complex because the crucial mechanisms of chronic pain in patients have not yet been described on a molecular level.

A variety of peripherally and centrally acting mechanisms can contribute to both acute and chronic pain conditions [16,47] (Fig. 1A). Animal and human pain models try to mimic these processes and thereby aim to produce a pain state that is comparable to the clinical condition. The different models have their limitations and virtues and cannot cover the entire clinical state in its complexity, and therefore studies in patients with chronic pain remain crucial. Animal models, but also human pain models and experimental models in pain patients, are therefore limited to investigating only certain aspects of clinical pain conditions (Fig. 1B). Regardless of species, the models have to be chosen according to the intended mechanism of action: if mechanisms related to neuronal injury are to be investigated, animal models are the only choice, whereas investigating qualitative sensory changes in acute central sensitization is more straightforward in human pain models.

In this chapter we will follow the pragmatic approach that has directed the development of pain models: initially, models and techniques were set up to test responses to *acute nociceptor activation* in the healthy state. These models cannot be expected to give information about the diseased state. However, they are of particular value when studying interaction of a candidate drug with its target (i.e., target engagement studies).

Many clinical pain states are linked to *sensitized nociceptive processing,* and therefore models were developed that induced neuronal sensitization at the site of injury or in the spinal cord. Paradigms for evoked nociceptive responses already developed for acute nociceptive testing are used to quantify the pain responses in the sensitized state. Classically, irritants were applied locally to incite an inflammatory process that renders the nociceptors hypersensitive. Later models have aimed at creating longer-lasting

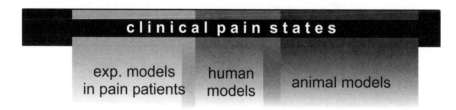

Fig. 1. Upper panel: Schematic view of neuronal changes leading to chronic pain and possible readout variables. DRG, dorsal root ganglion. Lower panel: Schematic view of aspects covered by human experimental models. Note that for structural changes and spontaneous pain there are no adequate human models.

neuronal sensitization (peripheral and central) without skin injury.

Neuropathic pain states are not linked to tissue inflammation, but rather to responses of the injured nervous system. Animal models were developed that initially focused on mechanical injury of a peripheral nerve to induce neuropathic pain. Human models of neuropathic pain are based on functional sensitization of spinal nociceptive processing.

Although nerve injury in preclinical models may simulate certain human pain conditions, our current understanding of the pathomechanisms of clinical pain suggest that the models do not mimic non-traumatic neuropathic pain. Thus, new animal models have been developed that use agents known to evoke chronic pain conditions clinically, such neuropathic pain following chemotherapy or herpes zoster viral infection, or inflammatory pain linked to bone cancer. These disease-related animal models are supposed to produce pain and hyperalgesia via the same (still unknown) mechanisms as in pain patients. A similar approach in the human is not possible, but additional information can be obtained using application of experimental pain models in pain patients.

Pain Models of Acute Nociceptor Activation

These models activate nociceptors mechanically, thermally, or chemically to induce pain *without* creating peripheral or central sensitization. Typically, mechanical and thermal pain thresholds are assessed by well-controlled stimuli of increasing intensity and behavioral or psychophysical readouts.

Human Psychophysics

A variety of standard methods are available for quantitative sensory testing (QST), using mechanical and thermal stimuli, to assess thresholds of pain detection and pain tolerance, as well as stimulus-response functions [56]. The most commonly used parameters include sensory thresholds and suprathreshold responses.

For both mechanical and thermal stimulation, slowly increasing stimulus ramps are commonly used to let the subjects indicate the stimulus intensity at which sensation is felt as just painful (*pain detection threshold*) or just bearable (*pain tolerance threshold*).

Suprathreshold mechanical or thermal stimulation can also be applied for a defined duration, while subjects rate the painfulness of the stimulation, most commonly on a 0–100 pain visual analogue scale (0 = "no pain" to 100 = "worst pain imaginable").

Thermal Stimulation

Most commonly, computer-controlled Peltier systems are used to deliver graded heat and cold stimuli. Thus, thresholds to cold and warm stimuli and to noxious heat and cold can be determined. The application of these systems is mainly restricted to the skin.

Mechanical Stimulation

Most widely used for mechanical stimulation of the skin are calibrated nylon filaments (von Frey hairs) or metal pins with identical tip diameter, but different weight [55]. For phasic mechanical pain, stimulators providing velocity-controlled impact stimuli have been developed [33]. In deeper tissues, pressure algometers with a greater contact surface are applied, whereas for visceral pain, balloons with controlled pressure are used.

For the cornea and nasal mucosa, combined mechanical, chemical, and temperature stimulators have been designed using different gases and air at different temperatures [12,42]. Flow of CO_2 causes pulses of low-pH-induced chemical pain, whereas heated or cooled air provides temperature stimuli and high-flow pulses produce mechanical stimulation.

Inflammatory Models Including Sensitization

Pain models can be classified according to which clinical condition they are presumed to simulate (nociceptive vs. neuropathic), the tissue involved (skin vs. muscle vs. viscera), and their time course (acute vs. subchronic). Models of neuronal sensitization can be categorized as peripheral or central sensitization. Peripheral sensitization implies that endogenous or exogenous mediators lower excitation thresholds and increase suprathreshold firing in the primary afferent nociceptors. Central sensitization implies that spinal processing of afferent information is sensitized such that normally nonpainful input is causing pain (allodynia) or normally slightly painful stimuli are felt more painful (hyperalgesia). Conceptually, the two forms of sensitization are strictly separated; however, most of the actual pain models are characterized by a combination of peripheral and central sensitization. As an example, topical

application of capsaicin will lead to primary sensitization to heat, evidenced by lowered heat pain thresholds within the stimulated skin (primary hyperalgesia). In addition, depending on its intensity, the nociceptive barrage to the spinal cord can induce central sensitization, evidenced by mechanical allodynia and hyperalgesia in an area surrounding the stimulation site (secondary hyperalgesia) (Fig. 2).

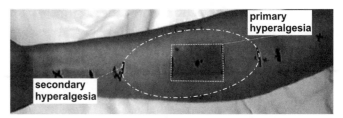

Fig. 2. Heat/capsaicin sensitization is induced on a rectangular stimulation site on the forearm by using the thermode to heat the skin to 45°C for 5 minutes, and the stimulation site is then treated with topical capsaicin cream for 30 minutes, leaving the stimulation site hyperalgesic for thermal stimulation ("primary hyperalgesia"). Cutaneous hyperalgesia can be maintained by heating the stimulation site to 40°C for 5 minutes (rekindling procedure) at 40-minute intervals. After each rekindling, areas of secondary hyperalgesia can be quantified with a 1-inch foam brush (the area of brush-evoked secondary hyperalgesia marked in the figure) and with a 26-g von Frey hair. The green channel from a color photograph is shown enhanced for contrast between normal skin and erythema.

Human Psychophysics

Acute Application of Algogens

Among the *exogenous mediators*, local capsaicin application is most commonly used. Capsaicin activates transient receptor potential, type V1 (TRPV1) receptors and sensitizes the local nociceptive endings to heat stimuli. A similar sensitization pattern can be induced by mustard oil application, which supposedly also excites TRPA1 receptors. In contrast, topical menthol application acting on TRPM8 receptors has been used to induce sensitization to cold and cold pain sensation [75]. The thermal sensitization induced in menthol models is extensive and robust; however, it is not clear which endogenous mechanism of sensitization is being modeled. Studies have shown reduction of menthol-induced cold hyperalgesia with tramadol, but not with gabapentin or ibuprofen [2].

Local Inflammation by Exogenous Irritants

Formalin, carrageenan, or Freund's adjuvants are not suited for use in humans. There are only case reports in which these substances have been applied inadvertently. Intravenously applied formalin caused acute pain at the injection site and coughing [66]. Freund's adjuvants inadvertently injected in human skin provoked a local inflammation combined with a transient heat hyperalgesia (lasting 2 weeks) and a very long-lasting mechanical hyperalgesia (lasting 8 weeks) [21]. Both examples confirm the activity of these agents in human and suggest similar pattern of hyperalgesia in animals and humans.

Local Inflammation by Endogenous Mediators

In order to avoid injection of irritants, human pain models have been developed that rely on the release of endogenous mediators. Tonic pressure of a skin fold provokes a local inflammatory response such that repetition of the pressure causes increased pain [19,29]. It is unclear as to whether the increased pain of pinching is a true mechanical hyperalgesia or a combination of mechanical stimulation and local ischemia [62]. Regardless, it is a simple and robust model to test analgesic effects of nonsteroidal anti-inflammatory drugs (NSAIDs) [19,29]. Interestingly, the pinch model is one of the few causing acute mechanical sensitization, whereas primary mechanical hyperalgesia in other models involving endogenous mediators develops gradually over several hours (e.g., ultraviolet B [UVB] burn [22,24,35] and the freeze lesion [30,39]). While irradiation with UVB does not cause pain per se, the application of the −20°C stimulus in the freeze model is painful. It is generally held that these inflammatory models mainly cause local sensitization of nociceptive endings (primary hyperalgesia) restricted to the inflamed tissue. However, with more intense stimulation or larger UVB burns, spontaneous activity in nociceptors can arise, leading to increased afferent input and central sensitization (see below) [22]. Mechanistically, among the endogenous inflammatory mediators, prostaglandin E_2 may be responsible for early heat hyperalgesia [41], whereas in longer-lasting mechanical hyperalgesia, nerve growth factor may be involved [8,9].

The freeze lesion leaves skin sites with pigmentations or depigmentations lasting for several months. UVB irradiation induces the well-known tanning response, and heat lesions may induce blisters, depending on the temperature protocol applied.

Mechanical hyperalgesia induced by endogenous mechanisms can also be provoked in skeletal muscle by controlled eccentric exercise leading to delayed-onset muscle soreness. The exact mechanism leading to hypersensitivity in this micro-injury model is unclear,

and controlled mechanical stimulation of the muscle requires more elaborate stimulation techniques. Moreover, pain adapts upon repetitive stimuli in this model, which is not the case in most clinical muscle pain states. This model has been used in pharmacological trials, with an analgesic effect being shown for NSAIDs and morphine [71].

Incision Model

Based on animal models of postoperative pain, experimental incisions of skin and muscle in humans have been developed [27,28]. Acute pain responses by the incisions have also been investigated by functional imaging [52]. The acute activation of nociceptors leads to the pain and flare response. The ensuing phase of inflammation and repair is linked to the development of mechanical hyperalgesia at the site of injury that lasts for about 2 days, similar to the results in rodents. In addition to the sensitization at the site of injury, the nociceptive barrage to the spinal cord also induces an area of punctate mechanical hyperalgesia around the incision as a sign of central sensitization (see below).

Neuropathic Pain Models

Human Psychophysics

In contrast to animal models that can induce sensitization functionally and by neuronal injury, human experimental models of neuropathic pain are limited to functional means; that is, peripherally applied nociceptive barrage to the spinal cord. As stated above, we describe inflammatory and neuropathic pain separately mainly for educational purposes; it is important to keep in mind that the two processes are intimately linked in clinical pain states and experimental models.

Several studies have suggested that in neuropathic pain, noxious input from injured nociceptors in the periphery drive or maintain the central sensitization process [16,47]. Indeed, secondary mechanical hyperalgesia to brushing (touch allodynia) or to punctate stimuli (pinprick hyperalgesia) has been shown to vary in spatial extent with the intensity of ongoing pain in neuropathic pain patients [34]. In healthy volunteers, activation of nociceptors can induce reversible central sensitization; various stimulation methods have been proposed using electrical [20,36], chemical [37,65], or heat stimuli [11,43,46,49]. As stimulation-induced lasting injury is a major concern, models were developed that limited tissue injury, but still induced central sensitization. The most commonly used model is injection of capsaicin, which not only can cause local sensitization to heating stimuli (peripheral sensitization; see above), but also provokes strong, but transient nociceptor activation, which in turn induces punctate hyperalgesia and touch allodynia as a result of central sensitization. Heating of the skin similarly activates nociceptors, and the noxious barrage to the spinal cord leads to central sensitization, depending on stimulus intensity and duration (in addition to the peripheral inflammation described above) [43]. Stimulation with heat at 47°C for 5 minutes leads to long-lasting sensitization, but about 25% of subjects develop blisters. The brief thermal sensitization (BTS) model (45°C for 3 minutes) provides short-lasting sensitization and can be induced 2–3 times at hourly intervals without skin injury. The heat/capsaicin sensitization model combines noninjurious levels of these two stimuli to induce long-lasting central sensitization [49]. In this model, heating of the skin to 45°C for 5 minutes activates and sensitizes peripheral nociceptors, and is sufficient to induce short-lasting central sensitization. This procedure is followed by immediate application of topical capsaicin (0.075%) to further activate and sensitize nociceptors so as to enhance and prolong the central sensitization. Then mild heating stimuli (40°C for 5 minutes) can be repeated every 40 minutes to activate the peripherally sensitized nociceptors and provoke a nociceptive barrage to the spinal cord sufficient to maintain the central sensitization for up to 4 hours.

Electrical stimuli would appear ideal to provoke nociceptor activation, but high current densities are required to excite the high threshold mechano-insensitive C-nociceptors, which are crucially involved in the induction of central sensitization [61]. Using stimulation at high current density, pain and central sensitization can be maintained at a stable level for a few hours [6,13,36,73].

Also, high-frequency stimulation at high current density for short bursts (five 1-second bursts at 100 Hz at 2 mA, 2 ms) has been used to induce secondary mechanical hyperalgesia [31]. Pharmacological tests in this model revealed antihyperalgesic effects of N-methyl-D-aspartate (NMDA) blockers against electrical stimulation, but not to pinprick hyperalgesia or touch allodynia [32].

All the models mentioned above involve painful stimulation of nociceptive afferent fibers for induction.

However, once hyperalgesia is induced, severe ongoing spontaneous pain, which is the main complaint of neuropathic pain patients, is no longer present in any of the models.

Nerve Growth Factor Injection

A new development of human pain models with aspects of peripheral and central sensitization without inflammation has emerged recently: intracutaneous injection of nerve growth factor (NGF) is known to produce mechanical and heat hyperalgesia lasting for several weeks [17]. Recent studies [58] more clearly characterized the mechanical hyperalgesia as being a combination of lasting static (but not dynamic) allodynia [45], cold hyperalgesia, and hyperalgesia to mechanical impact and punctate stimuli [58] (Fig. 3).

The sensitizing effects of NGF include phosphorylation, translocation, and upregulation of TRPV1 [67,79], which might be linked to heat hyperalgesia. The molecular mechanisms for mechanical and cold hyperalgesia remain unclear.

Positive reports of Phase 2 studies using anti-NGF strategies in osteoarthritis, but also lower back pain [10] have increased the interest in NGF-induced sensitization in humans. Interestingly, systemic application of NGF in humans has been reported to cause widespread muscle pain for weeks [50], whereas local intramuscular injections induce mechanical sensitization lasting for only a few days [3,68,69]. While the NGF human pain model appears to generate a combination of symptoms found in pain patients, the model still lacks the most relevant symptom of pain patients—spontaneous pain.

Limitations of Human Pain Models

Pain states that are associated with nerve injury and take time to develop cannot be modeled in healthy volunteers. Thus, if compounds are to be tested clinically in neuropathic pain, the main question is selection of the disease among possible options such as post-traumatic neuropathic pain, postherpetic neuralgia, or chemotherapy-induced neuropathic pain. Herpes zoster (HZ) can also be used as a "model system" for predicting efficacy in human neuropathic pain conditions. Advantages of using HZ as a model are its known etiology, a clear diagnosis with definite nerve injury and inflammation, the fact that it occurs in otherwise healthy individuals, and the ability to

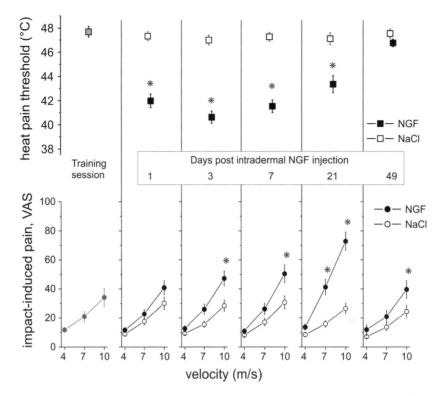

Fig. 3. Time course of hyperalgesia to heat (upper panel) and mechanical impact stimuli of different velocity (4–10 m/s) following intracutaneous injection of nerve growth factor (NGF) in a human study. Note that the peak of mechanical hyperalgesia (day 21) is delayed as compared to the peak of heat hyperalgesia (day 3).

study analgesic effects on acute neuropathic/inflammatory pain. Both HZ-associated pain and allodynia were reduced with a single oral dose of 900 mg gabapentin [7]. Potential challenges to this type of study include the recruitment of a sufficient number of subjects as the incidence of shingles declines through the increased penetration of the HZ vaccine. Moreover, given the evidence that both opioids and gabapentin are efficacious in relieving HZ pain, subjects may be less willing to participate in testing of compounds that are still in early development. Finally, designing studies of HZ pain is challenging given that in the majority of subjects, pain resolves rapidly over the first few weeks or months [72].

Experimental Pain Models in Patients

Given the limitations of pain models on one hand and the high variability of clinical pain conditions on the other, combining the two approaches appears useful. There are two main purposes of using experimental pain models in patients: improving drug testing by applying standardized painful stimuli in the patients, and improving knowledge about similarity of clinical and

experimental pain mechanisms. In this section, we will focus on attempts to employ experimental models of acute nociception and neuronal sensitization in patients who already suffer from chronic pain. Many studies have demonstrated altered pain perception in patients with a variety of chronic pain conditions, but only very few have simultaneously correlated drug effects on experimental and clinical pain. Most of these studies have included threshold determination with heat, cold, or mechanical stimulation or with the cold pressor model, and a few with neuronal sensitization [1,64]. Correlating drug effects in experimental and clinical pain may help in analgesic drug development and in studies of drug mechanism of action, as well as in studies aimed at understanding mechanisms underlying chronic pain.

Any experimental pain model used in patients must be safe in this population, which is generally older and with more comorbidities. To meet this requirement, models should be noninvasive and noninjurious, and it should be possible to terminate the stimulation upon the patient's request, as the subjects are already in pain. The model-related tasks required of the subjects must be kept simple and as nonaversive as possible, to avoid study dropouts.

Why Include a Pain Model in a Chronic Pain Clinical Trial?

Correlating Study Drug Effects on Experimental Pain and Chronic Pain

A matrix of possible correlations is presented in Table I. The first requirement is that the drug has been shown effective in experimental pain models in healthy volunteers using the same or a very similar pain model. If the treatment effects on experimental and chronic pain are correlated, the study shows that the study drug is effective and that experimental and chronic pain may share common mechanisms. This outcome would strongly support a "go-decision" for further development of the drug (Table IA).

If the drug is effective only in experimental, but not clinical, pain (Table IB), the study confirms the healthy volunteer data but suggests that the drug will not be useful for that that particular type of chronic pain. The drug may still be effective, but it should not be developed for that disease indication. It is possible that the clinical pain has a different underlying mechanism than the experimental pain, or that the subjects included simply do not represent the disease.

It becomes more difficult to interpret the results when the drug is effective in clinical, but not experimental, pain (Table IC). Possible interpretations include placebo response, expectations, or the possibility that the study drug is effective for the mechanisms underlying the chronic pain, but that these mechanisms were not simulated by the model (model failure). An example would be intravenous lidocaine, which is effective in chronic neuropathic pain, but not convincingly effective in human experimental pain models. The effect of lidocaine probably depends on neuronal injury that cannot be mimicked in human pain models. The effect of intravenous lidocaine on experimental and clinical pain has not been tested simultaneously in patients, however.

Table I
Interpretations of possible outcomes comparing drug effects on clinical pain and experimental pain (heat/capsaicin sensitization model)

	Clinical pain success	Clinical pain failure
Experimental pain success	(A) Efficacy validated	(B) Clinical failure
Experimental pain failure	(C) Expectations/placebo? Model failure?	(D) Study failure? Drug failure?

When the drug has no effect on experimental or clinical pain (Table ID), the reason may be true lack of drug effect or study failure. The results from Phase 1 studies can help guide interpretation. In this situation, no recommendation regarding further development can be made.

Analgesic Drug Development

Once an analgesic effect of the study drug has been demonstrated in a human experimental pain model or in a preclinical or Phase 1 study, the model can be used again in later studies at each stage of development. This model could take the place of a standard positive comparator drug and thereby simplify the study design because an additional control session with the comparator drug might be eliminated. The effects of the study drug on experimental and clinical pain can be correlated as demonstrated in Table I, which will aid in study interpretation along with Phase 1 results. Models can also be useful as an additional means of gathering data on the time course of analgesic effect by repeating model measures at different time points after dosing has started, either in a single-dose, single-session format, or during a multiple-dose study. Dose-response data can be gathered by comparing the effect on model measures after administering various doses (Fig. 4). The stimulus applied with the model is standardized across all subjects, whereas the injuries leading to chronic pain vary across subjects and diseases, possibly contributing to variations in drug response.

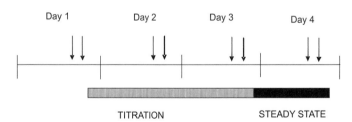

Fig. 4. Example of an experimental protocol combining assessment of clinical and experimental pain. Analgesic effects of cannabis are assessed in neuropathic pain patients by daily visual analogue scale (VAS) pain ratings (upper panel). In addition, experimental pain models (Heat/Capsaicin with 4 rekindling periods [RK1–RK4]) are employed repetitively for 4 days (lower panel). Medication is started after the first test. Systemic levels of the drug can then be correlated to clinical analgesic effects and to analgesia in the models.

Investigating Drug Mechanism of Action and Pain Mechanisms

The mechanisms underlying the sensory phenomena observed in the cutaneous sensitization models have been extensively studied. The addition of models in patient studies allow us to study the effect of the study drugs on model-related pain mechanisms and to relate the results to the drug's effects on chronic pain.

In a few cases, experimental pain models in patients can detect abnormal processing of noxious stimuli in the patients, and thereby give mechanistic information about the possible underlying pathophysiology. For example, using the model of electrically induced hyperalgesia, neurogenic protein extravasation was found in patients with complex regional pain syndrome (CRPS), but not in healthy controls [76]. In the same model, CRPS patients showed reduced activity of their endogenous pain inhibition [64].

Few studies have investigated compounds that are effective in chronic pain *and* in models in healthy volunteers, to test if efficacy in models and clinical pain correlate when the models are performed in patients (positive/negative controls). In one of the earliest studies using experimental pain stimulation in patients with low back pain, Price recorded sensory and affective visual analogue scale (VAS) ratings to noxious heat pulses and ongoing clinical pain during infusion of fentanyl. He suggested that opioid suppression of experimental noxious stimulation was correlated with relief of chronic pain [53,77].

In a more recent study, Abrams and colleagues [1] tested the effect of smoked marijuana on pain associated with human immunodeficiency virus (HIV)-induced neuropathy and experimental cutaneous sensitization. Adults with painful HIV-associated sensory neuropathy were randomly assigned to smoke either cannabis (3.56% tetrahydrocannabinol) or seemingly identical placebo cigarettes with the cannabinoids extracted three times daily for 5 days. Primary outcome measures were ratings of chronic pain and the percentage of patients achieving more than 30% reduction in pain intensity. In association with the first (day 1) and last cigarette (day 5), acute analgesic and antihyperalgesic effects of smoked cannabis were assessed simultaneously with chronic pain using a cutaneous heat stimulation procedure and the heat/capsaicin sensitization model (Fig. 5).

Use of marijuana in treatment of pain is controversial, and the study only included individuals with previous experience with smoked marijuana, which could potentially bias the results. The inclusion of the rigorous experimental pain model was an attempt to lessen the bias. The model-associated outcome measures were novel to each patient and were not strongly associated with expectations of relief of chronic pain. In addition, areas of secondary hyperalgesia were mapped by an investigator while the patient looked away. The hypothesis was that model-associated outcomes were less subjective than pain intensity ratings on a VAS. The study indeed demonstrated that smoked marijuana had analgesic effects on the acute central neuronal sensitization

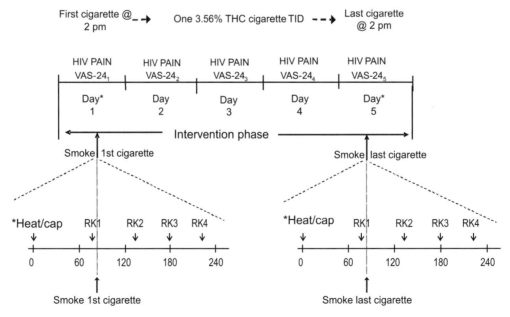

Fig. 5. Experimental protocol comparing analgesic effects of smoked cannabis on clinical and experimental pain is shown. In the intervention phase, clinical pain ratings are assessed on a visual analogue scale (VAS) in HIV neuropathy patients. In parallel, the heat/capsaicin (Heat/cap) model with four periods of rekindling (RK) is performed in association with the first intervention on day 1 and at steady state on day 5. THC, tetrahydrocannabinol.

induced by the heat/capsaicin sensitization model, as well as on the pain associated with HIV neuropathy. Table II provides a matrix of correlation of effect of cannabis on clinical and experimental outcomes, supporting a true analgesic effect, probably induced, at least partially, via reduction of central neuronal sensitization.

Table II
Contingency table comparing analgesic effects
on clinical and experimental pain for active
treatment vs. placebo [2]

P a i n m o d e l		Clinical pain	
	Active treatment	>30% relief	<30% relief
	>30% area reduction	10	1
	<30% area reduction	2	1
	Placebo	>30% relief	<30% relief
	>30% area reduction	2	1
	<30% area reduction	6	7

Investigating Opioid Analgesic Tolerance

In animals, near-complete analgesic tolerance can develop within 24 hours of continuous administration of opioids. Studies during management of postoperative pain suggest the development of acute tolerance, but they are difficult to interpret. Postoperative pain is a poor model for studying analgesic tolerance development because the underlying source of pain is not stable during the first 24 hours, and intraoperative analgesia regimens are complex. Human experimental pain models that are opioid responsive provide an ideal means for studying the development of opioid analgesic. The models anchor the assessment of opioid responsivity by supplementing subjective ratings of ongoing chronic pain with assessment of model-associated sensory changes and responses to standardized noxious stimuli.

Vinik and Kissin [74] showed in an unblinded preliminary study in eight healthy volunteers that 4 hour-long intravenous (i.v.) infusions of remifentanil had a nearly 75% loss of analgesic effect using cold immersion pain and mechanical pressure pain thresholds. However, acute opioid tolerance was not detected during a 3-hour infusion of remifentanil in 36 healthy volunteers using electrical- and heat-evoked pain and the cold pressor test [4].

The brief thermal stimulation model is noninvasive and tolerable in patients; it induces short-lasting areas of secondary hyperalgesia. The model has been repeated up to twice daily for five days in volunteers.

When twice-daily opioid versus placebo injections were given for 4 days, the reduction in the area of secondary hyperalgesia on the first morphine day was significant and robust in both groups. Morphine suppression of the painfulness of skin heating, and elevation of the heat pain detection threshold, were also significant. During the 4 days of injections, there was a trend toward a decline in the antihyperalgesic effects of morphine, but it did not reach statistical significance ($P = 0.06$) compared to placebo. The baseline areas of secondary hyperalgesia from BTS, as well as the baseline painfulness of the BTS model, were stable across the five study sessions, suggesting that neither residual morphine analgesia nor withdrawal hyperalgesia was present [48].

Chu and colleagues [15] used both a heat pain stimulus and the cold pressor test in a group of six patients with low back pain treated for 1 month with morphine. Target-controlled infusions of remifentanil were used to test for the development of opioid tolerance. Both opioid tolerance and hyperalgesia were found in the cold pressor test, but not in the case of heat stimulation. The correlation to the level of chronic pain was not analyzed.

In summary, few studies have incorporated experimental models of pain and neuronal sensitization in patients with chronic pain, especially when compared to the large number of experimental pain model studies in healthy volunteers. Including experimental pain models in patient studies can be beneficial in drug development and in studies of pain and drug mechanisms and development of tolerance. The cold pressor, heat stimuli, BTS, and heat/capsaicin models are all well tolerated in patients and appear to perform similarly in patients.

Translational Approaches: Best Shots

For the induction of primary inflammatory hyperalgesia, corresponding data for UVB radiation exist for mice [60,78], rats [9,59], pigs [57], and humans [8,14,18,23,24,70] (Fig. 6).

The common features of this model include local inflammation, along with heat and mechanical hyperalgesia for about 2 days. It can be regarded as the best-studied translational model of inflammatory hyperalgesia. The model has been used in humans to investigate drug effects on local mediator production [5] and on central activation patterns [40,63].

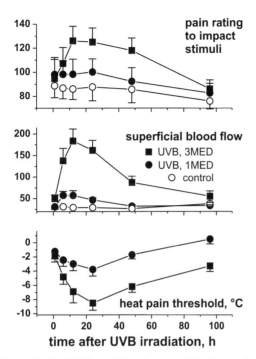

Fig. 6. Ultraviolet B (UVB) model in humans. The figure shows the time course of mechanical hyperalgesia (pain ratings on a 0–100 visual analogue scale), superficial blood flow as measured with a laser Doppler scanner (in arbitrary perfusion units), and heat hyperalgesia (heat pain thresholds in degrees Celsius). Note that the peak of the inflammatory vasodilation is found at 12–24 hours, and the peak hyperalgesia to mechanical and heat stimuli is slightly delayed at around 1–2 days.

NGF-induced hyperalgesia currently is the only experimental model to have produced a chronic (several weeks long) hyperalgesic state in humans (see Fig. 3). There is broad literature from rodents on NGF-induced sensitization [51]. NGF acutely lowers heat pain thresholds in humans [17] and rodents [38], by mechanisms that are already well described (see ref. [44] for review). Mechanical sensitization was observed following intracutaneous injection of NGF in humans [17]. Similarly, exogenous NGF elicited delayed mechanical sensitization in animals, via both peripheral and central mechanisms [25,26,38]. However, a single NGF injection into human skin elicited a long-lasting, but very localized, mechanical hyperalgesia at the injection site without signs of allodynia [58], suggesting a peripheral rather than central mechanism.

Pain Models: From Target Engagement Tools to Mechanistic Models

The most straightforward approach in pain models is the acute application of a known algogen, followed by inhibition of the response by potential antagonists under study (target engagement tools). This approach can help solve many basic questions of pharmacokinetics, dosing, and side effects. If, for example, a TRPV1 blocker does not inhibit capsaicin-induced pain, flare, and secondary hyperalgesia, the result would suggest pharmacokinetic problems of the compound. Target engagement studies are also helpful in dose-finding studies, and when interpreting negative clinical trials. However, while they confirm target engagement, they do not provide information on the role of the target in painful diseases.

The development of mechanistic models is much more problematic, as little is known about the molecular mechanisms of clinical pain conditions. Thus, experimental models of neuronal sensitization mimic only certain aspects of chronic pain conditions. The most commonly used models have been validated through both positive and negative control studies and are valuable in proof-of-concept studies. Ideally, models should match across preclinical and healthy volunteer models, should fully simulate the targeted clinical condition, and should have results that correlate with clinical efficacy. With regard to translational models for inflammatory pain, UVB irradiation has been investigated similarly in animal and human settings. In models of neuropathic pain models there is a disconnect, because preclinical models include nerve injury models in animals, whereas healthy volunteer models include only acute nociceptor excitation with capsaicin, heat, or electrical current. Moreover, in both animal and human models, the primary outcome is evoked hyperalgesia rather than spontaneous pain [54]. It is an open question as to whether "spontaneous" pain is based upon extreme sensitization such that even slight stimuli in the resting state would evoke nociceptor discharge (a possible example could be pain in osteoarthritis). Alternatively, the mechanisms of spontaneous discharge may be distinct from those that induce sensory sensitization (a possible example could be spontaneous activity generated in the dorsal root ganglia in neuropathic pain), and thus they should addressed separately.

The appropriate approach to this disconnect is to design experimental pain models that attempt to induce the actual disease in animals to model diseases such as chemotherapy and varicella zoster virus-associated pain. In parallel, a patient-centered approach using correlative studies of experimental pain models in patients should be followed to optimize translation between species and models. Despite all attempts to improve pain models and identify particular patient groups as disease "model systems" such as post-traumatic neu-ropathic pain, postherpetic neuralgia, or chemotherapy-induced neuropathic pain, clinical investigations of patients with the "real disease" remain the crucial step.

References

[1] Abrams DI, Jay CA, Shade SB, Vizoso H, Reda H, Press S, Kelly ME, Rowbotham MC, Petersen KL. Cannabis in painful HIV-associated sensory neuropathy: a randomized placebo-controlled trial. Neurology 2007;68:515–21.

[2] Altis K, Schmidtko A, Angioni C, Kuczka K, Schmidt H, Geisslinger G, Lotsch J, Tegeder I. Analgesic efficacy of tramadol, pregabalin and ibuprofen in menthol-evoked cold hyperalgesia. Pain 2009;147:116–21.

[3] Andersen H, Arendt-Nielsen L, Svensson P, Danneskiold-Samsoe B, Graven-Nielsen T. Spatial and temporal aspects of muscle hyperalgesia induced by nerve growth factor in humans. Exp Brain Res 2008;191:371–82.

[4] Angst MS, Chu LF, Tingle MS, Shafer SL, Clark JD, Drover DR. No evidence for the development of acute tolerance to analgesic, respiratory depressant and sedative opioid effects in humans. Pain 2009;142:17–26.

[5] Angst MS, Clark JD, Carvalho B, Tingle M, Schmelz M, Yeomans DC. Cytokine profile in human skin in response to experimental inflammation, noxious stimulation, and administration of a COX-inhibitor: a microdialysis study. Pain 2008;30:15–27.

[6] Angst MS, Koppert W, Pahl I, Clark DJ, Schmelz M. Short-term infusion of the mu-opioid agonist remifentanil in humans causes hyperalgesia during withdrawal. Pain 2003;106:49–57.

[7] Berry JD, Petersen KL. A single dose of gabapentin reduces acute pain and allodynia in patients with herpes zoster. Neurology 2005;65:444–7.

[8] Bishop T, Ballard A, Holmes H, Young AR, McMahon SB. Ultraviolet-B induced inflammation of human skin: characterisation and comparison with traditional models of hyperalgesia. Eur J Pain 2009;13:524–32.

[9] Bishop T, Hewson DW, Yip PK, Fahey MS, Dawbarn D, Young AR, McMahon SB. Characterisation of ultraviolet-B-induced inflammation as a model of hyperalgesia in the rat. Pain 2007;131:70–82.

[10] Cattaneo A. Tanezumab, a recombinant humanized mAb against nerve growth factor for the treatment of acute and chronic pain. Curr Opin Mol Ther 2010;12:94–106.

[11] Cervero F, Gilbert R, Hammond RGE, Tanner J. Development of secondary hyperalgesia following nonpainful thermal stimulation of the skin: a psychophysical study in man. Pain 1993;54:181–9.

[12] Chen XJ, Gallar J, Pozo MA, Baeza M, Belmonte C. CO_2 stimulation of the cornea: a comparison between human sensation and nerve activity in polymodal nociceptive afferents of the cat. Eur J Neurosci 1995;7:1154–63.

[13] Chizh BA, Gohring M, Troster A, Quartey GK, Schmelz M, Koppert W. Effects of oral pregabalin and aprepitant on pain and central sensitization in the electrical hyperalgesia model in human volunteers. Br J Anaesth 2007;98:246–54.

[14] Chizh BA, O'Donnell MB, Napolitano A, Wang J, Brooke AC, Aylott MC, Bullman JN, Gray EJ, Lai RY, Williams PM, Appleby JM. The effects of the TRPV1 antagonist SB-705498 on TRPV1 receptor-mediated activity and inflammatory hyperalgesia in humans. Pain 2007;132:132–41.

[15] Chu LF, Clark DJ, Angst MS. Opioid tolerance and hyperalgesia in chronic pain patients after one month of oral morphine therapy: a preliminary prospective study. J Pain 2006;7:43–8.

[16] Devor M. Pathophysiology of nerve injury. Handb Clin Neurol 2006;81:261-IV.

[17] Dyck PJ, Peroutka S, Rask C, Burton E, Baker MK, Lehman KA, Gillen DA, Hokanson JL, Obrien PC. Intradermal recombinant human nerve growth factor induces pressure allodynia and lowered heat pain threshold in humans. Neurology 1997;48:501–5.

[18] Eisenbarth H, Rukwied R, Petersen M, Schmelz M. Sensitization to bradykinin B1 and B2 receptor activation in UV-B irradiated human skin. Pain 2004;110:197–204.

[19] Forster C, Magerl W, Beck A, Geisslinger G, Gall T, Brune K, Handwerker HO. Differential effects of dipyrone, ibuprofen, and paracetamol on experimentally induced pain in man. Agents Actions 1992;35:112–21.

[20] Geber C, Fondel R, Kramer HH, Rolke R, Treede RD, Sommer C, Birklein F. Psychophysics, flare, and neurosecretory function in human pain models: capsaicin versus electrically evoked pain. J Pain 2007;8:503–14.

[21] Gould HJ, III. Complete Freund's adjuvant-induced hyperalgesia: a human perception. Pain 2000;85:301–3.

[22] Gustorff B, Anzenhofer S, Sycha T, Lehr S, Kress HG. The sunburn pain model: the stability of primary and secondary hyperalgesia over 10 hours in a crossover setting. Anesth Analg 2004;98:173–7.

[23] Gustorff B, Hoechtl K, Sycha T, Felouzis E, Lehr S, Kress HG. The effects of remifentanil and gabapentin on hyperalgesia in a new extended inflammatory skin pain model in healthy volunteers. Anesth Analg 2004;98:401–7.

[24] Hoffmann RT, Schmelz M. Time course of UVA- and UVB-induced inflammation and hyperalgesia in human skin. Eur J Pain 1999;3:131–9.

[25] Hoheisel U, Unger T, Mense S. Excitatory and modulatory effects of inflammatory cytokines and neurotrophins on mechanosensitive group IV muscle afferents in the rat. Pain 2005;114:168–76.

[26] Hoheisel U, Unger T, Mense S. Sensitization of rat dorsal horn neurons by NGF-induced subthreshold potentials and low-frequency activation. A study employing intracellular recordings in vivo. Brain Res 2007;1169:34–43.

[27] Kawamata M, Takahashi T, Kozuka Y, Nawa Y, Nishikawa K, Narimatsu E, Watanabe H, Namiki A. Experimental incision-induced pain in human skin: effects of systemic lidocaine on flare formation and hyperalgesia. Pain 2002;100:77–89.

[28] Kawamata M, Watanabe H, Nishikawa K, Takahashi T, Kozuka Y, Kawamata T, Omote K, Namiki A. Different mechanisms of development and maintenance of experimental incision-induced hyperalgesia in human skin. Anesthesiology 2002;97:550–9.

[29] Kilo S, Forster C, Geisslinger G, Brune K, Handwerker HO. Inflammatory models of cutaneous hyperalgesia are sensitive to effects of ibuprofen in man. Pain 1995;62:187–93.

[30] Kilo S, Schmelz M, Koltzenburg M, Handwerker HO. Different patterns of hyperalgesia induced by experimental inflammations in human skin. Brain 1994;117:385–96.

[31] Klein T, Magerl W, Hopf HC, Sandkuhler J, Treede RD. Perceptual correlates of nociceptive long-term potentiation and long-term depression in humans. J Neurosci 2004;24:964–71.

[32] Klein T, Magerl W, Nickel U, Hopf HC, Sandkuhler J, Treede RD. Effects of the NMDA-receptor antagonist ketamine on perceptual correlates of long-term potentiation within the nociceptive system. Neuropharmacology 2007;52:655–61.

[33] Kohlloffel LU, Koltzenburg M, Handwerker HO. A novel technique for the evaluation of mechanical pain and hyperalgesia. Pain 1991;46:81–7.

[34] Koltzenburg M, Torebjörk HE, Wahren LK. Nociceptor modulated central sensitization causes mechanical hyperalgesia in acute chemogenic and chronic neuropathic pain. Brain 1994;117:579–91.

[35] Koppert W, Brueckl V, Weidner C, Schmelz M. Mechanically induced axon reflex and hyperalgesia in human UV-B burn are reduced by systemic lidocaine. Eur J Pain 2004;8:237–44.

[36] Koppert W, Dern SK, Sittl R, Albrecht S, Schuttler J, Schmelz M. A new model of electrically evoked pain and hyperalgesia in human skin: the effects of intravenous alfentanil, S(+)-ketamine, and lidocaine. Anesthesiology 2001;95:395–402.

[37] LaMotte RH, Shain CN, Simone DA, Tsai EFP. Neurogenic hyperalgesia psychophysical studies of underlying mechanisms. J Neurophysiol 1991;66:190–211.

[38] Lewin GR, Rueff A, Mendell LM. Peripheral and central mechanisms of NGF-induced hyperalgesia. Eur J Neurosci 1994;6:1903–12.

[39] Lotsch J, Angst MS. The μ-opioid agonist remifentanil attenuates hyperalgesia evoked by blunt and punctuated stimuli with different potency: a pharmacological evaluation of the freeze lesion in humans. Pain 2003;102:151–61.

[40] Maihofner C, Ringler R, Herrndobler F, Koppert W. Brain imaging of analgesic and antihyperalgesic effects of cyclooxygenase inhibition in an experimental human pain model: a functional MRI study. Eur J Neurosci 2007;26:1344–56.

[41] Miller CC, Hale P, Pentland AP. Ultraviolet B injury increases prostaglandin synthesis through a tyrosine kinase-dependent pathway. Evidence for UVB-induced epidermal growth factor receptor activation. J Biol Chem 1994;269:3529–33.

[42] Mohammadian P, Hummel T, Loetsch J, Kobal G. Bilateral hyperalgesia to chemical stimulation of the nasal mucosa following unilateral inflammation. Pain 1997;73:407–12.

[43] Moiniche S, Dahl JB, Kehlet H. Time course of primary and secondary hyperalgesia after heat injury to the skin. Br J Anaesth 1993;71:201–5.

[44] Nicol GD, Vasko MR. Unraveling the story of NGF-mediated sensitization of nociceptive sensory neurons: ON or OFF the Trks? Mol Interv 2007;7:26–41.

[45] Ochoa JL, Yarnitsky D. Mechanical hyperalgesias in neuropathic pain patients: dynamic and static subtypes. Ann Neurol 1993;33:465–72.

[46] Pedersen JL, Kehlet H. Secondary hyperalgesia to heat stimuli after burn injury in man. Pain 1998;76:377–84.

[47] Petersen KL, Fields HL, Brennum J, Sandroni P, Rowbotham MC. Capsaicin evoked pain and allodynia in post-herpetic neuralgia. Pain 2000;88:125–33.

[48] Petersen KL, Meadoff T, Press S, Peters MM, Lecomte MD, Rowbotham MC. Changes in morphine analgesia and side effects during daily subcutaneous administration in healthy volunteers. Pain 2008;137:395–404.

[49] Petersen KL, Rowbotham MC. A new human experimental pain model: the heat/capsaicin sensitization model. Neuroreport 1999;10:1511–6.

[50] Petty BG, Cornblath DR, Adornato BT, Chaudhry V, Flexner C, Wachsman M, Sinicropi D, Burton LE, Peroutka SJ. The effect of systemically administered recombinant human nerve growth factor in healthy human subjects. Ann Neurol 1994;36:244–6.

[51] Pezet S, McMahon SB. Neurotrophins: mediators and modulators of pain. Annu Rev Neurosci 2006;29:507–38.

[52] Pogatzki-Zahn EM, Wagner C, Meinhardt-Renner A, Burgmer M, Beste C, Zahn PK, Pfleiderer B. Coding of incisional pain in the brain: a functional magnetic resonance imaging study in human volunteers. Anesthesiology 2010;112:406–17.

[53] Price DD, Harkins SW, Rafii A, Price C. A simultaneous comparison of fentanyl's analgesic effects on experimental and clinical pain. Pain 1986;24:197–203.

[54] Rice AS, Cimino-Brown D, Eisenach JC, Kontinen VK, Lacroix-Fralish ML, Machin I, Mogil JS, Stohr T. Animal models and the prediction of efficacy in clinical trials of analgesic drugs: a critical appraisal and call for uniform reporting standards. Pain 2008;139:243–7.

[55] Rolke R, Baron R, Maier C, Tolle TR, Treede RD, Beyer A, Binder A, Birbaumer N, Birklein F, Botefur IC, et al. Quantitative sensory testing in the German Research Network on Neuropathic Pain (DFNS): standardized protocol and reference values. Pain 2006;123:231–43.

[56] Rolke R, Magerl W, Campbell KA, Schalber C, Caspari S, Birklein F, Treede RD. Quantitative sensory testing: a comprehensive protocol for clinical trials. Eur J Pain 2006;10:77–88.

[57] Rukwied R, Dusch M, Schley M, Forsch E, Schmelz M. Nociceptor sensitization to mechanical and thermal stimuli in pig skin in vivo. Eur J Pain 2008;12:242–50.

[58] Rukwied R, Mayer A, Kluschina O, Obreja O, Schley M, Schmelz M. NGF induces non-inflammatory localized and lasting mechanical and thermal hypersensitivity in human skin. Pain 2010;148:407–13.

[59] Saade NE, Farhat O, Rahal O, Safieh-Garabedian B, Le BD, Jabbur SJ. Ultra violet-induced localized inflammatory hyperalgesia in awake rats and the role of sensory and sympathetic innervation of the skin. Brain Behav Immun 2008;22:245–56.

[60] Saade NE, Nasr IW, Massaad CA, Safieh-Garabedian B, Jabbur SJ, Kanaan SA. Modulation of ultraviolet-induced hyperalgesia and cytokine upregulation by interleukins 10 and 13. Br J Pharmacol 2000;131:1317–24.

[61] Schmelz M, Schmidt R, Handwerker HO, Torebjörk HE. Encoding of burning pain from capsaicin-treated human skin in two categories of unmyelinated nerve fibres. Brain 2000;123:560–71.

[62] Schmidt R, Schmelz M, Torebjörk HE, Handwerker HO. Mechano-insensitive nociceptors encode pain evoked by tonic pressure to human skin. Neuroscience 2000;98:793–800.

[63] Seifert F, Jungfer I, Schmelz M, Maihofner C. Representation of UV-B-induced thermal and mechanical hyperalgesia in the human brain: a functional MRI study. Hum Brain Mapp 2008;29:1327–42.

[64] Seifert F, Kiefer G, Decol R, Schmelz M, Maihofner C. Differential endogenous pain modulation in complex-regional pain syndrome. Brain 2009;132:788–800.

[65] Simone DA, Baumann TK, LaMotte RH. Dose-dependent pain and mechanical hyperalgesia in humans after intradermal injection of capsaicin. Pain 1989;38:99–107.

[66] Smedra-Kazmirska A, Zydek L, Barzdo M, Machala W, Berent J. [Accidental intravenous injection of formaldehyde.] Anestezjol Intens Ter 2009;41:163–5.

[67] Stein AT, Ufret-Vincenty CA, Hua L, Santana LF, Gordon SE. Phosphoinositide 3-kinase binds to TRPV1 and mediates NGF-stimulated TRPV1 trafficking to the plasma membrane. J Gen Physiol 2006;128:509–22.

[68] Svensson P, Cairns BE, Wang K, Arendt-Nielsen L. Injection of nerve growth factor into human masseter muscle evokes long-lasting mechanical allodynia and hyperalgesia. Pain 2003;104:241–7.

[69] Svensson P, Wang K, Arendt-Nielsen L, Cairns BE. Effects of NGF-induced muscle sensitization on proprioception and nociception. Exp Brain Res 2008;189:1–10.

[70] Sycha T, Gustorff B, Lehr S, Tanew A, Eichler HG, Schmetterer L. A simple pain model for the evaluation of analgesic effects of NSAIDs in healthy subjects. Br J Clin Pharmacol 2003;56:165–72.

[71] Tegeder I, Meier S, Burian M, Schmidt H, Geisslinger G, Lotsch J. Peripheral opioid analgesia in experimental human pain models. Brain 2003;126:1092–102.

[72] Thyregod HG, Rowbotham MC, Peters M, Possehn J, Berro M, Petersen KL. Natural history of pain following herpes zoster. Pain 2007;128:148–56.

[73] Troster A, Sittl R, Singler B, Schmelz M, Schuttler J, Koppert W. Modulation of remifentanil-induced analgesia and postinfusion hyperalgesia by parecoxib in humans. Anesthesiology 2006;105:1016–23.

[74] Vinik HR, Kissin I. Rapid development of tolerance to analgesia during remifentanil infusion in humans. Anesth Analg 1998;86:1307–11.

[75] Wasner G, Schattschneider J, Binder A, Baron R. Topical menthol: a human model for cold pain by activation and sensitization of C nociceptors. Brain 2004;127:1159–71.

[76] Weber M, Birklein F, Neundorfer B, Schmelz M. Facilitated neurogenic inflammation in complex regional pain syndrome. Pain 2001;91:251–7.

[77] Wolskee PJ, Gracely RH, Sayer MJ, Dubner R. Effect of morphine on experimental pain and measures of clinical pain in chronic pain patients. Pain 1981;11:S155.

[78] Zhang Q, Sitzman LA, Al-Hassani M, Cai S, Pollok KE, Travers JB, Hingtgen CM. Involvement of platelet-activating factor in ultraviolet B-induced hyperalgesia. J Invest Dermatol 2009;129:167–74.

[79] Zhuang ZY, Xu H, Clapham DE, Ji RR. Phosphatidylinositol 3-kinase activates ERK in primary sensory neurons and mediates inflammatory heat hyperalgesia through TRPV1 sensitization. J Neurosci 2004;24:8300–9.

Correspondence to: Professor Martin Schmelz, MD, Department of Anesthesiology and Intensive Care Medicine, Medical Faculty Mannheim, University of Heidelberg, Theodor-Kutzer-Ufer 1-3, 68167 Mannheim, Germany. Email: martin.schmelz@medma.uni-heidelberg.de.

The Logic of Animal Models

Gary J. Bennett, PhD

*Department of Anesthesia, Faculty of Dentistry, and the Alan Edwards Centre for Research on Pain,
McGill University, Montreal, Quebec, Canada*

Why Animals?

We use animal pain models for two reasons: to explore the basic physiological mechanisms that underlie pain and pain pathology and to develop analgesic drugs. In both cases, we have little or no interest in the animal. Instead, we are interested in understanding human pain and human analgesics; so why not use people? Of course, we do use people for some experiments. For example, there is now a very large research program devoted to mapping pain responses with brain imaging methods, and the efficacy of all new analgesics must be validated by a clinical trial in pain patients. But there are obvious ethical, safety, and cost reasons that preclude many types of experiments in human beings, and in such cases an animal is the alternative. Two questions arise from this practical necessity. First, is the animal alternative a valid source of knowledge about human pain or a waste of time? Second, if the animal alternative is valid, is it possible to measure pain in an animal?

The Similarity Principle

No one questions the validity of testing the efficacy of a new sunscreen on pig's skin, or investigating the pathophysiology of hypertension in a mouse. But pain is a phenomenon of the nervous system, and while nearly everyone is prepared to accept the hypothesis that our skin and our arteries are fundamentally identical to those of other mammals, we are all aware that it is our nervous system that most clearly differentiates us from the rest of the animal kingdom. It is obviously true that the human nervous system is not exactly the same as a rat's. We can say with equal certainty that the nervous system of a mouse is not exactly the same as a rat's; no two species will have exactly the same nervous systems.

But "exactly the same" misses the point: what we need to know is whether those regions of the nervous system that participate in the sensation of pain are similar in humans compared to rats (or mice or cats). If they are similar, then information from animal experiments will be useful to understanding the human case, and the degree of usefulness will be a function of the degree of similarity. I will refer to this as the "similarity principle." Our current knowledge is overwhelmingly supportive of the similarity principle, and it indicates that the degree of similarity is quite high for at least some aspects of human pain.

Consider the anatomy. Human brain imaging studies have found over a dozen regions of the brain that are activated by a noxious stimulus. Every single one of these areas was previously identified as pain-responsive in animal experiments; there are no "new" pain regions in humans. Or consider the pain inhibitory circuit involving neurons in the periaqueductal gray matter (PAG). Forty years ago, the PAG was an enigmatic region of the mid-brain with no known function. Reynolds [21] implanted a microelectrode into the PAG of a rat and observed that electrical stimulation of this region in the awake and unrestrained animal did not produce any obvious change in behavior; the rat continued to walk about its cage, eating, grooming, and so on. However, Reynolds found that during and for several minutes after PAG stimulation, the rat was completely unresponsive to incision of the abdomen. Mayer and colleagues [13], and subsequently many other laboratories, showed that this brain-stimulation-evoked analgesia was indeed specific to pain sensation, was blocked or reversed by the morphine antagonist, naloxone, and was due to activation of a pain-inhibiting system that included the PAG and the serotonergic raphe nuclei in the medulla. When neurosurgeons implanted an electrode in the PAG of patients with intractable cancer pain, they also found that stimulation produced analgesia both during and after stimulation and that this analgesia was also antagonized by naloxone (e.g., ref. [9]). Importantly, the effect in humans was also specific; that is, the patient's other sensations, movements, thinking, and feelings were not changed. Despite its efficacy, PAG stimulation did not prove to be a practical clinical method of pain relief. But the important point here is that electrical stimulation of an obscure region of the brain produces a specific and naloxone-reversible analgesia in both rats and humans. How could that be true if there were not fundamental similarities in the wiring of pain-related regions of the nervous system of humans and animals?

If the similarity principle is true for normal pain processing, then it follows that pain pathology will also be similar in humans and animals. The story of gabapentin highlights this idea. The analgesic efficacy of gabapentin for neuropathic pain was discovered accidentally. Two patients who had the misfortune of having both epilepsy and painful peripheral neuropathy had their epilepsy treatment switched to gabapentin, which was then a new antiepileptic drug. To their physician's surprise, gabapentin reduced the patients' neuropathic pain [14]. Subsequent work in the rat chronic constriction injury (CCI) and the spinal nerve injury (Chung) models of painful peripheral neuropathy confirmed that gabapentin inhibited allodynia and hyperalgesia [10,29], and subsequent randomized, placebo-controlled, double-blind clinical trials validated the clinical anecdote and the animal work. Additional animal work showed

that gabapentin's action was associated with its binding to the $\alpha_2\delta$ subunit of calcium channels. These channels were found to be located in the spinal cord dorsal horn and dorsal root ganglia of both rats and humans. A drug development program based on $\alpha_2\delta$ binding and screening in an animal neuropathic pain model yielded pregabalin (for review, see ref. [19]). Again, how could all of this be true if there were not fundamental similarities in the structure and function of pain-related regions of the nervous system of humans and animals?

The uniqueness of the human nervous system is most pronounced in the evolutionary expansion of the cerebral cortex. But more primitive parts of the brain, for example the brainstem, have changed relatively little. Pain is primitive. Even invertebrates respond to noxious stimuli. Pinch a worm and one observes a withdrawal reflex that is not very different from that evoked by pinching a person. Even bacteria will swim away from an environment that is injuriously hot or acidic. None of this is surprising, because pain has obvious survival value and as such will tend to be preserved as species evolve. The Darwinian perspective is thus strongly supportive of the similarity principle. Pain processing in the human nervous system is very similar to that in the rat or mouse nervous system because we have all evolved from the same primitive mammal.

Exceptions to the Similarity Principle?

We are well aware that the human pain experience is highly complex and not just a sensory phenomenon. At least some aspects of this complexity are certainly not present in lower animals. For example, only in the human being is pain influenced by its context. A new pain in the abdomen evokes a different experience in a normal person than in a cancer survivor, and the experience of passing one's first kidney stone is not the same as for one's second. It is likewise obviously true that the human brain is unique in its ability to extrapolate from experience. Thus, the back pain patient does not actually have to play a round of golf to know that it will make his pain worse. The modulation of pain by higher cognitive function is clearly observed developmentally. One might have to observe very carefully to see a pain response in an adult receiving an intramuscular injection (perhaps a slight flinch or grimace), but one can detect an infant's response from the other side of the room.

Between the simple behavioral responses to pain that are shared by humans and animals and the uniquely human pain factors due to higher cognitive function, there are very important aspects of the human pain experience that are probably shared with other mammals to a considerable, but difficult to quantify, extent. Pain evokes fear (anxiety), which has both emotional and motivational characteristics. We have a great deal of information about pain-evoked fear and anxiety, because animal models such as the passive avoidance test (which uses exposure to a painful electric shock) are routinely used to screen for antianxiety drugs. I would guess that every antianxiety drug on the market today was first shown to be active in a rat or mouse in the passive avoidance test or a similar test. The relationship between animal and human fear/anxiety is nicely paralleled by the animal-human pain relationship. Of course animals experience fear/anxiety and of course people do too, although the possession of higher cognitive functions makes human fear/anxiety a more complicated thing. The argument described above also applies to pain-evoked depression, but for depression there is a special difficulty with the pharmacological line of reasoning. A great deal of evidence suggests that at least some antidepressant medications (e.g., amitriptyline, duloxetine) have an analgesic effect that is independent of their direct effect on mood.

Prolonged pain, especially when it is severe, gives rise to what we would generally call "suffering," and the alleviation of suffering is of paramount concern to the clinician. Evidence from animals is limited here. There is near-universal agreement that it is unethical to induce animal suffering, and this principle has been codified in the ethical guidelines of the International Association for the Study of Pain, the U.S. National Institutes of Health, and government funding bodies in countries around the world.

History of the Similarity Principle

There was considerable debate among pain researchers in the 1970s as to whether animal pain was the same as human pain. The result of this debate was a sort of tie. The use of the phrase "painful stimulus" was prohibited and was replaced by "noxious stimulus." This was rather beside the point but nevertheless an improvement, since "painful stimulus" is simply sloppy language—pain is a property of the organism that is stimulated, not the stimulus.

On the main point, there was general acceptance of a change in nomenclature: humans had pain sensation, animals had nociception; noxious stimulation in humans evoked pain behaviors, noxious stimulation in animals evoked nociceptive behaviors. For many, this change was both accepted and taken as an official recognition of a fundamental difference between pain in animals and pain in humans. For others (for me at least), acceptance of the new nomenclature was actually acquiescence, and the human-animal distinction was understood to be provisional and awaiting more data. Nevertheless, no one abandoned animal pain research as an irrelevancy. Instead, the amount of such work continued to increase steadily, with a very notable shift from studies of the basis of acute pain in normal animals to the persistent pain seen with inflammation and the pathological pain seen with nerve injury [17].

We have much more data now than we had 40 years ago, and one rarely hears the argument that animal pain is fundamentally different from human pain. There are those who continue to stress that the total human pain experience is more complex than that found in an animal. But no one ever claimed that this was not so. However, it seems to me that a new debate has started. It side-steps the similarity principle and instead questions whether our current methods for measuring animal pain are valid in the human context [2,15,16,25,27].

Can We Measure Pain in an Animal?

If we accept the similarity principle it becomes appropriate to study animal pain, but the question remains as to whether it is possible to actually measure pain in an animal. It is instructive to begin thinking about this issue by considering how we measure pain in human beings.

Pain Is a Subjective Phenomenon

It is commonly said that one can never know what is happening in an animal's mind. That is certainly true. But it is equally true that one can never know what is in another person's mind. Mental states are inherently subjective; I have certain knowledge only of my own mental states (and only some of those!). One *infers* the existence of similar or identical mental states in other people, and one measures them by evoking a measurable behavior. Behavior is an objective phenomenon. As a matter of convenience, this behavior is usually the spoken word ("My pain is 6 on a 1–10 scale"), or a mark on a line representing pain severity, or the selection of certain words on a list such as the McGill Pain Questionnaire. We find a lawful (and hence useful) relationship between these human behaviors and variables of interest such as the potency of an analgesic drug. Indeed, such relationships between sensation and behavior have been studied for over 150 years, and they form the field of study known as psychophysics. It is well known that psychophysical relationships are not perfect. People make mistakes, are inattentive, uncooperative, and sometimes untruthful. In the United States during the Vietnam War, a draft-age young man could buy instructions and practice tapes to learn how to fail the Draft Board's psychophysical test for hearing acuity. Nevertheless, psychophysical tests are useful. Snell's eye chart for visual acuity, one of the most frequently used medical tests of all time, is a simple psychophysical test. My optician provided me with a very useful set of bifocals by using a simple psychophysical test (the Method-of-Limits with a set of lenses with different indices of refraction). The examination of human pain is a well-developed branch of psychophysics [5], and there is no evidence whatsoever that the psychophysical relationship between noxious stimuli and the pain that they evoke is in any significant way different than the relationships obtained with any other form of stimulation (touch, vision, hearing, etc.).

In conclusion, we may say that pain in a person and in an animal is a subjective phenomenon, but that this subjectivity has relatively little practical importance. We can measure pain in a person, albeit imperfectly, but undeniably in a useful way. Can we say the same of an animal?

Animal Pain Measures

We can ask an animal how much a stimulus hurts, but they never tell us, and they cannot complete a visual analogue scale (VAS) or answer the McGill questionnaire. It is of interest to note that the same problem sometimes occurs with people, for example, newborns [20].

Thus, we must test animal pain in a way that does not rely on language and abstract thinking (the concept of a scale of intensity). There are three possible choices: naturalistic measures, operant measures, and reflex measures.

Naturalistic Measures of Animal Pain

In animals, noxious stimuli evoke certain responses that are not learned (operant), yet are also not obviously reflexive. Many of these responses are shared by man, as Darwin discusses at length in *The Expression*

of the Emotions in Man and Animals [4]. For example, in a person, pain in and around the head (e.g., a toothache or headache), evokes a characteristic response on the side of the pain: the corrugator muscles contract (squeezing the eye shut and raising the corner of the mouth), the jaw clenches, the head tilts to the side, and the shoulder rises to meet the head. Very similar movements (for the face at least) have been described in mice that bear a mutation associated with migraine headaches [12]. Pinch a baby's toe and it cries out. Pinch a rat's toe and it also cries out, although you will not hear the cry because it is ultrasonic [11]. Rats will lick a cut if they can reach it, and if you or I get a cut on our finger we will almost certainly put in our mouth. This is an adaptive response because licking cleans the wound, and saliva is bactericidal.

Naturalistic responses have received relatively little attention (but see refs. [1,11,12]), and it remains to be seen whether they will be of practical use. One can anticipate several problems. For example, these responses are generally associated with pain of sudden onset (or a sudden exacerbation of background pain), and the probability of the response occurring after each stimulus appears to be relatively low (compared to a reflex).

Operant Measures of Animal Pain

It is not difficult for a rat to learn a particular behavioral response that will terminate its exposure to a noxious stimulus. For example, the animal can be placed in a box that has two compartments linked by a communicating doorway. The animal is placed in one compartment that has a temperature-controlled metal floor. When the floor temperature is brought into the noxious range, the animal learns to escape into the adjacent compartment whose floor is at an innocuous temperature [26]. This method gives satisfactory data. The latency to the escape response corresponds fairly well with the threshold for heat activation of nociceptive primary afferents, and the latency to escape decreases when the floor temperature is raised above the afferents' threshold.

This and other operant tests have potential problems. For example, when the animal is walking about on the floor, the exposure to the heat varies from moment to moment as the skin of the paws makes episodic contact with the floor. Moreover, the animal must remember where the door is, remember that exiting through it escapes the noxious stimulus, and be motivated to make the effort of exiting. Thus, a drug that reduces memory retrieval or produces euphoria will appear to be analgesic.

It is certain that operant responses are the result of activity at cortical levels of the neuraxis (motivation, decision making, memory retrieval, etc.). This is often cited as the reason why operant responses are especially relevant to human pain. This may be a weak argument because it pushes the similarity principle too far. It is the cerebral cortex that is most dissimilar in animals and humans. In any case, even if one accepts all of the arguments in favor of operant tests of pain, it is very clear that the method is much more time-consuming than the reflex methods.

The Pain-Related Withdrawal Reflex

Step on a tack and you will experience a withdrawal reflex. Experimentally, the reflex is usually evoked by noxious heat, cold, or mechanical stimulation applied to the tip of the animal's tail (the "tail-flick test") or to the plantar surface of the hind paw (the "paw-withdrawal test"). A very large majority of animal studies use the withdrawal reflex as the pain measure. All modern analgesic discovery programs are based on tests of an animal's withdrawal reflex.

The withdrawal reflex is often said to be a flexor response, and a flexor response is indeed what we often choose to measure, but withdrawal can also be an extensor reflex. For example, if the tack sticks the bottom of your big toe, then the digital and foot extensors will contract, while the flexor hamstrings will contract to lift your foot from the floor. If the pin sticks your heel, then the digital and plantar flexors will contract as well as the hamstring flexors. In both cases, the reflex has a clear purpose: to withdraw the affected body region away from the most likely direction of stimulation.

The withdrawal reflex is sometimes said to be a "simple" reflex. It is actually one of the most complex reflexes. Consider a truly simple reflex, the monosynaptic muscle stretch reflex evoked by tapping a tendon (e.g., the knee-jerk reflex). The afferent limb of the reflex consists of stretch-sensitive primary afferent neurons that innervate the tendon. These neurons enter the spinal cord and synapse directly and exclusively on the motor neurons whose axons innervate the muscle whose tendon has been tapped; no other motor neurons are involved. As described above, the withdrawal reflex usually involves multiple muscles (digit, foot, and thigh). It even evolves contralateral muscles: leg flexion

is accompanied by a crossed reflex of the opposite thigh extensors (which is why stepping on a tack does not cause us to fall down). Nociceptive primary afferents synapse in pools of interneurons, not directly on motor neurons, and these interneurons receive many other inputs, including inputs from the brain [6]. This is why one can consciously suppress the withdrawal reflex, but not a knee jerk. This is also why it is misleading to call the withdrawal reflex a "spinal" reflex. True, the essential components of the circuit are in the spinal cord, but there is considerable supraspinal modulation of the reflex via the interneuron pool.

Possible Dissociation between Pain and the Reflex

The nociceptor input that triggers the withdrawal reflex is the same nociceptor input that drives the transmission neurons whose signals reach the brain and produce pain sensation. But there is at least one clear difference in the connectivity. A-fiber nociceptors make monosynaptic contact with lamina I transmission neurons, and C-fiber nociceptors make monosynaptic contacts with lamina V transmission neurons. There is no evidence for monosynaptic nociceptor input to the motor neurons that evoke the reflex. However, the nociceptor input to transmission neurons, especially in the deeper laminae, is both monosynaptic and polysynaptic. The polysynaptic input comes via a pool of interneurons that receive both A-fiber and C-fiber input. The relation between the interneuron pool that innervates transmission neurons and the interneuron pool that innervates the withdrawal reflex motor neurons is not known. It seems safe to presume that they are at least partly overlapping, but at least some–and perhaps considerable–independence cannot be excluded on the basis of our current knowledge. This gives rise to the possibility of dissociation between the signals that drive the reflex and the signals that are transmitted to the brain.

Such a possibility is of particular concern in the context of testing pain-modifying drugs. A drug that influenced the interneuron pool driving the reflex motor neuron, but had little or no influence on the interneuron pool innervating the transmission neurons, might have an effect on the withdrawal reflex that was distinctly different than its effect on the perception of pain. It is certainly true that many drugs have effects on the motor system that are distinct from their effects on perception. The generally accepted solution to this problem is to select doses that have no effect in a demanding test of motor system function, the rotarod test. This is a valid test because it is known that at least part of the interneuron pool that drives the reflex is also involved in the control of voluntary locomotion [22]. Dissociative drug effects might also involve levels of the nervous system above the spinal interneuron pools. For example, many drugs produce sedation, and sedation is accompanied by hyporeflexia. The generally accepted solution here is to use drug doses that do not cause the animal to fall asleep in the testing environment.

While the existence of potentially confounding dissociative effects is a logical possibility, I know of no well-documented example where such dissociation has been proven to be the basis of an incorrect identification of analgesic efficacy.

Pain and the Withdrawal Reflex in Humans

It is sometimes said that the animal's withdrawal reflex is not a good measure of pain because it is just a reflex—"a reflex is not pain." It is certainly true that the withdrawal reflex is not pain itself. Of course, it is equally true that an operant response is also not pain itself, nor is a person's VAS response. In any case, the objection misses the point; no one has ever claimed that there is a perfect identity between a reflex measure and the subjective experience of pain. Again, the relevant point is the similarity principle: is the animal reflex a useful, albeit imperfect, correlate, or covariant, or indicator, or proxy for what we wish to understand—human pain? The strongest evidence that this is true comes from studies of the reflex in humans.

Noxious stimuli evoke withdrawal reflexes in both people and animals, and it is perfectly possible to measure the human withdrawal reflex and compare it directly to the same subject's report of his pain experience. We do not do this very often for the simple reason that it is inconvenient, but there is nevertheless an extensive literature on the subject (for reviews see refs. [18,22,28]).

A common procedure is to apply transcutaneous electric shocks to the sural nerve at the ankle and electromyographically (EM) record the activity of the flexor muscle in the thigh (note that this test involves the same afferents and muscles as the rat paw withdrawal). An electrical stimulus is of course unnatural,

but it has two advantages. First, its timing and intensity can be controlled with great precision. Second, different functional classes of sensory afferents have distinctly different thresholds for electrical activation. Proprioceptive and touch afferents with large myelinated axons (Aβ fibers) have very low electrical thresholds; the threshold for Aδ myelinated nociceptors is about five times greater than that of the Aβ fibers; and the threshold of unmyelinated C-fiber nociceptors is about 20 times greater.

At low stimulus intensities, the EM recording shows a response (called "RII") whose latency corresponds to a triggering input from large myelinated afferents; the subject reports that these stimulus intensities do not cause pain. Increasing the stimulus intensity into the range that is known to activate myelinated nociceptors evokes a second EM discharge ("RIII") whose latency corresponds to a triggering input from small myelinated nociceptors, and the subject reports that these stimuli do produce pain. Further increases in stimulus intensity produce larger RIII responses, and the subject reports increasingly severe pain. RIII is suppressed by the same interventions (e.g., morphine, diffuse noxious inhibitory controls) that cause the subject to report less pain.

In summary, the threshold stimulus intensity for the subject's reflex is very close to the threshold intensity that elicits the subject's report of pain, and in both cases this stimulus intensity is very close to the threshold for activation of nociceptors. The stimulus-response relationship between stimulus intensity and the subject's reflex magnitude, and the relationship between stimulus intensity and subject's report of pain intensity, are very similar. Analgesic interventions decrease both the subject's reflex magnitude and the intensity of the pain he or she experiences with very similar dose-response relationships. Thus, the human withdrawal reflex is very similar to the human sensation of pain. Why should this not be the same in an animal? While we do not (cannot) have an animal's pain report, it is indeed established that the magnitude of the withdrawal reflex in an unanesthetized rat has a clear relationship to stimulus intensity and that the reflex magnitude is decreased by morphine [3]. A stimulus-response relation even holds in the anesthetized rat [23]. Moreover, it has been shown that the threshold and latency of the rat's withdrawal reflex corresponds to triggering inputs from A-fiber and C-fiber nociceptors [30,31].

What about the NK1 Blockers?

Every discussion about animal pain models eventually gets around to someone citing the clinical failure of substance P receptor (NK1) antagonists as an example of the inadequacy of animal pain models [2,7,8]. This is usually part of a critique of animal models of painful peripheral neuropathy, apparently in ignorance of the fact that clinical trials have not supported preclinical findings of efficacy in postoperative, inflammatory, and neuropathic pain.

Critiques aimed specifically at the animal neuropathic pain models cite the failed clinical trails of Merck's NK1 blocker, MK-869 (previously named L754,030). This compound was designed to block the NK1 receptor found in the guinea pig, whose structure is close to that of the human NK1 receptor (the rat's NK1 receptor is not). It has been stated that MK-869 was never tested in the guinea pig neuropathic pain model [8,24]. I have not been able to find any published data showing that MK-869 was ever tested in a neuropathic pain model in the rat or any other animal. Hill [8] has responded to this issue by replying that: "Although this particular compound was not subjected to such experiments, we have shown that analogues of this compound were active in guinea-pig antinociception tests (see Fig. 2 in Ref. 6)." Ref. 6 in the quotation is to Boyce and Hill [2], in which their Fig. 2 shows the effects of the analogues L733,060 and L733,601 on carrageenan-evoked mechanohyperalgesia. This is not a neuropathic pain model. It is absurd to fault the predictive validity of an animal model if the drug was never tested in an appropriate animal model. Of course, clinical trials can fail for many reasons that have nothing to do with the validity of animal models. A cogent discussion of these issues can be found elsewhere [24]. It is sufficient to say that the NK1-antagonist story is anything but a definitive exception to the similarity principle.

Conclusions

1) Animal models of pain are valid for understanding human pain, pain pathology, and analgesia.

2) Both operant and reflex measures of animal pain give information that is useful in the human context. There is no evidence that either measure is fundamentally superior or more human-like.

3) Neither operant nor reflex measures are perfect (very few things are), and both have potential confounds that must be examined for proper interpretation of the data.

4) No animal model can mirror the entire complexity of the human pain experience. No one claims that they do.

References

[1]   Attal N, Jazat F, Kayser V, Guilbaud G. Further evidence for 'pain-related' behaviours in a model of unilateral peripheral mononeuropathy. Pain 1990;41:235–51.

[2]   Boyce S, Hill RG. Discrepant results from preclinical and clinical studies on the potential of substance P-receptor antagonist compounds as analgesics. In: Devor M, Rowbotham MC, Wiesenfeld-Hallin Z, editors. Proceedings of the 9th World Congress on Pain. Progress in pain research and management, vol. 16. Seattle: IASP Press; 2000. p 313–24.

[3]   Carstens E, Wilson C. Rat tail flick reflex: magnitude measurement of stimulus-response function, suppression by morphine and habituation. J Neurophysiol 1993;70:630–9.

[4]   Darwin C. The expression of the emotions in man and animals. London: John Murray; 1872.

[5]   Gracely RH. Pain measurement. Acta Anaesthesiol Scand 1999;43:897–908.

[6]   Grossman MS, Basbaum AI, Fields HL. Afferent and efferent connections of the rat tail flick reflex (a model used to analyze pain control mechanisms). J Comp Neurol 1982;206:9–16.

[7]   Hill R. NK1 (substance P) receptor antagonists: why are they not analgesic in humans? Trends Pharmacol Sci 2000;21:244–6.

[8]   Hill R. Reply: will changing the testing paradigms show that NK1 receptor antagonists are analgesic in humans? Trends Pharmacol Sci 2000;21:265.

[9]   Hosobuchi Y, Adams JE, Linchitz R. Pain relief by electrical stimulation of the central gray matter in humans and its reversal by naloxone. Science 1977;197:183–6.

[10] Hwang JH, Yaksh TL. Effect of subarachnoid gabapentin on tactile-evoked allodynia in a surgically induced neuropathic pain model in the rat. Reg Anesth 1997;22:249–56.

[11] Jourdan D, Ardid D, Chapuy E, Le Bars D, Eschalier A. Effect of analgesics on audible and ultrasonic pain-induced vocalization in the rat. Life Sci 1998;63:1761–8.

[12] Langford DJ, Bailey AL, Chanda ML, Clarke SE, Drummond TE, Echols S, Glick S, Ingrao J, Klassen-Ross T, LaCroix-Fralish ML, Matsumiya L, Sorge RE, Sotocinal SG, Tabaka JM, Wong D, van den Maagdenberg AMJM, Ferrari MD, Craig KD, Mogil JS. Coding of facial expressions of pain in the laboratory mouse. Nat Methods 2010; in press.

[13] Mayer DJ, Wolfle TL, Akil H, Carder B, Liebeskind JC. Analgesia from electrical stimulation in the brainstem of the rat. Science 1971;174:1351–4.

[14] Mellick LB, Mellick GA. Successful treatment of reflex sympathetic dystrophy with gabapentin. Am J Emerg Med 1995;13:96.

[15] Mogil JS. Animal models of pain: progress and challenges. Nat Rev Neurosci 2009;10:283–94.

[16] Mogil JS, Crager SE. What should we be measuring in behavioral studies of chronic pain in animals? Pain 2004;112:12–5.

[17] Mogil JS, Simmonds K, Simmonds MJ. Pain research from 1975 to 2007: a categorical and bibliometric meta-trend analysis of every research paper published in the journal, *Pain*. Pain 2009;142:48–58.

[18] Neziri AY, Andersen OK, Petersen-Felix S, Radanov B, Dickenson AH, Scaramozzino P, Arendt-Nielsen L, Curatolo M. The nociceptive withdrawal reflex: normative values of thresholds and reflex receptive fields. Eur J Pain 2010;14:134–41.

[19] Perret D, Luo ZD. Targeting voltage-gated calcium channels for neuropathic pain management. Neurotherapeutics 2009;6:679–92.

[20] Ranger M, Johnston CC, Anand KJ. Current controversies regarding pain assessment in neonates. Semin Perinatol 2007;31:283–8.

[21] Reynolds DV. Surgery in the rat during electrical analgesia induced by focal brain stimulation. Science 1969;164:444–5.

[22] Sandrini G, Serrao M, Rossi P, Romaniello A, Cruccu G, Willer JC. The lower limb flexion reflex in humans. Prog Neurobiol 2005;77:353–95.

[23] Tsuruoka M, Matsui A, Matsui Y. Quantitative relationship between the stimulus intensity and the response magnitude in the tail flick reflex. Physiol Behav 1988;43:79–83.

[24] Urban LA, Fox AJ. NK1 receptor antagonists: are they really without effect in the pain clinic? Trends Pharmacol Sci 2000;21:462–4.

[25] Vierck CJ, Hansson PT, Yezierski RP. Clinical and pre-clinical pain assessment: are we measuring the same thing? Pain 2008;135:7–10.

[26] Vierck CJ Jr, Kline R 4th, Wiley RG. Comparison of operant escape and innate reflex responses to nociceptive skin temperatures produced by heat and cold stimulation of rats. Behav Neurosci 2004;118:627–35.

[27] Villaneuva L. Is there a gap between preclinical and clinical studies of analgesia? Trends Pharmacol Sci 2000;21:461–2.

[28] Willer JC. Clinical exploration of nociception with the use of reflexologic techniques. Neurophysiol Clin 1990;20:335–56.

[29] Xiao WH, Bennett GJ. Gabapentin has an antinociceptive effect mediated via a spinal site of action in a rat model of painful peripheral neuropathy. Analgesia 1996;2:267–73.

[30] Yeomans DC, Pirec V, Proudfit HK. Nociceptive responses to high and low rates of noxious cutaneous heating are mediated by different nociceptors in the rat: behavioral evidence. Pain 1996;68:133–40.

[31] Yeomans DC, Proudfit HK. Nociceptive responses to high and low rates of noxious cutaneous heating are mediated by different nociceptors in the rat: electrophysiological evidence. Pain 1996;68:141–50.

Correspondence to: Gary J. Bennett, PhD, McIntyre Building, Room 1202, McGill University, 3655 Promenade Sir Wm. Osler, Montreal, Quebec, Canada H3G 1Y6. Email: gary.bennett@mcgill.ca.

Part 6

Basics, Management, and Treatment of Complex Regional Pain Syndrome

Complex Regional Pain Syndrome: A Neuropathic Disorder?

Ralf Baron, Dr med, Dennis Naleschinski, Dr med,
Philipp Hüllemann, Dr med, and Friederike Mahn, Dr med

*Division of Neurological Pain Research and Therapy, Department of Neurology,
University Hospital Schleswig-Holstein, Kiel, Germany*

Definition and Clinical Characteristics of Complex Regional Pain Syndrome

S. Weir Mitchell observed that about 10% of American Civil War patients with traumatic partial peripheral nerve injuries in the distal extremity had a dramatic clinical syndrome [31], which he named causalgia. These patients described prominent, distal, spontaneous burning pain, and their distal extremity showed considerable swelling, smoothness and mottling of the skin, and, in some cases, acute arthritis. Early in the 20th century, similar signs and symptoms were reported in a group of patients without detectable nerve injury [41]. This entity was later named reflex sympathetic dystrophy [13]. These two clinical pain syndromes, causalgia (CRPS-II) and reflex sympathetic dystrophy (CRPS-I), are now subsumed under the term "complex regional pain syndrome" (CRPS).

A U.S. population-based study on CRPS-I calculated an incidence of about 5.5 per 100,000 person-years at risk and a prevalence of about 21 per 100,000 [37]. In contrast, a European population-based study determined a much higher incidence of 26.2 for CRPS in general when using a different diagnostic approach [10].

In CRPS-I a trauma affecting the distal part of an extremity is the most common precipitating event—especially fractures, postsurgical conditions, contusions, and strains or sprains. Central nervous system (CNS) lesions, such as spinal cord injuries and cerebrovascular accidents, as well as cardiac ischemia, are less common. CRPS type II (causalgia) develops after injury to a major peripheral nerve.

In both forms patients develop asymmetric distal-extremity pain. They often report feeling burning spontaneous pain in the distal part of the affected extremity. Characteristically, the pain is disproportionate in intensity to the inciting event. The pain usually increases when the extremity is in a drooping position. Stimulus-evoked pain is a striking clinical feature. These sensory abnormalities often appear early, are most pronounced distally, and have no consistent spatial relationship to individual nerve territories or to the site of the inciting lesion. Typically pain can be elicited by movement of and pressure on the joints (deep somatic allodynia), even if the joints are not directly affected by the inciting lesion. *Autonomic abnormalities* include swelling and changes in sweating and skin blood flow [38,47]. The acute distal swelling of the affected limb depends very critically on aggravating stimuli. Since the swelling may diminish after sympathetic blocks it is likely that it is maintained by sympathetic activity. *Trophic changes* such as abnormal nail growth, increased or decreased hair growth, fibrosis, thin glossy skin, and osteoporosis may be present, particularly in chronic stages. Weakness of all muscles of the affected distal extremity is often present. Small accurate movements are characteristically impaired [26]. About half of the patients have a postural or action tremor representing an increased physiological tremor. In about 10% of cases, dystonia of the affected hand or foot develops [45].

Classification of CRPS

In the past few decades there has been absolutely no doubt that CRPS types I and II have to be classified as neuropathic pain disorders. The reasons were obvious. First, sensory signs and symptoms, in particular thermal and mechanical hyperalgesia, are very similar to other neuropathic pain disorders such as painful diabetic neuropathy and postherpetic neuralgia. Second, CRPS fits nicely into the 1994 International Association for the Study of Pain (IASP) definition of neuropathic pain, "pain initiated or caused by a primary lesion or dysfunction in the nervous system" [30], in which the abnormal sensory perceptions of the patients relate to the dysfunctional nervous system.

This situation dramatically changed, however, when a proposal to redefine neuropathic pain states was published recently in the journal *Neurology*. In this paper the authors suggest replacing the current definition of neuropathic pain with the following: "pain arising as a direct consequence of a lesion or disease affecting the somatosensory system" [42]. Importantly, they deleted the term "dysfunction" from this new definition. Furthermore, since a gold standard for the diagnosis of CRPS is still lacking, they proposed a clinical grading system of definite, probable, and possible neuropathic pain.

This new attempt to redefine neuropathic pain creates several problems in the classification of CRPS. By definition, in CRPS-II a peripheral nerve lesion is present, thus fulfilling the new definition of a neuropathic disorder. However, if the grading system of certainty for neuropathic pain is applied, CRPS-II fails to qualify as neuropathic pain because the pain, which is characteristically generalized in the distal extremity, does not have a distinct neuroanatomically plausible distribution (i.e., Criterion 1 is not fulfilled). Even more problematic is the situation with CRPS-I. In this entity a disease or lesion of a major peripheral nerve is not demonstrable, which does not match the new definition of neuropathic pain. In the grading system neither of the two major criteria, "pain with a distinct neuroanatomically plausible distribution" and "a history suggestive of

Table I
Revised diagnostic criteria for CRPS

Categories of Clinical Signs/Symptoms

1) Positive sensory abnormalities
     spontaneous pain
     mechanical hyperalgesia
     thermal hyperalgesia
     deep somatic hyperalgesia
2) Vascular abnormalities
     vasodilation
     vasoconstriction
     skin temperature asymmetries
     skin color changes
3) Edema, sweating abnormalities
     swelling
     hyperhidrosis
     hypohidrosis
4) Motor, trophic changes
     motor weakness
     tremor
     dystonia
     coordination deficits
     nail, hair changes
     skin atrophy
     joint stiffness
     soft tissue changes

Interpretation for Clinical Use

≥1 symptom of ≥3 categories each
AND ≥1 sign of ≥2 categories each
Sensitivity 0.85   Specificity 0.60

Interpretation for Research Use

≥1 symptom of 4 categories each
AND ≥1 sign of ≥2 categories each
Sensitivity 0.70   Specificity 0.96

a relevant lesion or disease affecting the peripheral or central somatosensory nervous system," are fulfilled, clearly excluding the presence of neuropathic pain in CRPS-I.

In fact, the exclusion of CRPS from neuropathic pain disorders was done on purpose. The authors argue that CRPS are not well-defined clinical entities, and their underlying pathophysiological mechanisms are largely unclear. Including these poorly understood entities into clinical studies might confuse the issue and obscure the results. Furthermore, the authors state that "controversy over whether diseases such as complex regional pain syndrome type I constitute neuropathic pain cannot be resolved by the process of formulating a definition. These issues must be decided on the basis of evidence from scientific research into the pathophysiology of these clinical entities. A definition of neuropathic pain, however, should include a set of rules on how such new scientific findings will lead to a decision one way or the other." The question arises, therefore, as to what scientific evidence already exists to help classifying CRPS as neuropathic or not.

Evidence for a Neuropathic Disorder

Similar Sensory Phenotypes— Similar Mechanisms?

As mentioned before, several sensory phenomena of CRPS-I patients are identical to those present in classical painful neuropathies—that is, postherpetic neuralgia or painful diabetic neuropathy—although in CRPS-I no overt nerve lesion is demonstrable. Based on numerous experimental findings in neuropathic animals with mechanical nerve lesions, spontaneous pain and various forms of hyperalgesia in CRPS are thought to be generated by processes of peripheral and central sensitization.

For example, the sensory symptom "cold hyperalgesia," which is very frequent in advanced stages of CRPS (affecting 30% of patients), is very likely to be caused by a combination of peripheral sensitization of cold-sensing C-fiber nociceptors and secondary central sensitization of second-order neurons. Patients have normal cold sensation, severe burning pain upon application of small amounts of menthol, a decreased threshold to painful cold stimuli, and a reduced threshold to punctate mechanical stimuli. An upregulation of cold- and menthol-sensitive transient receptor potential channels (TRPM8) may lead to peripheral sensitization of cold-sensitive C-fiber nociceptors. It is very likely that this mechanism may also play an important role in the pathophysiology of clinical cold pain and hyperalgesia in CRPS.

Mechanical nerve lesions in neuropathic animal models induce a pathological catecholamine sensitivity of afferent fibers, a mechanism that is thought to be the basis of sympathetically maintained pain (SMP). Clinical studies in CRPS patients support the idea that in CRPS-I, without a nerve lesion, nociceptors also may develop catecholamine sensitivity. We performed a study in patients with CRPS-I using physiological stimuli of the sympathetic nervous system. Cutaneous sympathetic vasoconstrictor outflow to the painful extremity was experimentally activated to the highest possible physiological degree by whole-body cooling. During the thermal challenge the affected extremity was clamped at 35°C in order to avoid thermal effects at the nociceptor level. The intensity as well as the area of spontaneous pain and mechanical hyperalgesia (dynamic and punctate) increased significantly in patients who had been classified as having SMP by positive sympathetic blocks but not in patients with sympathetically independent pain [3]. The experimental setup used in the study selectively alters sympathetic cutaneous vasoconstrictor activity without influencing other sympathetic systems innervating the extremities; that is, piloerector, sudomotor and muscle vasoconstrictor neurons. Therefore, the interaction of sympathetic and afferent neurons measured here is likely to be located within the skin.

The fact that there are aspects of the pain in CRPS (e.g., hyperalgesia, allodynia, and adrenergic sensitivity) similar to neuropathic pain in better-characterized neurological syndromes does not necessarily indicate identical underlying mechanisms. However, from a clinical point of view, it is hard to believe that the hyperalgesia in CRPS and postherpetic neuralgia do not share mechanistic similarities. As long as this distinction remains unclear, it might be appropriate for any clinical trial to separately analyze treatment effect for those pain disorders with a known neurological cause and those without.

CRPS and Small-Fiber Neuropathy

Although CRPS-I is defined by the absence of any major nerve lesion, recent studies indicate that in some of the patients, the nerve damage may be restricted to small afferent fibers in the periphery. Oaklander and colleagues studied 18 patients with CRPS-I affecting the arms and legs. They used skin punch biopsies to assess the afferent small-fiber innervation of the epidermis. They demonstrated a reduction of the axonal small-fiber density of 29% in the CRPS-affected skin sites as compared with the control skin sites, with a huge interindividual variance [32]. A second study by Albrecht and colleagues examined glabrous as well as hairy skin samples of the amputated upper and lower extremity in two CRPS-I patients. The authors found that the CRPS-affected skin areas showed an impressive change in the innervation of the different target tissues, as well as changes in the target itself [1].

Although these findings have not been received without controversy [4], both studies indicate that CRPS can be associated with pathological peripheral changes in the afferent innervation of the skin, and thus they support the concept that CRPS-I is a neuropathic condition.

Evidence for Non-Neuropathic Processes in CRPS

Some of the clinical features of CRPS, particularly in its early phase (i.e., heat, pain, redness, disturbance of function, and swelling), suggest that the pathological extremity is exhibiting an excessive inflammatory process. The idea of an inflammatory process, in particular in the deep somatic tissues, including bones, goes back to Sudeck, who believed that this syndrome is an inflammatory bone atrophy ("entzündliche Knochenatrophie") [41]. Clinical trials have shown that free-radical scavengers can reduce signs and symptoms of CRPS, indirectly suggesting that free radicals and increased oxidative stress are involved in the pathogenesis of the syndrome. Accordingly, levels of antioxidants are elevated in the serum and saliva of patients with CRPS [12]. There are now several lines of evidence supporting an inflammatory etiology in CRPS.

Immune-Cell-Mediated Inflammation and Cytokine Release

Several studies in CRPS patients address the extent to which an immune-cell-mediated inflammation is involved [5,43]. Skin biopsies in these patients show a striking increase in the number of Langerhans cells, which can release immune cell chemoattractants and proinflammatory cytokines. Moreover, in the fluid of artificially produced skin blisters, significantly higher levels of interleukin (IL)-6 and tumor necrosis factor-α (TNF-α), as well as tryptase (a measure of mast cell activity), were observed in the involved extremity compared with the uninvolved extremity [20]. In CRPS patients with hyperalgesia, higher levels of the soluble (TNF-α) receptor type I were found [27]. Accordingly, a significant increase in IL-1β and IL-6, but not TNF-α, was demonstrated in the cerebrospinal fluid of individuals afflicted with CRPS as compared with controls [2]. However, cytokine levels were not correlated with clinical features of CRPS [49]. The patchy osteoporosis that is found in more advanced CRPS cases may also be consistent with a regional inflammatory process in deep somatic tissues. Both IL-1 and IL-6 cause proliferation and activation of osteoclasts and suppress the activity of osteoblasts. Based on this concept, two case reports have described beneficial results with anti-TNF antibodies (infliximab) [6].

Autoimmunity in CRPS

Several other studies have focused on an autoimmune response in patients with CRPS. A recent study by Kohr and colleagues showed that about 30–40% of CRPS patients have surface-binding auto-antibodies against an inducible autonomic nervous system auto-antigen [8,23].

Neurogenic Inflammation and Nociceptor Sensitization

Because autoimmunity and infection have not been shown to account for the inflammatory reactions in CRPS, an exaggerated neurogenic inflammation has been proposed. Axon reflex vasodilatation was significantly increased on the affected side when measured with laser Doppler flowmetry after electrical C-fiber stimulation. Systemic calcitonin gene-related peptide (CGRP) levels were found to be increased in acute CRPS, but not in chronic stages [7]. Also, increased axon reflex sweating could be explained by nociceptor sensitization-related release of CGRP from nociceptive terminals acting on peripheral sweat glands [7].

In patients with acute, untreated CRPS-I, axon reflex activation was elicited by strong transcutaneous electrical stimulation of peptidergic unmyelinated afferents via intradermal microdialysis capillaries. Protein extravasation that was simultaneously assessed by the microdialysis system was only provoked on the affected extremity as compared with the normal side. The time course of electrically induced protein extravasation in the patients resembled that observed following application of exogenous substance P [48].

Plasma extravasation has also been demonstrated with other experimental techniques. Bone scintigraphy demonstrated periarticular tracer uptake in acute CRPS [24], and analysis of joint fluid and synovial biopsies in CRPS patients have shown an increase in protein concentration and synovial hypervascularity [35]. Furthermore, synovial effusion was enhanced in affected joints, as measured with magnetic resonance imaging (MRI) [18]. Scintigraphic investigations with radiolabeled immunoglobulins have shown extensive plasma extravasation [33].

A recent study using a retrospective case-control design examined the association between angiotensin-converting enzyme (ACE) inhibitors taken for cardiovascular indications and CRPS in a large cohort of Dutch subjects [11]. The background is that substance P can stimulate immunological responses, and when released from nerve endings in the dorsal horn, it mediates central sensitization. Another important peptide is bradykinin, which is involved in acute and chronic inflammatory responses as well as in peripheral nociceptor sensitization. Interestingly, ACE is one of the most important kinases involved in the inactivation of substance P and bradykinin. Therefore, ACE inhibitors would be able to increase the levels of these proinflammatory peptides. De Mos and colleagues found a positive dose- and duration-dependent association between ACE inhibitors and the risk of developing CRPS. The hypothesis is that ACE inhibitors may not affect the initiation of the neuro-inflammatory response, but rather develop the inflammatory response to a point where it becomes pathological [11].

Pharmacological Therapy for CRPS

Few evidence-based clinical trials for CRPS are available (Table II). In fact, three literature reviews of outcome studies found discouragingly little consistent information regarding the pharmacological agents and methods for treatment of CRPS [14]. Moreover, the methodology is often of low quality within the studies available. In the absence of more specific information about pathophysiological mechanisms and treatment of CRPS, we have to mainly rely on outcomes from treatment studies for other neuropathic pain syndromes.

Nonsteroidal Anti-Inflammatory Drugs

Nonsteroidal anti-inflammatory drugs (NSAIDs) have not been investigated in the treatment of CRPS thus far. However, from clinical experience it is clear that they can control mild-to-moderate pain.

Opioids

Opioids are clearly effective in postoperative, inflammatory, and cancer pain. The use of opioids in CRPS has not been studied. In other neuropathic pain syndromes, compounds such as tramadol, morphine, oxycodone, and levorphanol are clearly analgesic when compared to placebo. However, there are no long-term studies of the use of oral opioids for treatment of neuropathic pain, CRPS included. Even without solid scientific evidence, the expert opinion of pain clinicians is that opioids could be and should be used as a part of comprehensive pain

Table II
Evidence-based treatment of CRPS

Method	Evidence	Dose (Adults)	Comments
Bisphosphonates	↑↑		
Alendronate		40 mg/day for 8 weeks	In the morning, fasting
Pamidronate		60 mg i.v. single dose	
Clodronate		300 mg/day i.v. for 10 days	
Steroids	↑↑		
Prednisolone		100 mg/day	Taper over 2–3 weeks; no continuous therapy
Methylprednisolone		80 mg/day	
Anti-neuropathic pain drugs			
Gabapentin	↑	1200–2400 (3600) mg/day	
DMSO, topical	↔	50% cream, 5 times/day	Dermal irritations, garlic smell
Physiotherapy/occupational therapy (mirror therapy, motor learning)	↑	Every day, if possible	Must not hurt
Psychotherapy/relaxation techniques	↑		Use if there are signs of psychical comorbidity or chronicity
Sympathetic blocks	↔	2–3 times/week; max. number: 10–15	A series of sympathetic blocks should only be used after a positive diagnostic block
Spinal cord stimulation	↑		Use if there are signs for therapy—refractory pain—no substantial psychological comorbidity
Baclofen, intrathecal	↑		This therapy is advised for dystonia; implant the pump after a test injection; use if there is no substantial psychological comorbidity

treatment program. Given that some patients with neuropathic pain may obtain considerable pain relief, opioids should be prescribed immediately if other agents do not provide sufficient analgesia.

Antidepressants

Antidepressants (tricyclic antidepressants, serotonin-norepinephrine reuptake inhibitors) have been intensively studied in various neuropathic pain conditions, but not in CRPS.

Sodium-Channel-Blocking Agents

Lidocaine administered intravenously is effective in CRPS-I and -II against spontaneous and evoked pain [46]. Other agents of this class, such as carbamazepine and lamotrigine, have not been tested in CRPS.

GABA Agonists

Intrathecally administered baclofen is effective in the treatment of dystonia in CRPS [50]. Oral baclofen has been effective in the treatment of trigeminal neuralgia [15]. No further trials in CRPS are available, and there is no evidence for an analgesic effect of baclofen, valproic acid, vigabatrin, or benzodiazepines in CRPS or other neuropathic pain conditions.

Gabapentin

A randomized, double-blind, placebo-controlled trial demonstrated a mild effect of gabapentin on pain and a good effect on sensory symptoms in CRPS-I [29].

Steroids

Orally administered prednisone, 10 mg three times daily, has clearly demonstrated efficacy in the improvement of general clinical status by up to 75% in patients with acute CRPS (<13 weeks). In CRPS-I following a stroke, 40 mg prednisolone for 14 days improved significantly the signs and symptoms compared to piroxicam 20 mg daily [22].

Immune-Modulating Therapies

Two case reports have reported beneficial results with anti-TNF antibodies (infliximab) [6].

Immunoglobulins

In a case report, a pain reduction of more than 50% was demonstrated, accompanied by cessation of autonomic signs, after intravenous immunoglobulin treatments [21]. A prospective multiple-dose, open-label cohort study was conducted in patients who had a variety of chronic pain syndromes, including CRPS patients. Pain relief of about 70% was found in all major symptom groups when patients were treated with human pooled immunoglobulins. [17].

N-Methyl-D-Aspartate (NMDA) Receptor Blockers

Clinically available compounds that have NMDA receptor-blocking properties include ketamine, dextromethorphan and memantine. A pilot open-label study of the efficacy of subanesthetic ketamine in patients with refractory CRPS showed no effect on pain relief [9]. Another study that used ketamine as an adjuvant in sympathetic blocks for the management of central sensitization indicated relief of allodynia without significant neuropsychiatric side effects [44].

Calcium-Regulating Drugs

Calcitonin administered three times daily intranasally demonstrated a significant pain reduction in CRPS patients [16]. Clodronate 300 mg daily (i.v.) and alendronate 7.5 mg daily (i.v.) produced a significant improvement in pain, swelling, and range of motion in acute CRPS [28]. A recent meta-analysis critically assessed these results and came to the conclusion that further high-quality studies are necessary before such treatment can be generally recommended [19].

A non-placebo-controlled trial showed that calcitonin 200 IU/day together with physiotherapy had the same efficacy as the combination of acetaminophen (paracetamol) 1500 mg/day and physiotherapy [36]. The mode of action of these compounds in CRPS is unknown.

Free Radical Scavengers

A placebo-controlled trial was performed, using the free radical scavengers dimethylsulfoxide 50% (DMSO) topically or N-acetylcysteine (NAC) orally for the treatment of CRPS-I [34]. Both drugs were found to be equally effective, whereas DMSO seemed more favorable for "warm" and NAC for "cold" CRPS-I. The results were negatively influenced by a longer disease duration. A previous trial with DMSO failed to show a positive result in CRPS [51], whereas DMSO has been shown to be more effective than regional blocks with guanethidine in a small population of CRPS patients [25].

Other Agents

Transdermal application of the α_2-adrenoceptor agonist clonidine, which is thought to prevent the release of catecholamines by a presynaptic action, may be helpful when small areas of hyperalgesia are present.

Therapy Guidelines for CRPS

Treatment of CRPS should be immediate and, most importantly, should be directed toward restoration of full function of the extremity. This objective is best attained in a comprehensive interdisciplinary setting with particular emphasis on pain management and functional restoration [39,40]. The pain specialists should include neurologists, anesthesiologists, orthopedic surgeons, physiotherapists, psychologists, and the general practitioner.

The severity of the disease determines the therapeutic regime (Fig. 1). The reduction of pain is the precondition with which all other interventions have to comply. All therapeutic approaches must not cause any pain themselves. At the acute stage of CRPS, when patients still have severe pain at rest and

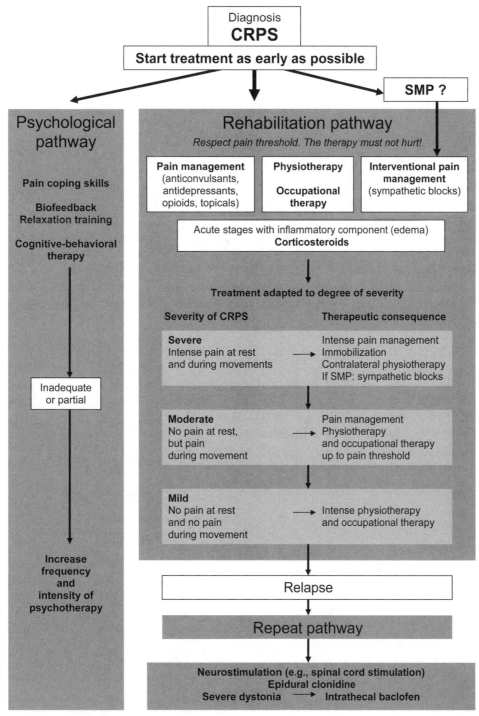

Fig. 1. Therapeutic regime for complex regional pain syndrome (CRPS), based on disease severity. SMP, sympathetically maintained pain.

during movements, it is mostly impossible to carry out intensive active therapy. Painful interventions and in particular aggressive physical therapy at this stage will often lead to deterioration. Therefore, immobilization and careful contralateral physical therapy should be the acute treatment of choice, and intense pain treatment should be initiated immediately. First-line analgesics and coanalgesics are opioids, antidepressants, gabapentin, pregabalin, and carbamazepine. Additionally, corticosteroids should be considered if inflammatory signs and symptoms are predominant. Sympatholytic procedures, preferably sympathetic ganglion blocks, should identify the component of the pain that is maintained by the sympathetic nervous system. For efficacy, a series should be perpetuated. Calcium-regulating agents can be used in cases of refractory pain. If resting pain subsides, at first passive physical therapy, and later active isometric training followed by active isotonic training should be performed in combination with sensory desensitization programs and mirror training until complete motor function is restored. Psychological treatment must accompany the regimen, to strengthen coping strategies and uncover contributing factors. In refractory cases, spinal cord stimulation and epidural clonidine could be considered. If refractory dystonia develops, intrathecal baclofen application is worth considering.

Conclusion

Many questions about CRPS are waiting to be answered. The first and most important step is to gain a deeper insight into the underlying pathophysiological mechanisms. The key questions to be asked in research are: What is the organizing principle leading to this complex syndrome? Can we combine central nervous system changes with neuropathic mechanisms in the periphery and in particular with the inflammatory processes? How does the autoimmune hypothesis fit into this picture? Do different patient subgroups exist that are characterized by a predominant neuropathic component or by a predominant inflammatory component? Do we have to treat these subgroups differently? Can we identify these patient groups in clinical practice?

As long as we do not have a clearer pathophysiological picture of these patients, and because of the obvious heterogeneity of signs, symptoms, and mechanisms, it would be wise to study CRPS separately from other classical neuropathic pain syndromes.

Thus, the new redefinition and grading system of neuropathic pain is an advance from previous guidelines and is likely to be useful for clinical trials. It remains to be seen, however, whether this redefinition will be as useful for the clinician. It is very important to reinforce the authors' statement that the "grading system is for communication among clinicians and researchers and not for medico-legal purposes" [42]. In addition, it would also be a disservice to patients for insurance providers and for those who make decisions on treatment coverage.

References

[1]   Albrecht PJ, Hines S, Eisenberg E, Pud D, Finlay DR, Connolly MK, Pare M, Davar G, Rice FL. Pathologic alterations of cutaneous innervation and vasculature in affected limbs from patients with complex regional pain syndrome. Pain 2006;120:244–66.

[2]   Alexander GM, van Rijn MA, van Hilten JJ, Perreault MJ, Schwartzman RJ. Changes in cerebrospinal fluid levels of pro-inflammatory cytokines in CRPS. Pain 2005;116:213–9.

[3]   Baron R, Binder A, Ulrich W, Maier C. [Complex regional pain syndrome. Reflex sympathetic dystrophy and causalgia]. Nervenarzt 2002;73:305–18; quiz 319.

[4]   Baron R, Janig W. Complex regional pain syndromes: how do we escape the diagnostic trap? Lancet 2004;364:1739–41.

[5]   Baron R, Sommer C, Tölle TR, Birklein F, Wasner G. Diagnostik und Therapie neuropathischer Schmerzen. In: Diener HC, Putzki N, editors. Leitlinien für Diagnostik und Therapie in der Neurologie. Thieme; 2008.

[6]   Bernateck M, Rolke R, Birklein F, Treede RD, Fink M, Karst M. Successful intravenous regional block with low-dose tumor necrosis factor-alpha antibody infliximab for treatment of complex regional pain syndrome 1. Anesth Analg 2007;1148–51.

[7]   Birklein F, Schmelz M, Schifter S, Weber M. The important role of neuropeptides in complex regional pain syndrome. Neurology 2001;57:2179–84.

[8]   Blaes F, Tschernatsch M, Braeu ME, Matz O, Schmitz K, Nascimento D, Kaps M, Birklein F. Autoimmunity in complex regional pain syndrome. Ann NY Acad Sci 2007;1107:168–73.

[9]   Correll GE, Maleki J, Gracely EJ, Muir JJ, Harbut RE. Subanesthetic ketamine infusion therapy: a retrospective analysis of a novel therapeutic approach to complex regional pain syndrome. Pain Med 2004;5:263–75.

[10] de Mos M, de Bruijn AG, Huygen FJ, Dieleman JP, Stricker BH, Sturkenboom MC. The incidence of complex regional pain syndrome: a population-based study. Pain 2007;129:12–20.

[11] de Mos M, Huygen FJ, Stricker BH, Dieleman JP, Sturkenboom MC. The association between ACE inhibitors and the complex regional pain syndrome: suggestions for a neuro-inflammatory pathogenesis of CRPS. Pain 2009;142:218–24.

[12] Eisenberg E, Shtahl S, Geller R, Reznick AZ, Sharf O, Ravbinovich M, Erenreich A, Nagler RM. Serum and salivary oxidative analysis in complex regional pain syndrome. Pain 2008;138:226–32.

[13] Evans JA. Reflex sympathetic dystrophy. Surg Clin North Am 1946;26:435–48.

[14] Forouzanfar T, Koke AJ, van Kleef M, Weber WE. Treatment of complex regional pain syndrome type I. Eur J Pain 2002;6:105–22.

[15] Fromm GH, Terrence CF, Chattha AS. Baclofen in the treatment of trigeminal neuralgia: double-blind study and long-term follow-up. Ann Neurol 1984;15:240–4.

[16] Gobelet C, Waldburger M, Meier JL. The effect of adding calcitonin to physical treatment on reflex sympathetic dystrophy. Pain 1992;48:171–5.

[17] Goebel A, Netal S, Schedel R, Sprotte G. Human pooled immunoglobulin in the treatment of chronic pain syndromes. Pain Med 2002;3:119–27.

[18] Graif M, Schweitzer ME, Marks B, Matteucci T, Mandel S. Synovial effusion in reflex sympathetic dystrophy: an additional sign for diagnosis and staging. Skeletal Radiol 1998;27:262–5.

[19] Hirschl MM, Binder M, Herkner H, Bur A, Brunner M, Seidler D, Stuhlinger HG, Laggner AN. Accuracy and reliability of noninvasive continuous finger blood pressure measurement in critically ill patients. Crit Care Med 1996;24:1684–9.

[20] Huygen FJ, De Bruijn AG, De Bruin MT, Groeneweg JG, Klein J, Zijlstra FJ. Evidence for local inflammation in complex regional pain syndrome type 1. Mediators Inflamm 2002;11:47–51.

[21] Huygen FJ, Niehof S, Zijlstra FJ, van Hagen PM, van Daele PL. Successful treatment of CRPS 1 with anti-TNF. J Pain Symptom Manage 2004;27:101–3.

[22] Kalita J, Vajpayee A, Misra UK. Comparison of prednisolone with piroxicam in complex regional pain syndrome following stroke: a randomized controlled trial. QJM 2006;99:89–95.

[23] Kohr D, Tschernatsch M, Schmitz K, Singh P, Kaps M, Schafer KH, Diener M, Mathies J, Matz O, Kummer W, Maihofner C, Fritz T, Birklein F, Blaes F. Autoantibodies in complex regional pain syndrome bind to a differentiation-dependent neuronal surface autoantigen. Pain 2009;143:246–51.

[24] Leitha T, Korpan M, Staudenherz A, Wunderbaldinger P, Fialka V. Five phase bone scintigraphy supports the pathophysiological concept of a subclinical inflammatory process in reflex sympathetic dystrophy. Q J Nucl Med 1996;40:188–93.

[25] Livingstone JA, Atkins RM. Intravenous regional guanethidine blockade in the treatment of post-traumatic complex regional pain syndrome type 1 (algodystrophy) of the hand. J Bone Joint Surg Br 2002;84:380–6.

[26] Maihofner C, Baron R, DeCol R, Binder A, Birklein F, Deuschl G, Handwerker HO, Schattschneider J. The motor system shows adaptive changes in complex regional pain syndrome. Brain 2007;130:2671–87.

[27] Maihofner C, Handwerker HO, Neundorfer B, Birklein F. Mechanical hyperalgesia in complex regional pain syndrome: a role for TNF-alpha? Neurology 2005;65:311–3.

[28] Manicourt DH, Brasseur JP, Boutsen Y, Depreseux G, Devogelaer JP. Role of alendronate in therapy for posttraumatic complex regional pain syndrome type I of the lower extremity. Arthritis Rheum 2004;50:3690–7.

[29] Mellick LB, Mellick GA. Successful treatment of reflex sympathetic dystrophy with gabapentin. Am J Emerg Med 1995;13:96.

[30] Merskey H, Bogduk N. Classification of chronic pain: descriptions of chronic pain syndromes and definition of terms, 2nd ed. Seattle: IASP Press; 1994.

[31] Mitchell S. Injuries of nerves and their consequences. New York: Dover; 1865.

[32] Oaklander AL, Rissmiller JG, Gelman LB, Zheng L, Chang Y, Gott R. Evidence of focal small-fiber axonal degeneration in complex regional pain syndrome-I (reflex sympathetic dystrophy). Pain 2006;120:235–43.

[33] Oyen WJ, Arntz IE, Claessens RM, Van der Meer JW, Corstens FH, Goris RJ. Reflex sympathetic dystrophy of the hand: an excessive inflammatory response? Pain 1993;55:151–7.

[34] Perez RS, Zuurmond WW, Bezemer PD, Kuik DJ, van Loenen AC, de Lange JJ, Zuidhof AJ. The treatment of complex regional pain syndrome type I with free radical scavengers: a randomized controlled study. Pain 2003;102:297–307.

[35] Renier JC, Arlet J, Bregeon C, Basle M, Seret P, Acquaviva P, Schiano A, Serratrice G, Amor B, May V, Delcambre B, D'Eshoughes JR, Vincent G, Ducastelle, Pawlotsky Y. [The joint in algodystrophy. Joint fluid, synovium, cartilage]. Rev Rhum Mal Osteoartic 1983;50:255–60.

[36] Sahin F, Yilmaz F, Kotevoglu N, Kuran B. Efficacy of salmon calcitonin in complex regional pain syndrome (type 1) in addition to physical therapy. Clin Rheumatol 2006;25:143–8.

[37] Sandroni P, Benrud-Larson LM, McClelland RL, Low PA. Complex regional pain syndrome type I: incidence and prevalence in Olmsted county, a population-based study. Pain 2003;103:199–207.

[38] Schattschneider J, Hartung K, Stengel M, Ludwig J, Binder A, Wasner G, Baron R. Endothelial dysfunction in cold type complex regional pain syndrome. Neurology 2006;67:673–5.

[39] Stanton-Hicks M, Baron R, Boas R, Gordh T, Harden N, Hendler N, Koltzenburg M, Raj P, Wilder R. Complex regional pain syndromes: guidelines for therapy. Clin J Pain 1998;14:155–66.

[40] Stanton-Hicks M, Burton AW, Bruehl SP, Carr DB, Harden RN, Hassenbusch SJ, Lubenow TR, Oakley JC, Racz GB, Raj PP, Rauck RL, Rezai AR. An updated interdisciplinary clinical pathway for CRPS: report of an expert panel. Pain Pract 2002;2:1–16.

[41] Sudeck P. Über die akute (trophoneurotische) Knochenatrophie nach Entzündungen und Traumen der Extremitäten. Dtsh Med Wochenschr 1902;28:336-342.

[42] Treede RD, Jensen TS, Campbell JN, Cruccu G, Dostrovsky JO, Griffin JW, Hansson P, Hughes R, Nurmikko T, Serra J. Neuropathic pain: redefinition and a grading system for clinical and research purposes. Neurology 2008;70:1630–5.

[43] Uceyler N, Eberle T, Rolke R, Birklein F, Sommer C. Differential expression patterns of cytokines in complex regional pain syndrome. Pain 2007;132:195–205.

[44] Ushida T, Tani T, Kanbara T, Zinchuk VS, Kawasaki M, Yamamoto H. Analgesic effects of ketamine ointment in patients with complex regional pain syndrome type 1. Reg Anesth Pain Med 2002;27:524–8.

[45] van Rijn MA, Marinus J, Putter H, van Hilten JJ. Onset and progression of dystonia in complex regional pain syndrome. Pain 2007;130:287–93.

[46] Wallace MS, Ridgeway BM, Leung AY, Gerayli A, Yaksh TL. Concentration-effect relationship of intravenous lidocaine on the allodynia of complex regional pain syndrome types I and II. Anesthesiology 2000;92:75–83.

[47] Wasner G, Schattschneider J, Heckmann K, Maier C, Baron R. Vascular abnormalities in reflex sympathetic dystrophy (CRPS I): mechanisms and diagnostic value. Brain 2001;124:587–99.

[48] Weber M, Birklein F, Neundorfer B, Schmelz M. Facilitated neurogenic inflammation in complex regional pain syndrome. Pain 2001;91:251–7.

[49] Wesseldijk F, Huygen FJ, Heijmans-Antonissen C, Niehof SP, Zijlstra FJ. Tumor necrosis factor-alpha and interleukin-6 are not correlated with the characteristics of complex regional pain syndrome type 1 in 66 patients. Eur J Pain 2008;12:716–21.

[50] Zuniga RE, Perera S, Abram SE. Intrathecal baclofen: a useful agent in the treatment of well-established complex regional pain syndrome. Reg Anesth Pain Med 2002;27:90–3.

[51] Zuurmond WW, Langendijk PN, Bezemer PD, Brink HE, de Lange JJ, van Loenen AC. Treatment of acute reflex sympathetic dystrophy with DMSO 50% in a fatty cream. Acta Anaesthesiol Scand 1996;40:364–7.

Correspondence to: Prof. Dr. med. Ralf Baron, Division of Neurological Pain Research and Therapy, Department of Neurology, University Hospital Schleswig-Holstein, Campus Kiel, Arnold-Heller-Str. 3, Haus 41, 24105 Kiel, Germany. Email: r.baron@neurologie.uni-kiel.de.

Movement Disorders in Complex Regional Pain Syndrome

Jacobus J. van Hilten, MD, PhD

Department of Neurology, Leiden University Medical Center, Leiden, The Netherlands

Complex regional pain syndrome (CRPS) is characterized by poorly controllable pain, swelling, and changes in skin blood flow and sweating that usually develop in the distal limbs [31]. The syndrome, which commonly is preceded by a minor-to-severe trauma or surgical intervention, occurs more frequently in women (~75%) and may occur at all ages [33]. Approximately 25% of patients with CRPS develop movement disorders including loss of voluntary control, bradykinesia, dystonia, myoclonus, and tremor. These disorders may occur very early in the disease course and may even precede the onset of pain and autonomic features of CRPS [53]. The prevalence of movement disorders increases as disease duration lengthens [54]. The recognition that these disorders are an important part of the clinical spectrum of CRPS has led experts to add this motor category to the new criteria set for CRPS [23], which is currently being evaluated in an international multicenter study.

A Role for Psychological Factors?

The neurological or psychiatric origin of the movement disorders that occur in a setting of peripheral tissue injury are still a matter of debate [53]. Several studies have tried to elucidate whether psychological issues may play role in CRPS patients with and without movement disorders. Research on psychological risk factors requires, at the least, a proper control group, along with reliable information regarding the period before onset. However, none of the studies featuring these assets have found differences in psychological characteristics between patients who did and did not develop CRPS after surgery or fractures [16,22,37]. A case-control study, in which patients who developed CRPS were compared with age- and sex-matched patients who did not develop CRPS after a similar trauma, showed that no psychological factors were associated with an increased chance of developing CRPS [33]. Cross-sectional studies in CRPS patients with [38,48] and without [8] dystonia did not find an association with distinct psychological characteristics either, and together these studies do not support the existence of a unique psychological risk profile for CRPS patients with dystonia.

Clinical Characteristics

Several movement disorders may be encountered in CRPS. Loss of voluntary control is frequently experienced by patients suffering weakness or dystonia in CRPS. Typically these patients report: "My mind tells my hand/foot to move, but it won't work" [42]. This feature has been reported in other causes of dystonia [3] and has been ascribed to both dysfunction of attention and abnormal motor function [1,18].

Bradykinesia or slowness of movement is also very common in CRPS patients, even in those who suffer only from pain [53]. Bradykinesia is evaluated by means of repetitive finger/hand or foot tapping. In CRPS patients the performance of these movements is typically slowed and is frequently associated with hesitancies.

Dystonia occurs in approximately 20% of patients with CRPS and is characterized by fixed flexion postures of the fingers (see Fig. 1), wrist, and feet that may vary in severity [42,52]. Patients with dystonia of the hands may show a relative sparing of the first two digits [52]. Dystonia of the lower extremity is usually characterized by inversion and/or plantar flexion of the foot, with or without clawing or scissoring of the toes [42,52]. Abnormal flexion postures that may develop because of structural changes in muscles, ligaments, and tendons (contractures), are a potential pitfall in diagnosing dystonia in CRPS. In dystonia in CRPS, however, passive stretching of affected digits provokes a contraction of the stretched muscle, suggesting stretch reflex hyperexcitability [46].

In patients with CRPS, electromyographic (EMG) monitoring of extremities affected by dystonia

revealed no abnormal EMG activity during rapid-eye-movement (REM) and non-REM sleep, whereas abnormal EMG activity immediately recurred at arousal during awakening [46].

The interval between the onset of CRPS and dystonia in the first affected extremity may vary from less than 1 week in 26% of patients to more than 1 year in 25% of patients [54]. Patients with CRPS and dystonia have a younger age at onset compared to CRPS patients without dystonia and have an increased risk of spread of dystonia to other extremities [54].

Myoclonus (involuntary, sudden, brief, jerk-like contraction of a muscle or muscle group) and tremor are frequently reported by CRPS patients with dystonia, but these dysfunctions rarely occur as the sole or predominant movement disorder [13, 34]. Jerks occur at rest, are aggravated during action, and are frequently associated with tremulousness or dystonia. Electromyography demonstrated a burst duration ranging from 25 to 240 ms, with burst frequencies varying from <1 jerk/second during rest to 20 jerks/second during action [34].

Mechanisms of Disease

Splitting the heterogeneous clinical spectrum of CRPS into clusters of features that are associated with different biological pathways facilitates our understanding of the coherence between the clinical profile and its pathophysiology. Over the last few years, knowledge of differentially involved mechanisms underlying inflammatory, vascular, sensory, and motor features of CRPS has gradually increased.

Tissue injury may excite C and Aδ fibers of sensory nerves and thereby induce neurogenic inflammation [6,24]. Several studies have now provided evidence implicating neurogenic inflammation in CRPS [4,5,29,57]. Because neurogenic inflammation is initiated by sensory nerves, which cannot account directly for the development of movement disorders, it remains unclear as to how peripheral extremity involvement in CRPS could induce these disorders. However, nociceptive neurons in the dorsal horns of the spinal cord may become sensitized (central sensitization) by peripheral tissue injury or inflammation, or by nerve lesions [59]. In central sensitization, the sensitivity of spinal neurons increases, despite a lack of change of afferent input. As a result, pain becomes chronic, and non-noxious stimuli become painful [58]. Central sensitization can be associated with cell death of spinal (inter)neurons and

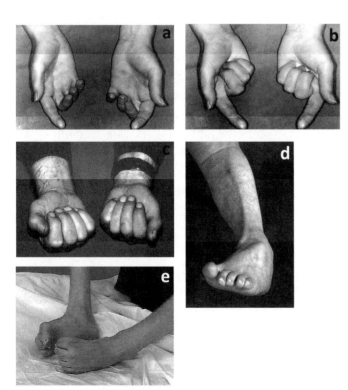

Fig. 1. This figure shows the variable severity of dystonia of the upper and lower limbs. Partial flexion of digits 3–5 (a), severe flexion of digits 3–5 (b), and severe flexion of digits 2–4 (c). Flexion-inversion of the foot (d) and flexion with some inversion of the foot and clawing of the toes (e).

prominent manifestations of neuroplasticity, including reorganization of afferent projections, sensitization of neurons, and changes in synaptic efficacy [58]. It would seem unlikely that central sensitization involves only those pathways that deal with perception of pain and not those that mediate a response to pain. Interestingly, the hazard of developing dystonia in subsequent extremities in patients with CRPS increases with the number of extremities already affected [54]. Apparently, once set into motion, the underlying mechanism of dystonia in CRPS has the capacity to facilitate the occurrence of dystonia in other body parts. This accelerated disease course is a characteristic that may point toward maladaptive neuronal plasticity, as has been documented for pain [60]. Ferguson et al. [15] found that spinal plasticity associated with central sensitization impairs motor behavior mediated by spinal cord circuitry. In line with this finding, patients with unilateral upper extremity CRPS may show bradykinesia and poorer execution of movement in a standardized drawing test of the unaffected extremity [39,42].

The cutaneous afferents responsible for neurogenic inflammation are linked to spinal interneuronal circuits that mediate nociceptive withdrawal reflexes (NWRs) [17]. Animal models of neurogenic inflammation have shown that substance P, released at the dorsal horn of the spinal cord, enhances NWRs [58]. In withdrawal reflexes, flexor muscles play a prominent role, and, interestingly, in dystonia of CRPS there is a conspicuous involvement of flexor postures, which may hint at involvement of spinal motor programs that mediate NWRs. Alterations of neurotransmission are an important consequence of neuroplasticity. Indeed, central sensitization is generally associated with a decrease of both tonic inhibitory and phasic actions of inhibitory interneurons [26]. Several studies have shown that disinhibition on a spinal and cortical level is a key neurophysiological characteristic in CRPS patients with and without dystonia [2,14,28,41,44]. Both substance P-sensitized NWRs in animal models and dystonia in CRPS patients respond to the γ-aminobutyric acid receptor B (GABA$_B$) agonist baclofen, which enhances spinal GABAergic inhibition [40,50,55]. Notably, intrathecal administration of glycine, a major neurotransmitter involved in central inhibition, had no influence on dystonia in CRPS [35]. Several studies have shown that the intravenous administration of ketamine, a potent N-methyl-D-aspartate (NMDA) receptor antagonist, is beneficial in decreasing pain severity in patients with CRPS [43,45]. However, in our experience, intravenous ketamine has no clear effect on dystonia in CRPS. Collectively, findings of interventional studies thus highlight a specific role of GABAergic mechanisms in CRPS patients with dystonia.

In the context of dystonia as a manifestation of impaired sensorimotor networks [32], the question remains whether the pathophysiology of movement disorders in CRPS is restricted only to spinal involvement. Two fMRI studies on CRPS patients with and without dystonia have shown prominent cortical changes in circuitry involved in voluntary and imaginary motor tasks [19,30]. Given the important role of supraspinal sensorimotor processing in the execution of movement, it is seems likely that to some extent these cortical changes contribute to the pathophysiology of movement disorders in CRPS. Alternatively, the cortical changes may occur secondary to the development of spinal central sensitization. A study by Maihöfner et al. [30] makes it clear that pain by itself is sufficient to develop such cortical abnormalities.

Genetic Factors

Knowledge about genes involved in CRPS and dystonia in CRPS may provide important information on biological pathways involved in the pathogenesis of the syndrome. Such information could potentially open up new avenues for diagnostics and therapeutic options.

Given that different mechanisms seem to underlie the inflammatory, vascular, sensory, and motor features of CRPS, different genetic factors are probably involved in each of these mechanisms. CRPS is associated with considerable clinical heterogeneity, which most likely reflects individual differences in susceptibility to each of the relevant mechanisms. Therefore, CRPS studies should focus on subtypes of the syndrome, because homogenous subgroups may lead to better coherency between clinical manifestations, pathophysiology, and genetic mechanisms.

Although on a population level the role of genetic factors in CRPS was found to be negligible, heritability of the syndrome substantially increased in young-onset cases [12]. CRPS may occur in a familial form, but a clear mode of inheritance could not be identified [10]. In comparison to sporadic patients with CRPS, patients with familial CRPS develop the syndrome at a younger age and are more likely to have multiple affected extremities and dystonia. Sporadic CRPS patients with a more severe phenotype (multiple affected extremities and dystonia) have a substantially younger age at onset compared with patients in whom the disease remits or stabilizes [54,56]. Collectively, these findings suggest a genetic predisposition to develop dystonia in patients in whom the syndrome develops at a young age.

One study failed to identify a genetic association between polymorphisms within the neutral endopeptidase (NEP) gene and CRPS [25]. Another study failed to identify mutations in the voltage-gated $Na_v1.7$ sodium channel, α_1 subunit gene, *SCN9A*, in CRPS patients with familial CRPS [11]. Several studies have found associations between CRPS and the human lymphocyte antigen (HLA) complex, but these studies generally lacked the power to draw meaningful conclusions [27,47,49,51]. The HLA complex comprises a gene family that has important immunological functions. A recent study investigated the role of HLA alleles (i.e., *HLA-A, HLA-B, HLA-DRB1,* and *HLA-DQB1*) in 150 CRPS patients, who also had fixed dystonia. Significant associations were found with CRPS and dystonia and *HLA-B62* and *HLA-DQ8* [10]. Because of the phenotype under study, it is not possible to indicate if the associations identified are related to susceptibility to develop CRPS or dystonia, or perhaps to processes underlying chronification of the syndrome. Given that HLA class I molecules have been implicated in non-immune roles, including synaptic development and plasticity in the central nervous system [7,20], the association with HLA-B62 (MHC class I) may indicate a role of HLA class I in maladaptive neuroplasticity in CRPS.

To date, at least 17 subtypes of dystonia can be distinguished on a genetic basis. For 10 of these subtypes, causative (*DYT*) genes involved in oxidative stress, aberrant inflammation, and/or aberrant neuroplasticity have been identified. A recent study sequenced all coding exons of the *DYT1, DYT5a, DYT5b, DYT6, DYT11, DYT12,* and *DYT16* genes for high-penetrant causal mutations in 44 CRPS patients with fixed dystonia, but no mutations were identified, indicating that these genes do not seem to play a major role in CRPS [21].

Treatment Options

There are no randomized controlled studies of physical therapy, occupational therapy, or pharmacotherapy in treatment of movement disorders in CRPS [36]. Splints or plaster casts have been used for the treatment of dystonic postures in CRPS, but they are often ineffective or may even worsen the dystonia. Five descriptive studies have reported on treatments of movement disorders in CRPS patients [36]. Three of them report that a small number of CRPS patients with dystonia/spasms benefit from treatment with benzodiazepines and high doses of baclofen. Few of the studies specify the extent of improvement. Anticholinergics, carbamazepine, and magnesium salts are also used in treating dystonia or spasms affecting CRPS patients, but there is no evidence to support their efficacy [36]. No controlled studies have examined the use of botulin toxin to treat dystonia in CRPS-I [36].

Intrathecal baclofen therapy (ITB), an invasive technique, has been evaluated in two studies on patients with CRPS-I and dystonia who failed to respond to oral drug treatments [50,55]. These studies used a double-blind placebo-controlled crossover and single-blind placebo-run-in dose-escalation design as a screening procedure, after which patients who fulfilled the responder criterion were implanted with a pump for continuous ITB and followed up over at least a year. Dystonia, pain, disability, and quality of life all improved on ITB, and treatment remained efficacious over a period of 1 year [55]. However, this treatment was also associated with a high complication rate; 89 adverse events occurred in 26 patients and were related to baclofen ($n = 19$) or to pump/catheter system defects ($n = 52$), or could not be specified ($n = 18$). The pump was removed in 6 out of 36 patients who entered the open follow-up phase. Unfortunately, the response in the dose-escalation study did not predict the response to ITB in the open-label study [55]. ITB should only be considered for patients with CRPS-I if dystonia is a major problem and conventional therapy has proven ineffective [36].

Acknowledgments

This work is part of TREND (Trauma RElated Neuronal Dysfunction; www.trendconsortium.nl), a knowledge consortium that integrates research on complex regional pain syndrome type I. This project is supported by a Dutch Government grant (BSIK03016).

References

[1]   Apkarian AV, Thomas PS, Krauss BR, Szeverenyi NM. Prefrontal cortical hyperactivity in patients with sympathetically mediated chronic pain. Neurosci Lett 2001;311:193–7.

[2]   Avanzino L, Martino D, van de Warrenburg BP, Schneider SA, Abbruzzese G, Defazio G, Schrag A, Bhatia KP, Rothwell JC. Cortical excitability is abnormal in patients with the "fixed dystonia" syndrome. Mov Disord 2008;23:646–52.

[3] Berardelli A, Rothwell JC, Hallett M, Thompson PD, Manfredi M, Marsden CD. The pathophysiology of primary dystonia. Brain 1998;121:1195–212.

[4] Birklein F, Schmelz M, Schifter S, Weber M. The important role of neuropeptides in complex regional pain syndrome. Neurology 2001;26:2179–84.

[5] Blair SJ, Chinthagada M, Hoppenstehdt D, Kijowski R, Fareed J. Role of neuropeptides in pathogenesis of reflex sympathetic dystrophy. Acta Orthop Belg 1998;64:448–51.

[6] Brain SD, Moore PK, editors. Pain and neurogenic inflammation. Basel: Birkhäuser; 1999.

[7] Corriveau RA, Huh GS, Shatz CJ. Regulation of class I MHC gene expression in the developing and mature CNS by neural activity. Neuron 1998;21:505–20.

[8] DeGood DE, Cundiff GW, Adams LE, Shutty MS Jr. A psychosocial and behavioral comparison of reflex sympathetic dystrophy, low back pain and headache patients. Pain 1993;54:317–22.

[9] de Rooij AM, de Mos M, van Hilten JJ, Sturkenboom MC, Gosso MF, van den Maagdenberg AM, Marinus J. Increased risk of complex regional pain syndrome in siblings of patients? J Pain 2009;10:1250–5.

[10] de Rooij AM, de Mos M, Sturkenboom MC, Marinus J, van den Maagdenberg AM, van Hilten JJ. Familial occurrence of complex regional pain syndrome. Eur J Pain 2009;13:171–7.

[11] de Rooij AM, Gosso MF, Alsina-Sanchis E, Marinus J, van Hilten JJ, van den Maagdenberg AM. No mutations in the voltage-gated Na1.7 sodium channel alpha1 subunit gene SCN9A in familial complex regional pain syndrome. Eur J Neurol 2010; Epub Jan 12.

[12] de Rooij AM, Gosso MF, Haasnoot GW, Marinus J, Verduijn W, Claas FH, van den Maagdenberg AM, van Hilten JJ. HLA-B62 and HLA-DQ8 are associated with Complex Regional Pain Syndrome with fixed dystonia. Pain 2009;145:82–5.

[13] Deuschl G, Blumberg H, Lucking CH. Tremor in reflex sympathetic dystrophy. Arch Neurol 1991;48:1247–52.

[14] Eisenberg E, Chistyakov AV, Yudashkin M, Kaplan B, Hafner H, Feinsod M. Evidence for cortical hyperexcitability of the affected limb representation area in CRPS: a psychophysical and transcranial magnetic stimulation study. Pain 2005;113:99–105.

[15] Ferguson AR, Crown ED, Grau JW. Nociceptive plasticity inhibits adaptive learning in the spinal cord Neuroscience 2006;141:421–31.

[16] Field J, Gardner FV. Psychological distress associated with algodystrophy. J Hand Surg (Br) 1997;22:100–1.

[17] Floeter MK, Gerloff C, Kouri J, Hallett M. Cutaneous withdrawal reflexes of the upper extremity. Muscle Nerve 1998;21:591–8.

[18] Galer BS, Jensen M. Neglect-like symptoms in complex regional pain syndrome: results of a self-administered survey. J Pain Symptom Manage 1999;18:213–7.

[19] Gieteling EW, van Rijn MA, de Jong BM, Hoogduin JM, Renken R, van Hilten JJ, Leenders KL. Cerebral activation during motor imagery in complex regional pain syndrome type 1 with dystonia. Pain 2008;134:302–9.

[20] Goddard CA, Butts DA, Shatz CJ. Regulation of CNS synapses by neuronal MHC class I. Proc Natl Acad Sci USA 2007;104:6828–33.

[21] Gosso MF, de Rooij AM, Alsina-Sanchis E, Kamphorst JT, Marinus J, van Hilten JJ, van den Maagdenberg AM. Systematic mutation analysis of seven dystonia genes in complex regional pain syndrome with fixed dystonia. J Neurol 2010; Epub Jan 12.

[22] Harden RN, Bruehl S, Stanos S, Brander V, Chung OY, Saltz S, Adams A, Stulberg SD. Prospective examination of pain-related and psychological predictors of CRPS-like phenomena following total knee arthroplasty: a preliminary study. Pain 2003;106:393–400.

[23] Harden NR, Bruehl SP. Diagnostic criteria: the statistical derivation of the four criterion factors. In: Wilson P, Stanton-Hicks M, Harden RN, editors. CRPS: current diagnosis and therapy. Progress in pain research and management, Vol. 32. Seattle: IASP Press; 2005. p. 45–58.

[24] Holzer P. Maggi CA. Dissociation of dorsal root ganglion neurons into afferent and efferent-like functions. Neuroscience 1998;86:389–98.

[25] Huehne K, Schaal U, Leis S, Uebe S, Gosso MF, van den Maagdenberg AM, Maihöfner C, Birklein F, Rautenstrauss B, Winterpacht A. Lack of genetic association of neutral endopeptidase (NEP) with complex regional pain syndrome (CRPS). Neurosci Lett 2010;472:19–23.

[26] Jones TL, Sorkin LS. Basic chemistry of central sensitisation. Semin Pain Med 2003;1:184–94.

[27] Kemler MA, van de Vusse AC, van den Berg-Loonen EM, Barendse GA, van Kleef M, Weber WE. HLA-DQ1 associated with reflex sympathetic dystrophy. Neurology 1999;53:1350–1.

[28] Krause P, Foerderreuther S, Straube A. Bilateral motor cortex disinhibition in complex regional pain syndrome (CRPS) type I of the hand. Neurology 2003;61:515–9.

[29] Leis S, Weber M, Isselmann A, Schmelz M, Birklein F. Substance-P-induced protein extravasation is bilaterally increased in complex regional pain syndrome. Exp Neurol 2003;183:197–204.

[30] Maihöfner C, Baron R, DeCol R, Binder A, Birklein F, Deuschl G, Handwerker HO, Schattschneider J. The motor system shows adaptive changes in complex regional pain syndrome. Brain 2007;130:2671–87.

[31] Merskey H, Bogduk N. Complex regional pain syndrome, type I (reflex sympathetic dystrophy). In: Classification of chronic pain: descriptions of chronic pain syndromes and definitions of pain terms, 2nd ed. Seattle: IASP Press; 1994. p. 41–2.

[32] Mink JW. Abnormal circuit function in dystonia. Neurology 2006;66:959.

[33] Mos de M, de Bruijn AG, Huygen FJ, Dieleman JP, Stricker BH, Sturkenboom MC. The incidence of complex regional pain syndrome: a population-based study. Pain 2007;129:12–20.

[34] Munts AG, van Rootselaar AF, van der Meer JN, Koelman JH, van Hilten JJ, Tijssen MA. Clinical and neurophysiological characterization of myoclonus in complex regional pain syndrome. Mov Disord 2008;23:581–7.

[35] Munts AG, van der Plas AA, Voormolen JH, Marinus J, Teepe-Twiss IM, Onkenhout W, van Gerven JM, van Hilten JJ. Intrathecal glycine for pain and dystonia in complex regional pain syndrome. Pain 2009;146:199–204.

[36] Netherlands Association of Posttraumatic Dystrophy Patients. EBGD guidelines CRPS type I 2006. Available at: http://pdver.atcomputing.nl/english.html.

[37] Puchalski P, Zyluk A. Complex regional pain syndrome type 1 after fractures of the distal radius: a prospective study of the role of psychological factors. J Hand Surg (Br) 2005;30:574–80.

[38] Reedijk WB, van Rijn MA, Roelofs K, Tuijl JP, Marinus J, van Hilten JJ. Psychological features of patients with complex regional pain syndrome type I related dystonia. Mov Disord 2008;23:1551–9.

[39] Ribbers GM, Mulder T, Geurts AC, den Otter RA. Reflex sympathetic dystrophy of the left hand and motor impairments of the unaffected right hand: impaired central motor processing? Arch Phys Med Rehabil 2002;83:81–5.

[40] Saito K, Konishi S, Otsuka M. Antagonism between Lioresal and substance P in rat spinal cord. Brain Res 1975;97:177–80.

[41] Schouten AC, van de Beek WJT, van Hilten JJ, van der Helm FCT. Proprioceptive reflexes in patients with reflex sympathetic dystrophy. Exp Brain Res 2003;151:1–8.

[42] Schwartzman RJ, Kerrigan J. The movement disorder of reflex sympathetic dystrophy. Neurology 1990;40:57–61.

[43] Schwartzman RJ, Alexander GM, Grothusen JR, Paylor T, Reichenberger E, Perreault M. Outpatient intravenous ketamine for the treatment of complex regional pain syndrome: a double-blind placebo controlled study. Pain 2009;147:107–15.

[44] Schwenkreis P, Janssen F, Rommel O, Pleger B, Völker B, Hosbach I, Dertwinkel R, Maier C, Tegenthoff M. Bilateral motor cortex disinhibition in complex regional pain syndrome (CRPS) type I of the hand. Neurology 2003;61:515–9.

[45] Sigtermans MJ, van Hilten JJ, Bauer MC, Arbous MS, Marinus J, Sarton EY, Dahan A. Ketamine produces effective and long-term pain relief in patients with Complex Regional Pain Syndrome Type 1. Pain 2009;145:304–11.

[46] van de Beek WJT, Vein A, Hilgevoord AAJ, van Dijk JG, van Hilten JJ. Neurophysiological aspects of patients with generalized or multifocal dystonia in reflex sympathetic dystrophy. J Clin Neurophysiol 2002;19:77–83.

[47] van de Beek WJ, Roep BO, van der Slik AR, Giphart MJ, van Hilten BJ. Susceptibility loci for complex regional pain syndrome. Pain 2003;103:93–7.

[48] van der Laan L, van Spaendonck K, Horstink M, Goris RJA. The symptom checklist-90 revised questionnaire: no psychological profiles in complex regional pain syndrome–dystonia. J Pain Symptom Manage 1999;17:357–62.

[49] Vaneker M, van der Laan L, Allebes WA, Goris RJ. Genetic factors associated with complex regional pain syndrome 1: HLA DRB and TNF alpha promotor gene polymorphism. Disabil Med 2002;2:69–74.

[50] van Hilten JJ, van de Beek WJT, Hoff JI, Voormolen JH, Delhaas EM. Intrathecal baclofen for the treatment of dystonia in patients with reflex sympathetic dystrophy. N Engl J Med 2000;343:625–30.

[51] van Hilten JJ, van de Beek WJ, Roep BO. Multifocal or generalized tonic dystonia of complex regional pain syndrome: a distinct clinical entity associated with HLA-DR13. Ann Neurol 2000;48:113–6.

[52] van Hilten JJ, van de Beek WJ, Vein AA, van Dijk JG, Middelkoop HA. Clinical aspects of multifocal or generalized tonic dystonia in reflex sympathetic dystrophy. Neurology 2001 26;56:1762–5.

[53] van Hilten JJ, Blumberg H, Schwartzman RJ. Factor IV: movement disorders and dystrophy—pathophysiology and measurement. In: Wilson P, Stanton-Hicks M, Harden RN, editors. CRPS: current diagnosis and therapy. Progress in pain research and management, Vol. 32. Seattle: IASP Press; 2005. p. 119–137.

[54] van Rijn MA, Marinus J, Putter H, van Hilten JJ. Onset and progression of dystonia in complex regional pain syndrome. Pain 2007;130:287–93.

[55] van Rijn MA, Munts AG, Marinus J, Voormolen JH, de Boer KS, Teepe-Twiss IM, van Dasselaar NT, Delhaas EM, van Hilten JJ. Intrathecal baclofen for dystonia of complex regional pain syndrome. Pain 2009;143:41–7.

[56] Veldman PH, Goris RJ. Multiple reflex sympathetic dystrophy. Which patients are at risk for developing a recurrence of reflex sympathetic dystrophy in the same or another limb? Pain 1996;64:463–6.

[57] Weber M, Birklein F, Neundorfer B, Schmeltz M. Facilitated neurogenic inflammation in complex regional pain syndrome. Pain 2001;91:251–7.

[58] Woolf C, Wiesenfeld-Hallin Z. Substance P and calcitonin gene-related peptide synergistically modulate the gain of the nociceptive flexor withdrawal reflex in the rat. Neurosci Lett 1986;66:226–30.

[59] Woolf CJ, Mannion RJ. Neuropathic pain: aetiology, symptoms, mechanisms, and management. Lancet 1999;353:1959–64.

[60] Woolf CJ, Salter MW. Neuronal plasticity: increasing the gain in pain. Science 2000;288:1765–9.

Correspondence to: Jacobus J. van Hilten, MD, PhD, Department of Neurology, Leiden University Medical Center, P.O. Box 9600, 2300 RC Leiden, The Netherlands. Email: J.J.van_Hilten@lumc.nl.

Rehabilitation of People with Chronic Complex Regional Pain Syndrome

G. Lorimer Moseley, PhD

Prince of Wales Medical Research Institute, Randwick, and The University of New South Wales, Sydney, New South Wales, Australia

If you have opened this particular chapter of the refresher course book, you most likely will already know that complex regional pain syndrome (CRPS) is difficult to treat once it "sets in." Each year, a whole new range of pathophysiological findings associated with CRPS are discovered, and we must open our minds wider and wider to the possible contributions, risk factors, and underlying biological mechanisms that cause this disease. For the scientist, this progress presents a cornucopia of interesting problems that are at once intriguing, perplexing, and exciting. For the clinician, all these so-called "advances" can seem intimidating and overwhelming. As a clinical scientist, I am as excited by the clinical opportunities that arise from the advances in our understanding of pathophysiology as I am by the advances themselves. In this chapter, I will outline an approach to the *rehabilitation* of CRPS that is based on a conceptual framework in which CRPS is considered an exaggerated protective response that is almost always triggered by tissue trauma but, once "set in," is maintained by central mechanisms. Aspects of the approach have various levels of supportive evidence, ranging from data from randomized controlled trials, to evidence from non-CRPS chronic pain patients, to biologically based propositions that have not been tested in robust clinical trials. The approach involves three components: (1) minimizing conceptual and psychosocial contributions to threat; (2) graded exposure to threats; and (3) correcting secondary pathophysiologies. I will briefly outline the rationale behind each component. Finally, I will present audit data that do not constitute empirical evidence but do permit the generation of informed hypotheses about the potential contribution of different components of the approach to outcomes.

The Conceptual Framework: CRPS as an Exaggerated Protective Response

Biological organisms are proficient at protecting themselves from threat. Seminal work more than a century ago clearly demonstrated that even unicellular organisms can propel themselves away from physical threat [21]. The sophistication with which organisms can protect themselves from threat seems to increase in line with the sophistication of the organism. Mammals are a fine case in point, with a protective armory that includes monosynaptic motor responses, coordinated polysynaptic motor responses, and sympathetic, endocrine, and local and systemic immune responses. The most sophisticated response, however—one that is particularly well-developed (and certainly well-studied) in humans—is a conscious experience that motivates the entire organism to take drastic protective action. This experience is called pain.

Pain is clearly a cardinal sign for CRPS, but the other characteristics of CRPS are consistent with protective responses in other systems—endocrine, immune, motor, and autonomic. That such a comprehensive multisystemic protective response can be triggered by minor injury, or perhaps with no tissue injury at all [18], still remains a mystery, although local and peripheral neural factors are probably important (see Dr. Baron's chapter in this section). This might be why, when in the acute stage, CRPS is fairly responsive to a range of pharmacological strategies, but when it "sets in," it is famously resistant to almost everything. I contend that this clearly suggests that if we are to effectively treat chronic CRPS, we need to think beyond drugs. One response is to "go back to the drawing board" and ask "Why do we hurt?"

Pain is a conscious event that emerges in association with a pattern of activity spread across multiple brain areas [66]. The exact areas and the pattern of activity within those areas are individually specific, although some areas are more commonly activated than others, which is why they have been termed the "pain matrix" [3], although recent evidence raises the possibility that much of the activation relates to salience rather than pain [50]. The individual pattern of activity can be called a pain neurosignature [30], or, colloquially perhaps, a pain neurotag [6]. A very large amount of research shows that activity of the pain neurotag can be modulated by a range of factors including cognitive, emotional, contextual, environmental, and nociceptive factors (for a review and lay-friendly explanation, see ref. [6]). Disappointingly, and somewhat surprisingly, this multifactorial aspect of pain has failed to overcome the dominant interpretation of pain, which regards pain as a perceptual equivalent of nociception. The folly of this position was elegantly noted over 20 years ago, by Wall and McMahon [68]—"the labelling of nociceptors as pain fibres was not an admirable simplification but an unfortunate trivialization"—and their observations remain fundamental to the current conceptual framework: "pain is an integrated package of analysed results related to meaning, significance and imperative action" (p. 255).

According to this conceptual framework, anything that changes the brain's implicit evaluation of threat to body tissue should affect pain. If it increases the perceived threat, it should increase pain. If it decreases the perceived threat, it should decrease pain. The magnitude of the effect will depend upon how important that issue is in the brain's evaluation of danger. This conceptualization accounts for the myriad findings

from experimental studies that modulate pain by manipulating contextual variables (e.g., ref. [40]) or that induce placebo analgesia (see refs. [8,39]). To conceptualize the neurobiology that underpins the multifactorial nature of pain, one can consider each factor as being represented by its own neurotag. All of these neurotags have synaptic connections with the pain neurotag, which means that they can influence its activation (Fig. 1). This conceptual framework can help guide management of chronic CRPS and underpins in particular the first component of the rehabilitation approach described here.

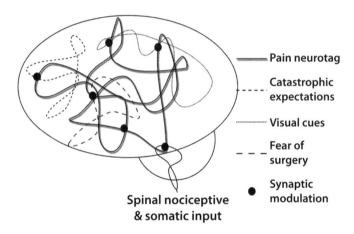

Fig. 1. Conceptual model of the modulation of pain by cognitive, emotional, and contextual factors. Clinically relevant examples are used. Each line denotes a network of brain cells that represent that factor. Filled circles denote a site of synaptic modulation of one neural network by another.

Minimizing Conceptual and Psychosocial Contributions to Threat

Conceptual Contributions to Threat

A conceptual contribution to threat means that the way an individual makes sense of signs and symptoms increases the perceived threat to body tissue. There has been a very large amount of research into the relationship between pain and the meaning of pain, which, by and large, tells us that the more heavily the patient's explanation of the pain emphasizes tissue damage, then the more it hurts [5,22,32,33,40,44,55,63,65]. With regard to CRPS, this issue is very important because, in chronic cases, the pain and the other signs and symptoms do not relate to the state of the tissues. However, many patients believe that tissue injury remains at the heart of their problem and of those who do not, most do not explain their condition in terms of nervous system dysfunction. What is more, many defiantly claim that they have been told that their condition is not real, that it is usually caused by personality defects or unresolved childhood problems. Obviously, such a view is contrary to the available evidence [11] and is inconsistent with current understandings of the pathophysiology of the condition.

As an illustration, according to unpublished clinical audit data, 69 patients with CRPS answered the question "How accurately do you think your symptoms reflect the amount of tissue damage in your (hand)?" by selecting a score from 1 to 5, where 1 = "not at all accurately," 3 = "reasonably accurately," and 5 = "completely accurately." The score (mean ± SD) was 3.6 ± 1.3. Eighty-four patients with CRPS completed a pain physiology knowledge true/false questionnaire. Higher scores reflect a belief that the nervous system is an important contributor to chronic pain [30]. The score was 56% ± 20%. When 59 patients with CRPS were asked about previous professional clinical advice regarding their condition, 59% reported that they had been told that CRPS was not real, 47% had been told that it was caused by unresolved childhood problems, 49% had been told that it was caused by personality characteristics and 10% had been told that it was a disease of the central nervous system.

The first component of rehabilitation then, is to explain to patients what we currently understand about the causes and mechanisms of CRPS. This process of reconceptualization is not a trivial one. In fact, it is considered a critical platform for the whole approach. "Explaining" goes beyond simply providing information. Rather, it integrates current thought from several learning-related disciplines, from basic animal studies that rely on aversive or pleasant stimuli to induce learning, to cognitive architecture theory that emphasizes the utility of metaphors that challenge old schema, along with precise instruction in order to implant a new schema [64]. Application of this interdisciplinary knowledge to pain rehabilitation has led to a three-stage conceptual change process that aims to shift the patient's explanation for the pain from an inaccurate or mysterious explanation to one that is consistent with the current understanding of the pathophysiology of the condition.

The first stage aims to challenge the current explanation in a nonconfrontational but emotionally engaging way, for example via stories that can be used as metaphors for important concepts [38]. Anecdotally, a comprehensive physical assessment can be a useful complement to this process; by fully examining the affected limb, a physical therapist or physician is able to reinforce, with credibility, that the tissues of the affected body part are not injured.

The second stage of the conceptual change process aims to implant the new conceptualization. For patients with CRPS, the key concepts are: (1) Pain is an output of the brain that depends upon an implicit evaluation of the danger to body tissue, not on an input to the brain from injured tissue. (2) The best available evidence clearly shows that personality issues, intelligence, level of education, and severity of injury do not cause CRPS. (3) The pattern of signs and symptoms that characterize CRPS result from a heightened protective system, which is maintained by dysfunction within the nervous system and brain. (4) There is no evidence that this dysfunction is associated with brain or nervous system damage, which is good because it leaves open the pathway to recovery, but it renders the nervous system very sensitive, which is bad because that sensitivity manifests in protective responses such as pain. (5) To overcome this disorder, we must address each contributing factor we can identify.

Our group has undertaken several clinical studies to evaluate the effects of explaining the biology of pain to patients with chronic pain. The majority of data relate to non-CRPS chronic pain, so they should be interpreted accordingly, but they clearly show a range of positive effects. For example, "explaining pain" (the material for which is described in full in Butler and Moseley [6]) increases pain threshold during provocative tasks [33], changes beliefs and attitudes about how to manage pain [44], and improves the outcome of activity-based rehabilitation [31,48]. Notably, most clinicians wrongly presume that the typical chronic pain patient is unable to grasp key concepts of modern pain biology [49], which may be why an old-fashioned, seductively simple Cartesian understanding of chronic pain seems to predominate, at least within the clinical community.

I contend that we may get better results by tailoring the reconceptualization aspect of rehabilitation to CRPS, instead of a broader "explain pain" approach. Clinical audit data support this contention. Data from over 200 consecutive patients suggest that "explaining CRPS" was associated with a decreased conviction that moving the affected area would make the condition worse (Fig. 2) and with a reduction in the frequency of flare-ups (Fig. 3).

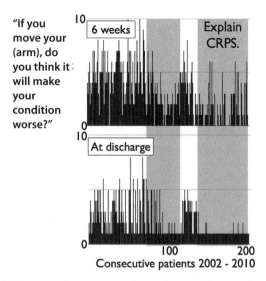

Fig. 2. Responses from consecutive patients to the question shown on the y-axis, using a single 0–11 numerical rating scale, anchored at left with "No, not at all" and at right with "Yes, absolutely." Top panel shows data obtained after 6 weeks of treatment. Bottom panel shows data obtained at discharge, the timing of which varied between patients. The shaded area denotes that "explain CRPS" was formally included in the rehabilitation program.

Psychosocial Contributions to Threat

A range of psychosocial issues have been linked to CRPS, for example catastrophizing, fear avoidance beliefs [10], depression [58], anxiety [58], and stressful life events [17,57]. Notably, however, there is no typical "psychosocial profile" that predisposes individuals to CRPS or maintains the condition [11]. Nonetheless, the guiding framework discussed here implies that psychosocial issues *can* contribute to the perceived threat to body tissues, and therefore, addressing these issues should modulate the disease. There is preliminary evidence to support this view—directly targeting fear of (re)injury in treatment can have a major impact on CRPS [10]—but further work is required to establish

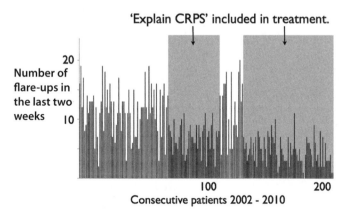

Fig. 3. Number of flare-ups during the last 2 weeks, reported 6 weeks after commencement of treatment. Shaded areas coincide with the inclusion of the "explain CRPS" component. Note that the frequency of flare-ups appears lower when "explain CRPS" is included.

the effects of psychological treatments. For the time being, there are sufficient data from other chronic pain disorders, and from cohorts that include CRPS patients, to suggest that rehabilitation should adhere to cognitive-behavioral principles, and that teaching people how best to cope with their pain [7,13,59] should be helpful. There is a great deal written on psychological approaches to chronic pain *management* (for example, ref. [51]), and in-depth discussion is beyond the scope of this chapter.

Graded Exposure to Threats

Graded exposure to threatening cues is a core theme of rehabilitation of psychological and physical disorders. In each case, the basic rule of thumb is to sufficiently expose the individual to the threatening cue to induce a physiological, physical, or functional adaptation, but not sufficiently to evoke the unwanted response. Over time, the system adapts and eventually returns to normal, at least theoretically. The enhanced sensitivity of the protective system in CRPS makes this approach difficult. For example, people with chronic CRPS of one hand report increased pain, and demonstrate increased swelling, when they imagine moving their affected arm, even when they do not move their arm nor demonstrate any detectable muscle activity in the arm [35,46]. Furthermore, visual input suggesting that the affected area has been touched is sufficient to elicit pain and swelling, even though the affected area has not in fact been touched [1].

We have attributed these two findings to a very sensitized nociceptive system: for imagined movements to provoke pain and swelling, we proposed that the command to move has become sufficient to evoke pain, possibly in part because of classical conditioning; the command has become the conditioned stimulus and pain the conditioned response. For pain provoked by *apparent* touch, we proposed that input from bimodal visuotactile brain cells is enough to "ignite" the pain neurotag, possibly via connections to primary somatosensory cells incorporated in the pain neurotag. Others propose that such findings are more likely to reflect a cortical protective response to the incongruence that each situation imparts: imagined movements do not evoke sensory feedback that is consistent with the movement command, and touching a nonpainful counterpart while you watch it in the mirror predicts tactile input from the opposite body part—tactile input that never arrives. The idea that such incongruence maintains or underpins pathological pains has been well described in the literature [15,19,26–28], but experimental data are conflicting (see refs. [41,43]). Such a discussion is perhaps more relevant to part three of the current approach, but insofar as both explanations depend upon the sensitized protective system, they both imply that the line between sufficient exposure to induce adaptation but not evoke pain is a very thin one, if it exists at all.

One response to this conundrum is to reconsider the conventional baseline of movement- or function-based rehabilitation. A range of experiments indicate that when we are shown a picture of a hand and are required to judge whether it is a left or right hand, we mentally maneuver our own hand to match the picture before responding (see ref. [52] for review). As such, left/right judgments of pictured limbs may provide an exposure to movement that is sufficient to induce adaptation but not sufficient to evoke pain. This idea formed the theoretical rationale for a randomized controlled trial (RCT) of graded motor imagery in people with chronic CRPS triggered by wrist fracture [34]. This study was followed by a second RCT that included a more heterogeneous group of CRPS patients (and patients with phantom limb pain from amputation or brachial plexus avulsion injury, since there is an established rationale for grouping such conditions together [2,15]). A systematic review of physical therapy interventions for CRPS concluded that there is good evidence to support the use of graded motor imagery in people with chronic CRPS [9]. The number needed to treat (NTT) for a 50% reduction in pain and disability is about 3, which compares favorably with other treatments that have been tested for chronic CRPS.

What Is Graded Motor Imagery?

Graded motor imagery is a three-stage program of graded exposure to movement. Stage 1 involves left/right judgments of pictured hands or feet, depending upon the affected body part. Clinicians can use their own photographs or line drawings, and there are commercially available on-line and hard copy versions that include clear instructions and have display, scoring, and data storage capacity (e.g., Recognise, Adelaide, Australia [www.noigroup.com/recognise]). In the RCTs, patients were encouraged to train for 5 minutes every waking hour for 2 weeks. Electronic diaries, which are more accurate than paper diaries

and have the added advantage of enhancing participation [37], yielded about 78% participation. The frequency and duration of training sessions during Stage 1 of graded motor imagery depends on symptoms, practical considerations (for example access to a computer), and level of interest. Anecdotally, every effort should be take to maximize the frequency of training. It may also be preferable to use a criteria-based progression, whereby patients move to Stage 2 when their performance on the task satisfies speed (depending on the picture bank and method used to present the pictures) and accuracy (>80% on both sides) benchmarks, rather than a time-based progression.

Stage 2 involves explicit motor imagery, or imagined movements. The duration and frequency of sessions, and the duration of this stage of the program, are similar to those used for Stage 1, but the objective is no longer to simply recognize the laterality of the pictured limb, but to intentionally imagine matching the position of the pictured hand with one's own hand, and then to imagine returning one's hand to its resting position. The same pictures or software can be used for Stages 1 and 2.

Executed movements are not commenced until Stage 3, at which time they are performed using a mirror. Within the context of graded motor imagery, the theoretical basis for using a mirror is that the visual input, which suggests that the limb looks healthy and is performing a graceful movement, overrides other proprioceptive and noxious input that would increase the perceived threat. Again, in RCTs, training duration and frequency, along with the duration of this stage of the graded motor imagery program, are similar to those for Stages 1 and 2, but anecdotally, a criteria-based progression, in which functional tasks are introduced in line with the principle of graded exposure without evoking the unwanted response, is probably more appropriate.

According to the guiding theory, the order in which the stages of the graded motor imagery program are implemented should be critical to the outcome. This prediction was tested in an RCT in which CRPS patients were randomly allocated to programs in which the component stages were in one of three orders [36]. That trial supported the prediction by clearly showing that if the order was modified, for example if imagined movements (Stage 2) preceded left/right judgments (Stage 1), there was no treatment effect. Notably, the design of that trial allows us to conclude that Stages 1 and 2 are important contributors to the overall effect, but it does not give us the same confidence concerning Stage 3 (mirror movements). There is a rapidly growing literature on the use of mirror movements alone in the rehabilitation of phantom limb pain, an approach that was pioneered 15 years ago [56] and later tested in people with CRPS by McCabe and colleagues [29]. By and large, for chronic CRPS, the bigger and more robust studies are less encouraging than the smaller and less robust ones, but it is not yet possible to unequivocally conclude for or against their efficacy in such conditions (see ref. [41] for a discussion on this topic).

How Does Graded Motor Imagery Work?

Graded motor imagery is based on a driving conceptual model: left/right judgments involve a smaller motor recruitment than imagined movements, which involve a smaller motor recruitment than mirror movements, which involve less threatening input than non-mirror movements and functional tasks. The clear order-dependent treatment effects seem to support that conceptual model. The idea that implicit motor imagery might involve premotor cells "priming" primary motor cells subthreshold has been applied to motor recovery after stroke [61] and would seem consistent, on a cellular level, with the systems-based guiding framework of exposure to threat (movement) without eliciting the unwanted response, which is pain.

However, empirical evidence to support this explanation is lacking, and other possible explanations should also be considered. First, and perhaps foremost, is that graded motor imagery has a purely psychocognitive exposure effect, or that the extensive practice induces better coping strategies and reduced fear or anxiety. Alternatively, perhaps graded motor imagery corrects disrupted cortical representations of the affected body part (see below), as has been proposed for mirror movements [29]. A very large amount of research is relevant to these questions, and full discussion is beyond the scope of this chapter. However, although it is tempting to lose steam in our pursuit of answers to these questions because the treatment clearly seems to work, our treatments still have substantial room for improvement.

Beyond Movement: Graded Exposure to Other Threats

Graded motor imagery lends itself to a very structured training program because one can increase exposure via the number of pictures, the type of pictures, the context

of the task, and the training load. A similar approach is taken for gradual exposure to all of the threatening cues that are identified as contributing to an individual's pain state. These cues are not confined to movements or tasks; they may be particular people, environmental or social contexts, sensory cues, or return to work or other duties. The practical implementation of this approach relies on a committed and persevering patient and clinical team, all of whom are "on message" with regard to the biological rationale. Full discussion of the practical implementation of this component is beyond the scope of this chapter. Usual principles of rehabilitation apply, but the guiding biological rationale implies that the graduations should be conservative by virtue of the sensitized system. For example, some patients increase work hours by minutes each day rather than hours each week or days each month, which would most likely be the case in a more conventional rehabilitation situation.

Correcting Secondary Pathophysiologies

Of the many pathophysiological changes that have been identified in people with CRPS, recent advances in rehabilitation focus on changes in the way the affected body part is represented in primary sensory cortex (S1). These changes in CRPS are well documented [23–25, 53,54,67] and can be summarized thus: the area of S1 neurons that are activated in response to tactile input from the affected body part becomes smaller, tactile acuity is reduced, and the precision with which the brain can localize a tactile stimulus to a particular cutaneous location is impaired. The extent of changes tends to relate to usual pain intensity. The mechanisms that underpin these changes may relate to a loss of normal intracortical inhibition, or *dis*inhibition [16,60]. Although the effects of such changes extend beyond the representation of the surfaces of the body, for example to an altered representation of peri-personal space [42], it is the altered representation of the surfaces of the body that raises obvious implications for treatment.

Cortical organization, and intracortical inhibition, can be trained, as has been established in human and animal studies in which the S1 representation of a particular body part has been shown to shift in response to use. Braille readers have a larger representation in S1 of their reading finger on weekdays than they do on the weekend [62], and string players have a larger representation of their left hand than they do of their right [12].

To induce changes in cortical organization, it is thought necessary to stimulate the skin of the relevant body part, preferably in a way that makes the characteristics of the stimuli important, for example reading Braille or playing the violin, or that makes the objective of the task important, for example unwrapping food [4,20,69]. In an elegant study that captured this requirement, amputees with chronic phantom limb pain (which shares commonalities in cortical changes with CRPS; ref. [2]) took part in a sensory discrimination protocol, every day for 10 days [14]. The researchers measured S1 organization and demonstrated that discrimination training, but not stimulation alone, led to normalization of S1 and reduction of phantom limb pain.

This finding was extended to people with CRPS of one limb [47]. In this replicated case series, which controlled for time but not for the order of conditions, patients undertook one to two sessions of tactile stimulation or tactile discrimination training each day for 2 weeks. (Not controlling for the order of conditions leaves open the possibility that, if the active treatment occurs after the control treatment, which was the case in this study, any effect of the active treatment is dependent on the prior occurrence of the control treatment.) Each session involved repeated stimulation with a random combination of probes of different widths, and at five different locations on the affected limb. In the discrimination condition, patients had to respond to each stimulus by judging its width and location. Tactile discrimination, but not tactile stimulation alone, led to significant improvements in pain, disability, and tactile acuity.

A subsequent randomized repeated-measures experiment evaluated the effect of visual input, and gaze direction, on the short-term effects (up to 48 hours) of a single 30-minute session of tactile discrimination training [45]. In order to capture visual input of the skin of the affected area, and gaze direction, without giving the patient a view of the limb, a mirror was used to "replace" the affected limb with a virtual counterpart. That work showed a clear advantage to training with a mirror.

A critical consideration for this component of the approach is that the objective is to induce changes in brain function. As such, practice is paramount. Clinically, patients are encouraged to see rehabilitation as though they have had a stroke and need to retrain their brain. Of course, the fact that they have not sustained any brain damage is emphasized, but so too is the need for a long and patient journey of at least twice-daily training sessions. Clinicians are thought of as coaches rather than therapists, and progress is documented over time to reassure patients that they are indeed making progress.

Outcomes and Evidence

The various components of the current approach to rehabilitation of people with chronic CRPS have different levels of empirical support. "Explaining CRPS" has only pilot data support, although "explaining pain" has empirical support for decreasing pain and disability from several RCTs; cognitive-behavioral pain management programs have systematic review-level evidence for decreasing disability in people with chronic pain, but CRPS-specific RCTs are lacking; graded motor imagery has systematic review-level evidence for decreasing pain and disability; tactile discrimination training, mirror therapy, and other physical therapy approaches not discussed here have preliminary support but are yet to be tested in robust RCTs. This chapter, however, outlines an approach to rehabilitation that includes each of these components. To my knowledge, such a multimodal approach has not been tested using empirical methods, and as such, its effectiveness is yet to be determined. Nevertheless, audit data from 244 consecutive patients permits comparison between different stages in the development of this approach and demonstrates a clear and positive trend toward better outcomes related to pain (Fig. 4) and disability (Fig. 5). Notably, the number of sessions

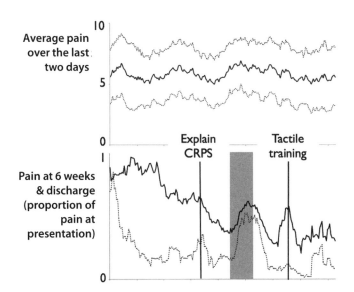

Fig. 4. Top panel: Pain over the last two days, rated at initial assessment. Solid line denotes mean, and broken lines indicate standard deviation, of previous 10 patients. Bottom panel: Pain 6 weeks after initial assessment (solid line) and at discharge (broken line), as a proportion of pain at initial assessment (1 = no change, 0 = complete pain relief). Data represent the average of the previous 10 patients.

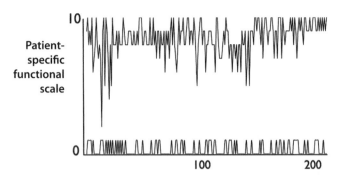

Fig. 5. Disability at initial assessment (lower line) and at discharge (upper line), as measured by a patient-specific functional scale. Patients select four tasks that they cannot do because of their CRPS and rate their ability to perform that task on a numeric rating scale, where 0 = completely unable to perform, and 10 = able to perform the task normally.

between initial assessment and discharge was reduced over the same period (Fig. 6). It is critical to note that these data do not constitute robust evidence for particular components, but they do suggest that, for whatever reason, patients with CRPS improve over the course of treatment and the degree to which they improve has increased in accordance with developments in the rehabilitation approach.

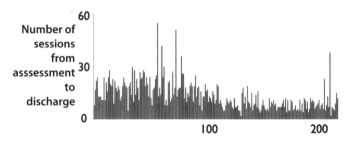

Fig. 6. Number of sessions from initial assessment to final discharge for 227 patients.

Summary

The current chapter has presented a pragmatic approach to rehabilitation of patients with chronic CRPS. The guiding framework considers CRPS to be an exaggerated protective response that is triggered by peripheral injury and maintained by nervous system dysfunction. The approach endorses a modern view of pain as an output of the brain that reflects the brain's evaluation of threat to body tissue. As such, conceptual and psychosocial contributions to perceived threats are considered as important as movement and function-related contributions to perceived threats. Rehabilitation integrates "explaining CRPS" with cognitive-behavioral strategies, graded motor imagery and functional exposure, and tactile discrimination training. Importantly, the exact components of rehabilitation are determined for each patient by application of the conceptual frameworks rather than via explicit prescriptive guidelines. The various components of rehabilitation have varying levels of evidence, and clearly, more research is required to optimize outcomes.

Acknowledgments

The author is supported by a Senior Research Fellowship from the National Health & Research Council of Australia.

References

[1] Acerra NE, Moseley GL. Dysynchiria: watching the mirror image of the unaffected limb elicits pain on the affected side. Neurology 2005;65:751–3.

[2] Acerra NE, Souvlis T, Moseley GL. Stroke, complex regional pain syndrome and phantom limb pain: can commonalities direct future management? J Rehabil Med 2007;39:109–14.

[3] Apkarian AV, Bushnell MC, Treede RD, Zubieta JK. Human brain mechanisms of pain perception and regulation in health and disease. Eur J Pain 2005;9:463–84.

[4] Braun C, Haug M, Wiech K, Birbaumer N, Elbert T, Roberts LE. Functional organization of primary somatosensory cortex depends on the focus of attention. Neuroimage 2002;17:1451–8.

[5] Bunketorp L, Lindh M, Carlsson J, Stener-Victorin E. The perception of pain and pain-related cognitions in subacute whiplash-associated disorders: its influence on prolonged disability. Disabil Rehabil 2006;28:271–9.

[6] Butler D, Moseley GL. Explain pain. Adelaide: NOI Group; 2003.

[7] Carson JW, Keefe FJ, Affleck G, Rumble ME, Caldwell DS, Beaupre PM, Kashikar-Zuck S, Sandstrom M, Weisberg JN. A comparison of conventional pain coping skills training and pain coping skills training with a maintenance training component: a daily diary analysis of short- and long-term treatment effects. J Pain 2006;7:615–25.

[8] Colloca L, Lopiano L, Lanotte M, Benedetti F. Overt versus covert treatment for pain, anxiety, and Parkinson's disease. Lancet Neurol 2004;3:679–84.

[9] Daly AE, Bialocerkowski AE. Does evidence support physiotherapy management of adult Complex Regional Pain Syndrome Type One? A systematic review. Eur J Pain 2009;13:339–53.

[10] de Jong JR, Vlaeyen JWS, Onghena P, Cuypers C, Hollander MD, Ruijgrok J. Reduction of pain-related fear in complex regional pain syndrome type I: the application of graded exposure in vivo. Pain 2005;116:264–75.

[11] de Mos M, Huygen F, Dieleman JP, Koopman J, Stricker BHC, Sturkenboom M. Medical history and the onset of complex regional pain syndrome (CRPS). Pain 2008;139:458–66.

[12] Elbert T, Pantev C, Wienbruch C, Rockstroh B, Taub E. Increased cortical representations of the fingers of the left hand in string players. Science 1995;270:305–7.

[13] Emery CF, Keefe FJ, France CR, Affleck G, Waters S, Fondow MDM, McKee DC, France JL, Hackshaw KV, Caldwell DS, Stainbrook D. Effects of a brief coping skills training intervention on nociceptive flexion reflex threshold in patients having osteoarthritic knee pain: a preliminary laboratory study of sex differences. J Pain Symptom Manage 2006;31:262–9.

[14] Flor H, Denke C, Schaefer M, Grusser S. Effect of sensory discrimination training on cortical reorganisation and phantom limb pain. Lancet 2001;357:1763–4.

[15] Flor H, Nikolajsen L, Jensen TS. Phantom limb pain: a case of maladaptive CNS plasticity? Nat Rev Neurosci 2006;7:873–81.

[16] Forderreuther S. Clinical, electrophysiological and imaging findings in patients suffering from complex regional pain syndrome (CRPS). Klin Neurophysiol 2004;35:237–42.

[17] Geertzen JH, de Bruijn-Kofman AT, de Bruijn HP, van de Wiel HB, Dijkstra PU. Stressful life events and psychological dysfunction in Complex Regional Pain Syndrome type I. Clin J Pain 1998;14:143–7.

[18] Grande LA, Loeser JD, Ozuna J, Ashleigh A, Samii A. Complex regional pain syndrome as a stress response. Pain 2004;110:495–8.

[19] Harris AJ. Cortical origin of pathological pain. Lancet 1999;354:1464–6.

[20] Jenkins WM, Merzenich MM, Ochs MT, Allard T, Guic-Robles E. Functional reorganization of primary somatosensory cortex in adult owl monkeys after behaviorally controlled tactile stimulation. J Neurophysiol 1990;63:82–104.

[21] Jennings HS. The interpretation of the behavior of the lower organisms. Science 1908;27:698–710.

[22] Jensen MP, Romano JM, Turner JA, Good AB, Wald LH. Patient beliefs predict patient functioning: further support for a cognitive-behavioural model of chronic pain. Pain 1999;81:95–104.

[23] Juottonen K, Gockel M, Silen T, Hurri H, Hari R, Forss N. Altered central sensorimotor processing in patients with complex regional pain syndrome. Pain 2002;98:315–23.

[24] Maihofner C, Handwerker HO, Neundorfer B, Birklein F. Patterns of cortical reorganization in complex regional pain syndrome. Neurology 2003;61:1707–15.

[25] Mailis-Gagnon A. Disrupted central somatosensory processing in CRPS: a unique characteristic of the syndrome? Pain 2006;123:3–5.

[26] McCabe CS, Blake DR. An embarrassment of pain perceptions? Towards an understanding of and explanation for the clinical presentation of CRPS type 1. Rheumatology 2008:47:1612–6.

[27] McCabe CS, Blake DR, Skevington SM. Cortical origins of pathological pain. Lancet 2000;355:318–9.

[28] McCabe CS, Haigh RC, Halligan PW, Blake DR. Simulating sensory-motor incongruence in healthy volunteers: implications for a cortical model of pain. Rheumatology 2005;44:509–16.

[29] McCabe CS, Haigh RC, Ring EFJ, Halligan PW, Wall PD, Blake DR. A controlled pilot study of the utility of mirror visual feedback in the treatment of complex regional pain syndrome (type 1). Rheumatology 2003;42:97–101.

[30] Melzack R. Phantom limbs and the concept of a neuromatrix. Trends Neurosci 1990;13:88–92.

[31] Moseley GL. Joining forces: combining cognition-targeted motor control training with group or individual pain physiology education: a successful treatment for chronic low back pain. J Man Manip Ther 2003;11:88–94.

[32] Moseley GL. Unravelling the barriers to reconceptualisation of the problem in chronic pain: the actual and perceived ability of patients and health professionals to understand the neurophysiology. J Pain 2003;4:184–9.

[33] Moseley GL. Evidence for a direct relationship between cognitive and physical change during an education intervention in people with chronic low back pain. Eur J Pain 2004;8:39–45.

[34] Moseley GL. Graded motor imagery is effective for long-standing complex regional pain syndrome: a randomised controlled trial. Pain 2004;108:192–8.

[35] Moseley GL. Imagined movements cause pain and swelling in a patient with complex regional pain syndrome. Neurology 2004;62:1644.

[36] Moseley GL. Is successful rehabilitation of complex regional pain syndrome due to sustained attention to the affected limb? A randomised clinical trial. Pain 2005;114:54–61.

[37] Moseley GL. Do training diaries affect and reflect adherence to home programs? Arthritis Care Res 2006;55:662–4.

[38] Moseley GL. Painful yarns. Metaphors and stories to help understand the biology of pain. Canberra: Dancing Giraffe Press; 2007.

[39] Moseley GL. Reconceptualising placebo. BMJ 2008;336:1086.

[40] Moseley GL, Arntz A. The context of a noxious stimulus affects the pain it evokes. Pain 2007;133:64–71.

[41] Moseley GL, Gallace A, Spence C. Is mirror therapy all it is cracked up to be? Current evidence and future directions. Pain 2008;138:7–10.

[42] Moseley GL, Gallace A, Spence C. Space-based, but not arm-based, shift in tactile processing in complex regional pain syndrome and its relationship to cooling of the affected limb. Brain 2009;132:3142–51.

[43] Moseley GL, Gandevia SC. Sensory-motor incongruence and reports of 'pain'. Rheumatology 2005;44:1083–5.

[44] Moseley GL, Nicholas MK, Hodges PW. A randomized controlled trial of intensive neurophysiology education in chronic low back pain. Clin J Pain 2004;20:324–30.

[45] Moseley GL, Wiech K. The effect of tactile discrimination training is enhanced when patients watch the reflected image of their unaffected limb during training. Pain 2009;144:314–9.

[46] Moseley GL, Zalucki N, Birklein F, Marinus J, von Hilten JJ, Luomajoki H. Thinking about movement hurts: the effect of motor imagery on pain and swelling in people with chronic arm pain. Arthritis Care Res 2008;59:623–31.

[47] Moseley GL, Zalucki NM, Wiech K. Tactile discrimination, but not tactile stimulation alone, reduces chronic limb pain. Pain 2008;137:600–8.

[48] Moseley L. Combined physiotherapy and education is efficacious for chronic low back pain. Aust J Physiother 2002;48:297–302.

[49] Moseley L. Unraveling the barriers to reconceptualization of the problem in chronic pain: the actual and perceived ability of patients and health professionals to understand the neurophysiology. J Pain 2003;4:184–9.

[50] Mouraux A, Iannetti GD. Nociceptive laser-evoked brain potentials do not reflect nociceptive-specific neural activity. J Neurophysiol 2009;101:3258–69.

[51] Nicholas MK, Siddal P, Tonkin L, Beeston L. Manage your pain. Sydney: ABC Books; 2002.

[52] Parsons LM. Integrating cognitive psychology, neurology and neuroimaging. Acta Psychol (Amst) 2001;107:155–81.

[53] Pleger B, Ragert P, Schwenkreis P, Forster AF, Wilimzig C, Dinse H, Nicolas V, Maier C, Tegenthoff M. Patterns of cortical reorganization parallel impaired tactile discrimination and pain intensity in complex regional pain syndrome. Neuroimage 2006;32:503–10.

[54] Pleger B, Tegenthoff M, Schwenkreis P, Janssen F, Ragert P, Dinse HR, Volker B, Zenz M, Maier C. Mean sustained pain levels are linked to hemispherical side-to-side differences of primary somatosensory cortex in the complex regional pain syndrome I. Exp Brain Res 2004;155:115–9.

[55] Rainville J, Ahern DK, Phalen L. Altering beliefs about pain and impairment in a functionally oriented treatment program for chronic low back pain. Clin J Pain 1993;9:196–201.

[56] Ramachandran VS, Rogers Ramachandran D, Cobb S. Touching the phantom limb. Nature 1995;377:489–90.

[57] Reedijk WB, van Rijn MA, Roelofs K, Tuijl JP, Marinus J, van Hilten JJ. Psychological features of patients with complex regional pain syndrome type I related dystonia. Mov Disord 2008;23:1551–9.

[58] Rommel O, Willweber-Strumpf A, Wagner P, Surall D, Malin JP, Zenz M. Psychological abnormalities in patients with complex regional pain syndrome (CRPS). Schmerz 2005;19:272–84.

[59] Sandstrom MJ, Keefe FJ. Self-management of fibromyalgia: the role of formal coping skills training and physical exercise training programs. Arthritis Care Res 1998;11:432–47.

[60] Schwenkreis P, Janssen F, Rommel O, Pleger B, Volker B, Hosbach I, Dertwinkel R, Maier C, Tegenthoff M. Bilateral motor cortex disinhibition in complex regional pain syndrome (CRPS) type I of the hand. Neurology 2003;61:515–9.

[61] Sharma N, Pomeroy VM, Baron JC. Motor imagery: a backdoor to the motor system after stroke? Stroke 2006;37:1941–52.

[62] Sterr A, Muller MM, Elbert T, Rockstroh B, Pantev C, Taub E. Perceptual correlates of changes in cortical representation of fingers in blind multifinger Braille readers. J Neurosci 1998;18:4417–23.

[63] Strong J, Ashton R, Chant D. The measurement of attitudes towards and beliefs about pain. Pain 1992;48:227–36.

[64] Sweller J. Evolution of human cognitive architecture. In: Ross B, editor. The psychology of learning and motivation, vol. 43. San Diego: Academic Press; 2003.

[65] Symonds TL, Burton AK, Tillotson KM, Main CJ. Do attitudes and beliefs influence work loss due to low back trouble? Occup Med (Lond) 1996;46:25–32.

[66] Tracey I. Imaging pain. Br J Anaesth 2008;101:32–9.

[67] Vartiainen NV, Kirveskari E, Forss N. Central processing of tactile and nociceptive stimuli in complex regional pain syndrome. Clin Neurophysiol 2008;119:2380–8.

[68] Wall P, McMahon S. The relationship of perceived pain to afferent nerve impulses. Trends Neurosci 1986;9:254–5.

[69] Wang X, Merzenich MM, Sameshima K, Jenkins WM. Remodelling of hand representation in adult cortex determined by timing of tactile stimulation. Nature 1995;378:71–5.

Correspondence to: G. Lorimer Moseley, PhD, Prince of Wales Medical Research Institute, Corner Easy and Barker Streets, Randwick, NSW 2031, Australia. Email: lorimer. moseley@gmail.com.

Part 7
Orofacial Pain and Headache

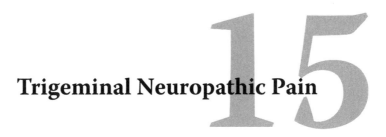

Trigeminal Neuropathic Pain

Joanna M. Zakrzewska, MD, FDSRCS, FFPMRCA

Facial Pain Unit, Eastman Dental Hospital, University College London Hospitals NHS Foundation Trust, London, United Kingdom

Trigeminal neuropathic pain is a feature of a group of conditions arising as a direct consequence of a lesion or disease affecting the somatosensory system. The most easily recognized condition is trigeminal neuralgia. Other forms of neuropathic facial pain include postherpetic neuralgia; glossopharyngeal neuralgia; and a condition variously called local facial neuralgia, trigeminal neuropathic pain, or atypical odontalgia. The etiologies of these conditions are variable, ranging from infection for postherpetic neuralgia to compression of the trigeminal nerve in trigeminal neuralgia. Another more frequently recognized group of conditions are the trigeminal autonomic cephalalgias, which include paroxysmal hemicrania, cluster headaches, SUNCT (short unilateral neuralgiform headache with conjunctival tearing), and SUNA (short unilateral neuralgiform headache with autonomic symptoms). These conditions are thought to have a different cause than the other types of neuralgic pain. Because of space limitations, this chapter will only cover trigeminal neuralgia and trigeminal neuropathic pain, focusing on their diagnosis and management.

Trigeminal Neuralgia

Definition

Trigeminal neuralgia is defined by the International Association for the Study of Pain (IASP) as a sudden, usually unilateral, severe, brief, stabbing, recurrent episode of pain in the distribution of one or more branches of the trigeminal nerve [16]. Trigeminal neuralgia is further divided into idiopathic and symptomatic types. Symptomatic trigeminal neuralgias are those much rarer cases where a primary cause is identified such as a benign or malignant tumor, demyelination such as that which occurs in multiple sclerosis, or the rarer arterial or vascular malformations. There has also been increasing awareness that not all trigeminal neuralgias present with the classic features as outlined in the International Headache Society (IHS) classification [1], and variations of this syndrome have been called atypical trigeminal neuralgia.

Epidemiology

In the 1990s most of the epidemiological studies on trigeminal neuralgia were carried out in the United States, and they were based on hospital cases. This research determined an annual incidence of trigeminal neuralgia of 4–5 cases per 100,000, with predominance in women and in persons between 50 and 70 years of age [28]. However, there have been two recent studies carried out in primary care based on general practice research databases both in the United Kingdom and in the Netherlands suggesting that the incidence of trigeminal neuralgia was approximately 28 cases per 1,000,000 [7,10]. However in a more careful study, where the diagnosis was validated by medical experts, the incidence rate was reported as 12.5 (95% CI: 10.4–14.9) [12], but initially when the data were first collected from the general practice databases, the authors reported an overall incidence of 21.7. All of these studies suggest that the condition is more common in women and that it first presents in middle age. Larger European studies looking at the burden of neuropathic pain across six European countries showed that 14% of neuropathic pain patients have trigeminal neuralgia [22]. Risk factors for trigeminal neuralgia include multiple sclerosis and hypertension, but data on prognosis are extremely limited. There is a general trend for an increasing number of relapses over time, but this pattern is not consistent.

Pathophysiology

The most commonly accepted theory as to the pathophysiology of trigeminal neuralgia is the "ignition" hypothesis put forward by Devor et al. [6]. There is some recent evidence to suggest that patients with more atypical forms of trigeminal neuralgia may in fact have more central changes, as they have been shown to have overactivation of central facilitation of trigeminal nociceptive processing rather than only peripheral changes [18].

Clinical Features

As with most pain conditions, diagnosis of trigeminal neuralgia relies heavily on the patient's medical history, which therefore needs to be taken with great care. Sometimes it is necessary to go over the history a second time at another date and potentially reconsider the diagnosis. The diagnostic criteria for trigeminal neuralgia have never been validated [26]. Once patients become branded with a diagnosis it is often difficult to remove it, and patients may receive inappropriate treatment if the wrong diagnosis has been made. While highlighting the key features of trigeminal neuralgia, I will use some patient narrative obtained through focus group work and e-mails used in writing a patient handbook entitled "Insights—Facts and Stories behind Trigeminal Neuralgia" [27]. The key features are shown in Fig. 1.

Diagnostic features are:
- pain described as electric shock-like, lightning, shooting
- pain comes in attacks that last for no more than 2 minutes
- a refractory period (when pain can no longer be provoked)
- a rapid rise and fall of pain intensity
- periods of remission
- pain provoked by light touch

Patients can have numerous attacks throughout the day, and these episodes can continue for weeks or months. Some patients, especially in the early stages, will go into periods of complete remission when they have no daily attacks and no longer need any medication. Some patients will report a burning, aching aftersensation when the main pain has disappeared, as illustrated by this patient's narrative: "The pain was sharp, stabbing, electrical shock-like pains that would last for only seconds; however, there would be a dull sensation after the pain subsided." This sensation gradually diminishes, and the patient is then free of pain between the attacks.

The most frequent location of the pain is in the second and third divisions of the trigeminal nerve. It is rare to see pain in only the first trigeminal division. If patients report pain in only the first division, then it is important to establish whether they truly have trigeminal neuralgia or whether it could be a trigeminal autonomic cephalalgia.

When the pain is extremely severe, eating becomes impossible, and patients will lose weight rapidly. Here is a patient's description: "It was a perfectly normal lovely day. Suddenly, a pain, the likes of which I have never before felt, sliced through the side of my left temple. A lightning bolt, the thwack of a sharp knife, the splintering of my skin, consciousness became pain. I stared into nothingness. I waited the 20 seconds or so it lasted; it filled the span of an eternity." Moreover, "the level-10 pain doubled me over the ground and I did not have control of my faculties … I could not have chewed or swallowed anything. Imagine toothache, only 10 times worse."

Many attacks of trigeminal neuralgia are evoked by light touch: "I had many trigger points that set my trigeminal neuralgia off, licking my lips, touching my face along my jaw around my ear or teeth, brushing my teeth was something I began to fear, forget flossing. At times I could not even swallow my own spit." Vibrations as well as cold winds will often be provoking stimuli. However, patients will also have spontaneous attacks of pain that do not seem to be associated with any of these triggers, as this patient describes: "After a while the pain didn't even seem to be triggered; it just came on by itself as if it had a mind of its own." Autonomic symptoms such as redness, tearing, and eye symptoms and signs are rare. Patients with trigeminal neuralgia like to keep still. Only about one-third of patients will be awoken at night by the pain.

Severe pain will often induce depression, and patients become extremely fearful of when they will get their next attack of pain and whether it will be more severe than previous episodes. Again it is useful to hear from the patients themselves about the loneliness and isolation; here are some of their reflections:

"The pain causes great fear of being out of control, and of course fear of the terrible pain."

"My husband reached over to try and calm me, and the touch made it even worse, and I had to push him away … don't touch me, don't touch me, and he feels rejected."

"The most frustrating is that you aren't understood or you feel as if no one understands how truly painful it is. You wish they could feel the pain for a day so they could understand just a little."

"Trigeminal neuralgia changes your identity. Suddenly you see how precious life can be, and it makes you reflect on what you are doing."

Examination may reveal no gross neurological abnormalities, except for the decreased corneal reflex or decreased sensation that is sometimes observed, and these patients are highly likely to have secondary causes for their trigeminal neuralgia. It is sometimes possible to trigger a pain attack during the examination by light touch on the trigger zones.

Differential Diagnosis

Any unilateral, episodic pain needs to be assessed as a potential symptomatic neuralgia, as not all such pain will be neuropathic initially. The other major class of conditions to consider are the trigeminal autonomic cephalalgias. Of particular importance are SUNCT, SUNA, and paroxysmal hemicrania. The major differentiating factor is that these pains tend to occur in the first division rather than in the second and third divisions of the trigeminal nerve. In patients with one of these conditions, each pain attack might be of longer duration. Attacks may not exhibit a refractory period and can be more numerous. Patients with these conditions are often restless and agitated, whereas patients with trigeminal neuralgia want to keep very still. Patients will report autonomic features including tearing, redness of the eye, meiosis, edema of the upper eyelids, stuffy nose or rhinorrhea, redness of the face, and a feeling of fullness in the ear. These patients should not undergo surgical treatments. Further details can be found in a series of articles [4], and they are summarized in Table I.

Investigations

Recently published international guidelines [5,9] now suggest that neurophysiological testing has high sensitivity and specificity to differentiate classical trigeminal neuralgia from symptomatic trigeminal neuralgia. Unfortunately, this type of testing is often only available in major academic institutions. Computed tomography (CT) scans and magnetic resonance imaging (MRI) will therefore be useful to identify cases of symptomatic trigeminal neuralgia. To detect neurovascular compression of the trigeminal nerve, high-quality, thin-cut MRIs are necessary. These scans must be focused on the posterior fossa and must be read by experienced neuroradiologists or neurosurgeons.

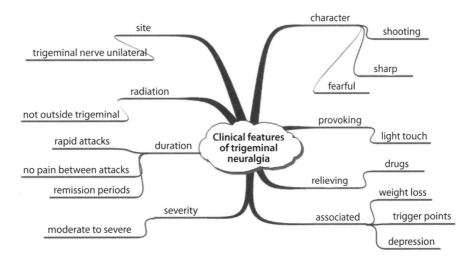

Fig. 1. Major clinical features of trigeminal neuralgia.

Table I
Principal diagnostic features of trigeminal neuralgias

Condition	Major Location and Radiation	Timing	Character/ Severity	Provoking Factors	Associated Factors
Trigeminal neuralgia (classical/typical)	Intra- or extraoral, in distribution of trigeminal nerve	Attacks last seconds to 2 minutes, with many attacks a day; remission periods last weeks to months	Sharp, shooting, moderate to very severe	Light touch: eating, washing, talking	Discrete trigger zones
Cluster headache (episodic, with pain-free periods; or chronic, with no remissions)	Trigeminal area, orbital, supraorbital, temporal	Attacks last 15–180 minutes to several hours, from 1 every other day to 8 per day; in episodic cases, remissions last one year or more	Hot, searing, tearing, penetrating, boring, sharp, burning, severe	Vasodilators (e.g., alcohol, high altitude)	Very pronounced conjunctival injection, lacrimation, nasal congestion, rhinorrhea, sweating, miosis, ptosis, eyelid edema, restlessness
Paroxysmal hemicrania	Eye, forehead; can radiate down the neck	Attacks last 2–30 minutes, 5–40 times daily, with remissions for months to years	Clawing, stabbing, throbbing, boring, severe	Head movements, alcohol; responds to indomethacin	Conjunctival injection, miosis, lacrimation, nasal stuffiness, rhinorrhea, facial edema, erythema
SUNCT (shorter-lasting, unilateral neuralgiform headache with conjunctival injection and tearing)	Ocular, periocular; may radiate to frontotemporal area, upper jaw, and palate	Attacks last up to 2 minutes, with 3–200 attacks daily, with remissions for months	Burning, electrical, stabbing, severe	Neck movements, light touch	Autonomic symptoms as for paroxysmal hemicrania, but short-lasting and mainly related to the eyes
SUNA (shorter-lasting, unilateral neuralgiform headache with autonomic features)	Ocular, periocular; may radiate to frontotemporal area, upper jaw, and palate	Attacks last from 1 to 600 seconds, once per day, with remissions for months	Burning, electrical, stabbing, severe	Light touch	Conjunctival injection and/or tearing, nasal congestion, and/or rhinorrhea, eyelid edema, ipsilateral sense of aural fullness or peri-aural swelling, ipsilateral forehead and facial sweating, ipsilateral miosis and/or ptosis

Management

The mainstay of management of trigeminal neuralgia are the antiepileptic drugs, which have been used since 1860. However it was the introduction of carbamazepine in 1962 that revolutionized the management of this condition, and this drug has remained the gold standard and the focus of three randomized control trials (RCTs). There have now been a variety of systematic reviews both within the Cochrane collaboration and elsewhere to evaluate the use of antiepileptic drugs, and international guidelines have been published [5,9,11,25].

The relative lack of robust, high-quality RCTs is related to several factors:

1) The rarity of the condition
2) Unpredictable remission periods
3) The lack of careful phenotyping
4) The lack of clear primary and secondary outcome measures
5) The difficulty of using a placebo control due to pain severity
6) The lack of power calculations

Medical Management

Table II provides a list of drugs that have been used in the management of trigeminal neuralgia and the evidence for their use.

Carbamazepine remains the drug of choice, but it is extremely important to begin with low doses and to gradually increase the dosage over a number of days. Patients need to learn to control the drug themselves. As the daily dosage rises, so does the possibility of side effects; all patients will report drowsiness, ataxia, and poor concentration at higher doses. Carbamazepine causes a rise in liver enzymes and has a high potential for drug interactions. Up to 7% of patients will develop an allergy, and this percentage is higher in some racial groups.

Oxcarbazepine is a keto derivative of carbamazepine that is excreted unchanged through the kidneys and therefore has decreased potential for drug interactions. In head-to-head comparisons with carbamazepine, it displays the same efficacy, but its tolerability is much higher. At higher dosage levels, patients may develop hyponatremia; this effect is more likely if patients are on diuretics.

Lamotrigine. The guidelines suggest that the next drug of choice should be either lamotrigine or baclofen. Lamotrigine has been evaluated in an RCT, but only as an additional medication rather than as a primary therapy. This drug can only be increased very slowly, and it is therefore of limited value in acute cases. It is the preferred drug for SUNCT and SUNA patients.

Baclofen has been evaluated in RCTs and has some efficacy, but not as high as that of carbamazepine. While not an antiepileptic drug, it could potentially be used in combination with carbamazepine to increase efficacy.

Gabapentin and pregabalin. These two drugs have been recommended for use in neuropathic pain because they have an additional action to that of the usual antiepileptic drugs, acting also on calcium channels.

Table II
Medical management of trigeminal neuralgia

Drug/Therapy	Daily Dose Range	Efficacy	Side Effects	Use
Evaluated in RCTs				
Carbamazepine	300–1000 mg; begin with 300 mg daily , raise dose by 200 mg every 3 days	Effective: NNT = 2.6 (range 2–4)	Drowsiness, ataxia, headaches, nausea, constipation, blurred vision, rash, poor concentration, hyponatremia in higher doses; long-term use can deplete folate levels; NNH = 3.4 (2.5–5.2) for side effects; NNH = 24 (13–110) for withdrawal	Use four times daily; high potential for drug interactions, especially with warfarin; sustained-release version useful, especially at night
Oxcarbazepine	300–1200 mg; begin with 300 mg daily; raise dose by 300 mg every 3 days	Effective (NNT not available)	Fatigue, dizziness, nausea, hyponatremia at high doses	Use four times daily; 300 mg oxcarbazepine equally potent as 200 mg carbamazepine; no major drug interactions
Lamotrigine	200–400 mg; begin with 25 mg daily, initially raising by 25 mg every 2 weeks	NNT = 2.1 (range 1.3–6.1) as add-on medication	Dizziness, drowsiness, constipation, ataxia, diplopia, irritability	Use twice daily; important to start very slowly to avoid rash; can use with carbamazepine
Baclofen	50–80 mg; begin with 10 mg daily and raise by 10 mg a week	Possibly effective: NNT = 1.4 (range 1–2.6); only 10 patients	Ataxia, lethargy, fatigue, nausea, vomiting	Use four times daily; useful as add-on therapy; beware rapid withdrawal
Gabapentin	1800–3600 mg; begin with 300 mg daily and increase every 3 days	NNT = 2.4 with injections	Ataxia, dizziness, drowsiness, nausea, headache, edema	Use three times daily; was used with weekly ropivacaine injections in the RCT; open studies have used higher doses than in the RCT
Commonly Used, but Not Evaluated in RCTs				
Clonazepam	4–8 mg; escalate very slowly	Low	Severe drowsiness in 60%; addictive	Use once daily; mainly used by neurologists
Phenytoin	200–300 mg; begin with 100 mg and increase by 100 mg every week	Good	Ataxia, lethargy, nausea, headache, behavioral changes, folate deficiency with prolonged use, gingival hypertrophy	Use three times daily; small margin for dose escalation; rarely used; used intravenously for immediate effect
Pregabalin	150–600 mg; begin with 150 mg and increase every 3 days	Good, 1 year cohort data	Ataxia, dizziness, drowsiness, nausea, headache, edema	Use twice daily; rapid escalation possible
Valproic acid	600–1200 mg; begin with 600 mg and increase every 3 days	Poor	Irritability, restlessness, tremor, confusion, nausea, rash, weight gain	Use twice daily; monitor liver function

Abbreviations: NNT, number needed to treat ; NNH, number needed to harm, RCT = randomized controlled trial.

There has been one small RCT using gabapentin combined with weekly ropivacaine injections into trigger areas [13]. The results looked promising, but it must be remembered that the patients had been relatively newly diagnosed with trigeminal neuralgia, and so they may have been at increased probability of going into a natural pain remission period. Pregabalin has been evaluated in a year-long cohort study and again showed potential [19].

Other drugs. A variety of other drugs have either been tested in very small RCTs (less than three patients) or have been evaluated as case-control studies. These compounds are often used when other drugs fail, rather than moving on to a potential surgical solution.

Medical versus Surgical Procedures

The published studies provide insufficient evidence to create robust guidelines on the timing of switching from medical to surgical management. Cohort studies have suggested that patients would have preferred earlier surgical interventions. A decision analysis study looking at hypothetical situations and asking 156 patients to comment on their choice of procedure showed that microvascular decompression would be the treatment of choice, with medical treatment being the least-preferred choice [20]. However, the differences were very small [20].

Surgical Treatments

Surgical treatments can be divided into two main categories. One category includes treatments that are destructive (ablative) and aim to reduce sensory input from the trigeminal nerve. The other major procedure is to decompress the nerve, encouraging remyelination and return to normal function. There are very few high-quality studies in this area, as has been shown by systematic reviews [21,30] and in the guidelines [5]. Some of the more recent reports are beginning to use independent observers to determine outcome measures and are attempting to use validated questionnaires. Procedures can be done at three levels: peripheral nerves, the Gasserian ganglion, and the posterior fossa. The types of surgeries currently in use are summarized in Table III.

Peripheral procedures. These procedures are all destructive and are aimed at delivering treatment at the level of a trigger point. Included in this group are cryotherapy, neurectomy, injection with substances such as streptomycin, radiofrequency thermocoagulation, and

laser therapy. Most of these procedures are done under local anesthesia.

Gasserian ganglion procedures. These procedures were until recently the most popular option, as they are easy to perform and can be done in most patients, even those who are medically unfit. Under heavy sedation, a needle is passed through the foramen ovale into the Gasserian ganglion. The needle's position is checked by imaging, and then a variety of procedures can be performed at this level. The nerve can be coagulated using temperatures of 60°C and 80°C (radiofrequency thermocoagulation), bathed in glycerol (glycerol rhizotomy), or compressed by a Fogarty catheter (balloon microcompression).

Posterior fossa procedures. These procedures deliver treatment at the root entry zone, which is the cisternal part of the trigeminal nerve just as it enters the pons. The most frequently performed procedure is microvascular decompression, a major neurosurgical procedure. After gaining entry into the skull, the surgeon identifies the vessels, especially the arteries, that are compressing the trigeminal nerve. The most frequently involved artery is the superior cerebellar artery. The offending vessels are either moved out of the way by the use of a vascular sling or by the interposition of pieces of Teflon. If no compression is found, some surgeons will perform a partial sensory rhizotomy, which of course involves damage to the sensory nerves.

The final procedure done at this level is gamma knife surgery, which is the least invasive of all the procedures. Using MRI technology, the trigeminal nerve in the area of the root entry zone, sometimes extending to the Gasserian ganglion, is irradiated using doses of 60–90 Gy.

Outcomes after Surgery

All procedures are subject to technical failures, but most patients can expect to obtain complete pain relief for at least a short period of time. The more peripheral the procedure, the quicker the time to recurrence of pain. Peripheral procedures on average give a 10-month period of complete pain relief. Gasserian ganglion procedures and gamma knife surgery give a pain-free period of 4 years for 50% of patients, whereas after microvascular decompression and partial sensory rhizotomy, 70% of patients can expect to still be pain free at 10 years [5,9].

Very few studies have measured the secondary outcome measures such as quality of life. The available

Table III
Surgical procedures used for trigeminal neuralgia

Procedure	Probability of Being Pain Free (%)	Mortality	Complications
Peripheral neurectomy, cryotherapy, alcohol, injection, acupuncture	22% at 2 years	None	Low: sensory loss, transient hematoma, edema
Radiofrequency thermorhizotomy (RFT)	50% at 5 years	Low	Related to trigeminal nerve (V): dysesthesia, anaesthesia dolorosa 4%, eye problems 4%, masticatory problems, sensory loss in over 50%
Percutaneous glycerol rhizotomy	45% at 5 years	Low	Complications as for RFT, but fewer cases of sensory loss
Balloon microcompression	45% at 5 years	Low	Complications as for RFT, fewer cases of sensory loss, but temporary masticatory problems common in 50%
Gamma knife surgery	45% at 5 years	None	Late onset of relief that may only be partial; 7% sensory loss up to 2 years post-treatment
Microvascular decompression	76% at 5 years	0.2–0.4%	Overall, 75% no complications; 16% perioperative complications; 2% transient dysfunction of cranial nerves IV, VI; 4% transient dysfunction of cranial nerve VIII, with 2% permanent deafness

studies found the highest improvement in quality of life in patients who have undergone microvascular decompression [31]. Patients receiving Gasserian ganglion and posterior fossa surgery are often able to discontinue all their medications. This degree of improvement is unlikely in patients who have had peripheral procedures.

Complications

As would be expected, the more peripheral the procedure, the fewer the complications. After posterior fossa surgery the risk of death is between 0.2 and 0.4%. Mortality is extremely low after Gasserian ganglion surgery and not reported after peripheral procedures.

Immediate postoperative complications. Complications of microvascular decompression include meningitis (mostly aseptic); cerebrospinal fluid leak, which in some cases requires readmission; and stroke, if a major vessel is injured. Hematomas are an immediate sequel of Gasserian ganglion procedures.

Other cranial nerve complications. Hearing loss can occur in up to 4% of patients, which in 2% is likely to be long-term. Eye problems are generally temporary.

Trigeminal nerve complications. Sensory loss is highly likely in patients undergoing ablative procedures of the Gasserian ganglion and in gamma knife surgery as well as partial sensory rhizotomy. After gamma knife surgery the sensory loss may be delayed and only manifest itself 6 months after treatment. The sensory loss can vary from very mild to severe, with associated pain and discomfort termed "anesthesia dolorosa." The likelihood of anesthesia dolorosa is highest after radiofrequency

thermocoagulation, especially if high temperatures have been used. Problems with mastication are most likely after microcompression, but they tend to gradually improve with time. Patients may get corneal anesthesia that can lead to keratitis.

Peripheral procedures are likely to give a much smaller area of anesthesia, and they may only result in local edema and bleeding after surgical exposure of the nerve.

Conclusions

Patients with trigeminal neuralgia need to be carefully diagnosed, and should then be treated with first-line drugs. If these drugs either fail to control the pain or cause considerable side effects, a surgical opinion should be sought. An early opportunity to meet a neurosurgeon is important because severe pain will limit patients' ability to comprehend the outcomes and potential complications of procedures. Of the surgical procedures, medically fit patients should be considered for microvascular decompression and others should be offered one of the ablative procedures at the level of the Gasserian ganglion.

A variety of support groups exist in English-speaking countries that can help patients meet fellow sufferers; get further advice by telephone, e-mail, or web forums; and participate in conferences. At such conferences they can meet a variety of health care professionals and make more informed decisions about the future management of their condition [29]. These groups host websites in the United States (www.tna-support.org), the United Kingdom (www.tna.org.uk), Australia (www.tnaaustralia.org.au), and Canada (www.tnac.org) and publish their own literature, such as *Striking Back* [24] and *Insights* [27].

Trigeminal Neuropathic Pain (Atypical Odontalgia)

Definition

It is increasingly being recognized that, like other nerves in the body, the trigeminal nerve can develop a painful neuropathy. It is thought that many patients previously labeled as having chronic idiopathic facial pain or atypical facial pain really have trigeminal neuropathic pain. Atypical odontalgia, which has been well-described by Scandinavian researchers as pain in a tooth-bearing area, may also represent a local form of trigeminal neuropathic pain [2,14].

Clinical Features

There is often a history of trauma to the trigeminal nerve, either gross trauma from facial injuries or related to dental extractions, endodontic procedures, and other intraoral surgical procedures. The pain is described as being burning, tingling, and like "pins and needles," and it is often continuous, although there may be severe exacerbations, which are described as shooting and sharp. The pain is localized in the area of nerve damage and does not have extensive radiation. It can vary from being mild to very severe, and it is often provoked by light touch. Examination may find areas of decreased sensitivity to light touch,

but there may also be allodynia. Often application of a local anesthetic in the form of an injection or topical cream can reduce many of these symptoms temporarily. Fig. 2 illustrates the key features of trigeminal neuropathic pain.

Management

If these patients fulfill the major criteria for neuropathic pain [23] using one of the neuropathic screening tools [3], then management is similar to that used for all neuropathic pain. A variety of guidelines have been published by the European Federation of Neurological Societies, the Canadian Pain Society, and the Special Interest Group on Neuropathic Pain of IASP.

All these guidelines have recently been reviewed by O'Connor et al. [17] and are fairly consistent. Where there is good evidence there is good agreement on treatments, whereas where there are fewer RCTs the recommendations vary. First-line drugs include the tricyclic antidepressants, especially nortriptyline, the serotonin-norepinephrine reuptake inhibitors (SNRIs) such as duloxetine, and two anticonvulsant ($\alpha_2\delta$) drugs, pregabalin and gabapentin. Second-line drugs include tramadol and other opioids. There is debate over the value of topical lidocaine in the form of patches, whereas lidocaine injections used in an RCT have not been found to be useful [15]. These treatments are summarized in Table IV.

Additional Management Considerations

As with all chronic pain, patients with trigeminal neuropathic pain also need considerable psychological

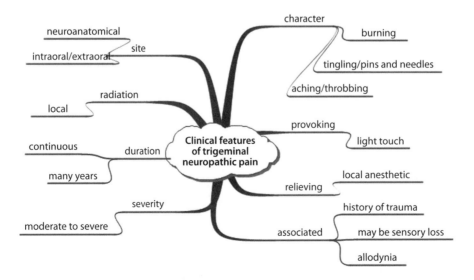

Fig. 2. Major clinical features of trigeminal neuropathic pain.

145

Table IV
Drugs used in neuropathic pain that could be used in trigeminal neuropathic pain

Drug	Daily Dose	Efficacy	Side Effects	Usage
Nortriptyline (tricyclic antidepressant)	50–150 mg Begin with 10 mg, raise weekly	Good	Sedation, dry mouth, weight gain	Use at night only; use with care in cardiac disease, glaucoma; can use lower doses with good response
Venlafaxine (SNRI)	75–225 mg Begin with 75 mg and raise dose weekly	Small RCT in atypical facial pain found no benefit	Nausea	Use once daily for 4–6 weeks
Gabapentin (acts on calcium channels)	600–3600 mg Begin with 300 mg daily and increase every 3 days	May be effective	Sedation, ataxia, dizziness, edema	Use three times daily; improves sleep; has few drug interactions; use care in renal dysfunction
Pregabalin	150–600 mg Begin with 150 mg and increase every 3 days	May be effective	Dizziness, tiredness, headaches, peripheral edema	Use twice daily; improves anxiety and sleep; use care in renal dysfunction
5% lidocaine patch (topical)	3 patches for a maximum of 12 hours	May be effective	Local erythema, rash	Use up to 12 hours at any one time; use only if extraoral pain and allodynia are present

Source: Based on a review of recent neuropathic pain treatment guidelines by O'Connor and Dworkin [17].
Abbreviations: RCT, randomized controlled trial; SNRI, serotonin norepinephrine reuptake inhibitor.

management. They need an explanation of their pain and reassurance that it is not going to progress to cancer. They need to take control of their pain and improve their outcomes by having a positive outlook, which may need to be achieved through sessions of cognitive-behavioral therapy [8]. Further surgical procedures must be avoided.

Acknowledgments

This work was undertaken at University College London (UCL)/UCLHT, which received a proportion of funding from the Department of Health's NIHR Biomedical Research Centre funding scheme. The author received an investigator-led grant from UCB Pharma for the study of levetiracetam.

References

[1] Anonymous. The International Classification of Headache Disorders, 2nd edition. Cephalalgia 2004;24(Suppl 1):9–160.
[2] Baad-Hansen L. Atypical odontalgia: pathophysiology and clinical management. J Oral Rehabil 2008;35:1–11.
[3] Bennett MI, Attal N, Backonja MM, Baron R, Bouhassira D, Freynhagen R, Scholz J, Tolle TR, Wittchen HU, Jensen TS. Using screening tools to identify neuropathic pain. Pain 2007;127:199–203.
[4] Cohen AS, Matharu MS, Goadsby PJ. Trigeminal autonomic cephalalgias: current and future treatments. Headache 2007;47:969–80.
[5] Cruccu G, Gronseth G, Alksne J, Argoff C, Brainin M, Burchiel K, Nurmikko T, Zakrzewska JM. AAN-EFNS guidelines on trigeminal neuralgia management. Eur J Neurol 2008;15:1013–28.
[6] Devor M, Amir R, Rappaport ZH. Pathophysiology of trigeminal neuralgia: the ignition hypothesis. Clin J Pain 2002;18:4–13.
[7] Dieleman JP, Kerklaan J, Huygen FJ, Bouma PA, Sturkenboom MC. Incidence rates and treatment of neuropathic pain conditions in the general population. Pain 2008;137:681–8.
[8] Dionne R, Newton-John T, Zakrzewska JM. Overall management of facial pain. In Zakrzewska JM, editor. Orofacial pain. Oxford: Oxford University Press; 2009. p. 53–68.
[9] Gronseth G, Cruccu G, Alksne J, Argoff C, Brainin M, Burchiel K, Nurmikko T, Zakrzewska JM. Practice parameter: the diagnostic evaluation and treatment of trigeminal neuralgia (an evidence-based review): report of the Quality Standards Subcommittee of the American Academy of Neurology and the European Federation of Neurological Societies. Neurology 2008;71:1183–90.
[10] Hall GC, Carroll D, Parry D, McQuay HJ. Epidemiology and treatment of neuropathic pain: the UK primary care perspective. Pain 2006;122:156–62.
[11] He L, Wu B, Zhou M. Non-antiepileptic drugs for trigeminal neuralgia. Cochrane Database Syst Rev 2006;3:CD004029.
[12] Koopman JS, Dieleman JP, Huygen FJ, de MM, Martin CG, Sturkenboom MC. Incidence of facial pain in the general population. Pain 2009;147:122–7.
[13] Lemos L, Flores S, Oliveira P, Almeida A. Gabapentin supplemented with ropivacaine block of trigger points improves pain control and quality of life in trigeminal neuralgia patients when compared with gabapentin alone. Clin J Pain 2008;24:64–75.
[14] List T, Leijon G, Helkimo M, Oster A, Dworkin SF, Svensson P. Clinical findings and psychosocial factors in patients with atypical odontalgia: a case-control study. J Orofac Pain 2007;21:89–98.
[15] List T, Leijon G, Helkimo M, Oster A, Svensson P. Effect of local anesthesia on atypical odontalgia—a randomized controlled trial. Pain 2006;122:306–14.
[16] Merskey H, Bogduk N. Classification of chronic pain. Descriptions of chronic pain syndromes and definitions of pain terms, 2nd ed. Seattle: IASP Press: 1994.
[17] O'Connor AB, Dworkin RH. Treatment of neuropathic pain: an overview of recent guidelines. Am J Med 2009;122(10 Suppl):S22–S32.
[18] Obermann M, Yoon MS, Ese D, Maschke M, Kaube H, Diener HC, Katsarava Z. Impaired trigeminal nociceptive processing in patients with trigeminal neuralgia. Neurology 2007;69:835–41.
[19] Obermann M, Yoon MS, Sensen K, Maschke M, Diener HC, Katsarava Z. Efficacy of pregabalin in the treatment of trigeminal neuralgia. Cephalalgia 2008;28:174–81.
[20] Spatz AL, Zakrzewska JM, Kay EJ. Decision analysis of medical and surgical treatments for trigeminal neuralgia: how patient evaluations of benefits and risks affect the utility of treatment decisions. Pain 2007;131:302–10.
[21] Tatli M, Satici O, Kanpolat Y, Sindou M. Various surgical modalities for trigeminal neuralgia: literature study of respective long-term outcomes. Acta Neurochir (Wien) 2008;150:243–55.
[22] Tolle T, Dukes E, Sadosky A. Patient burden of trigeminal neuralgia: results from a cross-sectional survey of health state impairment and treatment patterns in six European countries. Pain Pract 2006;6:153–60.

[23] Treede RD, Jensen TS, Campbell JN, Cruccu G, Dostrovsky JO, Griffin JW, Hansson P, Hughes R, Nurmikko T, Serra J. Neuropathic pain: redefinition and a grading system for clinical and research purposes. Neurology 2008;70:1630–5.

[24] Weigel G, Casey KF. Striking back: the trigeminal neuralgia handbook. Trigeminal Neuralgia Association; 2000.

[25] Wiffen P, Collins S, McQuay H, Carroll D, Jadad A, Moore A. Anticonvulsant drugs for acute and chronic pain. Cochrane Database Syst Rev 2005;3:CD001133.

[26] Zakrzewska JM. Diagnosis and differential diagnosis of trigeminal neuralgia. Clin J Pain 2002;18:14–21.

[27] Zakrzewska JM. Insights: facts and stories behind trigeminal neuralgia. Gainesville: Trigeminal Neuralgia Association; 2006.

[28] Zakrzewska JM, Hamlyn PJ. Facial pain. In: Crombie IK, Croft PR, Linton SJ, LeResche L, Von Korff M, editors. Epidemiology of pain. Seattle: IASP Press; 1999. p. 171–202.

[29] Zakrzewska JM, Jorns TP, Spatz A. Patient led conferences: who attends, are their expectations met and do they vary in three different countries? Eur J Pain 2009;13:486–91.

[30] Zakrzewska JM, Lopez BC. Quality of reporting in evaluations of surgical treatment of trigeminal neuralgia: recommendations for future reports. Neurosurgery 2003;53:110–22.

[31] Zakrzewska JM, Lopez BC, Kim SE, Coakham HB. Patient reports of satisfaction after microvascular decompression and partial sensory rhizotomy for trigeminal neuralgia. Neurosurgery 2005;56:1304–11.

Correspondence to: Prof. Joanna M. Zakrzewska MD, FDSRCS, FFPMRCA, Consultant in Oral Medicine, Facial Pain Unit, Eastman Dental Hospital, UCLH NHS Foundation Trust, 256 Gray's Inn Road, London WC1X 8LD, United Kingdom. Email: jzakrzewska@nhs.net.

16

Pain Associated with Temporomandibular Disorders and with Burning Mouth Syndrome

Antoon De Laat, DDS, PhD, Dr h.c.

Department of Oral and Maxillofacial Surgery, School of Dentistry, Oral Pathology and Maxillofacial Surgery, Catholic University of Leuven, Leuven, Belgium

Temporomandibular Disorders

Temporomandibular disorders (TMDs) comprise a number of clinical problems involving the structures of and around the temporomandibular joint (TMJ), the masticatory musculature, or both [16]. Pain is one of the most common complaints associated with TMDs, and can be clinically expressed as masticatory muscle pain (MMP) or as TMJ arthralgia (as in synovitis, capsulitis, or osteoarthritis) (for review see [3]). Pain can occur spontaneously or may be associated with joint function and loading (e.g., during chewing, yawning, or biting). TMDs may also include symptoms of dysfunction (limitation of movement, interference during movement, internal derangements of the TMJ, or locking of the joint). TMD pain can be, but is not necessarily, associated with such dysfunction.

Similar to the fact sheet that was recently produced on the occasion of the IASP Global Year Against Musculoskeletal Pain, this chapter will review current knowledge on epidemiology, diagnosis, classification, and management of pain associated with TMDs.

Epidemiology and Economic Impact

TMD pain is very common. It has been reported in 4–12% of the general population (especially in the 20–40-year age range), with a female-to-male ratio of 2:1 [32,48,77]. However, 1.4–7% seek treatment (four times as many females as males), and progression to severe and/or chronic pain is rare [60]. Development of chronic TMD pain is associated with more psychological disturbance and significantly affects an individual's quality of life, physical function, and socioeconomic state. TMD pain does not always get the attention it deserves. In prevalence studies on general musculoskeletal pain, or in the criteria for fibromyalgia/widespread muscle pain, the head area and the masticatory system often are not even included [74,91].

Pathophysiology

Many aspects of the etiology of TMDs are unclear. Where an occlusal/dental cause is not credible, there is definite support for a biopsychological and multifactorial background [39,82]. The occurrence of dysfunction and TMD pain is the result of a complex interaction between biological (e.g., hormonal, adrenergic) mechanisms [55,57,89], psychological states and traits [33,75,81], environmental or general health conditions [8,48], and (macro- or micro-) trauma [15,93].

In MMP, recent evidence suggests that ongoing overloading, (micro-)trauma, or local inflammation of the muscles releases neurotransmitters that sensitize the peripheral and central nervous system [2,84]. Typically, in the masticatory system, parafunctions such as tooth clenching and bruxism have been implicated (for review see [53]). More recently, daytime (low-level) tooth clenching was identified as a risk factor [12], and sleep bruxers with a low frequency of tooth grinding and clenching were more at risk of reporting pain than those with a high frequency of bruxing episodes [76]. In conjunction with altered pain-regulating mechanisms [57] and influenced by female hormones [86], this dysfunction may lead to localized or more generalized spread of muscle pain [17,27]. Recently, genetic factors (*COMT* gene haplotypes) have also been implicated in the onset of MMP [18,28].

TMJ arthralgia may be the consequence of trauma [15,93] or of intrinsic or extrinsic overloading of the TMJ (as in tooth clenching) that overcomes the adaptive capacity of the joint tissues (for review see [19]). This adaptive capacity of the TMJ may be reduced by intrinsic factors such as reduced blood supply and nutrition [65,66]. As in osteoarthritis, genes and gender have been identified as modulatory factors [35]. Free radicals, enzymes, bone morphogenetic proteins, and growth factors, together with nociceptive and proinflammatory neuropeptides, will mediate the inflammation, pain, and progressive tissue changes [59,65].

Both MMP and arthralgia should initially be considered nociceptive/inflammatory types of pain. However, development of chronicity and persistent pain may imply increased central sensitization and complication with neuropathic pain components.

Clinical Features

Masticatory muscle pain is reported as a dull, regional, aching pain, located in the jaw-closing muscles and around the ear. Pain can occur spontaneously and may be aggravated during function or stretching of the muscles (e.g., yawning). Some patients report more pain in the morning or the evening [14], but the pattern may be variable [34]. On a visual analogue scale, the intensity is rated 3–7/10. Patients often report associated symptoms such as limitation of movement, fullness of the ear, and neck pain and headache [3]. The specific relation between MMP and (tension-type) headache is unclear and a cause-and-effect relationship has not been established. MMP may be part of widespread musculoskeletal pain or fibromyalgia. The overlap between these conditions is significant [13,31,53].

TMJ arthralgia appears as sharp pain of moderate intensity, localized in or around the joint and often irradiating into the ear. Loading, movements of the joint, and stretching of the joint capsule during maximal mouth opening may aggravate the pain. As a result

of pain, mouth opening and joint function may be limited. TMJ pain is often associated with articular disk dysfunction (internal derangement of the joint), clinically expressed as clicking or locking of the TMJ. This dysfunction, of course, may also be a clear cause of limited or compromised jaw movements.

TMJ osteoarthritis may be part of a generalized arthritis and may be accompanied by crepitation. Whereas acute phases of arthritis typically are associated with increased pain, it is striking that a "settled" osteoarthrosis, even with significant radiological degeneration of the joint surfaces, often is characterized by increased crepitation without clinical pain complaints.

If chronic pain develops, both MMP and TMJ arthralgia may be accompanied by central sensitization [84] and by psychological problems such as depression, somatization, and anxiety [10].

Diagnostic Criteria

For the most common subgroups of TMD, research diagnostic criteria (RDC-TMD) were established [21] and were soon translated into a clinical classification [86]. Three subgroups have been distinguished:

1) Myofascial pain (masticatory muscle pain) with and without limitation of mouth opening, based upon a report of pain, confirmed by positive palpation of more than 3 out of 24 palpation sites and a cutoff for limitation at 40 mm between the incisors.

2) Anterior disk displacement, with reduction (clicking joints) or without reduction (closed lock). In the latter group a further distinction can be made based on the presence or absence of limitation of mouth opening, with a cutoff of 37 mm.

3) TMJ arthralgia, osteoarthritis, and osteoarthrosis, based upon the report of pain in the TMJ, the presence or absence of palpation pain, and the recording of coarse crepitus during mandibular movement.

Details and decision trees for these diagnoses, as well as numerous translations of the questionnaires and examination sheets, can be readily accessed at the RDC-TMD website (www.rdc-tmdinternational.org). Recently, and based upon extensive studies on the validity of the RDC-TMD, the diagnostic criteria have been refined, and steps are being taken to translate them into diagnostic criteria for TMD [68].

For MMP, the criteria are a complaint of muscle pain in the jaw, temple, face, or periarticular area, with pain/ tenderness on palpation or during jaw movement. For TMJ arthralgia, the criteria are pain in the face, jaw, temple, and in front of or in the ear, which changes during jaw movement and function, and report of pain upon palpation on or around the lateral pole of the TMJ or during dynamic testing of the range of motion. Psychosocial comorbidity in MMP or TMJ arthralgia is rated using the Graded Chronic Pain Scale and measurement scales for depression, anxiety, and nonspecific physical symptoms.

TMD pain is diagnosed from the history and clinical examination. Technical examinations (movement recording, electromyography, and occlusal analysis) have not been shown to be reliable and valid in the framework of pain diagnosis [36]. Imaging (radiographs, CT, or MRI) may be very helpful in the diagnosis of degenerative joint problems, intracapsular disease, and inflammation [56].

Management

Pain and other symptoms of temporomandibular disorders are usually self-limiting, with a benign natural course. Management aims at providing optimal circumstances for the body to adapt and heal. Concomitant with this adaptation process, pain will decrease, and most treatment approaches therefore, are reversible and fit into the biopsychosocial approach.

A primary and very important step is providing patients with information regarding the nature and natural course of TMD. Patients must be instructed in avoiding overload of the system (e.g., tooth clenching), and in active self-care, applying warmth and massage [64]. Temporarily, hard food or extreme jaw movements should be avoided.

Physical therapy is commonly used with reports of clinical success. Recent reviews, however, have not found any particular method to be superior, and more research is needed [63].

Intraoral occlusal appliances have a long tradition in the management of pain and dysfunction of the masticatory system. Several hypothesis regarding their observed clinical efficacy exist, none being solidly confirmed [50]. Most importantly, occlusal appliances—if used—should be designed in order to avoid irreversible changes in dental occlusion.

For a limited period of time, pain medication (analgesics, nonsteroidal anti-inflammatory drugs) can be used to overcome acute pain [20].

In patients with chronic TMD pain, these therapies must be accompanied by psychological support such as cognitive-behavioral therapy and relaxation therapy [71]. As in other chronic pain syndromes, low-dose tricyclic antidepressants or selective serotonin reuptake inhibitors can be considered [20]. A recent review [88] clearly stressed the need for psychological screening of TMD patients, in order to decide between simple or multimodal management (in case of major psychological problems).

In patients with persistent TMJ arthralgia, arthrocentesis of the joint might be considered [70]. TMJ surgery, aimed at optimizing the position of the joint structures, however, did not prove to be superior to medical management or conservative therapy in the case of internal derangement with locking [80].

Burning Mouth Syndrome

Also called stomatodynia (and glossodynia if the symptoms are confined to the tongue only), burning mouth syndrome (BMS) remains an ill-defined and poorly understood syndrome. Characterized by a spontaneous burning sensation in (parts) of the oral cavity, BMS is sometimes, but not always, accompanied by reports of dysgeusia (disturbed taste) and xerostomia (dry mouth) [42]. Scala et al. [79] proposed a classification into primary (idiopathic) BMS, without apparent organic cause and with a probable neuropathological cause, and secondary BMS, where the symptoms result from a local or systemic pathology, including mucosal disease, vitamin deficiency, diabetes, or medication side effects. Diagnostic criteria for BMS have been formulated, but not validated [69]. When patients present with symptoms of BMS, potential etiologic factors should first be ruled out and treated. This chapter will focus on primary BMS.

Epidemiology and Characteristics

Since no clear diagnostic criteria are available, the real prevalence of BMS in unknown. Available studies report BMS symptoms in 0.7% of the general population, and patients presenting in the clinic are predominantly peri- and postmenopausal women [6,7,58]. The sensation is described as burning, tingling, and sometimes numb; it can be accompanied by a feeling of dryness of the mouth and altered taste. The burning sensation is most prevalent in the evening, but it rarely occurs during sleep [37].

Pathophysiology

Local environmental factors, saliva composition, and mucosal blood flow have been reported to be different in BMS patients [38,45,51,67], but recent evidence favors neuropathic mechanisms in the etiology of BMS, in both the peripheral and central nervous system. For example, histological studies have found peripheral nerve damage corresponding to axonal degeneration [52,92]. Disturbed somatic sensations in the tongue (cold, heat, mechanical, and taste) were found in several controlled studies [30,38,43,83]. The coexistence of burning sensations and taste alterations suggests an interaction between the nociceptive and gustatory nervous system and inspired Femiano [24] to label BMS patients as "supertasters." Recently, evidence for chorda tympani hypofunction in BMS was presented [22]. Electrophysiological studies found that the nociceptive and tactile components of the blink reflex were disturbed [30,46]. Topical applications of neuroactive drugs (such as clonazepam or lidocaine) were effective in decreasing the burning pain [29,40]. In imaging studies (PET and fMRI), patients with BMS exhibited hypofunction in the dopaminergic system [45] and decreased volumetric activation of the whole brain during thermal stimulation [1].

However, it is unclear whether the underlying pathophysiological mechanisms are predominantly peripheral, central, or mixed. When the lingual nerve was anesthetized in BMS patients, some of them were completely pain-free, while others did not experience any therapeutic effect [41].

In addition to the emerging evidence indicating a trigeminal small-fiber neuropathy as the underlying etiology for BMS, a recent hypothesis implies steroid hormone dysregulation (as a consequence of chronic anxiety or post-traumatic stress) interfering with the synthesis of neuroactive steroids [90]. Given to the drastic hormonal changes in menopause, this line of thought would help to explain the typical overrepresentation of perimenopausal women in patient groups.

Psychosocial well-being is adversely affected by chronic pain, including BMS, which diminishes quality of life [4,51].

Management

Recent systematic reviews [7,72,94] have evaluated the reported efficacy of topical, systemic, and behavioral therapies. Clonazepam (1 mg) sucked 3 times daily for 3 minutes reduced pain intensity in two-thirds of the patients after 2 weeks [40]. Benzydamine mouthwash and topical lactoperoxidase were ineffective [23,78]. A single study indicated that amisulpride, paroxetine, and

sertraline over 8 weeks demonstrated beneficial effects in reducing pain intensity [62]. Multiple studies from a single center [23,26] on the efficacy of alpha-lipoic acid (600 mg daily over 2 months) were recently contradicted [9,11,60]. Systemic capsaicin (0.25% capsule, 3 times daily for 30 days) resulted in slight decrease in pain, but also gastrointestinal side effects [73]. Trazodone and bethanechol were ineffective [26,85].

Cognitive therapy sessions of 1 hour per week over 12 to 15 weeks had positive effects on the burning pain for up to half a year in one study [6], and in another study 2 months of psychotherapy also resulted in some improvement [24].

In addition to the evidence from controlled studies, medications regularly used for other neuropathic pains (systemic amitriptyline, clonazepam, selective serotonin reuptake inhibitors, duloxetine, pregabalin, gabapentin, and also topical capsaicin or lidocaine) have been used in clinical settings on a trial-and-error basis [7,72,94].

Conclusion

The etiology and natural course of burning mouth syndrome are still unclear. The pathophysiology points toward underlying neuropathic-like changes, but other hypotheses have been put forward. There is urgent need for testable diagnostic criteria and well-designed studies on the efficacy of medication used in other neuropathies on BMS.

References

[1] Albuquerque RJ, de Leeuw R, Carlson CR, Okeson JP, Miller CS, Anderson AH. Cerebral activation during thermal stimulation of patients who have burning mouth disorder: an fMRI study. Pain 2006;122:223–34.

[2] Arendt-Nielsen L, Graven-Nielsen T. Central sensitization in fibromyalgia and other musculoskeletal disorders. Curr Pain Headache Rep 2003;7:355–61.

[3] Benoliel R, Sharav Y. Masticatory myofascial pain, tension-type and chronic daily headache. In: Sharav Y, Benoliel R, editors. Orofacial pain and headache. Amsterdam: Elsevier; 2008. p. 109–28.

[4] Bergdahl J, Anneroth G, Perris H. Personality characteristics of patients with resistant burning mouth syndrome. Acta Odontol Scand 1995;53:7–11.

[5] Bergdahl J, Anneroth G, Perris H. Cognitive therapy in the treatment of patients with resistant burning mouth syndrome: a controlled study. J Oral Pathol Med 2004;33:213–5.

[6] Bergdahl M, Bergdahl J. Burning mouth syndrome: prevalence and associated factors. J Oral Pathol Med 1999;28:350–4.

[7] Buchanan J, Zakrzewska J. Burning mouth syndrome. Clin Evid 2005;14:1685–90.

[8] Burris JL, Evans DR, Carlson CR. Psychological correlates of medical comorbidities in patients with temporomandibular disorders. J Am Dent Assoc 2010;141:22–31.

[9] Carbone M, Pentenero M, Carrozzo M, Ippolito A, Gandolfo S. Lack of efficacy of alpha-lipoic acid in burning mouth syndrome: a double-blind, randomized, placebo-controlled study. Eur J Pain 2009;13:492–6.

[10] Carlson CR. Psychological considerations for chronic orofacial pain. Oral Maxillofac Surg Clin North Am 2008;20:185–95.

[11] Cavalcanti DR, da Silveira FR. Alpha lipoic acid in burning mouth syndrome: a randomized double-blind placebo-controlled trial. J Oral Pathol Med 2009;38:254–61.

[12] Chen CY, Palla S, Erni S, Sieber M, Gallo LM. Nonfunctional tooth contact in healthy controls and patients with myogenous facial pain. J Orofac Pain 2007;21:185–93.

[13] Cimino R, Michelotti A, Stradi R, Farinaro C. Comparison of clinical and psychologic features of fibromyalgia and masticatory myofascial pain. J Orofac Pain 1998;12:35–41.

[14] Dao TT, Lund JP, Lavigne GJ. Comparison of pain and quality of life in bruxers and patients with myofascial pain of the masticatory muscles. J Orofac Pain 1994;8:350–6.

[15] De Boever JA, Keersmaekers K. Trauma in patients with temporomandibular disorders: frequency and treatment outcome. J Oral Rehabil 1996;23:91–6.

[16] De Leeuw R. Orofacial pain: guidelines for assessment, diagnosis and management, 4th ed. The American Academy of Orofacial Pain. Quintessence; 2008.

[17] DeSantana JM, Sluka KA. Central mechanisms in the maintenance of chronic widespread noninflammatory muscle pain. Curr Pain Headache Rep 2008;12:338–43.

[18] Diatchenko L, Nackley AG, Slade GD, Bhalang K, Belfer I, Max MB, Goldman D, Maixner W. Catechol-O-methyltransferase gene polymorphisms are associated with multiple pain-evoking stimuli. Pain 2006;125:216–24.

[19] Dieppe PA, Lohmander LS. Pathogenesis and management of pain in osteoarthritis. Lancet 2005;365:965–73.

[20] Dionne RA, Berthold CW. Therapeutic uses of non-steroidal anti-inflammatory drugs in dentistry. Crit Rev Oral Biol Med 2001;12:315–30.

[21] Dworkin SF, LeResche L. Research diagnostic criteria for temporomandibular disorders: review, criteria, examinations and specifications, critique. J Craniomandib Disord 1992;6:301–55.

[22] Eliav E, Kamran B, Schaham R, Czerninski R, Gracely RH, Benoliel R. Evidence of chorda tympani dysfunction in patients with burning mouth syndrome. J Am Dent Assoc 2007;138:628–33.

[23] Femiano F. Burning mouth syndrome (BMS): an open trial of comparative efficacy of alpha-lipoic acid (thioctic acid) with other therapies. Minerva Stomatol 2002;51:405–9.

[24] Femiano F. Damage to taste system and oral pain: burning mouth syndrome. Minerva Stomatol 2004;53:471–8.

[25] Femiano F, Gombos F, Scully C. Burning mouth syndrome: open trial of psychotherapy alone, medication with alpha-lipoic acid (thioctic acid) and combination therapy. Med Oral 2004;9:8–13.

[26] Femiano F, Scully C. Burning mouth syndrome (BMS): double blind controlled study of alpha-lipoic acid (thioctic acid) therapy. J Oral Pathol Med 2002;31:267–9.

[27] Fernández-de-las-Peñas C, Galán-del-Río F, Fernández-Carnero J, Pesquera J, Arendt-Nielsen L, Svensson P. Bilateral widespread mechanical pain sensitivity in women with myofascial temporomandibular disorder: evidence of impairment in central nociceptive processing. J Pain 2009;10:1170–8.

[28] Fillingim RB, Wallace MR, Herbstman DM, Ribeiro-Dasilva M, Staud R. Genetic contributions to pain: a review of findings in humans. Oral Dis 2008;14:673–82.

[29] Formaker BK, Mott AE, Frank ME. The effects of topical anesthesia on oral burning in burning mouth syndrome. Ann NY Acad Sci 1998;855:776–80.

[30] Forssell H, Jääskeläinen S, Tenovuo O, Hinkka S. Sensory dysfunction in burning mouth syndrome. Pain 2002;99:41–7.

[31] Fricton JR. The relationship of temporomandibular disorders and fibromyalgia: implications for diagnosis and treatment. Curr Pain Headache Rep 2004;8:355–63.

[32] Gesch D, Bernhardt O, Alte D, Schwahn C, Kocher T, John U, Hensel E. Prevalence of signs and symptoms of temporomandibular disorders in an urban and rural German population: results of a population-based study of health in Pomerania. Quintessence Int 2004;35:143–50.

[33] Glaros AG. Temporomandibular disorders and facial pain: a psychophysiological perspective. Appl Psychophysiol Biofeedback 2008;33:161–71.

[34] Glaros AG, Williams K, Lausten L. Diurnal variation in pain reports in temporomandibular disorder patients and control subjects. J Orofac Pain 2008;22:115–21.

[35] Goldring MB, Goldring SR. Osteoarthritis. J Cell Physiol 2007;213:626–34.

[36] Gonzalez YM, Greene CS, Mohl ND. Technological devices in the diagnosis of temporomandibular disorders. Oral Maxillofac Surg Clin North Am 2008;20:211–20.

[37] Gorsky M, Silverman S Jr, Chinn H. Clinical characteristics and management outcome in the burning mouth syndrome. An open study of 130 patients. Oral Surg Oral Med Oral Pathol 1991;72:192–5.

[38] Granot M, Nagler RM. Association between regional idiopathic neuropathy and salivary involvement as the possible mechanism for oral sensory complaints. J Pain 2005;6:581–7.

[39] Greene CS. Concepts of TMD etiology: effects on diagnosis and treatment. In: Laskin DM, Greene CS, Hylander WL, editors. TMDs: an evidence-based approach to diagnosis and treatment. Quintessence; 2006. p. 219–28.

[40] Grémeau-Richard C, Woda A, Navez ML, Attal N, Bouhassira D, Gagnieu MC, Laluque JF, Picard P, Pionchon P, Tubert S. Topical clonazepam in stomatodynia: a randomised placebo-controlled study. Pain 2004;108:51–7.

[41] Grémeau-Richard C, Dubray C, Aublet-Cuvelier B, Ughetto S, Woda A. Effect of lingual nerve block on burning mouth syndrome (stomatodynia): a randomized crossover trial. Pain 2010;149:27–32.

[42] Grushka M, Epstein JB, Gorsky M. Burning mouth syndrome. Am Fam Physician 2002;65:615–20.

[43] Grushka M, Sessle BJ, Howley TP. Psychophysical assessment of tactile, pain and thermal sensory functions in burning mouth syndrome. Pain 1987;28:169–84.

[44] Hagelberg N, Forssell H, Rinne JO, Scheinin H, Taiminen T, Aalto S, Luutonen S, Någren K, Jääskeläinen S. Striatal dopamine D1 and D2 receptors in burning mouth syndrome. Pain 2003;101:149–54.

[45] Heckmann SM, Heckmann JG, Hilz MJ, Popp M, Marthol H, Neundörfer B, Hummel T. Oral mucosal blood flow in patients with burning mouth syndrome. Pain 2001;90:281–6.

[46] Jääskeläinen S, Forssell H, Tenovuo O. Abnormalities of the blink reflex in burning mouth syndrome. Pain 1997;73:455–60.

[47] Jääskeläinen SK, Rinne JO, Forssell H, Tenovuo O, Kaasinen V, Sonninen P, Bergman J. Role of the dopaminergic system in chronic pain: a fluorodopa-PET study. Pain 2001;15;90:257–60.

[48] Janal MN, Raphael KG, Nayak S, Klausner J. Prevalence of myofascial temporomandibular disorder in US community women. J Oral Rehabil 2008;35:801–9.

[49] King CD, Wong F, Currie T, Mauderli AP, Fillingim RB, Riley JL 3rd. Deficiency in endogenous modulation of prolonged heat pain in patients with irritable bowel syndrome and temporomandibular disorder. Pain 2009;143:172–8.

[50] Klasser GD, Greene CS. Oral appliances in the management of temporomandibular disorders. Oral Surg Oral Med Oral Pathol Oral Radiol Endod 2009;107:212–23.

[51] Lamey PJ, Freeman R, Eddie SA, Pankhurst C, Rees T. Vulnerability and presenting symptoms in burning mouth syndrome. Oral Surg Oral Med Oral Path Oral Radiol Endod 2005;99:48–54.

[52] Lauria G, Majorana A, Borgna M, Lombardi R, Penza P, Padovani A, Sapelli P. Trigeminal small-fiber sensory neuropathy causes burning mouth syndrome. Pain 2005;115:332–7.

[53] Lavigne GJ, Khoury S, Abe S, Yamaguchi T, Raphael K. Bruxism physiology and pathology: an overview for clinicians. J Oral Rehabil 2008;35:476–94.

[54] Leblebici B, Pektas ZO, Ortancil O, Hürcan EC, Bagis S, Akman MN. Coexistence of fibromyalgia, temporomandibular disorder and masticatory myofascial pain syndromes. Rheumatol Int 2007;27:541–4.

[55] LeResche L, Saunders K, Von Korff MR, Barlow W, Dworkin SF. Use of exogenous hormones and risk of temporomandibular disorder pain. Pain 1997;69:153–60.

[56] Lewis EL, Dolwick MF, Abramowicz S, Reeder SL. Contemporary imaging of the temporomandibular joint. Dent Clin North Am 2008;52:875–90.

[57] Light KC, Bragdon EE, Grewen KM, Brownley KA, Girdler SS, Maixner W. Adrenergic dysregulation and pain with and without acute beta-blockade in women with fibromyalgia and temporomandibular disorder. J Pain 2009;10:542–52.

[58] Lipton JA, Ship JA, Larach-Robinson D. Estimated prevalence and distribution of reported orofacial pain in the United States. J Am Dent Assoc 1993;124:115–21.

[59] Loeser RF. Molecular mechanisms of cartilage destruction in osteoarthritis. J Musculoskelet Neuronal Interact 2008;8:303–6.

[60] López-Jornet P, Camacho-Alonso F, Leon-Espinosa S. Efficacy of alpha lipoic acid in burning mouth syndrome: a randomized, placebo-treatment study. J Oral Rehabil 2009;36:52–7.

[61] Magnusson T, Egermark I, Carlsson GE. A prospective investigation over two decades on signs and symptoms of temporomandibular disorders and associated variables. A final summary. Acta Odontol Scand 2005;63:99–109.

[62] Maina G, Vitalucci A, Gandolfo S, Bogetto F. Comparative efficacy of SSRIs and amisulpride in burning mouth syndrome: a single-blind study. J Clin Psychiatry 2002;63:38–43.

[63] Medlicott MS, Harris SR. A systematic review of the effectiveness of exercise, manual therapy, electrotherapy, relaxation training, and biofeedback in the management of temporomandibular disorder. Phys Ther 2006;86:955–73.

[64] Michelotti A, de Wijer A, Steenks M, Farella M. Home-exercise regimes for the management of non-specific temporomandibular disorders. J Oral Rehabil 2005;32:779–85.

[65] Milam SB. Pathogenesis of degenerative temporomandibular joint arthritides. Odontology 2005;93:7–15.

[66] Milam SB. TMJ osteoarthritis. In: Laskin DM, Greene CS, Hylander WL, editors. TMDs: an evidence-based approach to diagnosis and treatment. Quintessence; 2006. p. 105–23.

[67] Nagler RN, Hershkovich O. Sialochemical and gustatory analysis in patients with oral sensory complaints. J Pain 2004;5:56–63.

[68] Ohrbach R, List T, Goulet JP, Svensson P. Workshop recommendations: convergence on an orofacial pain taxonomy. 2009. Available at: www.rdc-tmdinternational.org. Accessed February 8, 2010.

[69] Olesen J, Steiner TJ. The international classification of headache disorders, 2nd ed. (ICDH-II). J Neurol Neurosurg Psychiatry 2004;75:808–11.

[70] Onder ME, Tüz HH, Koçyiğit D, Kişnişci RS. Long-term results of arthrocentesis in degenerative temporomandibular disorders. Oral Surg Oral Med Oral Pathol Oral Radiol Endod 2009;107:e1–5.

[71] Orlando B, Manfredini D, Salvetti G, Bosco M. Evaluation of the effectiveness of biobehavioral therapy in the treatment of temporomandibular disorders: a literature review. Behav Med 2007;33:101–18.

[72] Patton LL, Siegel MA, Benoliel R, De Laat A. Management of burning mouth syndrome: systematic review and management recommendations. Oral Surg Oral Med Oral Pathol Oral Radiol Endod 2007;103(S39);e1–13.

[73] Petrussi M, Lauritano D, De Benedettis M, Baldoni M, Serpico R. Systemic capsaicin for burning mouth syndrome: a controlled study. J Oral Pathol Med 2004;33:111–4.

[74] Picavet HS, Schouten JS. Musculoskeletal pain in the Netherlands: prevalences, consequences and risk groups, the DMC(3)-study. Pain 2003;102:167–78.

[75] Reissmann DR, John MT, Wassell RW, Hinz A. Psychosocial profiles of diagnostic subgroups of temporomandibular disorder patients. Eur J Oral Sci 2008;116:237–44.

[76] Rompré PH, Daigle-Landry D, Guitard F, Montplaisir JY, Lavigne GJ. Identification of a sleep bruxism subgroup with a higher risk of pain. J Dent Res 2007;86:837–42.

[77] Rutkiewicz T, Könönen M, Suominen-Taipale L, Norblad A, Alanen P. Occurrence of clinical signs of temporomandibular disorders in adult Finns. J Orofac Pain 2006;20:208–17.

[78] Sardella A, Uglietti D, Demarosi F, Lodi G, Bez C, Carassi A. Benzydamine Hydrochloride oral rinses in management of burning mouth syndrome: a clinical trial. Oral Surg Oral Med Oral Pathol Radiol Endod 1999;88:683–6.

[79] Scala A, Checchi L, Montevecchi M, Marini I, Giamberardino MA. Update on burning mouth syndrome: overview and patient management. Crit Rev Oral Biol Med 2003;14:275–91.

[80] Schiffman EL, Look JO, Hodges JS, Swift JQ, Decker KL, Hathaway KM, Templeton RB, Fricton JR. Randomized effectiveness study of four therapeutic strategies for TMJ closed lock. J Dent Res 2007;86:58–63.

[81] Schmidt JE, Carlson CR. A controlled comparison of emotional reactivity and physiological response in masticatory muscle pain patients. J Orofac Pain 2009;23:230–42.

[82] Suvinen TI, Reade PC, Kemppainen P, Könönen M, Dworkin SF. Review of aetiological concepts of temporomandibular pain disorders: towards a biopsychosocial model for integration of physical disorder factors with psychological and psychosocial illness impact factors. Eur J Pain 2005;9:613–33.

[83] Svensson P, Bjerring P, Arendt-Nielsen L, Kaaber S. Sensory and pain thresholds to orofacial argon laser stimulation in patients with chronic burning mouth syndrome. Clin J Pain 1993;3:207–15.

[84] Svensson P, Graven-Nielsen T. Craniofacial muscle pain: review of mechanisms and clinical manifestations. J Orofac Pain 2001;15:117–45.

[85] Tammiala-Salonen T, Forssell H. Trazodone in burning mouth pain: a placebo-controlled double-blind study. J Orofac Pain 1999;13:83–8.

[86] Tousignant-Laflamme Y, Marchand S. Excitatory and inhibitory pain mechanisms during the menstrual cycle in healthy women. Pain 2009;146:47–55.

[87] Truelove EL, Sommers EE, LeResche L, Dworkin SF, Von Korff M. Clinical diagnostic criteria for TMD. New classification permits multiple diagnoses. J Am Dent Assoc 1992;123:47–54.

[88] Türp JC, Jokstad A, Motschall E, Schindler HJ, Windecker-Gétaz I, Ettlin D. Is there a superiority of multimodal as opposed to simple therapy in patients with temporomandibular disorders? A qualitative systematic review of the literature. Clin Oral Implants Res 2007;18(Suppl 3):138–50.

[89] Warren MP, Fried JL. Temporomandibular disorders and hormones in women. Cells Tissues Organs 2001;169:187–92.

[90] Woda A, Dao T, Grémeau-Richard C. Steroid dysregulation and stomatodynia (burning mouth syndrome). J Orofac Pain 2009;23:202–10.

[91] Wolfe F, Smythe HA, Yunus MB, et al. The American College of Rheumatology 1990 criteria for the classification of fibromyalgia. Arthritis Rheum 1990;33:160–72.

[92] Yilmaz Z, Renton T, Yiangou Y, Zakrzewska J, Chessell IP, Bountra C, Anand P. Burning mouth syndrome as a trigeminal small fibre neuropathy: increased heat and capsaicin receptor TRPV1 in nerve fibres correlates with pain score. J Clin Neurosci 2007;14:864–71.

[93] Yun PY, Kim YK. The role of facial trauma as a possible etiologic factor in temporomandibular joint disorder. J Oral Maxillofac Surg 2005;63:1576–83.

[94] Zakrzewska JM, Forssell H, Glenny AM. Interventions for the treatment of burning mouth syndrome. Cochrane Database Syst Rev 2005;CD002779.

Correspondence to: Antoon De Laat, DDS, PhD, Dr h.c., Department of Oral and Maxillofacial Surgery, School of Dentistry, Oral Pathology and Maxillofacial Surgery, Catholic University of Leuven, Kapucijnenvoer 7, B-3000 Leuven, Belgium. Email: antoon.delaat@med.kuleuven.be.

Primary Headache Disorders Presenting as Orofacial Pain

17

Peter J. Goadsby

Headache Group, Department of Neurology, University of California, San Francisco, California, USA

Headache is a remarkably common problem, so it is perhaps not surprising that its manifestations may involve the face, which is, of course, part of the head. Several books are devoted to primary headache disorders, and interested readers are directed to recent editions for more details [19,25,28,37,40]. The headache disorders are classified by the second edition of the International Classification of Headache Disorders [22] as being either primary, where the headache syndrome is itself the problem, or secondary, where the headache syndrome is driven by other pathological processes. This chapter will deal with primary headache disorders that often have a pain distribution in the face. Trigeminal neuropathies, trigeminal neuralgia, temporomandibular joint disorders, and fibromyalgic-type pains involving the face are covered in other chapters in this volume. In general, primary headache disorders tend to involve predominantly the ophthalmic (first) division of the trigeminal nerve, along with its physiological overlap with the high cervical input by way of the trigeminocervical complex [3]. However, many primary headache disorders also involve the face, in effect the second and third divisions of the trigeminal nerve, and are covered in this chapter. For coverage of the anatomy and physiology in detail, readers are referred to a recent review [17].

General Principles

It is a good general principle that all the common primary headache disorders can present with facial pain (Table I). This feature is less obviously a problem with a featureless, daily, not very disabling presentation, such as might be seen with tension-type headache, but it can be troublesome when migraine presents with facial pain, which has been called "facial migraine" in the past. I am aware of no difference in features, associations, or treatment response when migraine pain is localized in the second or third division of the trigeminal as opposed to the first, so the term "facial migraine" seems useless. Clinical clues include the associated features: photophobia, phonophobia or osmophobia, which are highly migrainous in this setting, or the very common feature of aggravation with movement. The former symptoms probably represent underlying migrainous biology, even when seen in the trigeminal autonomic cephalalgias (see below). The management of migraine has been recently reviewed and is outside the scope of this chapter [21]. Some particular headache disorders that may have facial pain presentations are discussed below.

Pain 2010—An Updated Review: Refresher Course Syllabus
edited by Jeffrey S. Mogil
IASP Press, Seattle, © 2010

153

Trigeminal Autonomic Cephalalgias

Cluster Headache

Cluster headache is a rare form of primary headache with a population frequency of approximately 0.1% [41]. It is perhaps the most painful condition that can occur in humans; in the cohort of more than 1,000 patients I have seen, not a single one has had a more painful experience, including childbirth, multiple fractures of the limbs, or renal stones. It is one of a group of conditions known now as trigeminal autonomic cephalalgias (TACs), and thus needs to be differentiated from other TACs [20] and from the short-lasting headaches without cranial autonomic symptoms, such as lacrimation or conjunctival injection (Table I).

The core feature of cluster headache is periodicity, be it circadian or in terms of active and inactive bouts over weeks and months (Table II). The typical cluster headache patient is male, with a 3:1 male : female predominance, with bouts of one to two attacks of relatively short duration, unilateral pain every day for 8–10 weeks a year. Patients are generally perfectly well between bouts. Patients with cluster headache tend to move about during attacks, pacing, rocking, or even rubbing their head for relief. The pain is usually retroorbital, boring, and very severe. It is associated with ipsilateral symptoms of cranial (parasympathetic) autonomic activation (a red or watering eye, the nose running or blocked) or cranial sympathetic dysfunction (eyelid droop). Cluster headache is likely to be a disorder involving central pacemaker regions of the posterior hypothalamus and perhaps other neurons of this region [32,33].

The TACs—cluster headache, paroxysmal hemicrania, and SUNCT (short-lasting unilateral neuralgiform headache attacks with conjunctival injection and tearing) syndrome—present a distinct group to be differentiated from short-lasting headaches that do not have prominent cranial autonomic syndromes, notably trigeminal neuralgia, idiopathic (primary) stabbing headache, and hypnic headache [16]. By determining the cycling pattern, length of attack, frequency of attacks, and timing of attacks, it is possible to usefully classify most patients. The importance of clinical classification of this group is threefold. First, the clinical phenotype determines the likely secondary causes that must be considered and the appropriate investigations that must be ordered. Second, the appropriate classification gives the patient a clear diagnosis and allows the physician to draw on available literature to comment on natural history. Third, the correct diagnosis determines therapy that can be very different in these conditions, being very effective if the diagnosis is correct but largely ineffective if it is not (Table III).

Managing Cluster Headache

Cluster headache is managed using acute attack treatments and preventive agents. Acute attack treatments are usually required by all cluster headache patients at some time, while preventives can seem almost life-saving for patients with chronic cluster headache and are often needed to shorten the active periods in patients with the episodic form of the disorder. Here I will review the principles of management; details of current strategies can be found elsewhere [18].

Preventive Treatments

The options for preventive treatment in cluster headache depend on the length of bouts. Patients with short bouts require medicines that act quickly but will not necessarily be taken for long periods, whereas those with long bouts or indeed those with chronic cluster headache require safe, effective medicines that can be taken for long periods. Verapamil is now widely considered as the first-line preventive treatment when the

Table I
Primary headache disorders presenting with facial pain

Section I/II	Section III	Section IV
	Trigeminal autonomic cephalalgias (TACs)*	Other headaches
Migraine Tension-type headache	Cluster headache Paroxysmal hemicrania SUNCT/SUNA† syndrome	Primary stabbing headache Hemicrania continua

Source: International Headache Society [22].
* Beware of pituitary tumor-related headache in the differential diagnosis of these TACs.
† Short-lasting unilateral neuralgiform headache attacks with conjunctival injection and tearing/cranial autonomic features.

Table II
Diagnostic criteria for cluster headache

3.1 Diagnostic Criteria

A. At least 5 attacks fulfilling B–D.

B. Severe or very severe unilateral orbital, supraorbital and/or temporal pain lasting 15 to 180 minutes if untreated.

C. Headache is accompanied by at least one of the following:

    1. ipsilateral conjunctival injection and/or lacrimation

    2. ipsilateral nasal congestion and/or rhinorrhea

    3. forehead and facial sweating

    4. ipsilateral eyelid edema

    5. ipsilateral forehead and facial sweating

    6. ipsilateral miosis and/or ptosis

    7. a sense of restlessness or agitation

D. Attacks have a frequency from 1 every other day to 8 per day.

E. Not attributed to another disorder.

3.1.1 Episodic Cluster Headache

Description: Occurs in periods lasting 7 days to one year separated by pain free periods lasting one month or more.

Diagnostic criteria:

A. All fulfilling criteria A–E of 3.1.

B. At least 2 cluster periods lasting from 7–365 days and separated by pain-free remissions of 1 month.

3.1.2 Chronic Cluster Headache

Description: Attacks occur for more than one year without remission or with remissions lasting less than 1 month.

Diagnostic criteria:

A. All alphabetical headings of 3.1.

B. Attacks recur over >1 year without remission periods or with remission periods of <1 month.

Source: International Headache Society [22].

bout is prolonged, or in chronic cluster headache. By contrast, limited courses of oral corticosteroids or methysergide can be very useful strategies when the bout is relatively short.

Verapamil has been suggested as a useful option for the last decade and compares favorably with lithium. What has clearly emerged from clinical practice is the need to use higher doses than had initially been considered, and certainly higher than those used in cardiological indications. Although most patients will start on doses as low as 40–80 mg twice daily, doses up to 960 mg daily are often required. Side effects, such as gingival hyperplasia, constipation, and leg swelling are recognized, as are cardiac dysrhythmias. Verapamil can cause heart block by slowing conduction in the atrioventricular (AV) node, monitored clinically by the P-R interval on the electrocardiogram (EKG). Given that the effects on the AV node take up to 10 days to manifest, 2-week intervals are recommended between dose changes on the first exposure, with EKGs prior to the next escalation, and routine semi-annual EKGs after the dose is established [13].

Acute Attack Treatment

Cluster headache attacks often peak rapidly and thus require a treatment with quick onset. Many patients with acute cluster headache respond very well to treatment with oxygen inhalation. This treatment should be given as 100% oxygen at 10–12 L/minute for 15–20 minutes [8]. It is important to have a high flow and high oxygen content. Injectable sumatriptan 6 mg is effective and rapid in onset [14] and shows no evidence of producing tachyphylaxis [15]. Nasal sprays of sumatriptan 20 mg [44] and zolmitriptan 5 mg [7,39] are effective in acute cluster headache in controlled trials, and they offer a useful option. Sumatriptan is not effective when given preemptively as 100 mg orally three times daily [35], and there is no evidence that it is useful when used orally in the acute treatment of cluster headache; indeed, it can be associated with medication overuse headache problems [38].

Surgical Treatment

The surgical treatment of cluster headache has been completely revolutionized with the introduction of neurostimulation therapies. Surgical treatment of cluster headache is reserved for the most refractory patients, typically those with chronic cluster headache. Destructive procedures have been used, such as pterygopalatinectomy or radiofrequency lesions of the trigeminal ganglion. The former procedure is without clear effects, and the latter are helpful, but often at

Table III
Differential diagnosis of short-lasting headaches

Feature	Cluster Headache	Paroxysmal Hemicrania	SUNCT/ SUNA*	Primary Stabbing Headache	Trigeminal Neuralgia
Gender	M > F 3:1	F = M	M > F	F > M	F > M
Pain type	Boring/ throbbing	Boring/ throbbing	Stabbing/ throbbing	Stabbing	Stabbing
Pain severity	Very severe	Very severe	Very severe	Severe	Very severe
Cranial location	Any	Any	Any	Any	V2/V3 > V1
Duration	15–180 min	2–30 min	5–600 s	Seconds–3 min	<5 seconds
Frequency	1–8 per day	1–40 per day	1 per day to 30 per hour	Any	Any
Autonomic	+	+	+	–	–
Alcohol	+	One-third	–	–	–
Cutaneous trigger for attacks?	–	–	+	–	+
Indomethacin	–	+	–	+	–

* SUNCT, short-lasting unilateral neuralgiform headache attacks with conjunctival injection and tearing; SUNA, short-lasting unilateral neuralgiform headache attacks with cranial autonomic symptoms. SUNCT/SUNA generally has no refractory period for triggering additional attacks—a feature that is common in trigeminal neuralgia.

significant cost, including ocular complications or anesthesia dolorosa. Trigeminal rhizotomy has also been employed, with all the complications of radiofrequency lesions and occasional death [23]. Set against these invasive approaches, the functional imaging work describing activations in the posterior hypothalamic region [33] have directly led to deep brain stimulation approaches in the same region that seem highly effective [26]. Occipital nerve stimulation is a further very promising and largely noninvasive approach to the management of intractable chronic cluster headache [4,5,29], which may become the surgical treatment of choice in this setting over the next 5–10 years.

Paroxysmal Hemicrania

Sjaastad and Dale [42] first reported eight cases of a frequent unilateral, severe but short-lasting headache without remission, coining the term "chronic paroxysmal hemicrania" (CPH). The mean daily frequency of attacks varied from 7 to 22, with the pain persisting from 5 to 45 minutes on each occasion. The site and associated autonomic phenomena were similar to those of cluster headache, but the attacks of CPH were suppressed completely by indomethacin.

The essential features of paroxysmal hemicrania that we have seen from a substantial cohort of patients are [6]:

• unilateral, very severe pain;
• short-lasting attacks, typically 20 minutes in length;

• very frequent attacks (usually more than five a day);
• marked autonomic features ipsilateral to the pain;
• robust, quick (less than 72 hours), and with excellent response to indomethacin.

The pathophysiology of paroxysmal hemicrania is marked by activations on positron emission tomography (PET) in the contralateral posterior hypothalamus and contralateral ventral midbrain [30]. The posterior hypothalamic activity is shared with cluster headache, SUNCT, and hemicrania continua, whereas the ventral midbrain activity is only seen in hemicrania continua, which remarkably is also an indomethacin-sensitive primary headache [9].

Treatment of paroxysmal hemicrania (PH) may be complicated by gastrointestinal side effects seen with indomethacin; topiramate may be helpful in preventing attacks in such patients [10]. Secondary PH is more likely if the patient requires high doses (>200 mg/day) of indomethacin, and raised cerebrospinal fluid (CSF) pressure should be suspected in apparent bilateral PH. It is worth noting that indomethacin reduces CSF pressure by an unknown mechanism [24]. It is appropriate to image patients, with magnetic resonance imaging (MRI) if practical, when a diagnosis of PH is being considered, particular with regard to pituitary pathology [27].

SUNCT/SUNA

Sjaastad and colleagues [43] reported three male patients whose brief attacks of pain in and around one eye were associated with sudden conjunctival injection and other autonomic features of cluster headache. The attacks lasted only 15–60 seconds but recurred 5–30 times per hour, and they could be precipitated by chewing or eating certain foods, such as citrus fruits. They were not abolished by indomethacin. Brain imaging has suggested that these attacks share with cluster headache and paroxysmal hemicrania the feature of involvement of the posterior hypothalamic region, as revealed by activation studies [34]. Among patients recognized with this problem, males dominate slightly. The paroxysms of pain may last between 5 and 300 seconds, although longer, duller interictal pains are recognized, as are longer attacks with a saw-tooth pattern [12]. The conjunctival injection seen with SUNCT is often the most prominent autonomic feature, and tearing may be very obvious. If either conjunctival injection or tearing is absent, or if neither feature is present but another cranial autonomic symptom is seen, the term "SUNA" is used. The two key clinical features of SUNCT/SUNA are the attacks being triggerable, with no refractory period to triggering. The latter feature serves as a very useful distinction between SUNCT/SUNA and trigeminal neuralgia. SUNCT/SUNA can be treated very often with lamotrigine, and if that is unhelpful, with topiramate or gabapentin [11]. Carbamazepine often has a useful but incomplete effect. Given what has been reported, cranial MRI with pituitary and posterior fossa views is highly recommended when SUNCT/SUNA is considered as a diagnosis.

Other Primary Headaches

Primary Stabbing Headache

Short-lived jabs of pain, defined by the Headache Classification Committee of The International Headache Society as primary stabbing headache [22] are well documented in association with most types of primary headache. The essential clinical features are:

1) Pain confined to the head, although it is rarely facial.

2) Stabbing pain lasting from one to many seconds and occurring as a single stab or a series of stabs.

3) Pain recurring at irregular intervals (hours to days).

These pains have been called ice-pick pains or "jabs and jolts." They generally respond to indomethacin (25–50 mg twice to three times daily). The symptoms tend to wax and wane, and after a period of control on indomethacin it is appropriate to withdraw treatment and observe the outcome. Most patients will not want treatment when the nature of the problem is explained and they are reassured that the attacks are not sinister in any way.

Hemicrania Continua

Two patients were initially reported with this syndrome, a woman aged 63 years and a man of 53, who developed unilateral headache without obvious cause. Both patients were relieved completely by indomethacin, whereas other nonsteroidal anti-inflammatory drugs (NSAIDs) were of little or no benefit. Newman and colleagues [36] reviewed the 24 previously reported cases and added 10 of their own, including some with pronounced autonomic features resembling cluster headache. They divided their case histories into remitting and unremitting forms. Of the 34 patients reviewed, 22 were women and 12 men with the age of onset ranging from 11 to 58 years. The symptoms were controlled by indomethacin 75–150 mg daily. The essential features of hemicrania continua are:

1) Unilateral pain.

2) Pain that is continuous but with exacerbations that may be severe.

3) Complete resolution of pain with indomethacin.

4) Exacerbations that may be associated with autonomic features.

Apart from analgesic overuse as an aggravating factor, and a report in an human immunodeficiency virus (HIV)-infected patient, the status of secondary hemicrania continua is unclear. Antonaci and colleagues [2] proposed the "indotest," by which the intramuscular injection of indomethacin 50 mg could be used as a diagnostic tool. In hemicrania continua, pain was relieved in 73 ± 66 minutes and the pain-free period was 13 ± 8 hours. A placebo-controlled modification of this test is preferred, where possible, to the open-label version. Studies using the latter method in conjunction with PET have shown that there is activation of the contralateral posterior hypothalamus and ipsilateral dorsal rostral pons in association with the headache of hemicrania continua, as well as activation of the ipsilateral ventrolateral midbrain [31]. The alternative is a trial of oral indomethacin, initially 25 mg three times daily, then 50 mg three times daily, and then 75 mg three times daily. One should allow up to 2 weeks for any dose to have a useful effect. Acute treatment with sumatriptan has been employed and reported to be of no benefit. Cyclooxygenase-2 (COX-2) antagonists seem effective, although undesirable now because of their toxicity, and topiramate is helpful in some patients [10], as is greater occipital nerve injection [1].

Conclusions

It is common for patients with primary headache disorders to present with facial pain. Here I have emphasized the trigeminal autonomic cephalalgias (TACs) where facial pain is very commonly a presenting feature. Migraine, which is the most common of the disabling headaches presenting to physicians in the United States, and probably in the world, can also manifest as facial pain, so it should always be considered. An understanding of the anatomy and physiology of the interaction between the branches of the trigeminal innervation of the head facilitates the accurate diagnosis and management of facial pain problems.

References

[1] Afridi SK, Shields KG, Bhola R, Goadsby PJ. Greater occipital nerve injection in primary headache syndromes: prolonged effects from a single injection. Pain 2006;122:126–9.

[2] Antonaci F, Pareja JA, Caminero AB, Sjaastad O. Chronic paroxysmal hemicrania and hemicrania continua. Parenteral indomethacin: the 'Indotest'. Headache 1998;38:122–8.

[3] Bartsch T, Goadsby PJ. Anatomy and physiology of pain referral in primary and cervicogenic headache disorders. Headache Currents 2005;2:42–8.

[4] Burns B, Watkins L, Goadsby PJ. Successful treatment of medically intractable cluster headache using occipital nerve stimulation (ONS). Lancet 2007;369:1099–106.

[5] Burns B, Watkins L, Goadsby PJ. Treatment of intractable chronic cluster headache by occipital nerve stimulation in 14 patients. Neurology 2009;72:341–5.

[6] Cittadini E, Matharu MS, Goadsby PJ. Paroxysmal hemicrania: a prospective clinical study of thirty-one cases. Brain 2008;131:1142–55.

[7] Cittadini E, May A, Straube A, Evers S, Bussone G, Goadsby PJ. Effectiveness of intranasal zolmitriptan in acute cluster headache. A randomized, placebo-controlled, double-blind crossover study. Arch Neurol 2006;63:1537–42.

[8] Cohen AS, Burns B, Goadsby PJ. High-flow oxygen for treatment of cluster headache: a randomized trial. JAMA 2009;302:2451–7.

[9] Cohen AS, Goadsby PJ. Functional neuroimaging of primary headache disorders. Expert Rev Neurother 2006;6:1159–72.

[10] Cohen AS, Goadsby PJ. Paroxysmal hemicrania responding to topiramate. J Neurol Neurosurg Psychiatry 2007;78:96–7.

[11] Cohen AS, Matharu MS, Goadsby PJ. Suggested guidelines for treating SUNCT and SUNA. Cephalalgia 2005;25:1200.

[12] Cohen AS, Matharu MS, Goadsby PJ. Short-lasting unilateral neuralgiform headache attacks with conjunctival injection and tearing (SUNCT) or cranial autonomic features (SUNA). A prospective clinical study of SUNCT and SUNA. Brain 2006;129:2746–60.

[13] Cohen AS, Matharu MS, Goadsby PJ. Electrocardiographic abnormalities in patients with cluster headache on verapamil therapy. Neurology 2007;69:668–75.

[14] Ekbom K, The Sumatriptan Cluster Headache Study Group. Treatment of acute cluster headache with sumatriptan. N Engl J Med 1991;325:322–6.

[15] Ekbom K, Waldenlind E, Cole JA, Pilgrim AJ, Kirkham A. Sumatriptan in chronic cluster headache: results of continuous treatment for eleven months. Cephalalgia 1992;12:254–6.

[16] Goadsby PJ. Pathophysiology of cluster headache: a trigeminal autonomic cephalgia. Lancet Neurol 2002;1:37–43.

[17] Goadsby PJ, Charbit AR, Andreou AP, Akerman S, Holland PR. Neurobiology of migraine. Neuroscience 2009;161:327–41.

[18] Goadsby PJ, Cohen AS, Matharu MS. Trigeminal autonomic cephalalgias: diagnosis and treatment. Curr Neurol Neurosci Rep 2007;7:117–25.

[19] Goadsby PJ, Dodick D, Silberstein SD. Chronic daily headache for clinicians. Hamilton: Decker; 2005.

[20] Goadsby PJ, Lipton RB. A review of paroxysmal hemicranias, SUNCT syndrome and other short-lasting headaches with autonomic features, including new cases. Brain 1997;120:193–209.

[21] Goadsby PJ, Sprenger T. Current practice and future directions in the management of migraine: acute and preventive. Lancet Neurol 2010;9:285–98.

[22] Headache Classification Committee of the International Headache Society. The International Classification of Headache Disorders (second edition). Cephalalgia 2004;24(Suppl 1):1–160.

[23] Jarrar RG, Black DF, Dodick DW, Davis DH. Outcome of trigeminal nerve section in the treatment of chronic cluster headache. Neurology 2003;60:1360–2.

[24] Jensen K, Ohrstrom J, Cold GE, Astrup J. The effects of indomethacin on intracranial pressure, cerebral blood flow and cerebral metabolism in patients with severe head injury and intracranial hypertension. Acta Neurochir (Wien) 1991;108:116–21.

[25] Lance JW, Goadsby PJ. Mechanism and management of headache. New York: Elsevier; 2005.

[26] Leone M, Franzini A, Broggi G, May A, Bussone G. Long-term follow-up of bilateral hypothalamic stimulation for intractable cluster headache. Brain 2004;127:2259–64.

[27] Levy M, Matharu MS, Meeran K, Powell M, Goadsby PJ. The clinical characteristics of headache in patients with pituitary tumours. Brain 2005;128:1921–30.

[28] Lipton RB, Bigal M. Migraine and other headache disorders. New York: Marcel Dekker; 2006.

[29] Magis D, Allena M, Bolla M, De Pasqua V, Remacle JM, Schoenen J. Occipital nerve stimulation for drug-resistant chronic cluster headache: a prospective pilot study. Lancet Neurol 2007;6:314–21.

[30] Matharu MS, Cohen AS, Frackowiak RSJ, Goadsby PJ. Posterior hypothalamic activation in paroxysmal hemicrania. Ann Neurol 2006;59:535–45.

[31] Matharu MS, Cohen AS, McGonigle DJ, Ward N, Frackowiak RSJ, Goadsby PJ. Posterior hypothalamic and brainstem activation in hemicrania continua. Headache 2004;44:747–61.

[32] May A, Ashburner J, Buchel C, McGonigle DJ, Friston KJ, Frackowiak RSJ, Goadsby PJ. Correlation between structural and functional changes in brain in an idiopathic headache syndrome. Nat Med 1999;5:836–8.

[33] May A, Bahra A, Buchel C, Frackowiak RS, Goadsby PJ. Hypothalamic activation in cluster headache attacks. Lancet 1998;352:275–8.

[34] May A, Bahra A, Buchel C, Turner R, Goadsby PJ. Functional MRI in spontaneous attacks of SUNCT: short-lasting neuralgiform headache with conjunctival injection and tearing. Ann Neurol 1999;46:791–3.

[35] Monstad I, Krabbe A, Micieli G, Prusinski A, Cole J, Pilgrim A, Shevlin P. Preemptive oral treatment with sumatriptan during a cluster period. Headache 1995;35:607–13.

[36] Newman LC, Gordon ML, Lipton RB, Kanner R, Solomon S. Episodic paroxysmal hemicrania: two new cases and a literature review. Neurology 1992;42:964–6.

[37] Olesen J, Tfelt-Hansen P, Ramadan N, Goadsby PJ, Welch KMA. The headaches. Philadelphia: Lippincott, Williams & Wilkins; 2005.

[38] Paemeleire K, Bahra A, Evers S, Matharu MS, Goadsby PJ. Medication-overuse headache in cluster headache patients. Neurology 2006;67:109–13.

[39] Rapoport AM, Mathew NT, Silberstein SD, Dodick D, Tepper SJ, Sheftell FD, Bigal ME. Zolmitriptan nasal spray in the acute treatment of cluster headache: a double-blind study. Neurology 2007;69:821–6.

[40] Silberstein SD, Lipton RB, Goadsby PJ. Headache in clinical practice. London: Martin Dunitz; 2002.

[41] Sjaastad O, Bakketeig LS. Cluster headache prevalence. Vaga study of headache epidemiology. Cephalalgia 2003;23:528–33.

[42] Sjaastad O, Dale I. A new (?) clinical headache entity "chronic paroxysmal hemicrania." Acta Neurol Scand 1976;54:140–59.

[43] Sjaastad O, Saunte C, Salvesen R, Fredriksen TA, Seim A, Roe OD, Fostad K, Lobben OP, Zhao JM. Shortlasting unilateral neuralgiform headache attacks with conjunctival injection, tearing, sweating, and rhinorrhea. Cephalalgia 1989;9:147–56.

[44] van Vliet JA, Bahra A, Martin V, Aurora SK, Mathew NT, Ferrari MD, Goadsby PJ. Intranasal sumatriptan in cluster headache: randomized placebo-controlled double-blind study. Neurology 2003;60:630–3.

Correspondence to: Professor Peter J. Goadsby, Headache Group, Department of Neurology, University of California, San Francisco, 1701 Divisadero Street, Suite 480, San Francisco, CA 94115, USA. Email: pgoadsby@headache.ucsf.edu.

Part 8
Pain Psychology for Non-Psychologists

Pain Psychology for Non-Psychologists

Amanda C. de C. Williams, PhD,[a] Francis J. Keefe, PhD,[b] and Johan W.S. Vlaeyen, PhD[c,d]

[a]Research Department of Clinical, Educational and Health Psychology, University College London, London, United Kingdom;
[b]Department of Psychiatry and Behavioral Sciences, Duke University Medical Center, Durham, North Carolina, USA; [c]Department
of Clinical Psychological Science, University of Maastricht, Maastricht, The Netherlands; [d]Pain and Disability Research Program,
Department of Psychology, University of Leuven, Leuven, Belgium

Over the past four decades, psychological assessment and treatment methods have become an integral component of pain management programs. This chapter provides an overview and update on psychological assessment and treatment methods. It covers the multimethod assessment of pain and pain disability, such as core issues in assessing subjective experiences, how pain disability/function scales are developed, and major problems that may arise. Furthermore, we discuss the route to follow from deciding on patients, treatment, and aims of intervention to selecting methods of evaluating pain and disability at baseline and as outcomes. We also provide the conceptual basis for psychosocial approaches to pain management, and give an overview of psychosocial intervention protocols, training protocols based on cognitive-behavioral principles, hypnosis, emotional disclosure protocols, acceptance-based treatments, and partner- and family-assisted approaches. Finally, and as an illustration, we focus on the role of pain-related fear, discuss the theoretical background of fear learning mechanisms in relation to persistent pain, give an overview of assessment methods/instruments for pain-related fear, and review available fear-reduction techniques. Finally, we explore the role of health care provider attitudes about chronic pain.

Psychological Approaches to Multimethod Assessment of Pain and Pain Disability

Measuring Subjective Variables

Older texts on measurement often start or end with apologies for the lack of objective instruments to measure pain, yet subjective measures developed in psychology provide uniquely relevant and powerful insights into internal states such as pain, often accounting for substantial variance in differences between populations and in changes with treatment. While there are necessarily limits on what can be consciously accessed and reported, support is emerging from neuroscientific research, particularly using functional magnetic resonance imaging (fMRI) [93], of consistent associations between some questionnaire measures and the extent of activation of particular brain areas. While there is no basis for the claims of "objective" measures of pain from such images, they add a further dimension to our understanding of what self-report, as the fundamental measure of pain, can tell us. Of course, instruments assessing subjective state by direct report are subject to momentary fluctuations, to larger fluctuations over the time scales of treatment and follow-up, and to bias according to contextual variables that can be overt or subtle [85] and can be minimized by good design. Trait measures by definition are more stable. Before describing the selection of the instruments themselves, we will explore some of the concerns behind the common statement that a measuring instrument is "reliable and valid."

First, conceptual clarity about the construct to be measured informs the choice of items and response options. It is easy to assume that a total score means what the title suggests, but too often it does not. Pain psychology has many overlapping concepts, only a few of which map well onto known processes with physiological and pathway correlates and evident evolutionary function, such as fear; others have conceptual coherence and heuristic value even though they cannot be mapped on to such processes.

Second, it is assumed that any construct has a linear structure, such that, for instance, between the poles of calm and anxiety is a finite number of states in a fixed order and relationship to one another. However, it is highly likely that the poles are not simple opposites, and that there are multiple different states with no stable order between the two extremes. Assumptions of linearity are necessary for constructing measurement instruments but may misrepresent the construct to a problematic degree. Psychological constructs represented linearly can at best only be ordinal, but they are commonly scored and analyzed as if they were interval scales (where, for instance, a score of 40 on an anxiety scale truly represents twice as much anxiety as does a score of 20—a convenient illusion). Additionally, relationships among items in such a scale often differ from one population to another, for instance, with ethnic or age differences [14].

Despite these concerns about how abstract constructs are represented by scales, psychological measuring instruments have performed well enough to extend our understanding of the pain experience, and to be able to generalize and predict across heterogeneous populations. Attention is routinely paid to maximizing reliability by ensuring that items in a scale correlate with one another and with the total, so that they are sampling within the same domain (internal reliability or consistency), and by minimizing other sources of systematic error. Different researchers will define the limits of the domain differently, and this applies particularly to measurement of disability, described below. High internal reliability may be achieved at the cost of discarding items with low correlation with others, although they may be clinically interesting. Inter-rater reliability and test-retest reliability are, respectively, consistency among raters (often trained to a particular criterion of agreement), and consistency across time (although often shorter than the interval between pre- and post-treatment measurement). A reliability coefficient is often considered "good" if it is at least 0.8, but even this figure implies that a third of the variance is random. Any reliability coefficient is a property of the instrument in the context of the population in which it was tested, so the more representative these samples are of the population of concern, the more confidently can the instrument be used. Validity is more an ongoing project than a property, because there is rarely if ever an external referent for incontrovertible authentication. Even with the best established concepts such as fear, not every patient who describes fear of the pain worsening will show autonomic responses of acute fear, even when faced with a pain-exacerbating task. So new measuring instruments are compared with old ones—the ones they aim to improve upon—and a high correlation is taken as evidence of construct validity: that the instrument is measuring what it purports to measure. Predictive validity is more impressive—the capacity to predict (in temporal not statistical terms) an outcome such as clinical improvement, or physical performance at a pain-relevant task—but even here, the question "how good is good enough prediction?" remains unresolved.

Selecting Domains of Assessment

There are many ways of defining the domains of interest in pain studies, but at least for clinical trials involving people with persistent pain, the IMMPACT (Initiative on Methods, Measurement, and Pain Assessment in Clinical Trials) project [94,95] output is valuable. A series of energetic consensus conferences involving clinicians and researchers from academia and industry arrived at a shortlist of domains: pain; physical functioning; emotional functioning; improvement and satisfaction from the patient's viewpoint; symptoms and adverse events; and process variables such attrition and reasons for it, as recommended in trial descriptions. Traditionally, an analgesic drug intervention entails more detailed assessment of symptoms, adverse events, adherence, and attrition than of emotional functioning, but both are relevant, just as they are for a trial of a psychological intervention.

The package of questionnaires presented to patients at assessment points is often referred to as a "battery," reflecting the risks of fatigue and boredom, both of which reduce reliability. The balance between comprehensiveness of measurement and the burden on the patient should be considered carefully. Ideally, potential or actual patients are involved in study design and measure selection. The most recent IMMPACT study sampled patients [98], and the outcomes endorsed by at least half of the sample were strikingly more diverse than those in widespread use. There was far more emphasis on participation in social and family life, on its enjoyment, and on associated problems of fatigue, weakness, sleep, and cognitive impairment, and far less on performance of particular movements, household chores, and employment. We even lack adequate measures for some of these outcomes, or do not have any pain-relevant norms for those measures we import from elsewhere. Perhaps the next decade will remedy these deficits.

Once the domains are decided, the shortlist of measures (see ref. [26]) needs to be scrutinized for fit with the populations of interest. Particular problems can be floor and ceiling effects, where a population that scores generally high or low on a measure (designed for a different range of responses) has little room to score better after intervention: for instance, when instruments designed for measuring depression severity in psychiatric populations are used for samples drawn from the community of largely nondistressed individuals.

Measuring Pain

Pain by definition is multidimensional, so one of the first decisions for the study designer is whether these dimensions should be measured separately, or whether a single rating of pain, with the dimensions contributing differently within and between people and assessment occasions, is sufficient. It is also entirely subjective: while pain experience also contributes to behavioral expression, analgesic intake, and other indirect measures of pain, it should not be expected to bear any simple relationship to them, at least without extensive control of many sources of variance complicating generalization of study findings to clinical or everyday settings.

Pain intensity, distress, and interference are the main dimensions of pain experience sampled, usually by a choice of the same metric for them all: a visual analogue scale on which the patient makes a mark such that distance between the labeled extremes represents amount; or a numerical rating scale, usually 0–10, with the extremes similarly labeled. Strangely, the labels for the endpoints of scales have been studied less than aspects of the scale itself such as color or orientation: simple ones such as "no pain" and "extreme pain" are preferable to complex formulations (such as "the worst pain you can imagine"). An alternative is categorical scales, using terms such as "none," "mild," "moderate," and "severe": while simple and acceptable, it may have too few categories to offer sensitivity to change, and in particular, the "severe" category may require subdivision [12]. Similarly, faces scales used for nonverbal subjects are categorical (see, e.g., ref. [47]). There is one widely used adjectival scale (the McGill Pain Questionnaire; MPQ [67]) from which are commonly derived subscales of sensory, affective, and evaluative scores, but the stability of these subscales is questionable across populations. It is usual in persistent pain to ask for average pain, since pain at that moment may be significantly higher or lower than on average. Other aspects of pain worth consideration are worst pain, which can, through the individual's attempts to avoid it, predict behaviors; pain on movement or effort; and whether there are pain-free episodes. Pain relief is usually directly measured by asking for a percentage, and this measure does not necessarily correspond with the proportional difference between pre- and post-treatment ratings.

The practice of single measurement points before and after an intervention, for instance, has begun to give way to cumulative (such as daily diary) measurement. However, pain is a reactive measure; that is, attention is directed to pain by the request to rate it, and this can, of course, alter the quality and salience of the pain and thus affect the rating. Electronic methods, which can prompt rating at irregular intervals and record when the pain rating was made, are superior to pen-and-paper diary methods, which are often completed retrospectively; electronic methods are also more acceptable to patients [89]. However, single retrospective average ratings provide data of reasonable quality [60], and they are more easily analyzed than diary records.

Measuring Disability

The domain of disability, or its corollary, function, can be taken to cover anything from a short list of specific activities (e.g., walking without aids) or movements (e.g., lifting the arms above the head) to more objective or at least verifiable complex behaviors such as working or training, no longer seeking health care for pain, or taking a vacation. Measuring instruments vary in their inclusiveness and focus, and sometimes they mix very different activities or mix subjective and objective items. A further distinction is that some require a yes/no response—"Can you climb stairs?"—whereas others ask how much pain interferes. People with pain differ in their appraisal of what they would do without pain, and in their realism; activities vary with factors such as age, socioeconomic status, and education, and even with wider contexts such as local unemployment rate [7]. The response to the question above may be "Only with a handrail or walking aid," or "Yes, on good days," or "I can go down but not up," none of which fits easily into yes/no response options. Further, the context of responding may affect the answer: being assessed for much-needed help or care will elicit a poorer disability score than being assessed for fitness to take part in an enjoyable activity. Widely used measures are described elsewhere [6,26,112].

Selecting Assessment Instruments for the Population of Interest

For most studies, consideration of the points discussed above will help to arrive at a shortlist of measures, whose length, cognitive demands, content, and psychometric properties will recommend them (or not) to the study authors. On occasion, there is no suitable instrument, and study authors must construct one (see, e.g., refs. [8,76]). Problems may arise over translation into other languages in order to include sections of the population without fluency in the native tongue. Views vary, from those who hold that there are profound differences in world view between language communities, and those who are satisfied with translation and back-translation without considering whether the target concept is culturally constructed [48]. An empirical approach that invites feedback from participants on ease or difficulty of using scales, and on unfamiliarity with content or apparent gaps in coverage, allows more confident interpretation as well as providing material of interest to fellow researchers. Of note is the Brief Pain Inventory [13], a measure of pain and of its interference with everyday life, which has been translated into many languages (e.g., ref. [83]).

Psychosocial Approaches to Pain Management

The focus of psychosocial approaches to pain management is not on directly altering pain, but rather on the patient's adjustment to pain. As depicted in Fig. 1, three key domains of adjustment to pain are particularly important: thoughts, feelings, and behaviors. Patients who have had pain for months or years often report a number of negative thoughts about themselves ("I am useless"), about others ("No one cares about me anymore"), and about the future ("I am going to become an invalid") [34]. They ruminate about these thoughts and find it very difficult to move their attention away from them. Such negative thoughts not only are a problem in themselves, but also foster dysfunctional behaviors (e.g., an overly sedentary lifestyle) and negative feelings (e.g., depression). Patients with persistent pain often report that their emotional life is dominated by negative feelings (e.g., depression, anger, or guilt) and that they rarely experience positive feelings (e.g., joy, love, gratitude). The impact of a negative feeling such as depression or guilt can be so profound that individuals focus all of their energies and self-help efforts on it. Unfortunately, patients may turn to short-term remedies for soothing emotions (e.g., eating high-fat or high-sugar foods, smoking cigarettes, or drinking too much alcohol) that only serve to increase their difficulties; for example, overeating leads to weight gain, smoking can increase pain, and drinking has a depressive effect. Negative feelings also reinforce negative thoughts that affect the patient's motivation: "Feeling this depressed, there is no way that I can start a treatment program, I will wait until I feel better." Changes in behavior patterns are a major complaint of patients who seek treatment for persistent pain conditions [11]. Seeking to reduce pain, patients decrease their activity level, spending more time at

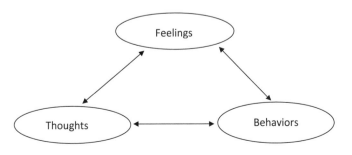

Fig. 1. A psychosocial model of adjustment to pain.

home in bed or in a recliner. The end result is less time spent in activities that give them a sense of mastery or purpose, and less time involved in pleasant interactions with family, friends, and coworkers. With this narrowing in the range of activities come feelings of boredom and less distraction from pain-related thoughts and feelings. Attempts to find a cure for their pain condition may lead to repeated failed trials of medical, surgical, and unproven treatments, all of which can have iatrogenic effects (e.g., dependence on pain medications, polypharmacy, or scar tissue) [61].

Over the past 20 years, a variety of psychosocial treatments have been developed to address such problems in adjusting to persistent pain. These approaches can be grouped into five broad categories: cognitive-behavioral therapy, emotional disclosure, hypnosis, acceptance-based treatments, and partner-based treatments. The approaches differ with respect to which of three domains of adjustment (i.e., thoughts, feelings, and behaviors) they focus on. In this section we provide a brief overview of each of these approaches. For each treatment approach, we describe its conceptual foundation, basic elements of treatment, and evidence of its efficacy, and highlight several key clinical issues. In separate sections, and by means of illustration, we will focus on a specific cognitive-behavioral treatment that is developed for chronic pain patients who report excessive pain-related fear and anxiety.

Cognitive-Behavioral Therapy

Conceptual Foundation

Cognitive-behavioral therapy (CBT) approaches to persistent pain first emerged in the late 1970s and early 1980s. The conceptual foundations of this approach included both the behavioral model of pain advanced by Fordyce [9] and the cognitive-behavioral model of pain advanced by Turk et al. [96]. From the behavioral model, CBT drew its emphasis on the role that learning can play on the development of problematic behavior patterns (e.g., an inactive lifestyle, overdependence on family, and excessive pain-avoidant posturing) and the notion that new patterns of behavior can be learned (e.g., regular exercise, becoming more independent, or relaxing during movement). From the cognitive-behavioral models, CBT drew its emphasis on the importance that the patient's thoughts can play in fostering or hindering self-management efforts. CBT models maintain that thought patterns, like other responses,

can be learned and that changes in thoughts can affect feelings and behavior. In sum, the conceptual foundations of CBT lie in both behavioral and cognitive-behavioral models of pain. CBT thus focuses on two key domains of adjustment (behavior and thoughts), with the notion that targeting these domains can lead to a cascade of improvements in thoughts, feelings, and behaviors (see Fig. 2A).

Basic Elements of Treatment

CBT protocols have three basic elements. First, there is a sharing conference in which the therapist provides a rationale for treatment. The rationale uses simple diagrams and give-and-take dialogue. The rationale helps patients understand how persistent pain has influenced their thoughts, feelings, and behaviors and how these have influenced their adjustment to pain. It also highlights the role that self-management efforts can play in changing adjustment. Simplified descriptions of theories of pain (e.g., the gate control or neuromatrix theories) are often used to underscore how thoughts, feelings, and behaviors can influence pain. Second, patients are trained in a variety of behavioral and cognitive coping skills to modify their adjustment to pain. Unlike early behavioral treatment interventions, which relied on specialized inpatient units where staff were taught to monitor and reinforce changes in behavior, the emphasis in CBT is on self-management. In CBT, patients are taught how to monitor their own behavior, set goals, and evaluate and reinforce their own progress, all important processes in self-management. Patients are trained in a variety of behavioral coping skills. One of the most common skills is an activity pacing approach (activity-rest cycling), in which patients learn to alternate periods of moderate activity with limited rest breaks in order to break the cycle of overactivity leading to pain-contingent rest, and to gradually build up the level of overall activity (and decrease the amount of rest). Patients also learn to use pleasant activity scheduling to help them better set and attain goals for expanding their range of activities. Finally, training in progressive relaxation training is often used to help patients learn to relax as they engage in daily activities (e.g., walking, transferring from one position to another, interacting with others socially, and decreasing pain-avoidant posturing). Using cognitive restructuring techniques adapted from the cognitive therapy literature, CBT teaches patients to identify overly negative thoughts (e.g., "I am worthless," "I can no longer do anything") and replace them with more realistic and helpful thoughts (e.g., "I may not be able to do some things I did in the past, but I am a valuable person") and to observe how the these thoughts affect their feelings. They are also taught skills designed to help them distract thinking away from pain (e.g., imagery, counting techniques, or use of a focal point). Finally, CBT provides training in strategies for maintaining the practice of learned coping skills (e.g., using simple forms or calendars to track and reinforce practice efforts, developing plans for dealing with setbacks or relapses in coping efforts).

Although the format by which CBT is delivered varies, treatment typically involves multiple sessions (often 6 to 10) conducted weekly (to allow time for skills practice) by a highly trained therapist (usually a psychologist). As with all psychosocial interventions, treatment is very interactive and patient-centered, with more emphasis on and time spent in give-and-take discussions and actual practice with skills than on transferring a lot of information through lectures, handouts, or video presentations.

Evidence of Efficacy

Numerous controlled studies of CBT have been conducted, and systematic reviews and meta-analyses summarizing their efficacy have been published. Recent meta-analyses have supported the efficacy of CBT for recurrent headache [77], chronic low back pain [42], arthritis pain [24], and cancer pain [1]. In general, these meta-analyses show that CBT produces improvements in a variety of indices of adjustment including pain, emotions (e.g., depression, anxiety), pain-related thoughts (e.g., pain catastrophizing, self-efficacy for pain), and behavior (e.g., activity level, medication intake).

Clinical Issues

CBT is currently the most widely used psychosocial treatment in the pain area. In clinical practice, several issues arise that are related to CBT. First, CBT is mainly available at specialized treatment centers or tertiary care clinics. Many patients who could potentially benefit from this treatment lack access to it. Home- and telephone-based CBT may provide an option for those patients, and ongoing research is examining other novel treatment delivery methods (e.g., via the Internet or a personal data assistant). Second, most studies of CBT have relied on psychologists having a solid background

of training in CBT, and a background in applying CBT with patients who have persistent pain. In practice, CBT is increasingly being delivered by nonpsychologists (including nurses and physical therapists) whose training and experience with CBT may be limited. The result can be lower-quality and less effective treatment. Clinicians who refer should be aware that practitioner skill and background are likely to be important factors influencing how well CBT will work for a given patient. Finally, CBT does not work for all patients. Because of its emphasis on self-management, CBT is not appropriate for patients who have significant memory problems or severe psychological problems (e.g., hallucinations).

Emotional Disclosure Interventions

Conceptual Foundation

Emotional disclosure interventions target the domain of feelings (see Fig. 2B). There are a number of reasons to believe that expressing one's feelings can improve one's adjustment to pain. First, excessive avoidance of emotional experiences is believed to make it difficult to process them and leads to poor outcomes. Second, when individuals work hard to suppress or inhibit emotions, they are more likely to experience unwanted intrusive thoughts, higher levels of anxiety, and chronic physiological arousal. Finally, clinical observations suggest that individuals who use emotional expression as a coping technique have better health outcomes.

Although emotional disclosure occurs in everyday situations, it can also be prompted by means of a formal, structured psychosocial intervention that encourages patients to write about (or talk about) their emotions. Emotional disclosure interventions can help in several ways [33], by enabling individuals to let go of unwanted emotions, helping them to confront and process negative emotions, and improving their skills in regulating emotions.

Basic Elements

In emotional disclosure protocols, participants typically are asked to privately write about (or talk into a tape recorder about) their feelings regarding very difficult, stressful experiences. The experiences focused on during the disclosure sessions may be pain-related or not. In particular, participants are encouraged to disclose difficult feelings that they have not discussed in detail before. The disclosures are typically conducted in three or four 20- to 30-minute sessions that are spaced at daily or weekly intervals.

Evidence of Efficacy

Controlled studies of emotional disclosure interventions have been conducted in several persistent pain disorders. Two studies of fibromyalgia patients have found that, compared to control conditions, emotional disclosure can lead to reductions in pain and improvements in function [9,35]. Among the functional improvements reported in these studies are increases in psychological well-being and decreases in pain interference, health care use, and physical disability. To date, a number of studies have examined the effects of emotional disclosure in rheumatoid arthritis patients. The first study [87] found that written emotional disclosure led to significant improvements in disease activity by the 4-month follow-up. Kelly et al. [52] found that emotional disclosure reduced emotional distress and improved performance during daily activities but did not affect joint function or pain. Other studies have reported that disclosure produced few or no benefits in patients with rheumatoid arthritis [20,50].

Studies conducted with other pain populations have found that the benefits of emotional disclosure are limited to particular subgroups of patients. For example, in a study of pelvic pain [74], emotional disclosure led to decreases in pain. However, improvements in disability were only evident in women who initially were ambivalent about expressing emotions, engaged in higher levels of pain catastrophizing, or were more prone to report negative emotions. A study of emotional disclosure carried out in undergraduates having migraine headaches [53] found that those who were more prone to discuss their feelings (i.e., used an emotional approach to coping) or who reported low self-efficacy for pain were much more likely to experience improvements following treatment.

Clinical Issues

Emotional disclosure interventions are clinically appealing because they target a domain that many patients with pain have difficulty with—expressing their emotions. The interventions used to promote emotional disclosure are simple, inexpensive, and can be integrated relatively easily into clinical practice. Emotional disclosure also is appealing because it seems to match what happens in clinical practice. Disclosure occurs often in clinical situations in which patients share their feelings about their condition with a doctor, nurse, or other health care professional. These naturally occurring disclosures, however, likely are different from the more intensive and prolonged disclosure interventions discussed above. Structured emotional disclosure protocols have not been found to yield many adverse effects, but many research studies have screened participants to ensure they have not had recent trauma and are not psychological unstable.

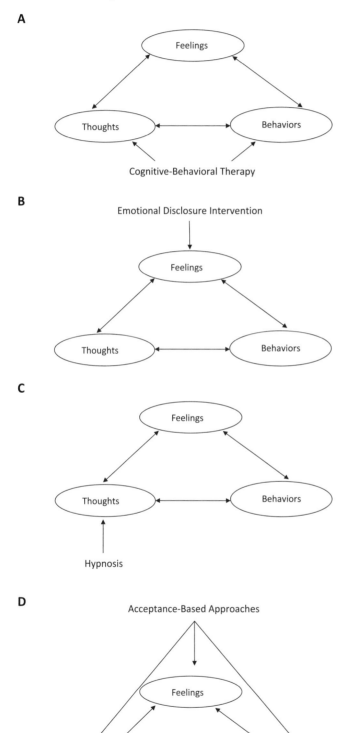

Fig. 2. Primary treatment targets for (A) cognitive-behavioral therapy, (B) emotional disclosure interventions, (C) hypnosis, and (D) acceptance-based treatments.

Perhaps the biggest drawback to implementing emotional disclosure interventions into practice is that the evidence as to their efficacy is mixed. The consensus emerging among researchers working in this area is that emotional disclosure interventions might work well for some patients, but that more work is needed before we pinpoint the patient subgroups most likely to benefit.

Hypnosis

Conceptual Foundation

Hypnosis has been used for pain control for centuries. Frequently used in the acute pain setting, hypnosis is now increasingly being used in patients with persistent pain [45]. Hypnosis involves a therapist guiding the patient through an induction that encourages patients to focus their attention. The induction is followed by suggestions on how to direct one's attention to images or experiences [45]. Although the focus of hypnosis is clearly on the domain of thoughts (see Fig. 2C), the suggestions used in persons with chronic pain may focus on the experience of pain (e.g., altering its unpleasantness), pain-related emotions (e.g., feeling more calm), and behavior (e.g., moving in a more relaxed and comfortable manner). Recently, there has been growing interest in hypnosis in pain management [46], in part because of evidence from brain imaging studies that hypnosis has effects on areas of the brain involved in pain—the thalamus, anterior cingulate cortex [ACC], insula, prefrontal cortex, parietal cortex. Studies by Rainville et al. [41,80], for example, have shown that hypnotic imagery focused on changing the unpleasantness of pain produced changes activity in the ACC (an area related to the emotional component of pain) but not activity in the primary somatosensory area, whereas imagery focused on changing the intensity of pain produced changes in brain regions related to processing of sensory information (the S1 cortex) but not in the ACC.

Basic Elements

Hypnosis protocols used with patients having persistent pain involve several basic steps [79]. First, an assessment is conducted to better understand the pain, the ways that the patient copes with pain, and the patient's pain-related images, thoughts, and words [79]. Second, an induction is carried out using techniques such as relaxation and guided imagery to help the patient to become comfortable and better focus his or her attention. Third, specific, individually tailored suggestions are provided for changing the pain experience and enhancing the patient's ability to relax [79]. These suggestions (with examples) might include: (1) pleasant imagery—imagining oneself in a favorite place (the beach, mountains, or a garden); (2) sensory substitution—imagining the pain as another sensation (cold or numbness); (3) hypnotic anesthesia—imagining turning down the volume of the pain; (4) decreased unpleasantness; (5) disassociation—imagining the painful area is not part of one's body; (6) displacement—moving the pain from one body area to another; or (7) incompatible emotive imagery—imagining scenes that evoke relaxation or joy. Fourth, patients are taught to practice hypnosis on their own to generalize learned skills and benefits.

Evidence of Efficacy

Several reviews of the literature on hypnosis in the treatment of chronic pain have appeared in the past 5 years (e.g., refs. [40,41]). Randomized controlled trials have been conducted on the effects of hypnosis in patients with headache, orofacial pain, multiple sclerosis, and chronic pain secondary to spinal cord injury. Taken together, the results of these studies indicate that patients trained in hypnosis report significantly greater improvements in pain than patients in control conditions. The effects of hypnosis, however, are not typically superior to other relaxation-based interventions such as progressive relaxation training or autogenic training [45,46].

Clinical Issues

Clinical observations and research studies suggest that patients with persistent pain vary in their response to hypnosis. Some report robust benefits across an array of outcomes, while others report little or no benefit. Individual differences in hypnotic suggestibility may be one of the reasons for these variations [45]. Simple hypnotizability scales are available and could be used in clinical settings to identify those patients most likely to respond to hypnosis. As with other psychosocial treatments, the efficacy of hypnosis depends on patients' motivation and willingness to practice their learned skills. Patients who practice more regularly are more likely to benefit from hypnosis. Many hypnotists incorporate techniques of motivational interviewing to enhance patients' expectations and willingness to practice [45].

Acceptance-Based Treatments

Conceptual Foundations

Acceptance-based treatments are designed to address the problems that arise when patients' attempts to control pain and pain-related thoughts and feelings begin to dominate their lives and cause them to avoid activities that are important to them [61]. Patients who report that they struggle to control pain have substantially higher levels of pain, psychological distress, and physical disability [61]. There is also evidence that people who struggle to control unwanted thoughts and feelings paradoxically experience a higher level of these thoughts and feelings [37,38]. Acceptance-based treatments are designed to help patients acknowledge and accept their unwanted thoughts and feelings (including pain sensations) while simultaneously engaging in valued behaviors. These treatments thus focus on all three domains of adjustment (see Fig. 2D).

Basic Elements

Acceptance-based treatments for pain are designed to increase a person's psychological flexibility [61] by focusing on several key processes: (1) acceptance—to foster acknowledgement of thoughts and feelings without struggling or evaluating them; (2) mindfulness—to enhance awareness of the present moment; (3) cognitive defusion—to help patients learn to label thoughts and feelings as just that, rather than as reality; (4) exploring values—to identify what is valued and meaningful; and (5) committed action—to set goals and encourage involvement in daily activities that match a person's true values. A variety of treatment techniques are used to promote these processes [107]. One set of techniques helps decrease avoidance of thoughts and feelings by having patients become aware of them in a nonevaluative fashion, typically through training in mindfulness meditation, yoga, or other meditation methods. These meditation techniques foster awareness and acceptance of a variety of thoughts and feelings. For example, patients might use meditation to become more aware of body sensations that arise during relaxation or physical exercise, emotions that occur during a flare of pain or after a failed trial of a new pain medication, or the thoughts and feelings they have about how others react to their pain. A second set of techniques helps patients identify and increase their level of meaningful activities. These activities vary but often include physical exercise (e.g., yoga, aerobic exercise) and behavioral experiments with activities one has been avoiding for fear of increased pain (e.g., resuming child care responsibilities, driving a car for a longer distance). To help identify activities that are meaningful, patients are often asked to rate how much they value activities across multiple domains (e.g., family, work, recreation, community, education, friends, intimate relationships, parenting, or self-care) [64] and to analyze prior unsuccessful efforts to accomplish these activities. To increase the level of commitment to meaningful activities, patients are also encouraged to set, state a commitment to, and record their attainment of specific behavioral goals.

Evidence of Efficacy

Several studies have reported that acceptance-based treatments can produce improvements in how patients with persistent pain adjust to pain (i.e., improvements in one or more of the following outcomes: pain, anxiety, depression, psychosocial disability, and physical functioning), though these studies lacked randomly assigned control groups [63,64,108,109,111]. Dahl et al. [19] have conducted one of the few randomized controlled studies of an acceptance-based intervention for persistent pain. A small sample ($N = 19$) of participants who were found to be at risk for early retirement due to persistent pain were randomly assigned to a four-session acceptance-based intervention or usual care. No differences in pain, stress, or quality of life were found following the treatment, although patients in the acceptance-based group had lower health care costs and took fewer sick days. Considered overall, the available research raises the possibility that acceptance-based approaches have merit. However, it is not possible to draw more definitive conclusions regarding this approach until a larger number of more rigorous, randomized clinical studies are conducted.

Clinical Issues

Patients vary in the degree to which they are willing to pursue approaches focused on acceptance. Some patients readily embrace this approach. Other patients (e.g., those with disease-related pain) may feel acceptance is not appropriate given that their medical treatment involves ongoing medical interventions designed to control and manage the underlying tissue damage that is causing their pain. Still other patients may balk at the term acceptance, considering it a form of resigning or giving up [61]. Acceptance-based approaches are clearly not for all patients. They may be particularly useful for patients whose struggles to control pain have become the central issue dominating their lives [61]. In such patients, acceptance based approaches may provide a means of helping them learn that they can engage in a meaningful life in spite of having persistent pain.

Partner-Based Treatments

Conceptual Foundation

Almost all psychosocial approaches to managing pain acknowledge the importance that significant others such as spouses/partners and family members can have in how individuals adjust to persistent pain. There is growing evidence that persistent pain has a major impact on partners and that the way that a partner responds to persistent pain can influence the patient's adjustment (see Somers et al. [88] for a recent review of this literature). Involving partners in treatment can benefit both partners (e.g., by reducing their distress and enhancing their confidence in their ability to support the patient) and patients (e.g., by increasing social support and improving communication), while also enhancing their relationship (e.g., improving dyadic satisfaction). Partner-based interventions focus on the social context of adjustment with the assumption that by altering that context, both the patient and persons in that context (i.e., a spouse or partner) will experience benefits.

Basic Elements

Baucom [4] has identified two major approaches that can be used to integrate others into psychosocial interventions for patients having persistent pain. The first is a partner-assisted approach in which the focus is clearly the patient, and the family member has an ancillary role; that is, to serve as a coach who assists the patient in learning symptom management skills. The second approach is a couples-based, disorder-specific approach [29]. In this couples-based approach, the focus is on the couple (the patient and his or her partner), and the role of the partner is that of an equal participant with the patient. The target of this approach is improving couples communication and interactions around a specific problem or disorder, such as pain.

Evidence of Efficacy

To date, there have not been enough studies of partner-based treatments for pain to warrant a meta-analysis. Several studies, however, have shown these interventions can be beneficial. For example, in our own laboratory we conducted a randomized controlled study testing the efficacy of a partner-assisted pain coping skills training protocol for osteoarthritis pain [51]. This study found that partner-assisted pain coping skills training produced significant benefits for patients, including reductions in pain, psychological disability, and pain behavior, and increases in marital adjustment and self-efficacy [51]. In a recent study of patients with pain due to gastrointestinal cancer, Porter et al. [79] compared a partner-assisted emotional disclosure intervention to an education/support intervention that involved patients and partners. The partner-assisted emotional disclosure intervention produced significant improvements in relationship quality and intimacy in couples where the patient was prone to hold back on discussing pain and other cancer-related concerns.

Couple-based interventions have been shown to be effective for treating a number of individual disorders including agoraphobia, depression, and alcohol abuse and dependence [8], but they have not yet been tested widely in pain conditions. In a recent randomized study, Baucom et al. [4] reported on the results of a study of a couples-based relationship enhancement intervention for women having breast cancer. The six-session intervention taught couples problem-solving skills and emotional expressiveness skills and then encouraged them to apply these skills to key relationship issues, including (1) the effects of breast cancer on intimacy and sexual functioning, (2) the meaning of the cancer for the couple, and (3) personal growth that may be occurring as a result of cancer. Compared to patients in a usual-care control condition, those who received the relationship enhancement intervention showed improvements in pain (effect size = 0.59) that were maintained at 1-year follow up (effect size = 0.53). Overall, the pattern of findings supported the efficacy of the couples-based intervention both at the post-treatment and 1-year follow up assessment points. Compared to the treatment-as-usual group, patients receiving the couples-based intervention showed improvements in measures of fatigue, other cancer symptoms, and well-being. Furthermore, both patients and partners receiving this intervention showed improvements in relationship satisfaction, personal growth, and psychological distress. Taken together, these findings support the notion that couples-based interventions focusing on relationship enhancement can be beneficial for patients having pain and other symptoms related to cancer.

Clinical Issues

Several issues need to be considered when using part-ner-based interventions in couples where one member has persistent pain [88]. First, these interventions may not be appropriate for highly distressed couples. In cases where couples are thinking of separating or di-vorcing, a referral for marital therapy is warranted and appropriate. Second, patients or partners may hold neg-ative attitudes or beliefs about psychosocial interven-tion that may undermine the efficacy of partner-based interventions. Providing a rationale and educational information about the benefits of the intervention is often sufficient to allay concerns that patients or part-ners may have. However, when one or both members of the dyad hold intractable, negative beliefs it is best not to proceed with intervention. Third, although we have focused on partner-based approaches in this section, many of the methods discussed could be used in the context of family-based treatment. Children and friends are often involved in trying to provide support to some-one with persistent pain, and including such individuals in interventions could be quite beneficial.

Psychological Assessment and Treatment of Pain-Related Fear and Avoidance

This section provides an overview of the role of pain-related fear in chronic pain and disability. This section is divided into three parts: empirical foundations, assess-ment methods, and intervention methods.

Empirical Foundations

Pain as a Biological Stimulus to Protect the Integrity of the Body

Pain is one of those biological stimuli with high rele-vance for survival. Indeed, pain informs the individual that there is an imminent threat or actual damage to the body. Interestingly, despite the salience of pain ex-periences, there is individual variation in the extent to which pain is experienced as aversive. First, pain is al-ways contextual, and when overall survival is at stake, pain may be suppressed. As Henry Beecher, a military surgeon who served in the U.S. army in 1941, pointed out more than half a century ago: "*There is no simple, direct relationship between the wound* per se *and the pain experienced. The pain is in very large part deter-mined by other factors, and of great importance here is*

the significance of the wound, i.e., reaction to the wound" (page 165, italics original) [5]. Much later, the concept of "pain catastrophizing" was introduced: an amplified negative interpretation of actual and anticipated pain experience [82,90]. For example, people with high levels of catastrophizing are more convinced that pain always means that their body is vulnerable and needs careful protection to prevent further harm as compared to low catastrophizers. An increasing number of studies have shown that there are important individual differences in pain catastrophizing. More importantly, pain cata-strophizing is associated with more emotional distress, higher levels of disability, and worse treatment outcome [91]. There is also evidence that pain catastrophizing is intricately associated with fear of pain and that it makes people more vulnerable to responding fearfully in the presence of painful stimuli. Fear is a hard-wired emo-tional response to an imminent and identifiable threat that is associated with a cascade of protective behav-iors. Pain-related fear is a specific fear of threat that is signaled by means of painful stimuli. In persistent pain, the time dimension in itself may heighten the threat value of pain, as in most cases pain is transient, ceasing after a few hours or days. The mismatch between what individuals expect (a rapid decrease) and what they ex-perience (persisting pain) might create suspicion about its cause and fuel increased worry.

Protective Responses Due to Fear

In response to the presence of threat and the activation of fear, protective behaviors arise that may have *cogni-tive, motivational,* and *physiological* features. Cognitive shifts occur to detect threat and narrow the attention-al focus upon potential threat cues (*hypervigilance*). Three distinct attentional processes can be distin-guished: (1) general hypervigilance, or the propensity to attend to any irrelevant stimuli being presented; (2) specific hypervigilance, or the inclination to attend se-lectively to pain-related stimuli; and (3) the difficulty of disengaging from the threat stimuli at the cost of ongo-ing tasks [16,27]. Pain captures attention to orient the individual to the source of threat and engage in behav-iors that in acute pain promote healing, such as *escape and avoidance behavior.* Although pain in itself cannot always be avoided, the activities assumed to increase pain or (re)injury may be avoidable. A number of stud-ies have shown an association between pain-related fear and decreased physical performance as assessed by range of motion [62], weight lifting [101,102], knee extension-flexion [17,18], lumbar extension [2], and lifting and carrying objects [10]. Besides escape and avoidance behavior, individuals may also engage in more subtle *safety-seeking behavior*, which is defined as behavior that prevents or minimizes a feared outcome while remaining in the feared situation (e.g., "I'd make sure that I don't lean forward when I'm holding something heavy because that might break my spine") [92]. Finally, fear-related physiological *arousal* may be associated with muscle contractions around the injured area; it is suggested that in acute pain these muscle contractions and the associated immobilization function to protect the body from further injury. In persistent pain, these contractions may be less adaptive [32].

Anticipating Harm through Learning

By virtue of its biological significance, pain is an important motivator in learning. Regardless of the threat value, people have the urge to reduce the impact of any aversive stimulus. This mechanism drives learning, since people search for stimuli that predict or signal the possible threat of the occurrence of the biologically relevant stimulus [30]. During associative learning, a former neutral stimulus becomes a conditioned stimulus (CS) and acquires a new meaning by being causally associated with a biologically relevant unconditioned stimulus (US) [40]. For example, a worker who experiences a shooting pain in the back during lifting may start avoiding lifting as a result of the learned association between lifting and the shooting pain. Through this learning, the thought of lifting elicits a conditioned response (CR), which usually is very similar to the protective responses elicited by the biologically relevant US. During learning, propositional knowledge about the US-CS relation are stored in long-term memory [21].

There are three ways in which propositional knowledge about the relationship between stimuli and pain can be acquired. The example about the worker who feels intense pain while lifting is an example of learning by *direct experience;* the person actually experiences the CS-US relation. In our own laboratory we recently showed that healthy subjects can become fearful of a joystick movement when this was followed by a painful electrocutaneous stimulus [69]. Research findings suggest that fear learning in chronic pain patients also occurs through *verbal threat information* [31]. Patients who contact health care providers may learn about the association between certain stimuli and pain through the diagnostic information, which

might be interpreted as being more threatening than intended by the medical specialist. Evidence shows that the beliefs and orientations of these providers can play a role in the acquisition of pain-related fear. Biomedically oriented health care providers often suggest that movement should be restricted, while those holding a more biopsychosocial orientation recommend high levels of activity despite pain, suggesting no relationship between activities and harm [43].

Olsson and Phelps found evidence for *observational learning* of the association between pain and fear [75]. They directly compared the three pathways to fear and found that a CS acquires its threat value through being paired with a painful shock (direct experience), with observed fear expression in another person or with the experimenter's verbal instructions. Skin conductance levels to the CS were lowest after verbal instruction, but were of comparable magnitude after experiential and observational learning. Likewise, healthy subjects can acquire pain-related fear by observing a human model performing a cold pressor task, in which orange or pink water indicated either pain or relaxation in the model's facial expression [39]. When tested themselves, the subjects fear and pain scores show that they had learned the associations they previously observed in the model, despite equal temperatures of both orange and pink cold pressor tasks.

In summary, pain-related fear in patients with chronic pain can be a learned, conditioned response that can be acquired through the three pathways. One of the difficulties is that through learning, individuals can remain engaged in protective behaviors, even when the source of threat had diminished. Fear responses may also generalize to similar stimuli that were never followed by pain or pain increase, thereby worsening the problem. Based on this and other observations, a cognitive-behavioral model of pain-related fear has been developed that postulates two opposing behavioral responses—confrontation and avoidance—and presents possible pathways by which injured patients can get caught in a downward spiral of increasing avoidance, disability, and pain [106] (see Fig. 3). The model identifies several ways by which pain-related fear can lead to disability: (1) there is a bidirectional association between negative appraisals about pain and its consequences and pain-related fear; (2) escape and avoidance behaviors occur in anticipation of pain rather than as a response to pain, so these behaviors may persist because there are fewer

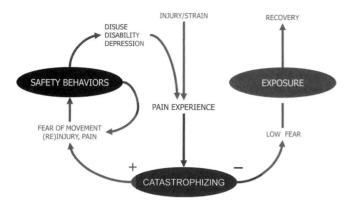

Fig. 3. The fear-avoidance model of chronic pain.

opportunities to correct the (inaccurate) expectancies and beliefs about pain; and (3) long-standing avoidance and physical inactivity can lead to disability and a withdrawal from essential reinforcers, leading to mood disturbances such as depression, irritability, and frustration. A number of prospective studies have provided support for this model [54].

Assessment of Fearful Beliefs about Pain

A semi-structured interview is useful to collect information about the antecedents of pain-related fear, its direct and indirect consequences, and other life stresses that may interfere with the patient's current functioning. Several issues may be relevant. First, beliefs of patients with chronic pain often reflect the acquired propositional knowledge about pain, such as "If I do this particular movement, pain will increase" or "If I feel pain, it means that my injury is getting worse." Often these forms of reasoning follow a confirmation bias in the sense that the "if … then" rule is seldom falsified. The selective search for confirming evidence and the lack of falsifying evidence reinforces the credibility of the false assumptions. Second, chronic pain patients do not always conceive their problem as a result of associative learning, nor may they frame their concerns in terms of fear. Therefore, it may help to paraphrase a patient's personal story in terms of perceived harmfulness (e.g., "You feel that it might be better not to do these activities," "I understand that you think that these activities might further harm your back") rather than using the words "fear" or "anxiety." Third, the interview may be supported by well-established questionnaires that have been developed to assess aspects of pain-related fear. The most frequently used are the Fear-Avoidance Beliefs Questionnaire (FABQ), focusing on patients' beliefs about how work and physical activity affect their low back pain [110]; the Pain Anxiety Symptoms Scale

(PASS) developed to measure cognitive anxiety symptoms, escape and avoidance responses, fearful appraisals of pain and physiological anxiety symptoms related to pain [65]; and the Tampa Scale for Kinesiophobia (TSK) [70,81], aimed at the assessment of fear of (re) injury due to movement. A limitation of these questionnaires, however, is that they do not provide information about which specific movements and activities (i.e., CSs) the patient fears or avoids. Therefore, pictorial assessment methods have been designed, each showing a person performing a specific movement or activity. Patients can organize photographs of various daily activities or movements in ascending order, based on the extent to which they believe that performing these activities is harmful. In this way, a personal hierarchy of fear-eliciting activities can be established that can also be used to guide exposure-based treatment (see below). Both sets have shown good test-retest reliability, stability over time, internal consistency, and construct validity [55,71,98].

Psychological Management Methods to Reduce Pain-Related Fear

Verbal Reassurance

Doctors can tell their patients that they do not have the particular disease they fear, often supported by showing them negative test results, and sometimes by providing an alternative non-disease explanation such as stress, muscle pain, or physical overuse. A surprisingly small number of studies have examined the effects of verbal reassurance, and the overall conclusion is that verbal reassurance does not reduce fears. In the long run, reassurance can even increase fear in some patients [25,66]. These results are not surprising because verbal reassurance does not activate the fear network (but rather attenuates it), and neither does it provide new information that disqualifies previous beliefs [57].

Education

Another way of reducing fear is to provide new information about the unlikelihood of the feared consequences. Verbal instruction may help in reconceptualizing pain as a common condition that can be self-managed, rather than as a serious disease or a condition that needs careful protection. One of the major goals of this informational session is to increase the willingness of patients to engage in activities they have been avoiding for a long time. A study by Moore et al. [71] examined the effects of a two-session educational group intervention for back pain patients in primary care. Besides the group meeting, there was also one individual meeting and telephone conversation with the group leader, and with a psychologist experienced in chronic pain management. The intervention was supplemented by educational materials (a book and videos) supporting active management of back pain. A control group received usual care. Participants assigned to the educational, self-care intervention showed significantly greater reductions in back-related worry and fear-avoidance beliefs than patients in the control group. In patients with chronic low back pain in tertiary care, however, education alone was not enough to change actual behavior; performance of relevant daily activities was not affected by the educational session and improved significantly only with exposure in vivo [23].

Graded Activity

Although most exercise and operant graded activity programs were not originally designed to reduce pain-related fear, these programs may have fear-reducing effects. Mannion et al. [59] conducted a study comparing three sorts of active treatment: (1) modern active physiotherapy, (2) muscle reconditioning on training devices, or (3) low-impact aerobics. After therapy, significant reductions were observed in pain intensity, frequency, pain disability, pain catastrophizing, and pain-related fear. These effects were maintained over the subsequent 6 months, with the exception of the patients receiving physiotherapy, who increased their levels of pain-related fear and disability. A subsequent study suggested that the improvements are probably a result of the positive experience of completing the prescribed exercises without undue harm [58]. Similar findings have been reported after an operant graded activity program [100].

Exposure in Vivo with Behavioral Experiments

Graded exposure to back-stressing movements has been tested as a treatment approach for back pain patients reporting substantial fear of movement/(re)injury. The idea is that extinction of fear and inhibition of fear responses occur when the individual observes the absence of the aversive pain stimulus when exposed to the CS [40]. Such a cognitive-behavioral fear reduction treatment usually consists of at least four steps: (1) defining functional (life) goals; (2) education about the paradoxical effects of safety-seeking behaviors; (3) establishing a fear hierarchy; and (4) exposure to activities with increasing levels perceived harmfulness, according

to the fear hierarchy. A detailed description of the treatment can be found elsewhere [105]. A series of studies using replicated single-case experimental designs revealed that decreases in pain-related fear occurred during the exposure module only. Additionally, these improvements were related to decreases in pain disability, pain vigilance, and an increase in physical activity [3]. In one study, patients with complex regional pain syndrome were able to take up desired functional activities after pain-related fear went down, but before pain levels decreased below 50%, suggesting that fear of pain is more disabling than the pain itself [22].

So far, the published randomized controlled trials on the effectiveness of exposure in chronic low back pain have found mixed results. Woods and Asmundson [113] randomly assigned 44 patients to graded exposure in vivo, graded activity, or a waiting-list control condition. They found that, in comparison with the graded activity condition, patients in the graded in vivo exposure condition demonstrated significantly greater improvements on measures of fear of pain/movement, fear avoidance beliefs, and pain-related anxiety, but only trend differences for pain-related disability and pain self-efficacy. When graded exposure in vivo was compared to the waiting-list control group, exposure showed significantly greater improvements on measures of fear-avoidance beliefs, fear of pain/movement, pain-related anxiety, pain catastrophizing, pain experience, anxiety, and depression. Over a 3-month follow up, the exposure group maintained improvements. Leeuw et al. [56] conducted a multicenter trial in which 85 participants were included in either a graded exposure or a graded activity program, with similar findings. Exposure resulted in a significantly decreased perceived harmfulness of activity, while the difference between both treatments in improved function almost reached statistical significance. A recent review on treatments available to address fear-avoidance beliefs in patients with chronic musculoskeletal pain suggests that graded exposure in vivo and acceptance and commitment therapy result in the best outcomes for treating fear-avoidance beliefs [3].

Challenges and Future Directions

Depression and Persistent Pain

The subject of depression in pain has been extensively described over several decades of pain research and treatment, and the interested reader is directed to reviews [11,97]. Rather than being characterized as a comorbidity, depressed mood is closely linked to pain on many levels [78], from experience and symptoms to common neurotransmitters [11]. It is more helpfully understood within a broader context that includes fears and restricted activity; persistent pain implies losses of role, of pleasant activities, and often of an anticipated active future, to the extent that the patient describes a changed identity [72]. Rehabilitation usually brings an improvement in mood with recovery of activities and of hopes [73], with emotional disengagement and acceptance curtailing rumination and "stuckness" [107].

An Affective-Motivational Approach

A number of authors have recently called for an expanded affective-motivational approach with a prominent focus on behavior in the context of multiple goals [99,104]. In their attempt to resume daily life activities, pain patients engage in various goals, some of which are directly related to dealing with pain, whereas others are unrelated. These multiple goals may facilitate each other, or they can be conflicting. For example, the goal to satisfy others by resuming work-related activities may conflict with the goal to protect bodily integrity by staying safely at home. Unfortunately, unresolved pain-related goal conflicts may fuel fear [49]. An emerging and intriguing question is whether cognitive-behavioral therapies aimed at the reevaluation of major life goals and at the resolution of enduring goal conflicts help to counter fear-driven and disabling avoidance behavior [99,104]. It would be worthwhile to examine whether the effects of fear-reduction treatments can be enhanced by adding a motivational component focused on the resolution of goal conflicts [84].

Persistence versus Avoidance

Finally, it is difficult to apply fear-avoidance principles to musculoskeletal pain syndromes associated with both task persistence and avoidance, and with frequent oscillation between the two extremes. Researchers and clinicians have observed that sometimes patients (e.g., those with work-related upper extremity pain) tend to persist in rather than escape/avoid physical activity, although the research on this topic is scarce. Novel paradigms are emerging, such as the mood-as-input model, of which the basic tenet is that task persistence is a function of the interaction between mood and the

stop-rule used [103]. Another approach is the avoidance-endurance model [36]. Although these novel approaches are quite promising, their validity in the field of pain needs further examination.

Using the Psychology of Pain in Clinical Encounters

Many of the characteristics of patients labeled "difficult" by clinicians—having multiple symptoms, having few signs that match the symptoms, and showing distress [44]—are true of many pain patients. Yet these characteristics can also be grasped as an opportunity to understand what most concerns patients and to engage them more fully in a joint plan for pain resolution or pain management. But until patients feel believed and properly assessed, it is hard for them to accept that there is no treatable problem at the root of the pain [86]. Unfortunately, patients may struggle to achieve a balance between representing their difficulties and distress with the attempt not to appear to be dramatizing or pathetic, and thus they present a confusing picture to the clinician. Too often their symptoms are assigned to a generic category of "psychological problem," under terms such as "somatization" or "medically unexplained symptoms," terms that are much misused in pain and are effectively rendered redundant by an integrated mind-body understanding of pain [15,68]. The risk of such misjudgments is greater where there is an ethnic or cultural difference between clinician and patient (for a review see Edwards et al. [28]). The issues outlined above provide alternative formulations to those proposing that the problems lie in the patient's character or rationality. In most cases, the patient's behavior can best be considered a "normal" response to an "unusual" situation of persistent pain.

References

[1] Abernethy AP, Keefe FJ, McCrory DC, Scipio CD, Matchar DB. Behavioral therapies for the management of cancer pain: a systematic review. In: Flor H, Kalso E, Dostrovsky JO, editors. Proceedings of the 11th World Congress on Pain. Seattle: IASP Press; 2006. p. 789–98.
[2] Al-Obaidi SM, Nelson RM, Al-Awadhi S, Al-Shuwaie N. The role of anticipation and fear of pain in the persistence of avoidance behavior in patients with chronic low back pain. Spine 2000;25:1126–31.
[3] Bailey KM, Carleton RN, Vlaeyen JW, Asmundson GJ. Treatments addressing pain-related fear and anxiety in patients with chronic musculoskeletal pain: a preliminary review. Cogn Behav Ther 2010; in press.
[4] Baucom DH, Porter LS, Kirby JS, Gremore TM, Wiesenthal N, Aldridge W, Fredman SJ, Stanton SE, Scott JL, Halford KW, Keefe FJ. A couple-based intervention for female breast cancer. Psychooncology 2009;18:76–83.
[5] Beecher HK. Pain in men wounded in battle. Ann Surg 1946;123:96–105.

[6] Beurskens AJ, de Vet HC, Koke AJ. Responsiveness of functional status in low back pain: A comparison of different instruments. Pain 1996;65:71–6.

[7] Blyth FM, March LM, Nicholas MK, Cousins MJ. Chronic pain, work performance and litigation. Pain 2003;103:41–7.

[8] Boynton PM, Greenhalgh T. Selecting, designing, and developing your questionnaire. BMJ 2004;328:1312–5.

[9] Broderick JE, Junghaenel DU, Schwartz JE. Written emotional expression produces health benefits in fibromyalgia patients. Psychosom Med 2005;67:326–34.

[10] Burns JW, Mullen JT, Higdon LJ, Wei JM, Lansky D. Validity of the pain anxiety symptoms scale (pass): prediction of physical capacity variables. Pain 2000;84:247–52.

[11] Campbell LC, Clauw DJ, Keefe FJ. Persistent pain and depression: a biopsychosocial perspective. Biol Psychiatry 2003;54:399–409.

[12] Caraceni A, Cherny N, Fainsinger R, Kaasa S, Poulain P, Radbruch L, De Conno F. Pain measurement tools and methods in clinical research in palliative care: recommendations of an expert working group of the European Association of Palliative Care. J Pain Symptom Manage 2002;23:239–55.

[13] Cleeland CS, Ryan KM. Pain assessment: global use of the Brief Pain Inventory. Ann Acad Med 1994;23:129–38.

[14] Cliff N, Keats JA. Ordinal measurement in the behavioral sciences. Mahwah, NJ: Lawrence Erlbaum; 2007.

[15] Crombez G, Beirens K, Van Damme S, Eccleston C, Fontaine J. The unbearable lightness of somatisation: a systematic review of the concept of somatisation in empirical studies of pain. Pain 2009;145:31–5.

[16] Crombez G, Van Damme S, Eccleston C. Hypervigilance to pain: an experimental and clinical analysis. Pain 2005;116:4–7.

[17] Crombez G, Vervaet L, Lysens R, Baeyens F, Eelen P. Avoidance and confrontation of painful, back-straining movements in chronic back pain patients. Behav Modif 1998;22:62–77.

[18] Crombez G, Vlaeyen JW, Heuts PH, Lysens R. Pain-related fear is more disabling than pain itself: evidence on the role of pain-related fear in chronic back pain disability. Pain 1999;80:329–39.

[19] Dahl J, Wilson KG, Nilsson A. Acceptance and commitment therapy and the treatment of persons at risk for long term disability resulting from stress and pain symptoms: a preliminary randomized trial. Behav Ther 2004;35:785–801.

[20] Danoff-Burg S, Agee JD, Romanoff NR, Kremer JM, Strosberg JM. Benefit finding and expressive writing in adults with lupus or rheumatoid arthritis. Psychol Health 2006;21:651–65.

[21] De Houwer J. The propositional approach to associative learning as an alternative for association formation models Learn Behav 2009;37:1–20.

[22] de Jong JR, Vlaeyen JW, Onghena P, Cuypers C, den Hollander M, Ruijgrok J. Reduction of pain-related fear in complex regional pain syndrome type I: the application of graded exposure in vivo. Pain 2005;116:264–75.

[23] de Jong JR, Vlaeyen JW, Onghena P, Goossens ME, Geilen M, Mulder H. Fear of movement/(re)injury in chronic low back pain: Education or exposure in vivo as mediator to fear reduction? Clin J Pain 2005;21:9–17.

[24] Dixon KE, Keefe FJ, Scipio CD, Perri LM, Abernethy AP. Psychological interventions for arthritis pain management in adults: a meta-analysis. Health Psychol 2007;26:241–50.

[25] Donovan JL, Blake DR. Qualitative study of interpretation of reassurance among patients attending rheumatology clinics: "Just a touch of arthritis, doctor?" BMJ 2000;320:541–4.

[26] Dworkin RH, Turk DC, Farrar JT, Haythornthwaite JA, Jensen MP, Katz NP, Kerns RD, Stucki G, Allen RR, Bellamy N, et al. Core outcome measures for chronic pain clinical trials: IMMPACT recommendations. Pain 2005;113:9–19.

[27] Eccleston C, Crombez G. Pain demands attention: a cognitive-affective model of the interruptive function of pain. Psychol Bull 1999;125:356–66.

[28] Edwards CL, Fillingim RB, Keefe F. Race, ethnicity and pain. Pain 2001;94:133–7.

[29] Epstein NB, Baucom DH. Enhanced cognitive-behavioral therapy for couples: a contextual approach. Washington, DC: American Psychological Association; 2002.

[30] Fanselow MS. From contextual fear to a dynamic view of memory systems. Trends Cogn Sci 2010;14:7–15.

[31] Field AP, Schorah H. The verbal information pathway to fear and heart rate changes in children. J Child Psychol Psychiatry 2007;48:1088–93.

[32] Flor H, Turk DC. Psychophysiology of chronic pain: do chronic pain patients exhibit symptom-specific psychophysiological responses? Psychol Bull 1989;105:215–59.

[33] Frattaroli J. Experimental disclosure and its moderators: a meta-analysis. Psychol Bull 2006;132:823–65.

[34] Gil KM, Williams DA, Keefe FJ, Beckham JC. The relationship of negative thoughts to pain and psychological distress. Behav Ther 1990:349–62.

[35] Gillis ME, Lumley MA, Mosley-Williams A, Leisen JC, Roehrs T. The health effects of at-home written emotional disclosure in fibromyalgia: a randomized trial. Ann Behav Med 2006:135–46.

[36] Hasenbring MI, Hallner D, Rusu AC. Fear-avoidance- and endurance-related responses to pain: development and validation of the Avoidance-Endurance Questionnaire (AEQ). Eur J Pain 2009;13:620–8.

[37] Hayes SC, Luoma JB, Bond FW, Masuda A, Lillis J. Acceptance and commitment therapy: model, processes and outcomes. Behav Res Ther 2006;44:1–25.

[38] Hayes SC, Wilson KG, Gifford EV, Follette VM, Strosahl K. Experiential avoidance and behavioral disorders: a functional dimensional approach to diagnosis and treatment. J Consult Clin Psychol 1996;64:1152–68.

[39] Helsen K, Kaelen S, De Peuter S, Goubert L, Vlaeyen J. Can pain-related fear be vicariously conditioned? Abstract presented at: "Pain in Europe," Lisbon, August 2009.

[40] Hermans D, Craske MG, Mineka S, Lovibond PF. Extinction in human fear conditioning. Biol Psychiatry 2006;60:361–8.

[41] Hofbauer RK, Rainville P, Duncan GH, Bushnell MC. Cortical representation of the sensory dimension of pain. J Neurophysiol 2001;86:402–11.

[42] Hoffman BM, Papas RK, Chatkoff DK, Kerns RD. Meta-analysis of psychological interventions for chronic low back pain. Health Psychol 2007;26:1–9.

[43] Houben RM, Ostelo RW, Vlaeyen JW, Wolters PM, Peters M, Stomp-van den Berg SG. Health care providers' orientations towards common low back pain predict perceived harmfulness of physical activities and recommendations regarding return to normal activity. Eur J Pain 2005;9:173–83.

[44] Jackson JL, Kroenke K. Difficult patient encounters in the ambulatory clinic: clinical predictors and outcomes. Arch Intern Med 1999;159:1069–75.

[45] Jensen MP. Hypnotic treatment of chronic pain. J Behav Med 2006;2006:95–124.

[46] Jensen MP. Hypnosis for chronic pain management: a new hope. Pain 2009;146:235–7.

[47] Jensen MP, Karoly P. Self-report scales and procedures for assessing pain in adults. In: Turk DC, Melzack R, editors. Handbook of pain assessment, 2nd edition, New York: Guilford Press; 2001. p. 15–34.

[48] Johnson TP. Methods and frameworks for cross-cultural measurement. Med Care 2006;44(11 Suppl 3):S17–20.

[49] Karoly P, Okun MA, Ruehlman LS, Pugliese JA. The impact of goal cognition and pain severity on disability and depression in adults with chronic pain: an examination of direct effects and mediated effects via pain-induced fear. Cogn Ther Res 2008;32:418–33.

[50] Keefe FJ, Anderson T, Lumley M, Caldwell D, Stainbrook D, McKee D, Watners SJ, Connelly M, Affleck G, Pope MS, et al. A randomized, controlled trial of emotional disclosure in rheumatoid arthritis: can clinician assistance enhance the effects? Pain 2008;137:164–72.

[51] Keefe FJ, Caldwell DS, Williams DA, Gil KM, Mitchell D, Robertson C, Martinez S, Nunley J, Beckham JC, Crisson JE, Helms M. Pain coping skills training in the management of osteoarthritic knee pain: a comparative study. Behav Ther 1990;21:49–62.

[52] Kelley JE, Lumley MA, Leisen JC. The health effects of emotional disclosure in rheumatoid arthritis. Health Psychol 1997;16:331–40.

[53] Kraft CA, Lumley MA, D'Souza PJ, Dooley JA. Emotional approach coping and self-efficacy moderate the effects of written emotional disclosure and relaxation training for people with migraine headaches. Br J Health Psychol 2008;13:67–71.

[54] Leeuw M, Goossens ME, Linton SJ, Crombez G, Boersma K, Vlaeyen JW. The fear-avoidance model of musculoskeletal pain: current state of scientific evidence. J Behav Med 2007;30:77–94.

[55] Leeuw M, Goossens ME, van Breukelen GJ, Boersma K, Vlaeyen JW. Measuring perceived harmfulness of physical activities in patients with chronic low back pain: the photograph series of daily activities—short electronic version. J Pain 2007;8:840–9.

[56] Leeuw M, Goossens ME, van Breukelen GJ, de Jong JR, Heuts PH, Smeets RJ, Koke AJ, Vlaeyen JW. Exposure in vivo versus operant graded activity in chronic low back pain patients: results of a randomized controlled trial. Pain 2008;138:192–207.

[57] Linton SJ, McCracken LM, Vlaeyen JW. Reassurance: help or hinder in the treatment of pain. Pain 2008;134:5–8.

[58] Mannion AF, Junge A, Taimela S, Muntener M, Lorenzo K, Dvorak J. Active therapy for chronic low back pain: Part 3. Factors influencing self-rated disability and its change following therapy. Spine 2001;26:920–9.

[59] Mannion AF, Muntener M, Taimela S, Dvorak J. A randomized clinical trial of three active therapies for chronic low back pain. Spine 1999;24:2435–48.

[60] Marty M, Rozenberg S, Legout V, Durand-Zaleski I, Moyse D, Henrotin Y, Perrot S. Influence of time, activities, and memory on the assessment of chronic low back pain intensity. Spine 2009;34:1604–9.

[61] McCracken LC, Carson JW, Eccleston C, Keefe FJ. Acceptance and change in the context of chronic pain. Pain 2004;109:4–7.

[62] McCracken LM, Gross RT, Sorg PJ, Edmands TA. Prediction of pain in patients with chronic low back pain: effects of inaccurate prediction and pain-related anxiety. Behav Res Ther 1993;31:647–52.

[63] McCracken LM, MacKichan F, Eccleston C. Contextual cognitive-behavioral therapy for severely disabled chronic pain sufferers: effectiveness and clinically significant change. Eur J Pain 2007;11:314–22.

[64] McCracken LM, Vowles KE, Eccleston C. Acceptance-based treatment for persons with complex, longstanding, chronic pain: a preliminary analysis of treatment outcome in comparison to a waiting phase. Behav Res Ther 2005;43:1335–46.

[65] McCracken LM, Zayfert C, Gross RT. The Pain Anxiety Symptoms Scale: development and validation of a scale to measure fear of pain. Pain 1992;50:67–73.

[66] McDonald IG, Daly J, Jelinek VM, Panetta F, Gutman JM. Opening Pandora's box: The unpredictability of reassurance by a normal test result. BMJ 1996;313:329–32.

[67] Melzack R. The Short-form McGill Pain Questionnaire. Pain 1987;30:191–7.

[68] Merskey H. Somatization: or another god that failed. Pain 2009;145:4–5.

[69] Meulders A, Vansteenwegen D, Vlaeyen JW. Unpredictable versus predictable pain: an experimental investigation on pain-related fear and pain intensity. Abstract presented at: 13th World Congress on Pain, Montreal, September 31–August 6, 2010.

[70] Miller RP, Kori SH, Todd DD. The Tampa Scale for Kinesophobia. Tampa, FL; 1991.

[71] Moore JE, Von Korff M, Cherkin D, Saunders K, Lorig K. A randomized trial of a cognitive-behavioral program for enhancing back pain self care in a primary care setting. Pain 2000;88:145–53.

[72] Morley S, Davies C, Barton S. Possible selves in chronic pain: self-pain enmeshment, adjustment and acceptance. Pain 2005;115:84–94.

[73] Morley S, Eccleston C, Williams A. Systematic review and meta-analysis of randomized controlled trials of cognitive behaviour therapy and behaviour therapy for chronic pain in adults, excluding headache. Pain 1999;80:1–13.

[74] Norman SA, Lumley MA, Dooley JA, Diamond MP. For whom does it work? Moderators of the effects of written emotional disclosure in a randomized trial among women with chronic pelvic pain. Psychosom Med 2004;66:174–83.

[75] Olsson A, Phelps EA. Social learning of fear. Nat Neurosci 2007;10:1095–1102.

[76] Onghena P, Edgington ES. Customization of pain treatments: single-case design and analysis. Clin J Pain 2005;21:56–68; discussion 69–72.

[77] Penzien DB, Rains JC, Andrasik F. Behavioral management of recurrent headache: three decades of experience and empiricism. Appl Psychophysiol Biofeedback 2002;27:163–81.

[78] Peters ML, Vlaeyen JW, van Drunen C. Do fibromyalgia patients display hypervigilance for innocuous somatosensory stimuli? Application of a body scanning reaction time paradigm. Pain 2000;86:283–92.

[79] Porter LS, Keefe FJ, Baucom DH, Hurwitz H, Moser B, Patterson E, Kim HJ. Partner-assisted emotional disclosure for patients with GI cancer: results from a randomized controlled trial. Cancer 2009;115:4326–38.

[80] Rainville P, Duncan GH, Price DD, Carrier B, Bushnell MC. Pain affect encoded in human anterior cingulated but not somatosensory cortex. Science 1997;227:968–71.

[81] Roelofs J, Goubert L, Peters ML, Vlaeyen JW, Crombez G. The Tampa Scale for Kinesiophobia: further examination of psychometric properties in patients with chronic low back pain and fibromyalgia. Eur J Pain 2004;8:495–502.

[82] Rosenstiel AK, Keefe FJ. The use of coping strategies in chronic low back pain patients: relationship to patient characteristics and current adjustment. Pain 1983;17:33–44.

[83] Saxena A, Mendoza T, Cleeland CS. The assessment of cancer pain in north India: the validation of the Hindi Brief Pain Inventory—BPI-H. J Pain Symptom Manage 1999;17:27–41.

[84] Schrooten MG, Vlaeyen JWS. Becoming active again? Further thoughts on goal pursuit in chronic pain. Pain 2010; Epub March 11.

[85] Schwarz N. Self-reports: how the questions shape the answer. Am Psychol 1999;54:93–105.

[86] Smith JA, Osborn M. Pain as an assault on the self: an interpretative phenomenological analysis of the psychological impact of chronic benign low back pain. Psychol Health 2007;22:517–34.

[87] Smyth JM, Stone AA, Hurewitz A, Kaell A. Effects of writing about stressful experiences on symptom reduction in patients with asthma or rheumatoid arthritis. JAMA 1999;281:1304–9.

[88] Somers TJ, Keefe FJ, Porter LS. Understanding and enhancing patient and partner adjustment to disease-related pain: a biopsychosocial perspective. In: Moore RJ, editor. Biobehavioral approaches to pain. New York: Springer; 2009.

[89] Stone AA, Broderick JE, Schwartz JE, Shiffman S, Litcher-Kelly L, Calvanese P. Intensive momentary reporting of pain with an electronic diary: reactivity, compliance, and patient satisfaction. Pain 2003;104:343–51.

[90] Sullivan MJ, Bishop SR, Pivik J. The pain catastrophizing scale: development and validation. Psychol Assess 1995;7:524–32.

[91] Sullivan MJ, Thorn B, Haythornthwaite JA, Keefe F, Martin M, Bradley LA, Lefebvre JC. Theoretical perspectives on the relation between catastrophizing and pain. Clin J Pain 2001;17:52–64.

[92] Tang NK, Salkovskis PM, Poplavskaya E, Wright KJ, Hanna M, Hester J. Increased use of safety-seeking behaviors in chronic back pain patients with high health anxiety. Behav Res Ther 2007;45:2821–35.

[93] Tracey I. Imaging pain. Br J Anaesth 2008;101:32–39.

[94] Turk DC, Dworkin RH, Allen RR, Bellamy N, Brandenburg N, Carr DB, Cleeland C, Dionne R, Farrar JT, Galer BS, et al. Core outcome domains for chronic pain clinical trials: IMMPACT recommendations. Pain 2003;106:337–45.

[95] Turk DC, Dworkin RH, Burke LB, Gershon R, Rothman M, Scott J, Allen RR, Atkinson JH, Chandler J, Cleeland C, et al. Developing patient-reported outcome measures for pain clinical trials: IMMPACT recommendations. Pain 2006;125:208–15.

[96] Turk DC, Meichenbaum D, Genest M. Pain and behavioral medicine: a cognitive-behavioral perspective. New York: Guilford Press; 1983.

[97] Turk DC, Okifuji A. Psychological factors in chronic pain: evolution and revolution. J Consult Clin Psychol 2002;70:678–90.

[98] Turk DC, Robinson JP, Sherman JJ, Burwinkle T, Swanson K. Assessing fear in patients with cervical pain: development and validation of the Pictorial Fear of Activity Scale-Cervical (PFACTS-C). Pain 2008;139:55–62.

[99] Van Damme S, Crombez G, Eccleston C. Coping with pain: a motivational perspective. Pain 2008;139:1–4.

[100] Van Den Hout JH, Vlaeyen JW, Heuts PH, Zijlema JH, Wijnen JA. Secondary prevention of work-related disability in nonspecific low back pain: does problem-solving therapy help? A randomized clinical trial. Clin J Pain 2003;19:87–96.

[101] van den Hout JH, Vlaeyen JW, Houben RM, Soeters AP, Peters ML. The effects of failure feedback and pain-related fear on pain report, pain tolerance, and pain avoidance in chronic low back pain patients. Pain 2001;92:247–57.

[102] Vlaeyen JW, Kole-Snijders AM, Boeren RG, van Eek H. Fear of movement/(re)injury in chronic low back pain and its relation to behavioral performance. Pain 1995;62:363–72.

[103] Vlaeyen JW, Morley S. Active despite pain: the putative role of stop-rules and current mood. Pain 2004;110:512–6.

[104] Vlaeyen JWS, Crombez G, Linton SJ. The fear-avoidance model of pain: we are not there yet. Comment on Wideman et al. "A prospective sequential analysis of the fear-avoidance model of pain" [Pain, 2009] and Nicholas "First things first: Reduction in catastrophizing before fear of movement" [Pain, 2009]. Pain 2009;146:222.

[105] Vlaeyen JWS, de Jong JR, Leeuw M, Crombez G. Fear reduction in chronic pain: graded exposure in vivo with behavioural experiments. In: Asmundson GJG, Vlaeyen JWS, Crombez G, editors. Understanding and treating fear of pain. Oxford: Oxford University Press; 2004.

[106] Vlaeyen JWS, Linton SJ. Fear-avoidance and its consequences in chronic musculoskeletal pain: a state of the art. Pain 2000;85:317–32.

[107] Vowles KE, McCracken LM. Acceptance and values-based action in chronic pain: a study of treatment effectiveness and process. J Consult Clin Psychol 2008;76:397–407.

[108] Vowles KE, McCracken LM, Eccleston C. Patient functioning and catastrophizing in chronic pain: the mediating effects of acceptance. Health Psychol 2008;27(2 Suppl):S136–43.

[109] Vowles KE, Wetherell JL, Sorrell JT. Targeting acceptance, mindfulness, and values-based action in chronic pain: findings of two preliminary trials of outpatient group-based intervention. Cogn Behav Pract 2009;16:49–58.

[110] Waddell G, Newton M, Henderson I, Somerville D, Main CJ. A fear-avoidance beliefs questionnaire (FABQ) and the role of fear-avoidance beliefs in chronic low back pain and disability. Pain 1993;52:157–68.

[111] Wicksell RK, Melon L, Olsson GL. Exposure and acceptance in the rehabilitation of adolescents with idiopathic chronic pain: a pilot study.
Eur J Pain 2007;11:267–74.

[112] Wittink H, Turk DC, Carr DB, Sukiennik A, Rogers W. Comparison of
the redundancy, reliability, and responsiveness to change among SF-36,
Oswestry Disability Index, and Multidimensional Pain Inventory. Clin J
Pain 2004;20(3):133–42.

[113] Woods MP, Asmundson GJ. Evaluating the efficacy of graded in vivo
exposure for the treatment of fear in patients with chronic back pain: a
randomized controlled clinical trial. Pain 2008;136:271–80.

Correspondence to: Johan W.S. Vlaeyen, PhD, Pain and Disability Research Program, Research Group Health Psychology, Department of Psychology, University of Leuven, 3000
Leuven, Belgium. Email: johannes.vlaeyen@psy.kuleuven.be.

Part 9

Persistent Postoperative Pain: Pathogenic Mechanisms and Preventive Strategies

Persistent Postoperative Pain: Pathogenic Mechanisms and Preventive Strategies

Henrik Kehlet, MD, PhD,[a] William A. Macrae, FRCA,[b] and Audun Stubhaug, MD, PhD[c]

[a]Section of Surgical Pathophysiology, Rigshospitalet, Copenhagen University, Denmark; [b]The Pain Service, Department of Clinical Neurosciences, Ninewells Hospital and Medical School, Dundee, Scotland, United Kingdom; [c]Pain Center, Oslo University Hospital, Oslo, Norway

During the last decade, increased attention has been paid to persistent pain complaints after almost any surgical operation, with reported incidences ranging between 5% and 50%. These chronic pain problems represent a major humanitarian and socioeconomic burden. The pathogenic mechanisms are multiple, and they can be grouped into preoperative, intraoperative, and postoperative factors (see Table I). This chapter will discuss recent developments with regard to the epidemiology of persistent postoperative pain and the different preoperative, intraoperative, and postoperative risk factors. Based on selected procedure-specific data, we will discuss the current status of knowledge and future strategies for prevention and treatment.

Epidemiology of Persistent Postoperative Pain

Epidemiology is the study of the distribution and determinants of diseases and the application of the findings to the control of health problems. It can also help us to understand the natural history of a disease and learn about causes and risk factors, which allows us to develop and test strategies for prevention.

In order to study a given disease, we need a definition of the disease and a valid set of diagnostic criteria. This prerequisite has been a major problem in chronic pain as a whole, and in chronic pain after

surgery in particular. Many studies have reported on the prevalence of chronic pain after surgery. (Prevalence is the number of cases of a given disease in a given population at a designated time. Incidence is the number of new cases arising during a given period in a specified population.) The results of these studies vary widely, because different populations were studied and different diagnostic criteria used. Most studies do not attempt a definition. In 1999, Macrae and Davies [51] proposed the following definition: (1) The pain developed after a surgical procedure. (2) The pain is of at least 2 months' duration. (3) Other causes for the pain should have been excluded (e.g., continuing malignancy or chronic infection). (4) The possibility that the pain is continuing from a preexisting problem must be explored and exclusion attempted. (There is an obvious gray area here in that surgery may simply exacerbate a preexisting condition, but attributing escalating pain to the surgery is clearly not possible because natural deterioration cannot be ruled out.)

There are many problems with this simplistic definition. The first problem is the diversity of the syndromes. Following breast surgery, for example, patients complain of a range of unpleasant symptoms after operations, including tingling, numbness, sensitivity, and swelling as well as pain [68,88]. The type of pain also varies: phantom pain [21,46], neuropathic pain caused by damage to the intercostobrachial nerve [92], or scar

Table I
Factors considered to be important for the
development of persistent postoperative pain

Preoperative Factors

Demographic factors
Psychosocial
Nociceptive function
Other pain syndromes
Pain in the planned surgical area
Genetic factors

Intraoperative Factors

Type of anesthesia
Perioperative medication
Type of incision
Nerve-sparing techniques
Nerve injury
Nerve identification
Surgical procedure (e.g., mesh implantation,
  minimally invasive surgery)

Postoperative Factors

Acute postoperative pain
Pain treatment (type, dose)
Chemotherapy and radiotherapy
Disease recurrence (e.g., malignancy, hernia)

pain [33]. After thoracotomy, patients may have musculoskeletal pain from rib resection or spreading of the ribs (in order to gain access to the chest). Neuropathic pain may result from damage to the intercostal nerves, and damage to organs may cause visceral pain. Chest drains can be a source of pain. Patients often find it difficult to differentiate between the symptoms: for example, after amputation some patients cannot easily separate phantom pain, stump pain, and other unpleasant sensations [31].

The question of the timeline is also difficult. If a patient has an operation for varicose veins and the saphenous nerve is injured, then he or she will probably have pain immediately after the operation. This pain may persist from the time of the operation and may possibly be permanent, as it is a neuropathic pain. When does it become chronic?

Another problem is that pain may have been the symptom that the patient presented with prior to surgery. In patients with right upper quadrant pain, the preexisting pain will confuse the issue because many patients continue to complain of pain after cholecystectomy [6]. This does not necessarily mean the surgery was responsible. Some patients present at the pain clinic with chronic pain that they attribute to an operation, but further questioning may reveal that the pain predates the surgery. Many patients have inappropriate

operations—for example, those with irritable bowel syndrome or many of those with back pain. Many of these patients continue to have the same pain after the operation, and in many cases their pain will be more severe.

Research on chronic pain after surgery is usually carried out on large populations, using questionnaires. This method relies on the patients' own reports of their symptoms and sensations, meaning that in some cases the quality and reliability of the data may be questionable. Studies in this area are difficult due to the expense of conducting individual interviews and examinations, and they always involve a compromise between adequate sample size and valid and objective data.

Preoperative Risk Factors

Psychosocial Factors

It has long been acknowledged that psychosocial factors are important for the transition from acute to chronic pain. A number of instruments have been used in the search for predictive factors. In a recent systematic review, Hinrichs-Rocker et al. [32] carefully reviewed the evidence for psychosocial predictors and correlates for chronic postsurgical pain. The authors scored a total of 50 studies that they considered relevant. They quantified the grade of association and found evidence for an association with chronic postsurgical pain (CPSP) for depression, psychological vulnerability, stress and late return to work. No conclusion of association was possible for anxiety, self-control, vitality, marital status, or social support, partly because of conflicting results and partly because of lack of replication. Neuroticism, female gender, employment, and education were surprisingly considered unlikely to be associated with CPSP. Major problems with any review of these matters based on the existing literature are small studies, the study of too many factors, the use of different instruments, and a general diversity of study designs and interventions.

Given the bidirectional nature of relationship between pain and mood disorders, it is quite obvious that data collection must start before surgery and that the interaction with preoperative pain should be elucidated. Standardized instruments should be used, such as Beck's Depression Inventory [7], the State-Trait Anxiety Index [84], the Hospital Anxiety and Depression Scale [99], and the Pain Catastrophizing Scale [87]. Hopefully, it will be possible to identify a few simple instruments that will help identify patients at risk before the intervention.

Genetic Factors

The huge interindividual variation in pain sensitivity has been well acknowledged by clinicians. In pain research, the variability has been generally looked upon as "noise," rather than as a topic for study. The recent findings from twin studies, showing that a major part of the variability can be explained by genetic factors [59,62], have led to increased hope that genes increasing risk for both acute and chronic pain can be identified.

So far, only candidate genes have been studied. Several genes have tentatively been found to affect pain sensitivity and chronic pain in humans. Genes affecting transduction of noxious stimuli, nociceptor conduction, synaptic transmission, and modulation of pain in humans have been reported, although the findings have seldom been replicated (for review, see Foulkes and Wood [26] and LaCroix-Fralish and Mogil [47]). No genes have been identified that specifically predispose individuals to the transition from acute to chronic postsurgical pain. However, the *GCH1* gene (encoding guanine triphosphate [GTP] cyclohydrolase) has been associated with chronic radiculopathy following diskectomy [90]. However, in the human part of the study, statistical power was low, and notably, all patients had preoperative pain due to disk herniation.

It is not unlikely that some of the several genes involved in pain sensitivity and different chronic pain states also affect the risk of persistent postsurgical pain. So far, the gene encoding human catechol-*O*-methyltransferase (*COMT*) has received special interest [19,20,58,100]. The *COMT* gene [69,70], the *OPRM1* gene [74], the *CYP2D6* gene [28], the *MC1R* gene [47], and the gene encoding cyclooxygenase-2 (COX-2) [49] have also been linked to analgesic efficacy which may modulate persistent pain. But again, except for *CYP2D6*, contradictory findings are frequent. The lack of clean phenotypes and adequately sized studies has been a limiting factor for progress.

Now, as technology makes genome-wide association studies (GWAS) possible, more than one million single-nucleotide polymorphisms (SNPs) from each subject can be mapped, and new candidate genes and new mechanisms may be found. But the crucial need for adequately sized studies becomes even more important [57]. For GWAS studies, 1,000–3,000 carefully phenotyped subjects are likely to be needed to gain adequate power [55]. This means that large multicenter trials may be the only way forward.

Nociceptive Function

In addition to investigation of the specific role of genetic and psychosocial factors, efforts have been made to preoperatively quantify the functional status of the nociceptive function by different nociceptive stimuli (heat, electricity, cold, etc.) [29,42,94]. The summary of these studies have clearly indicated that the pain response to such preoperative stimuli may to some extent predict the *acute* pain response to an operation, and in a few studies the risk for *persistent* pain as well. In a recent large prospective trial in inguinal and laparoscopic herniorrhaphy, the preoperative pain-related functional complaints and the pain response to 47°C heat stimulation were the most significant preoperative risk factors for the development of significant chronic pain complaints 6 months postoperatively [98], although *intra*operative factors (choice of surgical technique with different risks of nerve injury) were also important [98]. However, the preoperative nociceptive function tests continued to be an independent risk factor for chronification. Other studies have focused on the predictive role of the diffuse noxious inhibitory controls (DNIC) system [98] for acute and chronic post-thoracotomy pain.

In summary, it is indisputable that future studies should include a detailed *pre*operative assessment of the pain response to a nociceptive stimulus to define the relative role of pre-, intra-, and postoperative pathogenic factors for chronification [43].

Intraoperative Risk Factors

In most patients, persistent postoperative pain demonstrates features of neuropathic pain [42], and the highest incidences of these complaints have been reported from procedures where major nerves cross the surgical field (amputation, thoracotomy, breast surgery, and groin hernia repair). However, differentiation of neuropathic from non-neuropathic causes has been difficult, because signs of neurological damage have been reported following many procedures, in patients both with and without persistent pain [1,2,4,42]. Thus, intraoperative nerve injury may be a significant risk factor, but additional factors may determine whether a patient with nerve injury will eventually present with neuropathic pain or not. The interpretation of the few detailed studies with postoperative quantitative sensory testing has demonstrated a heterogenic pattern of nerve dysfunctions in the skin [1,2,42]. However, unfortunately, no study has looked at neurophysiological function in deeper anatomical layers, which obviously also may be a cause of persistent pain.

Based on the many clinical data demonstrating that nerve injury is probably the most important factor for chronification, nerve-sparing techniques via specific nerve identification, dissection, avoidance of involvement in sutures, mesh inflammation, and so on, and specific minimally invasive nerve-sparing techniques should be further developed and defined in well-designed prospective studies. So far, the only large, detailed prospective study has demonstrated that a laparoscopic groin hernia repair leads to less nerve injury and less chronic pain [3], although *pre*operative function of the nociceptive system remains an independent risk factor, even in laparoscopic procedures with a smaller risk of nerve damage [3].

Postoperative Risk Factors

Analgesia

Several prospective studies have shown that postoperative pain intensity is a risk factor for persistent pain [14,30,39,77]. Thus, we may hope to reduce the prevalence and severity of persistent postsurgical pain by optimal management of acute postoperative pain. However, no large, well-designed, randomized study has shown such a direct effect of generally improved analgesia. One reason may be that plasticity in the nervous system is central to the pathogenesis of persistent postsurgical pain [14], but most analgesic drugs may have only a minor effect on nervous system plasticity, and they may not help reversing sensitization that is already established. This consideration is particularly relevant in patients with *pre*operative pain. On the other hand, some drugs that are only weak analgesics may be effective in controlling central sensitization and the transition from acute to chronic pain. Alpha-2-agonists, *N*-methyl-D-aspartate (NMDA)-receptor antagonists, sodium channel blockers (local anesthetics and others), glucocorticoids, and drugs that modify functions of calcium channels and release of excitatory transmitters are candidates for further clinical research in this area [86].

Preemptive analgesia is still a controversial topic in humans. The idea is to prevent central sensitization. However, in major surgery in humans it is obvious that sensitization can occur both during surgery and postoperatively, as long as there is a sensitizing stimulus. This explains why a single intervention during surgery has only a minor effect on postoperative pain and hyperalgesia. Obviously, in clinical practice, the sensitizing stimulus continues after surgery and must be treated both intra- and postoperatively.

The original concept of preemptive analgesia, in which pretreatment was expected to have a lasting effect after surgery, has been proven by numerous studies to be futile [40]. This realization has led to the introduction of *preventive analgesia* as a more pragmatic concept compared with preemptive analgesia: we have to start inhibiting noxious input and central sensitization as soon as surgery starts, and continue during surgery and for as long after surgery as the pain impulses are strong [12,66].

To test whether a perioperative treatment is effective, we need adequately sized trials where patients are randomized to different treatment regimes and followed prospectively for a minimum of 6 months. The intensity and time course of postoperative pain must be assessed together with the later occurrence of chronic pain symptoms.

Although no perfect study in humans has been published yet, some evidence is accumulating. Regional techniques may make a difference [35], and there is some support for the use of drugs such as ketamine [48], glucocorticoids [73], and gabapentinoids [13,24,25,80,81].

Secondary Prevention?

Patients who have severe pain and abnormal sensory changes 4–6 weeks after surgery are high-risk patients for persistent pain [14,77]. Thus, it may be an interesting approach to use more aggressive treatment for patients with severe acute postoperative pain and signs of neuropathic components 1–3 weeks after surgery, at a time when pain subsides in most patients. Because the same pain mechanism can give rise to different symptoms, and one symptom may arise from different mechanisms, it seems prudent to study the use of a sodium channel blocker (lidocaine, topically and intravenously), a calcium-channel-modifying drug (gabapentin or pregabalin), glucocorticoids, and amitriptyline, clonidine, and ketamine.

The most important aim is to reduce severe and disabling CPSP, not only reduce minor discomfort. Because disabling CPSP occurs in only a small percentage of patients, large groups are needed to prove the efficacy of an intervention. We must stop conducting inconclusive small studies, but rather form research networks doing large multicenter trials in carefully chosen populations. Good suggestions for design of such studies exist [43] and should be followed.

Adjuvant Therapy

Many patients who have surgery will also receive other treatments. For patients who have cancer, radiotherapy and chemotherapy will form part of their treatment plan. Both of these treatments undoubtedly have a role in the management of breast cancer, but both have the potential to produce side effects and complications [15,23,27].

Radiotherapy can cause damage to tissues directly, as well as through free radical formation. Problems can arise early, particularly in skin, mucosa, and bone marrow, but later changes can affect connective tissue and cause vascular damage. In breast cancer survivors, the brachial plexus can be affected by both direct damage, causing demyelination and fibrosis around the plexus, as well as edema. The effects can be similar to those caused by local recurrence in the axilla.

Some cytotoxic drugs used in chemotherapy, such as the vinca alkaloids, are known to cause neuropathies, which may be painful. It is clear that in patients receiving several modalities of treatment, there may be several potential causes of nerve injury and pain, which complicates research in this area.

The evidence on the influence of concomitant treatments such as radiotherapy and chemotherapy is contradictory [27]. Some studies have shown that adjuvant treatments increase the risk of chronic pain [82,88,89], but others have shown no difference [46,75]. A study by Poleshuck et al. [67] included detailed pre- and postoperative assessment of multiple factors. The type of surgery and the use of radiation therapy independently increased the risk of chronic pain after breast cancer surgery: this finding persisted after adjustment for age, preoperative and acute pain, and other factors. Smith et al. [83] point out the difficulties in unraveling the relationship between the different treatments and pain because of confounding factors such as age. In a study from the Mayo Clinic looking at children having limb amputations for either trauma or cancer, Smith and Thompson [82] showed that chemotherapy increased the risk of phantom pain considerably.

Procedure-Specific Data

Inguinal Hernia

There is now general agreement among hernia surgeons that chronic pain after the common minor operation for a groin hernia is probably the most important outcome; such pain occurs in about 5–8% of patients with an influence on daily life functions [41]. The functional consequences and neurophysiological aspects are reasonably well characterized [1,41] and it is unquestionable that nerve injury in the region carries a considerable risk, as demonstrated in several studies with detailed quantitative sensory testing [1–4]. However, many pain-free patients also have demonstrable signs of nerve injury [4]. Several efforts have been made to reduce the risk of nerve injury and persistent pain, including the laparoscopic approach, intraoperative nerve identification and sparing or transection, and the use of less traumatic mesh fixation methods [41]. The conclusion from these studies is that the laparoscopic approach probably reduces the risk of nerve injury and persistent pain by about 50% [3,41]. However, the significant influence of the mesh fixation techniques (where tacks and staples should be avoided or placed outside the nerves at risk) needs to be further explored [2,41]. In this context, glue mesh fixation techniques may be promising, although again, more detailed studies are required to quantify the potential risk reduction. Finally, the mesh material used may have some influence, because heavy-weight meshes may cause a more pronounced inflammatory response, which may affect nearby nerves, with a subsequent risk of neuropathic pain [41].

During an open groin hernia repair, identification of the nerves at risk is an important measure that will probably lead to a reduction of persistent pain, based on preliminary studies, whereas preemptive transection of one of the nerves has not been demonstrated to reduce pain (or increase the risk) [54,63,95]. Further reduction of the risk of persistent pain may also depend on surgical expertise, although the available studies have not specifically demonstrated the importance of this factor.

In summary, inguinal herniorrhaphy is the operation in which we have most information about the relative role of pre-, intra-, and postoperative factors. This operation has little influence on psychological factors and no problems with malignancy or adjuvant therapy. The results so far have demonstrated the importance of both preoperative factors (nociceptive function) and intraoperative nerve injury.

Breast Surgery

Although cancer is the commonest reason for breast surgery, recent research has revealed considerable morbidity in patients having cosmetic breast surgery [77,91,93]. Most patients with cancer will have surgery, which in the past was usually mastectomy, with or without axillary clearance. Breast conservation surgery with sentinel node sampling or axillary clearance is now becoming increasingly common. Many patients will also receive radiotherapy and/or chemotherapy. The quality of publications on outcomes after breast surgery has improved in recent years: only 30 years ago pain after breast cancer treatment was thought to be rare [97].

The frequency of pain after breast surgery varies according to the type of pain, the surgery [93], other treatments given [89], and the methodology used in the study [21]. Patients may have many types of pain following breast surgery, including phantom pain [21,46], scar pain [46], and neuropathic pain [83]. A review paper by Jung et al. [33] examined neuropathic pain following breast cancer surgery and suggested that about half of all patients who have breast surgery for cancer will have chronic pain 1 year after surgery. This comprehensive paper is recommended because it discusses the complexity of the problem, risk factors, and mechanisms and proposes a classification scheme to assist future research. It is important to acknowledge that pain is not the only symptom that may be bothersome for patients after breast surgery; swelling, numbness, and other symptoms are commonly reported [68,88,89]. The need for clean distinctions between syndromes for research purposes is not reflected in the clinical reality. Many patients present to pain clinics with complex problems and many different symptoms. Developing valid and reliable data collection tools to improve the accuracy of detection and classification of syndromes remains a challenge.

As mentioned earlier, chronic pain has also been reported in significant numbers of patients who do not have cancer, for example those receiving breast reduction and augmentation [77,91,93]. These operations are often performed for cosmetic rather than medical reasons, and in our experience, patients are seldom informed about the risk of chronic pain prior to the surgery. Most of these patients probably will not face any medical consequences if they do not have the operation, and full disclosure of the risks might prevent many patients from unnecessary suffering by discouraging them from having surgery.

Amputation

Persistent pain is particularly common after amputation, with a reported incidence of 30–80% [42]. Whereas the majority of patients have phantom sensations, a smaller proportion have phantom pain that very often comes and goes. Stump pain is present in 30–50% of patients.

Most types of postsurgical pain seem to diminish with time [50], but a recent study found that both phantom pain and stump pain were present in 43% of upper limb amputees an average of 50 years after surgery [18].

Preemptive treatment was reported to prevent postamputation pain [5], and was in use for many years, but a randomized study could not reproduce the findings [60]. Still, recent studies confirm that both pre-amputation pain and early postoperative pain are risk factors [30].

Recent years have seen some interest in how surgical technique might influence persistent pain. After all, most surgical techniques are similar to the way nerves are treated in animal models of neuropathic pain [72].

A recent study found fewer pain reports in subjects with knee disarticulation compared with patients having femur or tibia amputation. This finding could be due to the simpler surgery, but also to less use of prostheses that could induce stump irritation and pain [8].

Thoracotomy

Considering what is involved in a thoracotomy, it is no surprise that many patients experience chronic pain afterwards. To gain access to the chest, the surgeon has to either spread the ribs or resect a part of a rib, which inevitably causes mechanical trauma. The intercostal nerves lie behind the lower border of the ribs and are easily injured. It is not surprising, therefore, to find that patients experience a wide range of symptoms after thoracotomy.

Early studies of pain after thoracotomy reported incidences of 5% [16], 11% [44], 44% [37], and 54% [17]. The wide variation in the reported incidence reflects differences in the design of the studies and methods of data collection as well as differences in surgical procedure. More recent studies would support an incidence of around 50% [53,65]. The incidence after open thoracotomy may be the same as after video-assisted thoracoscopy [85,96]. Acute postoperative pain correlates with long-term pain [37,39,98]. The severity of pain before the operation also correlates with the incidence of chronic pain [44]. Damage to the intercostal nerves has been assumed to be a major cause of chronic pain after thoracotomy, and Richardson et al. [75] found a point prevalence of post-thoracotomy neuralgia of 22% at 2 months and 14% at 12 months. An interesting series of papers from Nottingham confirmed that neuropathic pain was common and caused significant morbidity [53] and found that all patients who have rib retraction during thoracotomy sustain intercostal nerve damage [76]. However, the investigators did not find an association between nerve injury measured at the time of thoracotomy and chronic pain or altered sensation 3 months after surgery [52]. This finding suggests a more complicated etiology for neuropathic post-thoracotomy pain than injury to the intercostal nerve alone.

How much of the pain is neuropathic is controversial: many authors have assumed that most patients' pain is neuropathic, and there is evidence to support this assumption [45], but a questionnaire study of 243 patients in the Netherlands found that up to half the chronic pain after thoracotomy may not be neuropathic [85]. A more recent study found that 22% had positive results on a neuropathic pain score (using the Leeds Assessment of Neuropathic Symptoms and Signs [S-LANSS]) at 3 months, and this finding could be predicted to some extent by using the S-LANSS in the immediate postoperative period [79]. Another study investigating the prediction of chronic post-thoracotomy pain assessed the efficiency of patients' DNIC and found that this system influenced chronic but not acute pain after thoracotomy, an efficient DNIC predicting lower risk of chronic pain [98]. Emotional factors may also play a role [38].

Whether the reason for surgery is a risk factor is controversial. Richardson et al. [75] showed a higher incidence of chronic pain after operations for benign esophageal disease than after surgery for lung cancer, but other studies have shown no difference [37,64].

Chronic pain after sternotomy has been the subject of several studies, which showed similar results, with 28% of patients having pain that had a significant impact on their lives [36,56].

In summary, chronic post-thoracotomy pain remains a serious challenge, and controversy remains as to the etiology, mechanisms, and management of the pain [96]. More specific studies on perioperative risk factors are needed, including studies that make use of quantitative sensory testing.

Hysterectomy and Cesarean Section

Persistent pain is reported in 5–32% of women after hysterectomy [11]. In a large register-based study, risk factors for chronic pain were preoperative pelvic pain, previous cesarean delivery, pain as the main indication for surgery, and pain problems elsewhere [10].

A small prospective study in 90 patients confirmed the importance of preoperative pain: 15 women had pain 4 months after surgery, and in 11 of these women, the pain resembled the preoperative pain [9]. In a retrospective study of women after cesarean section, 12% reported pain after 3 months, and 6% of these women had pain daily or almost daily [61]. In this study, spinal anesthesia seemed to protect against persistent pain. If replicated in randomized trials, this finding would be a strong indication for spinal anesthesia, and not only in gynecology. A recent Finnish survey of women undergoing either vaginal delivery or cesarean section found that 18% had pain 1 year later following cesarean section compared with 10% after vaginal delivery. Risk factors were similar to those reported for hysterectomy: previous pain, previous back pain, and any chronic disease were significant risk factors [34]. In summary, chronic pain after hysterectomy and cesarean section is most likely multifactorial, calling for further studies investigating all perioperative risk factors.

Future Strategies

To move forward, future studies on persistent postoperative pain must be prospective, and their design must be improved compared to almost all previous studies. All known or potential pre-, intra-, and postoperative factors must be assessed (see Table II) [22,43,78]. Such studies would have potential major implications for the understanding of other chronic pain states. Obviously, clinical studies must be adjusted according to increased understanding of persistent pain, predominantly neuropathic pain, on the basis of experimental studies [78]. The optimized design would include relevant functional outcomes and the effect of improved perioperative analgesia [22,43].

Table II
The "ideal" study design for persistent postsurgical pain

Preoperatively

Pain (locally and remote) and functional consequences, nociceptive function, neurophysiological and psychosocial assessment, "pain genes," demographic factors

Intraoperatively

Incision, handling of nerves and muscles, disease data, anesthetic technique, perioperative medication

Early Postoperatively

Pain intensity and character, treatment modality, neurophysiological assessment

Late Postoperatively

Pain intensity and character and psychosocial consequences, neurophysiological assessment

Results from such improved studies would form a natural basis for procedure- and disease-specific preventive techniques or therapy in established persistent pain. Finally, there is a need for prospective cohort studies to define the natural history of persistent postoperative pain on a procedure-specific basis. Thanks to increased attention on this problem, including interest from government authorities [71], the improved understanding of the mechanisms for persistent postoperative pain may reduce the clinical significance of this common burden.

References

[1] Aasvang EK, Brandsborg B, Christensen B, Jensen TS, Kehlet H. Neurophysiological characterization of postherniorrhaphy pain. Pain 2008;137:173–81.

[2] Aasvang EK, Brandsborg B, Jensen TS, Kehlet H. Heterogenous sensory processing in persistent postherniotomy pain. Pain 2010; in press.

[3] Aasvang EK, Gmähle E, Hansen JB, Gmähle B, Bittner R, Kehlet H. Predictive factors for persistent postoperative pain. Anesthesiology 2010;112:957–69.

[4] Aasvang EK, Kehlet H. Persistent sensory dysfunction in pain-free patients after groin hernia repair. Acta Anaesthesiol Scand 2010;54:291–8.

[5] Bach S, Noreng MF, Tjellden NU. Phantom limb pain in amputees during the first 12 months following limb amputation, after preoperative lumbar epidural blockade. Pain 1988;33:297–301.

[6] Bates T, Mercer JC, Harrison M. Symptomatic gall stone disease: before and after cholecystectomy. Gut 1984;24:579–80.

[7] Beck AT, Ward CH, Mendelson M, Mock J, Erbaugh J. An inventory for measuring depression. Arch Gen Psychiatry 1961;4:561–71.

[8] Behr J, Friedly J, Molton I, Morgenroth D, Jensen MP, Smith DG. Pain and pain-related interference in adults with lower-limb amputation: comparison of knee-disarticulation, transtibial, and transfemoral surgical sites. J Rehabil Res Dev 2009;46:963–72.

[9] Brandsborg B, Dueholm M, Nikolajsen L, Kehlet H, Jensen TS. A prospective study of risk factors for pain persisting 4 months after hysterectomy. Clin J Pain 2009;25:263–8.

[10] Brandsborg B, Nikolajsen L, Hansen CT, Kehlet H, Jensen TS. Risk factors for chronic pain after hysterectomy: a nationwide questionnaire and database study. Anesthesiology 2007;106:1003–12.

[11] Brandsborg B, Nikolajsen L, Kehlet H, Jensen TS. Chronic pain after hysterectomy. Acta Anaesthesiol Scand 2008;52:327–31.

[12] Brennan TJ, Kehlet H. Preventive analgesia to reduce wound hyperalgesia and persistent postsurgical pain: not an easy path. Anesthesiology 2005;103:681–3.

[13] Buvanendran A, Kroin JS, la Valle CJ, Kari M, Moric M, Tuman KJ. Perioperative oral pregabalin reduces chronic pain after total knee arthroplasty: a prospective, randomized, controlled trial. Anesth Analg 2010;110:199–207.

[14] Callesen T, Bech K, Kehlet H. Prospective study of chronic pain after groin hernia repair. Br J Surg 1999;86:1528–31.

[15] Clarke M, Collins R, Darby S, Davies C, Elphinstone P, Evans E, Godwin J, Gray R, Hicks C, James S, et al. Effects of radiotherapy and of differences in the extent of surgery for early breast cancer on local recurrence and 15-year survival: an overview of the randomised trials. Lancet 2005;366:2087–106.

[16] Conacher ID. Therapists and therapies for post-thoracotomy neuralgia. Pain 1992;48:409–12.

[17] Dajczman E, Gordon A, Kreisman H, Wolkove N. Long-term postthoracotomy pain. Chest 1991;99:270–4.

[18] Desmond DM, Maclachlan M. Prevalence and characteristics of phantom limb pain and residual limb pain in the long term after upper limb amputation. Int J Rehabil Res 2010; Epub Jan 22.

[19] Diatchenko L, Nackley AG, Slade GD, Bhalang K, Belfer I, Max MB, Goldman D, Maixner W. Catechol-O-methyltransferase gene polymorphisms are associated with multiple pain-evoking stimuli. Pain 2006;125:216–24.

[20] Diatchenko L, Slade GD, Nackley AG, Bhalang K, Sigurdsson A, Belfer I, Goldman D, Xu K, Shabalina SA, Shagin D, et al. Genetic basis for individual variations in pain perception and the development of a chronic pain condition. Hum Mol Genet 2005;14:135–43.

[21] Dijkstra PU, Rietman JS, Geertzen JH. Phantom breast sensations and phantom breast pain: a 2-year prospective study and a methodological analysis of literature. Eur J Pain 2007;11:99–108.

[22] Dworkin RH, McDermott MP, Raja SN. Preventing chronic postsurgical pain: how much of a difference makes a difference? Anesthesiology 2010;112:516–8.

[23] Early Breast Cancer Triallists' Collaborative Group. Effects of chemotherapy and hormonal therapy for early breast cancer on recurrence and 15-year survival: an overview of the randomised trials. Lancet 2005;365:1687–717.

[24] Fassoulaki A, Melemeni A, Stamatakis E, Petropoulos G, Sarantopoulos C. A combination of gabapentin and local anaesthetics attenuates acute and late pain after abdominal hysterectomy. Eur J Anaesthesiol 2007;24:521–8.

[25] Fassoulaki A, Stamatakis E, Petropoulos G, Siafaka I, Hassiakos D, Sarantopoulos C. Gabapentin attenuates late but not acute pain after abdominal hysterectomy. Eur J Anaesthesiol 2006;23:136–41.

[26] Foulkes T, Wood JN. Pain genes. PLoS Genet 2008;4:e1000086.

[27] Gartner R, Jensen M-B, Nielsen J, Ewertz M, Kroman N, Kehlet H. Prevalence of and factors associated with persistent pain following breast cancer surgery. JAMA 2009;302:1985–92.

[28] Gasche Y, Daali Y, Fathi M, Chiappe A, Cottini S, Dayer P, Desmeules J. Codeine intoxication associated with ultrarapid CYP2D6 metabolism. N Engl J Med 2004;351:2827–31.

[29] Granot M. Can we predict persistent postoperative pain by testing preoperative experimental pain? Curr Opin Anaesthesiol 2009;22:425–30.

[30] Hanley MA, Jensen MP, Smith DG, Ehde DM, Edwards WT, Robinson LR. Preamputation pain and acute pain predict chronic pain after lower extremity amputation. J Pain 2007;8:102–9.

[31] Hill A. Phantom limb pain: a review of the literature on attributes and potential mechanisms. J Pain Symptom Manage 1999;17:125–42.

[32] Hinrichs-Rocker A, Schulz K, Jarvinen I, Lefering R, Simanski C, Neugebauer EA. Psychosocial predictors and correlates for chronic postsurgical pain (CPSP): a systematic review. Eur J Pain 2009;13:719–30.

[33] Jung BF, Ahrendt GM, Oaklander AL, Dworkin RH. Neuropathic pain following breast cancer surgery: proposed classification and research update. Pain 2003;104:1–13.

[34] Kainu JP, Sarvela J, Tiippana E, Halmesmaki E, Korttila KT. Persistent pain after caesarean section and vaginal birth: a cohort study. Int J Obstet Anesth 2010;19:4–9.

[35] Kairaluoma PM, Bachmann MS, Rosenberg PH, Pere PJ. Preincisional paravertebral block reduces the prevalence of chronic pain after breast surgery. Anesth Analg 2006;103:703–8.

[36] Kalso E, Mennander S, Tasmuth T, Nilsson E. Chronic post-sternotomy pain. Acta Anaesthesiol Scand 2001;45:935–9.

[37] Kalso E, Perttunen K, Kaasinen S. Pain after thoracic surgery. Acta Anaesthesiol Scand 1992;36:96–100.

[38] Katz J, Asmundson GJ, McRae K, Halket E. Emotional numbing and pain intensity predict the development of pain disability up to one year after lateral thoracotomy. Eur J Pain 2009;13:870–8.

[39] Katz J, Jackson M, Kavanagh BP, Sandler AN. Acute pain after thoracic surgery predicts long-term post-thoracotomy pain. Clin J Pain 1996;12:50–5.

[40] Katz J, McCartney CJ. Current status of preemptive analgesia. Curr Opin Anaesthesiol 2002;15:435–41.

[41] Kehlet H. Chronic pain after groin hernia repair. Br J Surg 2008;95:135–6.

[42] Kehlet H, Jensen TS, Woolf CJ. Persistent postsurgical pain: risk factors and prevention. Lancet 2006;367:1618–25.

[43] Kehlet H, Rathmell JP. Persistent postsurgical pain: The path forward through better design of clinical studies. Anesthesiology 2010;112:514–5.

[44] Keller SM, Carp NZ, Levy MN, Rosen SM. Chronic post thoracotomy pain. J Cardiovasc Surg (Torino) 1994;35:161–4.

[45] Kristensen AD, Pedersen TA, Hjortdal VE, Jensen TS, Nikolajsen L. Chronic pain in adults after thoracotomy in childhood or youth. Br J Anaesth 2010;104:75–9.

[46] Kroner K, Knudsen UB, Lundby L, Hvid H. Long-term phantom breast syndrome after mastectomy. Clin J Pain 1992;8:346–50.

[47] Lacroix-Fralish ML, Mogil JS. Progress in genetic studies of pain and analgesia. Annu Rev Pharmacol Toxicol 2009;49:97–121.

[48] Lavand'homme P, De KM, Waterloos H. Intraoperative epidural analgesia combined with ketamine provides effective preventive analgesia in patients undergoing major digestive surgery. Anesthesiology 2005;103:813–20.

[49] Lee YS, Kim H, Wu TX, Wang XM, Dionne RA. Genetically mediated interindividual variation in analgesic responses to cyclooxygenase inhibitory drugs. Clin Pharmacol Ther 2006;79:407–18.

[50] Macdonald L, Bruce J, Scott NW, Smith WC, Chambers WA. Long-term follow-up of breast cancer survivors with post-mastectomy pain syndrome. Br J Cancer 2005;92:225–30.

[51] Macrae WA, Davies HTO. Chronic postsurgical pain. In: Crombie IK, Linton S, Croft P, von Korff M, LeResche L, editors. Epidemiology of pain. Seattle: IASP Press; 1999. p. 125–42.

[52] Maguire MF, Latter JA, Mahajan R, Beggs FD, Duffy JP. A study exploring the role of intercostal nerve damage in chronic pain after thoracic surgery. Eur J Cardiothorac Surg 2006;29:873–9.

[53] Maguire MF, Ravenscroft A, Beggs D, Duffy JP. A questionnaire study investigating the prevalence of the neuropathic component of chronic pain after thoracic surgery. Eur J Cardiothorac Surg 2006;29:800–5.

[54] Malekpour F, Mirhashemi SH, Hajinasrolah E, Salehi N, Khoshkar A, Kolahi AA. Ilioinguinal nerve excision in open mesh repair of inguinal hernia: results of a randomized clinical trial: simple solution for a difficult problem? Am J Surg 2008;195:735–40.

[55] Max MB, Stewart WF. The molecular epidemiology of pain: a new discipline for drug discovery. Nat Rev Drug Discov 2008;7:647–58.

[56] Meyerson J, Thelin S, Gordh T, Karlsten R. The incidence of chronic post-sternotomy pain after cardiac surgery: a prospective study. Acta Anaesthesiol Scand 2001;45:940–4.

[57] Mogil JS. Are we getting anywhere in human pain genetics? Pain 2009;146:231–2.

[58] Nackley AG, Tan KS, Fecho K, Flood P, Diatchenko L, Maixner W. Catechol-O-methyltransferase inhibition increases pain sensitivity through activation of both β2- and β3-adrenergic receptors. Pain 2007;128:199–208.

[59] Nielsen CS, Stubhaug A, Price DD, Vassend O, Czajkowski N, Harris JR. Individual differences in pain sensitivity: genetic and environmental contributions. Pain 2008;136:21–9.

[60] Nikolajsen L, Ilkjaer S, Christensen JH, Kroner K, Jensen TS. Randomised trial of epidural bupivacaine and morphine in prevention of stump and phantom pain in lower-limb amputation. Lancet 1997;350:1353–7.

[61] Nikolajsen L, Sorensen HC, Jensen TS, Kehlet H. Chronic pain following Caesarean section. Acta Anaesthesiol Scand 2004;48:111–6.

[62] Norbury TA, MacGregor AJ, Urwin J, Spector TD, McMahon SB. Heritability of responses to painful stimuli in women: a classical twin study. Brain 2007;130:3041–9.

[63] Pappalardo G, Frattaroli FM, Mongardini M, Salvi PF, Lombardi A, Conte AM, Arezzo MF. Neurectomy to prevent persistent pain after inguinal herniorrhaphy: a prospective study using objective criteria to assess pain. World J Surg 2007;31:1082–6.

[64] Perttunen K, Tasmuth T, Kalso E. Chronic pain after thoracic surgery: a follow-up study. Acta Anaesthesiol Scand 1999;43:563–7.

[65] Pluijms WA, Steegers MA, Verhagen AF, Scheffer GJ, Wilder-Smith OH. Chronic post-thoracotomy pain: a retrospective study. Acta Anaesthesiol Scand 2006;50:804–8.

[66] Pogatzki-Zahn EM, Zahn PK. From preemptive to preventive analgesia. Curr Opin Anaesthesiol 2006;19:551–5.

[67] Poleshuck EL, Katz J, Andrus CH, Hogan LA, Jung BF, Kulick DI, Dworkin RH. Risk factors for chronic pain following breast cancer surgery: a prospective study. J Pain 2006;7:626–34.

[68] Polinsky ML. Functional status of long-term breast cancer survivors: demonstrating chronicity. Health Soc Work 1994;19:165–73.

[69] Rakvag TT, Klepstad P, Baar C, Kvam TM, Dale O, Kaasa S, Krokan HE, Skorpen F. The Val158Met polymorphism of the human catechol-O-methyltransferase (COMT) gene may influence morphine requirements in cancer pain patients. Pain 2005;116:73–8.

[70] Rakvag TT, Ross JR, Sato H, Skorpen F, Kaasa S, Klepstad P. Genetic variation in the catechol-O-methyltransferase (COMT) gene and morphine requirements in cancer patients with pain. Mol Pain 2008;4:64.

[71] Rappaport BA, Cerny I, Sanhai WR. ACTION on the prevention of chronic pain after surgery: public-private partnerships, the future of analgesic drug development. Anesthesiology 2010;112:509–10.

[72] Rasmussen S, Kehlet H. Management of nerves during leg amputation: a neglected area in our understanding of the pathogenesis of phantom limb pain. Acta Anaesthesiol Scand 2007;51:1115–6.

[73] Rasmussen S, Krum-Moller DS, Lauridsen LR, Jensen SE, Mandoe H, Gerlif C, Kehlet H. Epidural steroid following discectomy for herniated lumbar disc reduces neurological impairment and enhances recovery: a randomized study with two-year follow-up. Spine 2008;33:2028–33.

[74] Reyes-Gibby CC, Shete S, Rakvag T, Bhat SV, Skorpen F, Bruera E, Kaasa S, Klepstad P. Exploring joint effects of genes and the clinical efficacy of morphine for cancer pain: OPRM1 and COMT gene. Pain 2007;130:25–30.

[75] Richardson J, Sabanathan S, Mearns AJ, Sides C, Goulden CP. Post-thoracotomy neuralgia. Pain Clinic 1994;7:87–97.

[76] Rogers ML, Henderson L, Mahajan RP, Duffy JP. Preliminary findings in the neurophysiological assessment of intercostal nerve injury during thoracotomy. Eur J Cardiothorac Surg 2002;21:298–301.

[77] Romundstad L, Breivik H, Roald H, Skolleborg K, Romundstad PR, Stubhaug A. Chronic pain and sensory changes after augmentation mammoplasty: long term effects of preincisional administration of methylprednisolone. Pain 2006;124:92–9.

[78] Scholz J, Yaksh TL. Preclinical research on persistent postsurgical pain: what we don't know, but should start studying. Anesthesiology 2010;112:511–3.

[79] Searle RD, Simpson MP, Simpson KH, Milton R, Bennett MI. Can chronic neuropathic pain following thoracic surgery be predicted during the postoperative period? Interact Cardiovasc Thorac Surg 2009;9:999–1002.

[80] Sen H, Sizlan A, Yanarates O, Emirkadi H, Ozkan S, Dagli G, Turan A. A comparison of gabapentin and ketamine in acute and chronic pain after hysterectomy. Anesth Analg 2009;109:1645–50.

[81] Sen H, Sizlan A, Yanarates O, Senol MG, Inangil G, Sucullu I, Ozkan S, Dagli G. The effects of gabapentin on acute and chronic pain after inguinal herniorrhaphy. Eur J Anaesthesiol 2009;26:772–6.

[82] Smith J, Thompson JM. Phantom limb pain and chemotherapy in pediatric amputees. Mayo Clin Proc 1995;70:357–64.

[83] Smith WC, Bourne D, Squair J, Phillips DO, Chambers WA. A retrospective cohort study of postmastectomy pain syndrome. Pain 1999;83:91–5.

[84] Spielberger CD, Gorsuch RL, Lushene RE. Manual for the State-Trait Anxiety Inventory. Palo Alto, CA: Consulting Psychologists Press; 1970.

[85] Steegers MA, Snik DM, Verhagen AF, van der Drift MA, Wilder-Smith OH. Only half of the chronic pain after thoracic surgery shows a neuropathic component. J Pain 2008;9:955–61.

[86] Stubhaug A, Breivik H. Prevention and treatment of hyperalgesia and persistent neuropathic pain after surgery. In: Breivik H, Shipley M, editors. Pain: best practice and research compendium. Amsterdam: Elsevier; 2007. p. 281–6.

[87] Sullivan CD, Bishop SR, Pivik J. The Pain Catastrophizing Scale: development and validation. Psychol Assess 1995;7:524–32.

[88] Tasmuth T, Blomqvist C, Kalso E. Chronic post-treatment symptoms in patients with breast cancer operated in different surgical units. Eur J Surg Oncol 1999;25:38–43.

[89] Tasmuth T, von SK, Hietanen P, Kataja M, Kalso E. Pain and other symptoms after different treatment modalities of breast cancer. Ann Oncol 1995;6:453–9.

[90] Tegeder I, Costigan M, Griffin RS, Abele A, Belfer I, Schmidt H, Ehnert C, Nejim J, Marian C, Scholz J, et al. GTP cyclohydrolase and tetrahydrobiopterin regulate pain sensitivity and persistence. Nat Med 2006;12:1269–77.

[91] van Elk N, Steegers MA, van der Weij LP, Evers AW, Hartman EH, Wilder-Smith OH. Chronic pain in women after breast augmentation: prevalence, predictive factors and quality of life. Eur J Pain 2009;13:660–1.

[92] Vecht CJ, Van de Brand HJ, Wajer OJ. Post-axillary dissection pain in breast cancer due to a lesion of the intercostobrachial nerve. Pain 1989;38:171–6.

[93] Wallace MS, Wallace AM, Lee J, Dobke MK. Pain after breast surgery: a survey of 282 women. Pain 1996;66:195–205.

[94] Werner MU, Mjöbo HN, Nielsen PR, Rodin Å. Prediction of postoperative pain: a systematic review of predictive experimental pain studies. Anesthesiology 2010; in press.

[95] Wijsmuller AR, van Veen RN, Bosch JL, Lange JF, Kleinrensink GJ, Jeekel J, Lange JF. Nerve management during open hernia repair. Br J Surg 2007;94:17–22.

[96] Wildgaard K, Ravn J, Kehlet H. Chronic post-thoracotomy pain: a critical review of pathogenic mechanisms and strategies for prevention. Eur J Cardiothorac Surg 2009;36:170–80.

[97] Wood KM. Intercostobrachial nerve entrapment syndrome. South Med J 1978;71:662–3.

[98] Yarnitsky D, Crispel Y, Eisenberg E, Granovsky Y, Ben-Nun A, Sprecher E, Best LA, Granot M. Prediction of chronic post-operative pain: preoperative DNIC testing identifies patients at risk. Pain 2008;138:22–8.

[99] Zigmond AS, Snaith RP. The Hospital Anxiety and Depression Scale. Acta Psychiatr Scand 1983;67:361–70.

[100] Zubieta JK, Heitzeg MM, Smith YR, Bueller JA, Xu K, Xu Y, Koeppe RA, Stohler CS, Goldman D. COMT val158met genotype affects mu-opioid neurotransmitter responses to a pain stressor. Science 2003;299:1240–3.

Correspondence to: Henrik Kehlet, MD, PhD, Rigshospitalet, Section of Surgical Pathophysiology 4074, Blegdamsvej 9, DK-2100 Copenhagen, Denmark. Email: henrik.kehlet@rh.dk.

Part 10

Clinical Pharmacology: Evidence-Based Guidelines and Defining the Proper Outcome

Clinical Pharmacology of Antidepressants and Anticonvulsants for the Management of Pain

Ian Gilron, MD, MSc, FRCPC

*Clinical Pain Research and Departments of Anesthesiology and Pharmacology & Toxicology,
Queen's University and Kingston General Hospital, Kingston, Ontario, Canada*

Following development and clinical investigation of dibenzazepine derivatives such as imipramine for the treatment of depression in the 1950s [3], several such antidepressant drugs were observed to also relieve neuropathic [109] and rheumatic [55] pain. Subsequent evidence demonstrating analgesia with antidepressant drugs in neuropathic pain patients without clinical depression [106] provided evidence of analgesic mechanisms of these drugs independent of their antidepressant effects. Since these early clinical investigations, analgesic efficacy of antidepressants has been evaluated in dozens of randomized controlled trials. Other than anti-inflammatory drugs and opioids, antidepressants have since become the next most widely used class of drugs for the treatment of pain [65,107].

Pharmacological approaches to the treatment of seizures and epilepsy in the early 1900s [96] have led to the introduction of a diverse group of anticonvulsant drugs into clinical practice. Initial observations of pain reduction with phenytoin in the treatment of trigeminal neuralgia [6] have led to extensive preclinical and clinical investigation into the impact of anticonvulsant drugs on pain [17,110]. As research efforts have continued, important applications of anticonvulsant drugs have been demonstrated in a wide variety of pain conditions.

This chapter will review the clinical pharmacology of antidepressants and anticonvulsants in the setting of pain management with the exclusion of headache disorders, which are discussed elsewhere.

Pharmacological Classification and Analgesic Mechanisms

Antidepressants

Antidepressant drugs include a wide array of chemical agents that can be characterized by chemical structure and/or major pharmacological mechanism. These drugs broadly include the older tricyclic antidepressants (TCAs), selective serotonin reuptake inhibitors (SSRIs), serotonin and norepinephrine reuptake inhibitors (SNRIs), monoamine oxidase inhibitors (MAO-Is), and others (see Table I). Regardless of specific molecular mechanisms discussed below, the clinical rationale for using antidepressants in the management of chronic pain may include treatment of comorbid depression and sleep disturbance as well as reduction of pain intensity [99]. A large body of preclinical research has pointed to several putative analgesic mechanisms of antidepressant drugs (see Table II). These include increased supraspinal availability of norepinephrine (thought to enhance descending inhibitory bulbospinal control), activation of endogenous mu- and delta-opioid receptors, sodium channel blockade, and *N*-methyl-D-aspartate (NMDA) receptor inhibition, among others [73].

Table I
Pharmacological classification of antidepressant drugs

Tricyclic Antidepressants

Tertiary Amine

Amitriptyline
Clomipramine
Doxepin
Imipramine
Trimipramine

Secondary Amine

Nortriptyline
Desipramine
Maprotiline
Protriptyline
Amoxapine

Serotonin-Norepinephrine Reuptake Inhibitors

Venlafaxine
Duloxetine
Milnacipran
Desvenlafaxine
Reboxetine
Sibutramine
Viloxazine
Bicifadine

Selective Serotonin Reuptake Inhibitors

Fluoxetine
Paroxetine
Fluvoxamine
Citalopram
Escitalopram
Sertraline
Lofepramine
Dapoxetine
Zimeldine

Monoamine Oxidase Inhibitors

Phenelzine
Tranylcypromine
Iproniazid
Isocarboxazid
Nialamide
Moclobemide
Selegiline
Pirlindole

Other Antidepressants

Trazodone
Nefazodone
Mirtazapine
Bupropion
Atomoxetine
Mianserin

Note: This list is not exhaustive. The above pharmacological classifications are not clearly delineated and some compounds also may be considered members of another drug subclass.

Anticonvulsants

Drugs that suppress experimental and clinical seizures, defined as anticonvulsant or antiepileptic drugs, are classified as "first-generation" anticonvulsants (e.g., benzodiazepines, carbamazepine, ethosuximide, phenobarbital, phenytoin, primidone, and valproic acid), which were introduced between 1910 and 1970, and "second-generation" anticonvulsants (e.g., felbamate, gabapentin, lamotrigine, levetiracetam, oxcarbazepine, pregabalin, tiagabine, topiramate, vigabatrin, and zonisamide), which were introduced more recently [60]. In addition to reduction in pain intensity, some anticonvulsants have also been shown to improve sleep [82] and reduce anxiety [79], which are of important clinical relevance to the management of chronic pain. Multiple pharmacological mechanisms (see Table III; Fig. 1) have been elucidated for most anticonvulsant drugs including sodium channel blockade, calcium channel blockade, suppression of glutamatergic transmission, and/or γ-aminobutyric acid (GABA)ergic modulation [17].

Trial-Based Evidence of Analgesic Efficacy

Attempts to describe efficacy of a given treatment often involve systematic review of available high-quality clinical trials (randomized controlled trials; RCTs) and meta-analysis in order to estimate the number needed to treat (NNT) to obtain at least 50% pain relief in one patient as compared to placebo (such that a lower NNT suggests better efficacy), or a mean difference between treatment and placebo across multiple trials using a common continuous outcome measure [71]. Several obstacles to the interpretation of NNT data and their generalizability to clinical practice include heterogeneity of trial design (e.g., the specific pain condition and size of population studied, control groups, parallel vs. crossover design, outcome measures, publication bias), the short-term nature of most RCTs and limited consideration for other important outcomes (e.g., disability, quality of life). However, since relatively few trials are available that directly compare one active treatment to another [108], meta-analyses currently are the most suitable approach to evaluating a given therapeutic intervention in the context of other available treatment options. Given data suggesting that pain reductions of as little as 30% are reported as clinically meaningful by trial patients [22], more recent meta-analyses have also been using 30% pain relief as an outcome of relevance in addition to the more traditional 50% relief yardstick. However, for consistency of reporting, this review reports meta-analysis results based on 50% pain reduction.

Several recent meta-analyses (see Tables IV and V) indicate that antidepressants have been studied in multiple high-quality placebo-controlled trials of neuropathic pain, fibromyalgia, and low back pain and that anticonvulsants have been studied in multiple high-quality placebo-controlled trials of neuropathic pain, fibromyalgia, and postsurgical pain.

Table II
Putative analgesic mechanisms of antidepressant drugs

Pain Mechanisms	Comments	Antidepressant
5-HT mediated	5-HT availability	
	Blockade of neural reuptake	TCAs, SNRIs, SSRIs
	Inhibition of MAO	IMAOs
	5-HT$_{1A}$ receptors	SNRI: venlafaxine; atypical: trazodone
	5-HT$_2$ receptors	TCAs: imipramine, nortriptyline, maprotiline; SNRI: milnacipran; SSRIs: fluoxetine, fluvoxamine; NRI: nisoxetine
	5-HT$_3$ receptors	TCAs: imipramine; atypical: trazodone
Noradrenergic	Norepinephrine availability	
	Blockade of neural reuptake	NRIs, TCAs, SNRIs
	Inhibition of MAO	IMAOs
	α_2-adrenoceptors	TCAs: amitriptyline, imipramine, dothiepin; SNRIs: milnacipran, venlafaxine; NRIs: reboxetine, (+)-oxaprotiline, (−)-oxaprotiline; SSRI: paroxetine; atypical: mirtazapine; IMAO: moclobemide
	α_1-adrenoceptors	TCAs: imipramine, nortriptyline, maprotiline; SNRI: milnacipran; NRI: nisoxetine
	β_1- and β_2-adrenoceptors	TCAs: desipramine, nortriptyline
Dopaminergic	Dopamine availability	
	Blockade of neural reuptake	DNRIs
	D$_2$-receptor activation	DNRI: nomifensine
Opioid-mediated	Activation of opioid endogenous system: δ-opioid receptors (supraspinal level) and μ-opioid receptors (spinal level)	TCAs: amitriptyline, clomipramine, desmethylclomipramine, imipramine, desipramine, maprotiline, nortriptyline, amoxapine, dothiepin; SNRI: venlafaxine; SSRI: paroxetine; NRIs: (+)-oxaprotiline, viloxazine; DNRI: nomifensine; atypical: nefazodone, mirtazapine, mianserin
Na$^+$ channels	Blockade	TCAs: amitriptyline, imipramine, trimipramine, desipramine, doxepin
K$^+$ channels	Activation	TCAs: amitriptyline, clomipramine
Ca^{2+} channels	Inverse correlation between increase in Ca^{2+} channel density and analgesic effect; Ca^{2+}-uptake inhibition	TCAs: amitriptyline, clomipramine, imipramine, trimipramine, desipramine, doxepin; SSRI: citalopram; NRI: oxaprotiline
Adenosine	Adenosine availability; local release of adenosine; activation of adenosine A$_1$ receptor	TCA: amitriptyline
NMDA receptors	Central level: inhibits NMDA-induced spinal hyperalgesia	TCAs: amitriptyline, desipramine
	Peripheral level: potentiated by NMDA-receptor antagonists	TCAs: clomipramine, desipramine
GABA$_B$ receptors	GABA$_B$ receptor function	TCAs: amitriptyline, desipramine; SSRI: fluoxetine
Substance P	Substance-P-induced behavior; production of substance P	TCAs: imipramine, clomipramine; SSRI: fluoxetine
P2X receptors	Peripheral modulation	TCA: amitriptyline
Inflammatory and immune parameters	Prostaglandin-E$_2$-like activity	TCAs: amitriptyline, clomipramine; SSRI: fluoxetine
	NO release	TCA: amitriptyline; SSRI: fluoxetine
	Migration of macrophages	TCA: clomipramine
	Production of TNF-α	TCA: amitriptyline

Source: Adapted with permission from: Micó et al. [73].
Abbreviations: DNRI, dopamine and norepinephrine reuptake inhibitor; IMAO, monoamine oxidase inhibitor; NO, nitric oxide; NRI, norepinephrine reuptake inhibitor; SNRI, serotonin and norepinephrine reuptake inhibitor; TCA, tricyclic antidepressant; TNF-α, tumor necrosis factor alpha.

Table III
Pharmacological classification of anticonvulsant drugs

Anticonvulsant Drug	Mechanism Relevant to Pain Treatment		
	Na+ Channel Blockade	Ca2+ Channel Blockade	Glutamate Suppression
1st Generation			
Benzodiazepines	–	–	–
Carbamazepine	++	+	+
Ethosuximide	–	+	?
Phenobarbital	–	–	–
Phenytoin	++	?	+
Primidone	–	–	–
Valproic acid	?	+	+
2nd Generation			
Felbamate	++	+	+
Gabapentin	?	+	+
Lamotrigine	++	++	+
Levetiracetam	–	+	?
Oxcarbazepine	++	+	+
Pregabalin	–	+	+
Tiagabine	–	–	–
Topiramate	++	+	+
Vigabatrin	–	–	–
Zonisamide	++	++	?

Source: Modified from Perucca [81].
Note: Question marks (?) denote that it is currently unclear whether this mechanism is involved.

Neuropathic Pain

Neuropathic pain, initially defined in 1994 as "pain initiated or caused by a primary lesion or dysfunction in the nervous system" [59], comprises a diverse group of clinical conditions such as cervical or lumbar radiculopathy, diabetic neuropathy, cancer-related neuropathy, postherpetic neuralgia, HIV-related neuropathy, spinal cord injury, trigeminal neuralgia, post-traumatic/postsurgical neuropathic pain, and complex regional pain syndrome type II, among others [31]. A very large proportion of

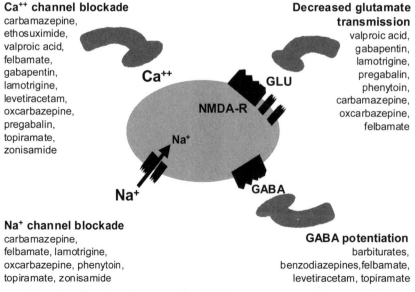

Ca++ channel blockade
carbamazepine,
ethosuximide,
valproic acid,
felbamate,
gabapentin,
lamotrigine,
levetiracetam,
oxcarbazepine,
pregabalin,
topiramate,
zonisamide

Decreased glutamate transmission
valproic acid,
gabapentin,
lamotrigine,
pregabalin,
phenytoin,
carbamazepine,
oxcarbazepine,
felbamate

Na+ channel blockade
carbamazepine,
felbamate, lamotrigine,
oxcarbazepine, phenytoin,
topiramate, zonisamide

GABA potentiation
barbiturates,
benzodiazepines, felbamate,
levetiracetam, topiramate

Fig. 1. Pharmacological mechanisms of anticonvulsants relevant to pain treatment. Modified from Gilron [27].

clinical drug trials in neuropathic pain have been conducted specifically in patients with painful diabetic neuropathy and postherpetic neuralgia [23], leaving other prevalent neuropathic pain conditions such as lumbar radiculopathy relatively understudied [51].

Antidepressants for Neuropathic Pain

Results from over a dozen RCTs of tricyclic antidepressants support their efficacy for neuropathic pain conditions including diabetic neuropathy (e.g., [66]), postherpetic neuralgia (e.g., [85]), and central poststroke pain (e.g., [57]), with recently estimated NNTs of 2.2 for imipramine, 2.6 for desipramine, and 3.1 for amitriptyline (see Table IV). However, it is important to note that high-quality RCTs failed to demonstrate efficacy of tricyclic antidepressants in HIV-related neuropathy [52,95] or in lumbar radiculopathy [51]. SSRIs have been less extensively studied in neuropathic pain. An estimated NNT of 6.8 for SSRIs [23] suggest that they are less effective than TCAs, a result also reported by a head-to-head comparison of paroxetine versus imipramine [97]. SNRIs such as venlafaxine and duloxetine have been evaluated more recently and shown to be superior to placebo in several RCTs with NNT estimates of 5.5 to 6.0 (see Table IV). Of interest because of its distinct pharmacological actions, the dopamine-norepinephrine reuptake blocker, bupropion, showed promising results in a single RCT involving mixed neuropathic pain conditions [93]; however, these results have not

since been replicated, and a subsequent RCT in mostly non-neuropathic low back pain failed to show a bupropion versus placebo difference [45]. Analgesic interactions between antidepressants and other drugs in the treatment of neuropathic pain have been evaluated in several combination trials. Graff-Radford et al. [38] observed no benefit of combining amitriptyline with the neuroleptic, fluphenazine, in the setting of postherpetic neuralgia, and Khoromi et. al. [51] reported the lack of efficacy of nortriptyline, either alone or in combination with morphine, for the treatment of lumbar radiculopathy. However, Gilron et al. [30] conducted an RCT that demonstrated that combining nortriptyline with gabapentin provided greater reductions in pain and sleep interference versus either drug alone.

Anticonvulsants for Neuropathic Pain

Reports of multiple high-quality neuropathic pain RCTs are available for carbamazepine, gabapentin, lamotrigine, phenytoin, pregabalin, topiramate, and valproate (see Table V). In the setting of trigeminal neuralgia, meta-analysis of multiple positive carbamazepine RCTs resulted in NNT estimates of 1.7 [23] to 1.9 [110]. Gabapentin has been evaluated in several RCTs of patients with diabetic neuropathy, postherpetic neuralgia, and other neuropathic conditions. Although previous meta-analyses of gabapentin have yielded NNT estimates ranging from 4.3 [110] to 4.7 [23], an updated systematic review is currently underway [111] in light of recent

Table IV
Systematic reviews of antidepressant drugs for pain relief

Condition	Reference	Study Drug (No. Trials/No. Participants)	NNT (95% CI)	SMD (95% CI)
Various neuropathic conditions	Saarto and Wiffen [89]	Amitriptyline (10/588*)	3.1 (2.5–4.2)	
		Desipramine (2/100*)	2.6 (1.9–4.5)	
		Imipramine (3/114*)	2.2 (1.7–3.2)	
Various neuropathic conditions	Finnerup et al. [23]	TCAs	3.1 (2.7–3.7)	
		SSRIs	6.8 (3.4–441)	
		SNRIs	5.5 (3.4–14)	
Diabetic neuropathy	Lunn et al. [61]	Duloxetine (3/1139)	6.0 (5.0–10.0)	
Fibromyalgia	Häuser et al. [42]	Several antidepressants (18/1427)		−0.43 (−0.55 to −0.30)
Low back pain	Salerno et al. [90]	Several antidepressants (9/287)		−0.41 (−0.22 to −0.61)
Low back pain	Urquhart et al. [102]	Several antidepressants (10/376)	No significant effect on pain or depression	

Abbreviations: 95% CI, 95% confidence interval; NNT, number needed-to-treat (relative to placebo); SMD, standardized mean difference vs. placebo; SSRIs, selective serotonin reuptake inhibitors; SNRIs, serotonin-norepinephrine reuptake inhibitors; TCAs, tricyclic antidepressants.
* Asterisks indicate the number of participants receiving active medication.

Table V
Systematic reviews of anticonvulsant drugs for pain relief

Condition	Reference	Study Drug (No. Trials/No. Participants)	NNT (95% CI)	Mean Difference (95% CI)
Various neuropathic conditions	Finnerup et al. [23]	Carbamazepine (7/235)	2.0 (1.6–2.5)	
		Phenytoin (2/50)	2.1 (1.5–3.6)	
		Lamotrigine (7/494)	4.9 (3.5–8.1)	
		Valproate (5/196)	2.8 (2.1–4.2)	
		Gabapentin/pregabalin (15/2381)	4.7 (4.0–5.6)	
		Topiramate (2/1582)	7.4 (4.3–28)	
Trigeminal neuralgia	Wiffen et al. [110]	Carbamazepine (2/47)	1.9 (1.4–2.8)	
Postherpetic neuralgia	Moore et al. [74]	Pregabalin, 300–600 mg (8/1453*)	3.9–5.3† (3.1–8.1)	
Diabetic neuropathy	Moore et al. [74]	Pregabalin, 300–600 mg (17/3833*)	5–11† (4–54)	
Central neuropathic pain	Moore et al. [74]	Pregabalin, 600 mg (2/176*)	5.6 (3.5–14)	
Fibromyalgia	Moore et al. [74]	Pregabalin, 300–600 mg (11/3872)	9.8–14 (7–33)	
Fibromyalgia	Häuser et al. [41]	Gabapentin/pregabalin (6/2422)		−0.28‡ (−0.36 to −0.20)
Postsurgical pain	Ho et al. [43]	Gabapentin, 1200 mg preoperatively (6/143)		−14.17§ (−21.11 to −7.22)
Postsurgical pain	Moore et al. [74]	Pregabalin (6/273)	"homogeneity insufficient for pooled analysis"	

Abbreviations: NNT, number needed-to-treat (relative to placebo); 95% CI, 95% confidence interval;
* Asterisks indicate the number of participants receiving active medication.
† NNT values (for 50% pain reduction) are lower at higher doses.
‡ SMD, standardized mean difference vs. placebo (0–10 pain scale).
§ WMD, weighted mean difference vs. placebo (0–100 pain scale).

controversy surrounding publication bias and selective outcome reporting [103]. Pregabalin, a more recent congener of the $\alpha_2\delta$ calcium channel ligand, gabapentin, has been studied in several large RCTs conducted in the settings of diabetic neuropathy, postherpetic neuralgia, and central neuropathic pain. A recent meta-analysis reported variable results depending on daily pregabalin doses ranging from 300 to 600 mg/day (i.e., with higher doses associated with lower NNTs) with NNTs of 3.9 to 5.3 for postherpetic neuralgia and 5 to 11 for diabetic neuropathy [74]. Two central neuropathic pain RCTs both involving daily doses of 600 mg yielded an NNT estimate of 5.6 [74]. Analgesic interactions between anticonvulsants and other drugs in the treatment of neuropathic pain have been evaluated in several combination trials. In two randomized controlled crossover trials, Gilron and colleagues reported that combining gabapentin with morphine [29] or with nortriptyline [30] resulted in superior analgesic efficacy in comparison with each respective monotherapy. Further support of the efficacy of a gabapentinoid-opioid combination is suggested by an open-label study suggesting that an oxycodone-pregabalin combination was superior to either drug alone [26].

Fibromyalgia

Fibromyalgia is a complex multisystem disorder characterized by a constellation of symptoms including chronic widespread pain, sleep disturbance, fatigue, irritable bowel syndrome, depressed mood, and cognitive dysfunction, which is reflected in functional disability and impaired quality of life [114]. Fibromyalgia is highly prevalent, affecting 3–5% of the general population, with female predominance [39,113]. Over the past 30 years, hundreds of randomized controlled trials have evaluated a wide variety of pharmacological interventions (e.g., nonsteroidal anti-inflammatory drugs, antidepressants, opioids and anticonvulsants) for the treatment of various aspects of fibromyalgia [34].

Antidepressants for Fibromyalgia Pain

A recent meta-analysis of 18 RCTs of antidepressants (including amitriptyline, nortriptyline, paroxetine, fluoxetine, citalopram, duloxetine, milnacipran, moclobemide, and pirlindole) support the variable efficacy of this broad class of drugs for fibromyalgia pain but also for depressed mood, fatigue, sleep disturbance, and quality of life (see Table IV). Of note, estimated effect sizes for pain reduction were noted to be large for

TCAs, medium for MAOIs, and small for SSRIs/SN-RIs. Analgesic interactions involving antidepressants in the treatment of fibromyalgia have received little attention. However, in one previous trial, Goldenberg et al. [33] reported that combining the TCA, amitriptyline, with the SSRI, fluoxetine, was more effective than either drug alone.

Anticonvulsants for Fibromyalgia Pain

Aside from early studies of certain benzodiazepines, anticonvulsants have not been widely studied in fibromyalgia until the more recent introduction of gabapentin and pregabalin [72]. Since then, several RCTs have demonstrated efficacy of gabapentinoids in patients suffering from fibromyalgia with such improvements as reduced pain, improved sleep, and improved quality of life. One recent fibromyalgia meta-analysis involving RCTs of gabapentin and pregabalin (see Table V) yielded a modest standardized mean difference of −0.28 for pain (based on a 0–10 numerical rating scale) and another meta-analysis involving only pregabalin RCTs reported NNT dose-dependent results ranging from 9.8 to 14 for doses between 300 to 600 mg/day (see Table V). To date, no combination trials have been published involving anticonvulsants for the treatment of fibromyalgia. However, an interesting rationale for combining pregabalin with the NMDA antagonist, memantine, has been suggested [86].

Back Pain

Back pain—due to a multitude of causes [16]—is perhaps the most common, as well as difficult to treat, chronic pain disorder with an estimated point prevalence of 28% and a lifetime prevalence of 84% [12]. It is thus not surprising that over a thousand RCTs involving back pain have been published to date, reflecting the continued challenge of identifying optimal treatment interventions for this devastating problem. While back pain may be related to a variety of different anatomical structures (e.g., vertebrae, ligaments, facet joints, intervertebral disks, and spinal nerve roots), may occur in different temporal patterns (e.g., acute recurring vs. chronic) and may manifest in various settings (e.g., occupational, sports-related, or degenerative), analgesic pharmacotherapy is often considered as one possible treatment option in most of these circumstances [10].

Antidepressants for Back Pain

Nearly a dozen RCTs of antidepressants have been published to date that are heterogeneous with respect to etiology of back pain and/or the presence of concomitant depression. Whereas one previous back pain review reported a modest yet statistically significant effect of antidepressants on the symptom of pain (see Table IV), a more recent meta-analysis that included two newer RCTs concluded that this class of drugs demonstrated no significant effect on pain or depression (see Table IV). Furthermore, this more recent meta-analysis excluded the negative nortriptyline trial by Khoromi et. al. [51] because it included only patients with lumbar radiculopathy.

Anticonvulsants for Back Pain

Although a few small back pain trials of the anticonvulsants topiramate [50,77], gabapentin [115], and pregabalin [88] have been recently published, no systematic reviews have been published to date, and there are not currently enough data to make any conclusions about the efficacy of these agents for the treatment of back pain.

Early Postsurgical Pain

Early postsurgical pain—occurring for periods of days to weeks and generally thought to parallel the temporal profile of postsurgical tissue inflammation—is perhaps the most predictable acute pain condition [47]. With over 40 million surgeries per year performed in North America alone and moderate to severe pain known to occur in over half of these procedures, postsurgical pain remains an important public health problem [98]. Limited efficacy and dose-related toxicities of commonly used opioids, local anesthetics, and nonsteroidal anti-inflammatory drugs have led to the study of other pharmacological agents for the treatment of pain after surgery [92], including some antidepressants and anticonvulsants.

Antidepressants for Postsurgical Pain

Evaluations of the impact of antidepressant drugs on postoperative pain and/or opioid efficacy in the early postoperative period have received relatively little attention. While two trials suggested that desipramine enhanced postoperative opioid analgesia [36,58] after third molar extraction, other investigations failed to show any effects of desipramine [67] or amitriptyline [49]. In the absence of additional trials, it remains unclear whether the two oral surgery studies yielded positive results because of the 3 to 7 days of preoperative study drug pretreatment or whether the two negative trial results might be attributed to more invasive surgery including major orthopedic procedures. Of note, a third oral surgery study reported no analgesic effect of the SSRI, fluoxetine, and further noted that this drug actually shortened the apparent duration of morphine action [35].

Anticonvulsants for Postsurgical Pain

Despite earlier disappointing results with valproate [63] and lamotrigine [8], recent enthusiasm has been expressed for the evaluation of gabapentin and pregabalin for the treatment of postsurgical pain [28]. A meta-analysis based on six gabapentin RCTs reported a significant weighted mean difference favoring gabapentin over placebo for reduction of pain [43]. Given that additional postoperative gabapentin trials have since been published, an updated systematic review is anticipated [75]. A recent systematic review of six postoperative pregabalin RCTs reporting mixed results concluded that this group of trials was too heterogeneous with respect to a number of important factors (e.g., surgical procedure, pregabalin dose, and timing of administration) to allow for a pooled analysis [74].

Prevention of Chronic Pain

Over the past 20 years, increasing attention has been devoted to studying the potential for analgesic interventions to prevent, or at least modify, the pathogenesis of chronic pain following acute tissue or nerve injury be it surgical, traumatic, or otherwise [19,37,78,105]. In the setting of surgery, certain procedures may cause chronic pain—that is, pain persisting beyond 3–6 months after surgery. Previous studies evaluating patients over time have identified various surgical procedures that are associated with a high incidence (proportion of operated patients) of chronic postsurgical pain including limb amputation (30–50%), breast cancer surgery (20–30%), thoracotomy (30–40%), and coronary bypass surgery (30–50%) [80]. Other situations where a rather predictable and discrete insult may lead to the development of chronic pain include varicella-zoster virus reactivation ("shingles") and its occasional progression to postherpetic neuralgia [19], as well as the administration of cancer chemotherapies that may lead to chemotherapy-induced peripheral neuropathic pain [112]. Given that well-established chronic pain is often resistant to therapy, investigative efforts are expanding to identify and evaluate potentially preventive treatments including antidepressants and anticonvulsants.

Antidepressants for Preventing Chronic Pain

To date, no completed RCTs of antidepressants for the prevention of chronic pain after surgery have been published. In the setting of varicella-zoster reactivation, Bowsher [9] published a double-blind placebo-controlled trial that reported that 90 days of amitriptyline (25 mg daily) administration, initiated soon after rash onset, significantly reduced the prevalence of postherpetic neuralgia pain 6 months after onset. However, this trial has been criticized for the potential confounding effects of allowing study physicians to decide whether or not study patients were to receive early antiviral therapy or not [18].

Anticonvulsants for Preventing Chronic Pain

The potential for gabapentin and pregabalin to prevent and/or treat chronic pain after surgery has been studied in over a dozen trials that have yielded mixed results to date. With continued research occurring in this area, at least one ongoing systematic review is anticipated [32]. In the setting of chemotherapy-induced neuropathy, one group reported promising results from a small study on the preventive effects of oxcarbazepine [1] whereas a different group observed no effect of carbamazepine [104] on the development of oxaliplatin-induced neuropathy. Thus, it is premature to draw conclusions on the potential impact of anticonvulsants on chemotherapy-induced neuropathic pain. In the setting of varicella-zoster reactivation, a small, open-label comparison suggested a substantially higher rate of postherpetic neuralgia in patients treated with oral carbamazepine versus those receiving oral prednisolone [46]. Although gabapentin has not been evaluated for prevention of postherpetic neuralgia, favorable results from a single-dose study of gabapentin in acute herpes zoster [7] support the feasibility of conducting such an investigation.

Other Pain Conditions

Although this chapter largely focuses on pain conditions where antidepressants and anticonvulsants have been extensively evaluated, it should be noted that these drug classes have received some research attention in other painful disorders. For example, the TCA, trimipramine [62], exhibited analgesic efficacy for rheumatoid arthritis pain, and the SNRIs, venlafaxine [100] and duloxetine [13], were reported to be effective in osteoarthritis. However, the anticonvulsant, phenytoin, was inferior to gold therapy in another rheumatoid arthritis trial [87], and results from a previous pregabalin trial in osteoarthritis (see [22]) are not available for review. Some favorable outcomes have been reported with gabapentin [4,91] in contrast to less promising results with amitriptyline [25,91] in the setting of chronic pelvic pain conditions. Although pain is one of several different symptoms associated with irritable bowel syndrome, it is worth mentioning a positive systematic review of TCA trials [84] as well as some promising early findings with gabapentin [56] and pregabalin [44] for the treatment of irritable bowel syndrome symptoms. In the setting of facial pain, small trials suggest the analgesic efficacy of the SNRI, venlafaxine [24], and the anticonvulsant, gabapentin [53].

Pain Treatment Guidelines

Developing and disseminating a clinical guideline or recommendation is a very complex process that involves the assembly and collaboration of appropriate individuals with proficiency in informatics, epidemiology, biostatistics, health services research, scientific communication, and, of course, clinical expertise in the area of interest [94]. The process of treatment guideline development starts with careful examination of available RCT evidence with respect to its validity, generalizability, and, of course, the nature of efficacy, tolerability, and other relevant results. Reviewed evidence may be categorized over a range from "Ia" (meta-analysis of multiple, high-quality RCTs) down to "IV" (expert opinion), and strength of recommendations can range from "A" (based on category I evidence) down to "D" (based on category IV evidence) [94]. Furthermore, other treatment-related factors may be incorporated

including treatment cost, ease of administration and, in some cases, regulatory and other social issues (e.g., opioids, cannabinoids, etc.). Given their complexity and broad-reaching implications, both the "producers" and "consumers" of treatment guidelines need to be acutely aware of possible conflicts of interest that may affect their development and potentially misguide the best possible patient care (see [15]).

Pain Treatment Guidelines Regarding Antidepressant Drugs

In the setting of neuropathic pain (with the exception of HIV neuropathy), tricyclic antidepressants have been recommended as first-line therapy by the European Federation of Neurological Societies (EFNS), the Canadian Pain Society (CPS), and the IASP Neuropathic Pain Special Interest Group (NeuPSIG) (see Table VI). Whereas the Canadian and European guidelines recommended SNRI antidepressants as second-line therapy because of estimates suggesting somewhat lesser efficacy than TCAs, the most recent IASP NeuPSIG guidelines consider them as first-line, possibly due to a more favorable side-effect profile. In 2007, the European League Against Rheumatism (EULAR) recommended antidepressants (indicating specifically amitriptyline, fluoxetine, duloxetine, milnacipran, moclobemide, and pirlindole) for the treatment of fibromyalgia with "A" strength recommendation based on category "Ib" evidence (see Table VI). Also, the German Interdisciplinary Association of Pain Therapy (DIVS) recommended, with strong consensus, the antidepressants amitriptyline, fluoxetine, paroxetine, and sertraline for fibromyalgia (see Table VI). However, these same guidelines notably "non-recommended," with strong consensus,

Table VI
Pain treatment guidelines regarding antidepressant drugs

Condition	Reference	Drug	Treatment Recommendation
Neuropathic pain	Dworkin et. al. [20]	Secondary amine TCAs; SNRIs	First-line
	Moulin et. al. [76]	TCAs	First-line
		SNRIs	Second-line
	Attal et. al. [2]	TCAs	First-line
		SNRIs	Second-line
Fibromyalgia	Carville et. al. [11]	Various antidepressants	"A" strength recommendation
	Häuser et. al. [41]	SSRIs; SNRIs	Strong consensus
Low back pain	Chou et al. [14]	TCAs	"Good evidence" (small to moderate benefit)

Abbreviations: SSRIs, selective serotonin reuptake inhibitors; SNRIs, serotonin-norepinephrine reuptake inhibitors; TCAs, tricyclic antidepressants.

moclobemide, pirlindole, and citalopram. The 2007 American Pain Society (APS)/American College of Physicians (ACP) guidelines on medications for low back pain concluded that good evidence exists for small to moderate benefit with tricyclic antidepressants in chronic low back pain (see Table VI).

Pain Treatment Guidelines Regarding Anticonvulsant Drugs

Gabapentin and pregabalin have been recommended as first-line therapy by the EFNS, CPS, and IASP NeuPSIG for neuropathic pain (with the exception of trigeminal neuralgia), and the EFNS and CPS recommended carbamazepine as first-line therapy for trigeminal neuralgia (see Table VII). For the treatment of fibromyalgia, both EULAR and DIVS have recommended pregabalin with "A" strength or strong consensus (see Table VII). The 2007 APS/ACP guidelines on medications for low back pain found only fair evidence for gabapentin in spinal radiculopathy (see Table VII). In the setting of postsurgical pain, the Internet-based "Procedure-Specific Postoperative Pain Management" working group (PROSPECT: http://www.postoppain.org) has made a grade A recommendation for gabapentin for the reduction of postoperative opioid use and nausea specifically in the setting of abdominal hysterectomy (see Table VII).

Pharmacokinetics, Safety, and Dosing

Given the diversity of drugs in these two classes and the complexity of their pharmacokinetics and pharmacodynamics in different clinical situations, prescribers are strongly encouraged to review relevant details (especially potential drug-drug interactions) of individual drugs before prescribing them. Patients with neuropathic pain in particular frequently receive many other medications and often suffer from other coexisting medical problems. Consideration of such comorbidities in the setting of chronic pain treatment has recently been reviewed [40].

Antidepressants

Generally, antidepressants are well absorbed when taken orally with apparent volumes of distribution of up to 10 to 50 L/kg, and most are inactivated and eliminated over periods of several days [3]. Metabolism of TCAs involves oxidation by hepatic microsomal enzymes and then conjugation with glucuronic acid [3]. The antidepressants, desipramine and nortriptyline, are active metabolites of their parent compounds, imipramine and amitriptyline, respectively. Liver metabolism of antidepressant drugs largely involves the cytochrome P450 family of isoenzymes such that most tricyclics are substrates for CYP1A2; citalopram and imipramine for CYP2C19; atomoxetine, duloxetine, mirtazapine, paroxetine, trazodone, and some tricyclics for CYP2D6; and some tricyclics and SSRIs for CYP3A3/4 [3]. As well as being substrates, some antidepressants also *inhibit* the metabolic activity of cytochrome P450 isoenzymes, including fluvoxamine (which inhibits CYP1A2, 2C9, and 2C19), fluoxetine (CYP2C9 and 2D6) and paroxetine (CYP2D6) [3]. These aspects of antidepressant drug metabolism give rise to the potential for multiple drug-drug interactions [40]. TCAs may cause several important adverse effects including cardiac conduction block, sedation, orthostatic hypotension, confusion, weight gain, and anticholinergic effects such as dry mouth, constipation, urinary retention, and blurred vision [40]. The potential for these complications warrants caution (e.g., electrocardiogram screening) or even precludes their use in patients with

Table VII
Pain treatment guidelines regarding anticonvulsant drugs

Condition	Reference	Drug	Treatment Recommendation
Neuropathic pain	Dworkin et al. [20]	Gabapentin; pregabalin	First-line
	Moulin et al. [76]	Gabapentin; pregabalin	First-line
		Carbamazepine	First-line (for trigeminal neuralgia only)
	Attal et al. [2]	Gabapentin; pregabalin	First-line
		Carbamazepine	First-line (for trigeminal neuralgia only)
Fibromyalgia	Carville et al. [11]	Pregabalin	"Should be considered"
	Häuser et. al. [41]	Pregabalin	Strong consensus
Low back pain	Chou et al. [14]	Gabapentin	Only "fair evidence" for radiculopathy
Abdominal hysterectomy pain	PROSPECT [83]	Gabapentin/pregabalin	Grade A recommendation for reducing postoperative opioid use and nausea

Table VIII
Prescribing recommendations for antidepressants and anticonvulsants in chronic pain management.

Drug	Starting Dosage	Titration	Maximum Dosage	Duration of Adequate Trial
Tricyclic Antidepressants				
Secondary amine TCAs: Nortriptyline*, desipramine* (use a tertiary amine TCA only if a secondary amine TCA is not available)	25 mg at bedtime	Increase by 25 mg daily every 3–7 days as tolerated	150 mg daily; if blood level of active medication and its metabolite is below 100 ng/mL (mg/mL), continue titration with caution	6–8 weeks with at least 2 weeks at maximum tolerated dosage
SNRI Antidepressants				
Duloxetine	30 mg once daily	Increase to 60 mg once daily after 1 week	60 mg twice daily	4 weeks
Venlafaxine	37.5 mg once or twice daily	Increase by 75 mg each week	225 mg daily	4–6 weeks
Anticonvulsants				
Gabapentin*	100–300 mg at bedtime or 100–300 mg three times daily	Increase by 100–300 mg three times daily every 1–7 days as tolerated	3600 mg daily (1200 mg three times daily); reduce if impaired renal function	3–8 weeks for titration plus 2 weeks at maximum dosage
Pregabalin*	50 mg thrice daily or 75 mg twice daily as tolerated	Increase to 300 mg daily after 3–7 days, then by 150 mg/day every 3–7 days as tolerated	600 mg daily (200 mg three times or 300 mg twice daily); reduce if renal function is impaired	4 weeks
Carbamazepine†	100–200 mg daily	Increase weekly by 100–200 daily	1600 mg daily	6–8 weeks

Source: Modified from Dworkin et al. [21].
Abbreviations: SNRI, serotonin norepinephrine reuptake inhibitor; TCA, tricyclic antidepressant.
* Consider lower starting dosages and slower titration in geriatric patients.
† Recommended only for treatment of trigeminal neuralgia.

certain conditions including recent myocardial infarction, heart block of any degree, prostatic hypertrophy, and narrow angle glaucoma [40]. The SNRIs duloxetine and venlafaxine are generally better tolerated, with fewer and less serious adverse effects than TCAs [40]. However, possible associations between venlafaxine and increased blood pressure [68] contraindicate the use of SNRIs in patients with uncontrolled hypertension. Serotonin syndrome is a potentially fatal condition associated with several TCAs, SSRIs, SNRIs, and MAOIs, as well as tramadol and several opioids, and is manifest as a spectrum of toxicity ranging from agitation to diaphoresis, hyperthermia, myoclonus, tremor, and confusion [101]. Although fatal cases of serotonin syndrome have been mostly attributed to combinations of MAOIs with other serotonergic drugs, concerns about serotonin syndrome suggest using extreme caution when combining any two or more serotonergic agents in the setting of pain management [40]. Recommendations for starting dosage, titration, maximum dosage, and duration of adequate individual drug trials are listed in Table VIII for TCAs and for the SNRIs duloxetine and venlafaxine.

Anticonvulsants

Whereas the oral absorption of pregabalin is quite fast (approximately 1 hour to maximal absorption), and oral bioavailability remains dose-independently high [5], absorption of gabapentin is slightly slower (2–3 hours to maximal absorption) and occurs through a saturable transport system in the gastrointestinal tract such that bioavailability decreases with increasing doses [70]. Therefore, gabapentin dose increases in higher dose ranges should be expected to lead to incrementally smaller increases in plasma drug concentrations (i.e., nonlinear pharmacokinetics). The lack of hepatic enzyme inhibition or induction and the lack of clinically important drug interactions are major perceived advantages of gabapentin and pregabalin. However, oral antacids are known to diminish the bioavailability of gabapentin by 20–30% [69]. As with other sedating drugs, gabapentin and pregabalin can potentiate the effects of other sedatives such as ethanol and benzodiazepines. Doses of both drugs should be reduced proportional to creatinine clearance in the presence of renal insufficiency, since they are normally excreted unchanged in the urine [5,69]. Relatively frequent adverse effects of gabapentin and pregabalin include sedation, dizziness, weight gain, peripheral edema, and blurry vision; these effects are generally dose-related and reversible.

Although carbamazepine is recommended as first-line therapy only for trigeminal neuralgia, some pharmacological details are presented here. Bioavailability of carbamazepine is variable, and its pharmacokinetics also change (reduced half-life) over the first few weeks of treatment due to auto-induction of CYP3A4-mediated metabolism [54]. Carbamazepine-induced induction is also responsible for potential drug interactions with various antidepressants, opioids, and other drugs [40]. Toxicities of carbamazepine include adverse effects such as somnolence, dizziness, headache, ataxia, nystagmus, diplopia, blurred vision, nausea, rash, hyponatremia, leukopenia, thrombocytopenia, and hepatotoxicity, thus necessitating frequent clinical biochemical monitoring.

Recommendations for starting dosage, titration, maximum dosage, and duration of adequate individual drug trials are listed in Table VIII for gabapentin, pregabalin, and carbamazepine.

Conclusions

Although initially developed for other conditions, a wide variety of antidepressant and anticonvulsant drugs have been extensively studied for their efficacy in treating pain. In light of accumulating evidence, these two classes of agents play an important role in the clinical management of pain. Continued investigation of currently available as well as novel antidepressants and anticonvulsants is expected to advance our knowledge about the mechanisms and management of pain.

Acknowledgments

This work was supported, in part, by funding from CIHR Grant #85649 and Queen's University Grant #383-861 to Dr. Ian Gilron.

References

[1] Argyriou AA, Chroni E, Polychronopoulos P, Iconomou G, Koutras A, Makatsoris T, Gerolymos MK, Gourzis P, Assimakopoulos K, Kalofonos HP. Efficacy of oxcarbazepine for prophylaxis against cumulative oxaliplatin-induced neuropathy. Neurology 2006;67:2253–5.

[2] Attal N, Cruccu G, Haanpää M, Hansson P, Jensen TS, Nurmikko T, Sampaio C, Sindrup S, Wiffen P; EFNS Task Force. EFNS guidelines on pharmacological treatment of neuropathic pain. Eur J Neurol 2006;13:1153.

[3] Baldessarini RJ. Drugs and the treatment of psychiatric disorders: depression and anxiety disorders. In: Brunton L, Lazo J, Parker K, editors. Goodman and Gilman's the pharmacological basis of therapeutics, 11th ed. McGraw-Hill; 2006.

[4] Ben-David B, Friedman M. Gabapentin therapy for vulvodynia. Anesth Analg 1999;89:1459–60.

[5] Ben-Menachem E: Pregabalin pharmacology and its relevance to clinical practice. Epilepsia 2004;45(Suppl 6):13–8.

[6] Bergouignan M. Cures hereuses de neuralgies essentielles par le diphenyl-bydantionate de soude. Rev Laryngol Otol Rhinol 1942;63:34–41.

[7] Berry JD, Petersen KL. A single dose of gabapentin reduces acute pain and allodynia in patients with herpes zoster. Neurology 2005;65:444–7.

[8] Bonicalzi V, Canavero S, Cerutti F, Piazza M, Clemente M, Chió A. Lamotrigine reduces total postoperative analgesic requirement: a randomized double-blind, placebo-controlled pilot study. Surgery 1997;122:567–70.

[9] Bowsher D. The effects of pre-emptive treatment of postherpetic neuralgia with amitriptyline: a randomized, double-blind, placebo-controlled trial. J Pain Symptom Manage 1997;13:327–31.

[10] Carragee EJ. Clinical practice. Persistent low back pain. N Engl J Med 2005;352:1891–8.

[11] Carville SF, Arendt-Nielsen S, Bliddal H, Blotman F, Branco JC, Buskila D, Da Silva JA, Danneskiold-Samsøe B, Dincer F, Henriksson C, et al.; EULAR. EULAR evidence-based recommendations for the management of fibromyalgia syndrome. Ann Rheum Dis 2008;67:536.

[12] Cassidy JD, Carroll LJ, Côté P. The Saskatchewan health and back pain survey. The prevalence of low back pain and related disability in Saskatchewan adults. Spine (Phila Pa 1976) 1998;23:1860–6.

[13] Chappell AS, Ossanna MJ, Liu-Seifert H, Iyengar S, Skljarevski V, Li LC, Bennett RM, Collins H. Duloxetine, a centrally acting analgesic, in the treatment of patients with osteoarthritis knee pain: a 13-week, randomized, placebo-controlled trial. Pain 2009;146:253–60.

[14] Chou R, Huffman LH; American Pain Society; American College of Physicians. Medications for acute and chronic low back pain. Ann Intern Med 2007;147:505.

[15] Cosgrove L, Bursztajn HJ, Krimsky S. Developing unbiased diagnostic and treatment guidelines in psychiatry. N Engl J Med 2009;360:2035–6.

[16] Deyo RA, Weinstein JN. Low back pain. N Engl J Med 2001;344:363–70.

[17] Dickenson AH, Matthews EA, Suzuki R. Neurobiology of neuropathic pain: mode of action of anticonvulsants. Eur J Pain 2002;6(Suppl A):51–60.

[18] Dworkin RH. Prevention of postherpetic neuralgia. Lancet 1999;353:1636–7.

[19] Dworkin RH, Perkins FM, Nagasako EM. Prospects for the prevention of postherpetic neuralgia in herpes zoster patients. Clin J Pain 2000;16(2 Suppl):S90–100.

[20] Dworkin RH, O'Connor AB, Audette J, Baron R, Gourlay GK, Haanpää ML, Kent JL, Krane EJ, Lebel AA, Levy RM, et al. Recommendations for the pharmacological management of neuropathic pain: an overview and literature update. Mayo Clin Proc 2010;85(3 Suppl):S3–14.

[21] Dworkin RH, O'Connor AB, Backonja M, Farrar JT, Finnerup NB, Jensen TS, Kalso EA, Loeser JD, Miaskowski C, Nurmikko TJ, et al. Pharmacologic management of neuropathic pain: evidence-based recommendations. Pain 2007;132:237.

[22] Farrar JT, Young JP Jr, LaMoreaux L, Werth JL, Poole RM. Clinical importance of changes in chronic pain intensity measured on an 11-point numerical pain rating scale. Pain 2001 Nov;94:149–58.

[23] Finnerup NB, Otto M, McQuay HJ, Jensen TS, Sindrup SH. Algorithm for neuropathic pain treatment: an evidence based proposal. Pain 2005;118:289–305.

[24] Forssell H, Tasmuth T, Tenovuo O, Hampf G, Kalso E. Venlafaxine in the treatment of atypical facial pain: a randomized controlled trial. J Orofac Pain 2004;18:131–7.

[25] Foster HE Jr, Hanno PM, Nickel JC, Payne CK, Mayer RD, Burks DA, Yang CC, Chai TC, Kreder KJ, Peters KM, et al.; Interstitial Cystitis Collaborative Research Network. Effect of amitriptyline on symptoms in treatment naïve patients with interstitial cystitis/painful bladder syndrome. J Urol 2010;183:1853–8.

[26] Gatti A, Sabato AF, Occhioni R, Baldeschi GC, Reale C. Controlled release oxycodone and pregabalin in the treatment of neuropathic pain: results of a multicenter Italian study. Eur Neurol 2009;61:129–37.

[27] Gilron I. The role of anticonvulsant drugs in postoperative pain management: a bench-to-bedside perspective. Can J Anaesth 2006;53:562–71.

[28] Gilron I. Gabapentin and pregabalin for chronic neuropathic and early postsurgical pain: current evidence and future directions. Curr Opin Anaesthesiol 2007;20:456–72.

[29] Gilron I, Bailey JM, Tu D, Holden RR, Weaver DF, Houlden RL. Morphine, gabapentin, or their combination for neuropathic pain. N Engl J Med 2005;352:1324–34.

[30] Gilron I, Bailey JM, Tu D, Holden RR, Jackson AC, Houlden RL. Nortriptyline and gabapentin, alone and in combination for neuropathic pain: a double-blind, randomised controlled crossover trial. Lancet 2009;374:1252–61.

[31] Gilron I, Watson CP, Cahill CM, Moulin DE. Neuropathic pain: a practical guide for the clinician. CMAJ 2006;175:265–75.

[32] Gilron I, Moore RA, Wiffen PJ, McQuay HJ. Pharmacotherapy for the prevention of chronic pain after surgery in adults (Protocol). Cochrane Database Syst Rev 2010;1:CD008307.

[33] Goldenberg D, Mayskiy M, Mossey C, Ruthazer R, Schmid C. A randomized, double-blind crossover trial of fluoxetine and amitriptyline in the treatment of fibromyalgia. Arthritis Rheum 1996;39:1852–9.

[34] Goldenberg DL, Burckhardt C, Crofford L. Management of fibromyalgia syndrome. JAMA 2004;292:2388–95.

[35] Gordon NC, Heller PH, Gear RW, Levine JD. Interactions between fluoxetine and opiate analgesia for postoperative dental pain. Pain 1994;58:85–8.

[36] Gordon NC, Heller PH, Gear RW, Levine JD. Temporal factors in the enhancement of morphine analgesia by desipramine. Pain 1993;53:273–6.

[37] Gottschalk A, Raja SN. Severing the link between acute and chronic pain: the anesthesiologist's role in preventive medicine. Anesthesiology 2004;101:1063–5.

[38] Graff-Radford SB, Shaw LR, Naliboff BN. Amitriptyline and fluphenazine in the treatment of postherpetic neuralgia. Clin J Pain 2000;16:188–92.

[39] Gran JT. The epidemiology of chronic generalized musculoskeletal pain. Best Pract Res Clin Rheumatol 2003;17:547–61.

[40] Haanpää ML, Gourlay GK, Kent JL, Miaskowski C, Raja SN, Schmader KE, Wells CD. Treatment considerations for patients with neuropathic pain and other medical comorbidities. Mayo Clin Proc 2010;85(3 Suppl):S15–25.

[41] Häuser W, Arnold B, Eich W, Felde E, Flügge C, Henningsen P, Herrmann M, Köllner V, Kühn E, Nutzinger D, et al. Management of fibromyalgia syndrome: an interdisciplinary evidence-based guideline. Ger Med Sci 2008;6:14.

[42] Häuser W, Bernardy K, Uçeyler N, Sommer C. Treatment of fibromyalgia syndrome with antidepressants: a meta-analysis. JAMA 2009;301:198–209.

[43] Ho KY, Gan TJ, Habib AS. Gabapentin and postoperative pain: a systematic review of randomized controlled trials. Pain 2006;126:91–101.

[44] Houghton LA, Fell C, Whorwell PJ, Jones I, Sudworth DP, Gale JD. Effect of a second-generation alpha2delta ligand (pregabalin) on visceral sensation in hypersensitive patients with irritable bowel syndrome. Gut 2007;56:1218–25.

[45] Katz J, Pennella-Vaughan J, Hetzel RD, Kanazi GE, Dworkin RH. A randomized, placebo-controlled trial of bupropion sustained release in chronic low back pain. J Pain 2005;6:656–61.

[46] Keczkes K, Basheer AM. Do corticosteroids prevent post-herpetic neuralgia? Br J Dermatol 1980;102:551–5.

[47] Kehlet H, Dahl JB. Anaesthesia, surgery, and challenges in postoperative recovery. Lancet 2003;362:1921–8.

[48] Kehlet H, Jensen TS, Woolf CJ. Persistent postsurgical pain: risk factors and prevention. Lancet 2006;367:1618–25.

[49] Kerrick JM, Fine PG, Lipman AG, Love G. Low-dose amitriptyline as an adjunct to opioids for postoperative orthopedic pain: a placebo-controlled trial. Pain 1993;52:325–30.

[50] Khoromi S, Patsalides A, Parada S, Salehi V, Meegan JM, Max MB. Topiramate in chronic lumbar radicular pain. J Pain 2005;6:829–36.

[51] Khoromi S, Cui L, Nackers L, Max MB. Morphine, nortriptyline and their combination vs. placebo in patients with chronic lumbar root pain. Pain 2007;130:66–75.

[52] Kieburtz K, Simpson D, Yiannoutsos C, Max MB, Hall CD, Ellis RJ, Marra CM, McKendall R, Singer E, Dal Pan GJ, Clifford DB, Tucker T, Cohen B. A randomized trial of amitriptyline and mexiletine for painful neuropathy in HIV infection. AIDS Clinical Trial Group 242 Protocol Team. Neurology 1998;51:1682–8.

[53] Kimos P, Biggs C, Mah J, Heo G, Rashiq S, Thie NM, Major PW. Analgesic action of gabapentin on chronic pain in the masticatory muscles: a randomized controlled trial. Pain 2007;127:151–60.

[54] Kudriakova TB, Sirota LA, Rozova GI, Gorkov VA. Autoinduction and steady-state pharmacokinetics of carbamazepine and its major metabolites. Br J Clin Pharmacol 1992;33:611–5.

[55] Kuipers RK. Imipramine in the treatment of rheumatic patients. Acta Rheumatol Scand 1962;8:45–51.

[56] Lee KJ, Kim JH, Cho SW. Gabapentin reduces rectal mechanosensitivity and increases rectal compliance in patients with diarrhoea-predominant irritable bowel syndrome. Aliment Pharmacol Ther 2005;22:981–8.

[57] Leijon G, Boivie J. Central post-stroke pain: a controlled trial of amitriptyline and carbamazepine. Pain 1989;36:27–36.

[58] Levine JD, Gordon NC, Smith R, McBryde R. Desipramine enhances opiate postoperative analgesia. Pain 1986;27:45–9.

[59] Loeser JD, Treede RD. The Kyoto protocol of IASP basic pain terminology. Pain 2008;137:473–7.

[60] Loscher W. Current status and future directions in the pharmacotherapy of epilepsy. Trends Pharmacol Sci 2002;23:113–8.

[61] Lunn MP, Hughes RA, Wiffen PJ. Duloxetine for treating painful neuropathy or chronic pain. Cochrane Database Syst Rev 2009;4:CD007115.

[62] Macfarlane JG, Jalali S, Grace EM. Trimipramine in rheumatoid arthritis: a randomized double-blind trial in relieving pain and joint tenderness. Curr Med Res Opin 1986;10:89–93.

[63] Martin C, Martin A, Rud C, Valli M. [Comparative study of sodium valproate and ketoprofen in the treatment of postoperative pain]. Ann Fr Anesth Reanim 1988;7:387–92.

[64] Max MB, Culnane M, Schafer SC, Gracely RH, Walther DJ, Smoller B, Dubner R. Amitriptyline relieves diabetic neuropathy pain in patients with normal or depressed mood. Neurology 1987;37:589–96.

[65] Max MB, Gilron I. Antidepressants, muscle relaxants, and NMDA receptor antagonists. In: Loeser JD, Turk D, Chapman CR, Butler S, editors. Bonica's management of pain, 3rd ed. Williams & Wilkins; 2001.

[66] Max MB, Lynch SA, Muir J, Shoaf SE, Smoller B, Dubner R. Effects of desipramine, amitriptyline, and fluoxetine on pain in diabetic neuropathy. N Engl J Med 1992;326:1250–6.

[67] Max MB, Zeigler D, Shoaf SE, Craig E, Benjamin J, Li SH, Buzzanell C, Perez M, Ghosh BC. Effects of a single oral dose of desipramine on postoperative morphine analgesia. J Pain Symptom Manage 1992;7:454–62.

[68] Mbaya P, Alam F, Ashim S, Bennett D. Cardiovascular effects of high dose venlafaxine XL in patients with major depressive disorder. Hum Psychopharmacol 2007;22:129–33.

[69] McLean MJ. Clinical pharmacokinetics of gabapentin. Neurology 1994;44:S17–22.

[70] McLean MJ, Gidal BE. Gabapentin dosing in the treatment of epilepsy. Clin Ther 2003;25:1382–406.

[71] McQuay HJ, Kalso E, Moore RA, editors. Systematic reviews in pain research: methodology refined. Seattle: IASP Press; 2008.

[72] Mease PJ, Choy EH. Pharmacotherapy of fibromyalgia. Rheum Dis Clin North Am 2009;35:359–72.

[73] Micó JA, Ardid D, Berrocoso E, Eschalier A. Antidepressants and pain. Trends Pharmacol Sci 2006;27:348–54.

[74] Moore RA, Straube S, Wiffen PJ, Derry S, McQuay HJ. Pregabalin for acute and chronic pain in adults. Cochrane Database Syst Rev 2009;3:CD007076.

[75] Moore RA, Derry S, Wiffen PJ, McQuay HJ, Straube S. Single dose oral gabapentin for acute postoperative pain in adults (Protocol). Cochrane Database Syst Rev 2010;1:CD008183.

[76] Moulin DE, Clark AJ, Gilron I, Ware MA, Watson CP, Sessle BJ, Coderre T, Morley-Forster PK, Stinson J, Boulanger A, et al.; Canadian Pain Society. Pharmacological management of chronic neuropathic pain: consensus statement and guidelines from the Canadian Pain Society. Pain Res Manag 2007;12:13.

[77] Muehlbacher M, Nickel MK, Kettler C, Tritt K, Lahmann C, Leiberich PK, Nickel C, Krawczyk J, Mitterlehner FO, Rother WK, Loew TH, Kaplan P. Topiramate in treatment of patients with chronic low back pain: a randomized, double-blind, placebo-controlled study. Clin J Pain 2006;22:526–31.

[78] Olesen LL, Jensen TS. Prevention and management of drug-induced peripheral neuropathy. Drug Saf 1991;6:302–14.

[79] Pande AC, Crockatt JG, Feltner DE, Janney CA, Smith WT, Weisler R, Londborg PD, Bielski RJ, Zimbroff DL, Davidson JR, Liu-Dumaw M. Pregabalin in generalized anxiety disorder: a placebo-controlled trial. Am J Psychiatry 2003;160:533–40.

[80] Perkins FM, Kehlet H. Chronic pain as an outcome of surgery. A review of predictive factors. Anesthesiology 2000;93:1123–33.

[81] Perucca E. An introduction to antiepileptic drugs. Epilepsia 2005;46(Suppl 4):31–7.

[82] Placidi F, Diomedi M, Scalise A, Marciani MG, Romigi A, Gigli GL. Effect of anticonvulsants on nocturnal sleep in epilepsy. Neurology 2000;54(Suppl 1):S25–32.

[83] PROSPECT: procedure-specific postoperative pain management. Available at: http://www.postoppain.org. Accessed April 2010.

[84] Rahimi R, Nikfar S, Rezaie A, Abdollahi M. Efficacy of tricyclic antide-pressants in irritable bowel syndrome: a meta-analysis. World J Gastro-enterol 2009;15:1548–53.

[85] Raja SN, Haythornthwaite JA, Pappagallo M, Clark MR, Travison TG, Sabeen S, Royall RM, Max MB. Opioids versus antidepressants in postherpetic neuralgia: a randomized, placebo-controlled trial. Neurol-ogy 2002;59:1015–21.

[86] Recla JM, Sarantopoulos CD. Combined use of pregabalin and meman-tine in fibromyalgia syndrome treatment: a novel analgesic and neuro-protective strategy? Med Hypotheses 2009;73:177–83.

[87] Richards IM, Fraser SM, Hunter JA, Capell HA. Comparison of phe-nytoin and gold as second line drugs in rheumatoid arthritis. Ann Rheum Dis 1987;46:667–9.

[88] Romanò CL, Romanò D, Bonora C, Mineo G. Pregabalin, celecoxib, and their combination for treatment of chronic low-back pain. J Or-thop Traumatol 2009;10:185–91.

[89] Saarto T, Wiffen PJ. Antidepressants for neuropathic pain. Cochrane Database Syst Rev 2007;4:CD005454.

[90] Salerno SM, Browning R, Jackson JL. The effect of antidepressant treatment on chronic back pain: a meta-analysis. Arch Intern Med 2002;162:19–24.

[91] Sator-Katzenschlager SM, Scharbert G, Kress HG, Frickey N, Ellend A, Gleiss A, Kozek-Langenecker SA. Chronic pelvic pain treated with ga-bapentin and amitriptyline: a randomized controlled pilot study. Wien Klin Wochenschr 2005;117:761–8.

[92] Schug SA, Manopas A. Update on the role of non-opioids for postop-erative pain treatment. Best Pract Res Clin Anaesthesiol 2007;21:15–30.

[93] Semenchuk MR, Sherman S, Davis B. Double-blind, randomized trial of bupropion SR for the treatment of neuropathic pain. Neurology 2001;57:1583–8.

[94] Shekelle PG, Woolf SH, Eccles M, Grimshaw J. Clinical guidelines: de-veloping guidelines. BMJ 1999;318:593–6.

[95] Shlay JC, Chaloner K, Max MB, Flaws B, Reichelderfer P, Wentworth D, Hillman S, Brizz B, Cohn DL. Acupuncture and amitriptyline for pain due to HIV-related peripheral neuropathy: a randomized controlled trial. Terry Beirn Community Programs for Clinical Research on AIDS. JAMA 1998;280:1590–5.

[96] Shorvon SD. Drug treatment of epilepsy in the century of the ILAE: the first 50 years, 1909–1958. Epilepsia 2009;50(Suppl 3):69–92.

[97] Sindrup SH, Gram LF, Brøsen K, Eshøj O, Mogensen EF. The selective serotonin reuptake inhibitor paroxetine is effective in the treatment of diabetic neuropathy symptoms. Pain 1990;42:135–44.

[98] Strassels SA, Chen C, Carr DB. Postoperative analgesia: economics, resource use, and patient satisfaction in an urban teaching hospital. Anesth Analg 2002;94:130–7.

[99] Sullivan MD, Robinson JP. Antidepressant and anticonvulsant medica-tion for chronic pain. Phys Med Rehabil Clin N Am 2006;17:381–400.

[100] Sullivan M, Bentley S, Fan MY, Gardner G. A single-blind placebo run-in study of venlafaxine XR for activity-limiting osteoarthritis pain. Pain Med 2009;10:806–12.

[101] Sun-Edelstein C, Tepper SJ, Shapiro RE. Drug-induced serotonin syn-drome: a review. Expert Opin Drug Saf 2008;7:587–96.

[102] Urquhart DM, Hoving JL, Assendelft WW, Roland M, van Tulder MW. Antidepressants for non-specific low back pain. Cochrane Database Syst Rev 2008;1:CD001703.

[103] Vedula SS, Bero L, Scherer RW, Dickersin K. Outcome reporting in industry-sponsored trials of gabapentin for off-label use. N Engl J Med 2009;361:1963–71.

[104] von Delius S, Eckel F, Wagenpfeil S, Mayr M, Stock K, Kullmann F, Obermeier F, Erdmann J, Schmelz M, Quasthoff S, Adelsberger H, Bredenkamp R, Schmid RM, Lersch C. Carbamazepine for prevention of oxaliplatin-related neurotoxicity in patients with advanced colorectal cancer: final results of a randomised, controlled, multicenter phase II study. Invest New Drugs 2007;25:173–80.

[105] Wall PD. The prevention of postoperative pain. Pain 1988;33:289–90.

[106] Watson CP, Evans RJ, Reed K, Merskey H, Goldsmith L, Warsh J. Amitriptyline versus placebo in postherpetic neuralgia. Neurology 1982;32:671–3.

[107] Watson CPN, et. al. Antidepressant analgesics: a systematic review and comparative study. In: McMahon SB, Koltzenburg M, editors. Wall and Melzack's textbook of pain. London: Elsevier; 2006. p. 481.

[108] Watson CP, Gilron I, Sawynok J. A qualitative systematic review of head-to-head randomized controlled trials of oral analgesics in neuro-pathic pain. Pain Res Manage 2010; in press.

[109] Webb HE, Lascelles RG. Treatment of facial and head pain associated with depression. Lancet 1962;1:355–6.

[110] Wiffen P, Collins S, McQuay H, Carroll D, Jadad A, Moore A. Anticon-vulsant drugs for acute and chronic pain. Cochrane Database Syst Rev 2005;3:CD001133.

[111] Wiffen PJ, Moore RA, Derry S, McQuay HJ. Gabapentin for chronic neuropathic pain in adults (Protocol). Cochrane Database Syst Rev 2009;3:CD007938.

[112] Wolf S, Barton D, Kottschade L, Grothey A, Loprinzi C. Chemother-apy-induced peripheral neuropathy: prevention and treatment strate-gies. Eur J Cancer 2008;44:1507–15.

[113] Wolfe F, Ross K, Anderson J, Russell IJ, Hebert L. The prevalence and characteristics of fibromyalgia in the general population. Arthritis Rheum 1995;38:19–28.

[114] Wolfe F. Fibromyalgia wars. J Rheumatol 2009;36:671–8.

[115] Yaksi A, Ozgönenel L, Ozgönenel B. The efficiency of gabapentin therapy in patients with lumbar spinal stenosis. Spine (Phila Pa 1976) 2007;32:939–42.

Correspondence to: Ian Gilron, MD, MSc, FRCPC, Director, Clinical Pain Research, Departments of Anesthesiology and Pharmacology & Toxicology, Queen's University, Kingston General Hospital, 76 Stuart Street, Kingston, ON K7L 2V7, Canada. Email: gilroni@queensu.ca.

Clinical Pharmacology of Opioids in the Treatment of Pain

Eija Kalso, MD, DMedSci

*Department of Pain Medicine, University of Helsinki, Institute of Clinical Medicine; Pain Clinic,
Department of Anesthesiology, Intensive Care Medicine, Emergency Medicine and Pain Medicine,
Helsinki University Central Hospital, Helsinki, Finland*

Opioids are still important analgesics in the management of acute and chronic pain. They can be very effective and also safe if they are used wisely, with a thorough understanding of their pharmacology. Opioids have highly variable individual effects. Recent advances in pharmacogenetics have significantly increased our understanding of these differences. Several opioids and different routes of administration are available today for clinical use. Opioids often cause adverse effects that can be serious. In order to improve the efficacy of opioid analgesia, new strategies have been introduced. These strategies include increased use of analgesic drug combinations. This chapter will discuss the use of opioids in acute and chronic pain. It will provide up-to-date information regarding the pharmacokinetic and pharmacogenetic differences among opioids and provide examples of how these differences can lead to rare but potentially serious complications or lack of efficacy. This chapter will also discuss guidelines that have been introduced to improve patient selection and follow-up for chronic opioid administration.

The endogenous opioid networks are involved in regulating a multitude of physiological functions, from mood to guts. It is essential to understand what kinds of effects opioids may have in both acute and in chronic administration. Respiratory depression and nausea are important adverse effects when opioids are used to treat acute pain, whereas constipation, cognitive impairment, hormonal effects, addiction, and tolerance are relevant concerns in chronic opioid administration.

Pain and opioid effects show significant interindividual variation. Recent advances in the genetics of opioid receptors and peptides, and in the pharmacokinetics of opioids, have increased our understanding of this variation. This information can be used to improve effective and safe use of opioids in the management of pain, and it also offers possibilities for improving opioid efficacy and reversing opioid tolerance.

Endogenous Opioid Systems

Opioid receptors are G-protein-coupled receptors. They and their endogenous ligands modulate numerous physiological functions such as nociception, mood, reward, learning, stress response, hormonal functions, appetite, sleep, immune function, and gastrointestinal function. Three receptor classes—mu (MOR), delta (DOR), and kappa (KOR)—have been described by pharmacological approaches. These receptors have been cloned, and their genes have been characterized in both mice and humans. A homologous receptor, ORL-1, is considered to be part of an anti-opioid system involved, for example, in the development of tolerance.

Studies with MOR-deficient mice [22] indicate that MOR is the major molecular target for morphine in vivo, mediating analgesia, place preference (reward), physical dependence, respiratory depression, and immunosuppression. DOR activity has been shown to affect mood states (DOR-deficient mice show more anxiety and depression), whereas KORs have a prominent role in the perception of visceral pain.

Opioid receptors are located throughout the central and peripheral nervous system. Opioid receptors in the dorsal horn of the spinal cord have a central role in the modulation of pain, which is also the basis for spinal administration of opioids to produce segmental analgesia. Opioid receptors in the brainstem are involved in the regulation of arousal, respiration, and both anti- and pronociceptive effects. Opioid receptors are found almost everywhere in the cerebral cortex and cerebellum. In the periphery, opioids are involved in the regulation of gastrointestinal function. Activation of MORs in the gut leads to increased absorption of water from the stools and spasticity of the gut. Opioid receptors in the peripheral nervous system are regulated by inflammation and by the immune system.

Opioids in the Clinic: Alleviation of Acute and Chronic Pain

Opioids remain the main analgesics in the treatment of moderate-to-severe acute pain and cancer pain. They have a restricted role in the management of other chronic pains.

Acute Postoperative and Other Trauma-Related Pain

Opioids are usually added to nonopioid analgesics such as acetaminophen (paracetamol) and nonsteroidal anti-inflammatory drugs (NSAIDs). Other adjuvant analgesics such as corticosteroids [56], ketamine [4], and gabapentin or pregabalin [64] are increasingly used to improve analgesia and reduce opioid-related adverse effects as part of a multimodal analgesia strategy. Short-acting opioids (e.g., remifentanil, sufentanil, fentanyl, and alfentanil) are usually administered intravenously (i.v.) perioperatively. Patient-controlled analgesia (PCA) can be used postoperatively to optimize analgesia because interindividual variation is considerable. Oral administration is preferred when feasible. Mild-to-moderate pain can be alleviated with codeine combinations or tramadol. Oral oxycodone and morphine are available for moderate-to-severe pain. Tapentadol is a new mu-opioid receptor agonist

and norepinephrine reuptake inhibitor that was approved by the U.S. Food and Drug Administration in 2008 for the treatment of moderate-to-severe acute pain [68]. Several other opioids are also used (e.g., ketobemidone, piritramide), but these more unusual opioids will not be discussed in this chapter.

Spinal opioid analgesia is used for major surgery. Morphine is used both for subarachnoid and epidural administration, whereas fentanyl is used to improve epidural analgesia with local anesthetic agents. Opioids are also administered locally, even though the effectiveness of this method has not been confirmed [25].

Cancer-Related Pain

Opioids are the main analgesics in cancer pain, even though other drugs (e.g., NSAIDs in bone-related pain and inflammation) and drugs that are used to treat neuropathic pain have an important role as well. Controlled-release formulations (e.g., morphine, oxycodone, oxymorphone, and hydromorphone orally and fentanyl/buprenorphine transdermally) are used to provide stable pain relief. Faster-acting formulations of oral morphine or oxycodone and very fast-acting transmucosal fentanyl formulations (lozenges, buccal tablets, and intranasal sprays) are used for breakthrough pain [66]. If oral administration is not feasible, opioids can be administered transdermally or subcutaneously. Spinal opioids can also be used. The use of opioids in cancer-related pain is mostly empirical and is based on guidelines provided by the World Health Organization (WHO) and expert panels [20]. Most clinical studies on opioids in cancer pain are equivalence trials [5].

Opioids for Chronic Noncancer Pain

Most of the increase in the worldwide consumption of opioids has been in chronic noncancer pain, even though this is the most controversial indication. Several systematic reviews have indicated short-term efficacy of opioids (for up to 3 months) in both osteoarthritis-related and neuropathic pain [2,27,15]. Both weak and strong opioids outperformed placebo for pain and function in all types of pain [16]. Mean pain relief with strong opioids in these studies was about 30% in both neuropathic and osteoarthritis pain when mean daily doses of 40 mg of oxycodone and 80–100 mg of morphine were used [27]. Interindividual variation has been considerable, and these randomized and controlled short-term studies can be considered to represent the best that can be achieved with opioids in an ideal patient population. Musculoskeletal pains other than osteoarthritis have not shown long-term benefit from opioids [34]. Opioids may be efficacious for short-term pain relief for back pain, whereas their long-term efficacy is unclear. Aberrant medication-taking behaviors have reported to occur in up to 24% of back pain patients [43].

The biggest hurdle in the long-term management of chronic pain with opioids is risk-benefit estimation and analysis; some risks, such as opioid addiction, are rare but difficult to predict and hard to treat. Several risk assessment tools have been developed for opioid misuse by chronic pain patients [65].

Guidelines regarding the role of opioids in the treatment of various chronic painful conditions [1,58] or chronic opioid treatment in general [8,10,26] have been published. They have been written by expert panels that have used the evidence available.

Basic Pharmacology of Opioids: Relevance for Clinical Use

Opioid Receptor-Binding Profiles and Nonopioid Effects

Morphine, oxycodone, oxymorphone, methadone, and fentanyl are all MOR agonists in doses that are commonly used to treat pain in the clinic (see Table I). Differences exist, however, among these opioids in their capacity to activate the MORs in different parts of the brain and spinal cord [62]. For example, oxycodone poorly activates the MORs in the spinal cord [37],

which may explain why it is not an effective analgesic when administered spinally [3,54].

Some opioids have nonopioid effects that are relevant for their analgesic profile. Racemic methadone is commonly used in the clinic. It consists of two enantiomers (l- and d-), both of which have been described to be noncompetitive N-methyl-D-aspartate (NMDA)-receptor antagonists, using the same binding site as MK-801. It is l-methadone that is responsible for the MOR effects, whereas d-methadone is only a weak opioid agonist. The activation of the NMDA-receptor/channel complex at the spinal level and in the brain is related to the activation of the excitatory glutamatergic nociceptive pathway.

Tramadol is also used as a racemate. The parent compound has only very weak affinity to the MOR. Weak opioid analgesia is mediated by the M1 (O-desmethyltramadol) metabolite, which has a 200-fold greater affinity to the MOR than tramadol and also inhibits the reuptake of both norepinephrine and serotonin [13].

Tapentadol binds with a 10-fold greater affinity to the rat MOR compared with DOR and KOR receptors, but morphine has a 50 times greater affinity to the MOR than tapentadol [66]. At the human recombinant MOR, tapentadol had a similar K_i of 0.16 mM as at the native rat MOR. In the human MOR [^{35}S]GTPγS binding assay, tapentadol showed agonistic efficacy that was 88% relative to that of morphine. Tapentadol is also a norepinephrine reuptake inhibitor. Its binding affinity in the human recombinant monoamine transporter binding assay is similar to that of venlafaxine but only about 1/600 of that of duloxetine [66].

Table I
Competitive displacement (Ki) of [^{3}H]-diprenorphine from its binding to membranes prepared from cultured cells expressing MOR, DOR, and KOR subtypes by oxycodone, oxymorphone, and morphine, and opioid receptor subtype-specific ligands (DAMGO for MOR, DPDPE for DOR, and U50.488 for KOR)

| Ligand | [^{3}H]-Diprenorphine Displacement (K_i) (nmol/L) | | | [^{35}S]GTPγS Binding to hMOR1 | |
	hMOR1	mDOR1	hKOR1	EC$_{50}$ (nmol/L)	E$_{max}$ (%)
Oxycodone	16.0 ± 2.9	>1000	>1000	343 ± 7.9	234
Oxymorphone	0.36 ± 0.01	118 ± 20	148 ± 17	42.8 ± 0.8	261
Morphine	3.19 ± 0.43			94.2 ± 1.9	252
DAMGO	0.21 ± 0.03			96.6 ± 1.4	315
DPDPE		2.0 ± 0.8			
U50,488			0.78 ± 0.31		
Fentanyl*	0.67 ± 0.19	91.6 ± 3.89	77.2 ± 6.38		
Methadone*	1.89 ± 0.3	76.1 ± 1.73	299.8 ± 66.7		

Source: Adapted from [35] and [70].
Abbreviations: DOR, delta-opioid receptor; EC$_{50}$, half-maximal effective concentration; h, human; KOR, kappa-opioid receptor; m, mouse; MOR, mu-opioid receptor.
* Mouse only, with a different experimental design.

Pharmacokinetic Aspects

Physicochemical Properties, Absorption, and Transport

Two factors—the relative lipophilicity and the degree of ionization at physiological pH—affect the rate and extent of transmembrane flux and binding to receptors. The pKa controls the extent of ionization at a particular pH; it varies from 76% for morphine to 99% for methadone. Table II shows that fentanyl is highly lipophilic, whereas morphine is hydrophilic. Thus, fentanyl passes through lipid-rich membranes more easily than morphine. This property explains why fentanyl is readily absorbed through the skin and mucous membranes and why morphine has a long half-life in the cerebrospinal fluid after a subarachnoid injection. It also explains why i.v. fentanyl is better for rapid titration of analgesia in severe pain compared with morphine: the peak effect of i.v. morphine may take several minutes because the transfer of morphine across the blood-brain barrier takes several minutes. The potential for overdosing may arise if the long lag period is not appreciated [39].

Table II
The calculated logarithmic octanol/water
partition coefficients (C$_{log}$D) of opioids at 25°C

	C$_{log}$D		
	pH 7.0	pH 7.4	pH 8.0
Morphine	-0.85	-0.49	-0.04
Oxymorphone	0.19	0.47	0.72
Oxycodone	0.98	1.26	1.52
Fentanyl	1.86	2.27	2.79
Sufentanil	2.12	2.52	2.94

Source: Modified from [38].

Several other factors can affect the absorption of drugs through different membranes. Transdermal administration requires a lipophilic opioid (fentanyl or buprenorphine). Fentanyl is absorbed from a patch in relation to its surface area. A fentanyl depot is formed in the upper layers of the skin (the stratum corneum), from which the drug then passively diffuses into the dermis, where it is taken up into the microcirculation to finally reach the systemic circulation. Any factors that increase skin perfusion (e.g., fever, sauna) will increase absorption of fentanyl, whereas the opposite is true when skin perfusion is reduced (cachexia, hypovolemia, or vasoconstriction). In cancer patients, absorption from fentanyl patches has varied from 18% to

100% [60]. In cachectic patients, absorption of fentanyl is decreased by 50% compared with patients who have a normal body mass index [23].

Opioids can be transported across membranes by various transporter proteins such as P-glycoprotein (MDR1a). The substrates of P-glycoprotein include morphine, fentanyl, and methadone [63,69]. In the intestine, P-glycoprotein limits the absorption of substrate drugs by transporting them back from enterocytes into the gut lumen. In the brain, the P-glycoprotein transport system sends a wide range of pharmacologically active compounds to the systemic circulation. Animal studies have shown that inhibition of P-glycoprotein markedly enhances the antinociceptive effects of morphine [69]. Morphine, methadone, and fentanyl also induced greater antinociception in P-glycoprotein knockout mice compared with wild-type mice [63]. Controversy exists regarding the role of P-glycoprotein in oxycodone pharmacokinetics [7,21]. In humans, the relevance of P-glycoprotein modulation is unclear. No clinically relevant changes in the pharmacodynamics of morphine, methadone, or fentanyl have been shown in various studies, even though plasma opioid concentrations have significantly increased [29,30,59]. However, these studies were performed in healthy volunteers using low doses of opioids. Several drugs (e.g., itraconazole, cyclosporine A, verapamil, and HIV protease inhibitors) are relatively potent inhibitors of P-glycoprotein and could potentially increase the effects of morphine and methadone. P-glycoprotein inhibition could thus, at least in theory, be used to improve morphine efficacy. Certain pathological states can also affect P-glycoprotein. The proinflammatory cytokine tumor necrosis factor has upregulated P-glycoprotein in cerebral endothelial cells, resulting in reduced cellular uptake of drugs [71].

Active transport through the blood-brain barrier has been suggested as one explanation as to why oxycodone has good analgesic efficacy, even though it is a relatively weak MOR agonist compared with morphine. Concentrations of oxycodone are higher in the brain compared to the plasma, whereas the reverse is true with morphine [7].

Metabolism, Excretion, and Drug Interactions

The main pharmacokinetic parameters of some commonly used opioids are shown in Table III. The clearance of most opioids is high, and hepatic blood flow is important for the rate of metabolism. For these opioids,

Table III
Pharmacokinetic aspects of opioids

Opioid	Terminal Half-Life (h)	Clearance (L/min)	Oral Bio-availability (%)	Main Metabolic Pathway	Active Metabolites
Morphine	2–4	0.8–1.2	19–47	UGT1A1;2B7	M6G
Methadone	4–130	0.1–0.3	60–90	CYP 3A4/5;2D6;1A2;2B6;2C19	None
Fentanyl	4–8	0.7–1.5	<2/90 (t.d.)	CYP 3A4/5	None
Oxycodone	3.5 ± 0.8	0.4–1.1	40–130	CYP 3A4/5;2D6	Oxymorphone
Hydromorphone	2–4	0.4	35–80	UGT1A1;2B7	None
Codeine	3–4	0.6–0.9	60–90	CYP 2D6;3A4/5	Morphine
Tramadol	5–6		75	CYP 2D6;3A4/5	M1
Buprenorphine	20–25		70 (s.l.)	CYP3A4/5 and UGT1A1;2B7	

Abbreviations: s.l. = sublingual; t.d. = transdermal.

hepatic function must be severely compromised before their pharmacokinetics are influenced. The clearance of methadone is much lower (see Table III); therefore, its metabolism can be either stimulated or inhibited by other drugs that influence CYP3A4 activity (see below). Elimination half-life is an important parameter as it will indicate, for example, when a steady state is reached with the drug. As five half-lives are needed for steady state, it can be calculated that for morphine it will take from 10 to 20 hours to reach a steady state, whereas for methadone it may take anywhere between 20 and 650 hours.

Most opioids are metabolized in the liver by glucuronidation and/or demethylation (dealkylation) catalyzed by CYP450 isoenzymes, mainly 2D6 and 3A4. At least for morphine, hydromorphone, and buprenorphine, glucuronidation is a major metabolic pathway. Human UDP-glucuronosyltransferases (e.g., UGT1A1 and UGT2B7, which are relevant in morphine and buprenorphine metabolism) are polymorphic but not inducible. Evidence for reduced morphine glucuronidation in the presence of UGT2B7-840G was recently shown in a population of sickle cell patients with a high frequency of this variant allele (0.7) [11].

The CYP2D6 isoenzyme is polymorphic and under genetic control. The clinical relevance of this fact is that poor metabolizers will not metabolize codeine to the active metabolite morphine, and thus they do not experience analgesia from codeine [53]. On the other hand, ultrarapid metabolizers produce morphine efficiently, which can lead to overdosing, particularly in the presence of other factors such as kidney failure [17]. Analgesia from tramadol is reduced in poor metabolizers and if CYP2D6 is inhibited by

paroxetine. There is another important reason why paroxetine and fluoxetine should not be coadministered with tramadol. Tramadol increases the availability of serotonin (and norepinephrine), whereas its main metabolite M1 (CYP2D6) is responsible for its opioid activity. The selective serotonin reuptake inhibitors fluoxetine and paroxetine are potent inhibitors of CYP2D, and they have a long half-life. The combination of either of these drugs with tramadol will inhibit the metabolism of tramadol and increase its serotonergic activity, potentially leading to serotonin syndrome (tremors, restlessness, fever, and confusion). This interaction is also possible with other drugs that increase the availability of serotonin, but the likelihood is reduced unless other drugs or pharmaco-genetic factors cause an additional risk [42].

CYP3A4 is inducible. Induction of CYP3A4 by rifampicin, carbamazepine, or protease inhibitors (lopinavir/ritonavir) [44] will increase the metabolism of methadone and thus reduce its efficacy. Higher doses of methadone would be needed to maintain analgesia. On the other hand, inhibition of CYP3A4 by drugs such as ciprofloxacin can lead to serious methadone toxicity [24]. Similar interactions could be anticipated with buprenorphine, which is also a CYP3A4 substrate [45].

The main (90%) metabolic pathway of oxycodone is through N-demethylation catalyzed by CYP3A4 to noroxycodone, which is inactive. CYP3A4 inhibitors such as itraconazole and grapefruit will increase the exposure to oxycodone [49,57], whereas induction of CYP3A4 by rifampicin, for example, will reduce oxycodone's efficacy [48]. Less than 10% of the drug's metabolism is through O-demethylation catalyzed by CYP2D6 to oxymorphone, which is several times more potent as an analgesic than oxycodone. However, because of the very small amount of oxymorphone produced, it is unlikely that blocking CYP2D6 would change oxycodone analgesia [22,35].

Opioids undergo extensive hepatic biotransformation, and their metabolites are excreted renally. If these metabolites are active (such as morphine-6β-glucuronide), compromised renal function may lead to opioid toxicity. In patients with significantly reduced renal function, lipophilic opioids that do not have active metabolites, such as buprenorphine, fentanyl, and methadone, should be considered, whereas hydrophilic opioids like morphine and codeine that have active metabolites should be avoided. Tramadol, hydromorphone, and oxycodone can be used only with caution and close monitoring of the patient [14,50].

Pharmacogenetics and Interindividual Variability in Opioid Response

Several polymorphisms of genes have been shown to affect opioid efficacy [38]. The best-known clinically relevant polymorphisms include those modulating the activity of MOR (*OPRM1* gene variant 118A>G). The effects of opioids have been shown to be decreased in carriers of the variant 118G allele. This effect has been shown, for example, with morphine and morphine-6β-glucuronide [60], and with levomethadone [41].

Cancer patients who carried the variant of the catechol-*O*-methyl transferase (*COMT*) gene coded by the 472G>A single-nucleotide polymorphism (SNP) needed less morphine than patients who did not carry this variant [55]. The 472G>A SNP leads to a low-function *COMT* along with higher dopamine tone and upregulation of opioid receptors, which has been suggested to explain the difference in morphine consumption.

The functional impairment of P-glycoprotein transport may result in increased bioavailability of orally administered opioids or may increase their brain concentrations, as was described above. A diplotype of three SNP positions in the *ABCB1* gene that encodes P-glycoprotein was associated with clinically relevant increased effects of fentanyl [51]. A combination of two polymorphisms, both of which affect the pharmacokinetics of morphine, may have a robust effect on morphine analgesia. In a study on morphine

analgesia in cancer pain patients, SNP 3435C>T of the *ABCB1* gene and 80A>G of the *OPRM1* gene both caused significant variability in morphine responses. When the extreme genotypes of both genes (associated with either good or poor morphine analgesia) were combined, the association between patient polymorphism and pain relief was strong enough to allow the detection of strong responders, responders, and nonresponders [9].

Variants of the *CYP2D6* gene may have significant effects on the analgesic efficacy of opioids that are metabolized via this enzyme pathway. The analgesic efficacy of codeine (a prodrug) depends on its *O*-demethylation to morphine. Ultrarapid metabolizers who have a *CYP2D6* gene duplication form higher amounts of morphine and can have an exaggerated opioid effect, whereas poor metabolizers who lack CYP2D6 activity have poor analgesia from codeine [32]. Ultrarapid metabolism of codeine to morphine can lead to life-threatening opioid intoxication with low daily doses (75 mg) of codeine if other enzymatic pathways are concomitantly inhibited and the patient has renal insufficiency [11]. The effects of CYP2D6 activity on oxycodone metabolism are minor. Some effect has been shown in experimental pain models [72], whereas no effect was seen in postoperative analgesia by oxycodone [73].

CYP2D6 genotyping should be considered in patients who have unexpected responses to drugs that are metabolized via CYP2D6 (e.g., codeine, tramadol, and many antidepressants) and if drug combinations with potential for adverse effects such as serotonin syndrome are considered.

Modes and Routes of Administration

Different physicochemical and other properties of opioids can be considered when designing opioids for special routes and modes of administration. Morphine and noroxymorphone [38] are hydrophilic opioids that stay for a long time in the compartment where they have been administered. Both morphine and noroxymorphone are suitable for intrathecal administration, as they will stay in the subarachnoid space and will not escape into the blood circulation, unlike lipophilic opioids such as fentanyl. Loperamide is another example of a hydrophilic opioid that penetrates the blood-brain barrier very poorly. It can thus be used as an antidiarrheal agent because it has virtually no central nervous system effects.

Lipophilic drugs such as fentanyl can be administered through various membranes (skin and mucous membranes). As its first-pass metabolism is very high, and consequently its oral bioavailability is very low (see Table III), it cannot be taken orally. Transdermal administration has been developed to enable slow onset with stable concentrations for nearly 3 days [19]. As analgesic concentrations are first achieved after 12–16 hours, this mode of administration should be used only when stable known doses of opioids are indicated. Buprenorphine is another lipophilic opioid that can be administered transdermally [33]. Transdermal buprenorphine is available in patches (5–20 μg/h) that provide stable concentrations over 7 days.

Pharmaceutical technology has developed various sustained- or modified-release formulations that provide fairly stable plasma concentrations with once- or twice-daily oral dosing. Such formulations have been developed for morphine, oxycodone, oxymorphone, hydromorphone, and tramadol. Usually the time to maximum plasma drug concentration (T_{max}) is 2–4 hours [18]. Normal- or immediate-release formulations are used if faster onset is needed, with a T_{max} of 30–60 minutes.

Transmucosal administration has been developed for rapid relief of breakthrough pain and procedural pain. Hardened lozenge formulations of fentanyl have been available for several years, whereas buccal fentanyl tablets were introduced more recently [12]. The fastest onset of effect is, however, achieved with intranasal fentanyl sprays [47].

Treatment of Opioid-Induced Adverse Effects

As described at the beginning of this chapter, opioids regulate many physiological functions and can therefore cause various adverse effects. Titrating the dose—balancing between analgesia and adverse effects—is the challenge for managing pain with opioids.

Acute administration of opioids can cause respiratory depression, sedation, nausea, and vomiting. Pain stimulates the respiratory center, and opioids counterbalance this adverse effect if titration of the dose is successful. Patients who have central sleep apnea have increased sensitivity to opioid-induced respiratory depression [6]. In the absence of pain, tolerance usually develops to opioid-induced respiratory depression. Respiratory depression, like all opioid-mediated effects, can be reversed with opioid-receptor antagonists such as naloxone.

Nausea and vomiting are often the dose-limiting adverse effects of opioids, particularly in the treatment of acute pain. Opioids can cause emesis by direct stimulation of the chemoreceptor trigger zone (CTZ) or the vestibular apparatus, and through inhibition of gut motility [52]. The CTZ is stimulated by opioid receptor activation, and signaling to the vomiting center occurs primarily via dopamine D_2 receptors. Butyrophenones such as haloperidol and droperidol act as antiemetics by blocking D_2 receptors. The vestibular apparatus is stimulated directly by opioids, and the sensory input to the vomiting center occurs via the histamine H_1 and cholinergic ACh_m pathways. This explains why antihistamines and anticholinergic agents are effective against nausea that is aggravated by movement. Inhibition of gut motility causes emesis through serotonergic signaling to the vomiting center. This can be blocked by $5HT_3$-receptor antagonists.

Tolerance does not usually develop to constipation, which is a major problem, particularly in long-term opioid administration. The fact that opioids cause constipation mainly through peripheral opioid receptors offers the possibility of treating constipation by blocking peripheral opioid receptors in the gut, by means of an opioid antagonist that either does not penetrate the blood-brain barrier (methylnaltrexone) or that is efficiently metabolized during first-pass metabolism in the liver (naloxone) [46].

Opioids have significant effects on the endocrine system. The effects are reversible after acute use, but they persist and may cause serious symptoms if they are not diagnosed and treated in chronic opioid administration [28]. Long-term opioid therapy can cause hypogonadism via central suppression of hypothalamic secretion of gonadotropin-releasing hormone, decreased pituitary luteinizing hormone, decreased adrenal dehydroepiandrosterone and testosterone, decreased estradiol and progesterone in women, and decreased testicular testosterone in men. Symptoms of opioid-induced hypogonadism include loss of libido, infertility, fatigue, depression, anxiety, loss of muscle strength and mass, osteoporosis, impotence, and menstrual irregularities. Monitoring of hormone levels and hormone supplementation when indicated should be considered in chronic opioid therapy.

Conclusions

Even though the currently available opioids are mu-opioid receptor agonists, they have significant differences in their pharmacokinetic parameters that need to be considered relative to the individual features of pain patients. Pharmaceutical design has produced alternative routes of administration that enable tailor-made opioid analgesia for the treatment of acute and chronic pain. Good understanding of basic clinical pharmacology of opioids is necessary for the effective and safe use of these possibilities for the benefit of our patients.

References

[1] Attal N, Cruccu G, Baron R, Haanpää M, Hansson P, Jensen TS, Nurmikko T. FENS guidelines on the pharmacological treatment of neuropathic pain: 2009 revision. Eur J Neurol 2010; Epub Apr 9.

[2] Avouac J, Gossec L, Dougados M. Efficacy and safety of opioids for osteoarthritis: a meta-analysis of randomized controlled trials. Osteoarthritis Cartilage 2007;15:957–65.

[3] Backlund M, Lindgren L, Kajimoto Y, Rosenberg PH. Comparison of epidural morphine and oxycodone for pain after abdominal surgery. J Clin Anesth 1997;9:30–5.

[4] Bell RF, Dahl JB, Moore RA, Kalso E. Perioperative ketamine for acute postoperative pain. A quantitative systematic review. Acta Anaesthesiol Scand 2005;49:1405–28.

[5] Bell RF, Wisløff T, Eccleston C, Kalso E. Controlled clinical trials in cancer pain. How controlled should they be? A qualitative systematic review. Br J Cancer 2006;94:1559–67.

[6] Bernards CM, Knowlton SL, Schmidt DF, DePaso WJ, Lee MK, McDonald SB, Bains OS. Respiratory and sleep effects of remifentanil in volunteers with moderate obstructive sleep apnea. Anesthesiology 2009;110:41–9.

[7] Boström E, Simonsson USH, Hammarlund-Udenaes M. In vivo blood-brain barrier transport of oxycodone in the rat: indications for active influx and implications for pharmacokinetics/pharmacodynamics. Drug Metab Dispos 2006;34:1624–31.

[8] British Pain Society with Royal College of Psychiatrists and Royal College of General Practitioners. Opioids for persistent pain: good practice (2010). Available at: http://britishpainsociety.org/pub_professional.htm.

[9] Campa D, Gioia A, Tomei A, Poli P, Barale R. Association of ABCB1/MDR1 and OPRM1 gene polymorphisms with morphine pain relief. Clin Pharmacol Ther 2008;83:559–66.

[10] Chou R, Fanciullo GJ, Fine PG, Adler JA, Ballantyne JC, Davies P, Donovan MI, Fishbain DA, Foley KM, Fudin J, et al.; American Pain Society-American Academy of Pain Medicine Opioids Guidelines Panel. Clinical guidelines for the use of chronic opioid therapy in chronic noncancer pain. J Pain 2009;10:113–30.

[11] Darbari DS, van Schaik RHN, Capparelli EV, Rana S, McCarter R, van den Anker J. UGT2B7 promoter variant -840g>A contributes to the variability in hepatic clearance of morphine in patients with sickle cell disease. Am J Hematol 2008;83:200–2.

[12] Darwish M, Kirby M, Robertson P, Tracewell W, Jiang JG. Absolute and relative bioavailability of fentanyl buccal tablet and oral transmucosal fentanyl citrate. J Clin Pharmacol 2007;47:343–50.

[13] Dayer P, Desmeules J, Collart L. Pharmacologie du tramadol. Drugs 1997;53:18–24.

[14] Dean M. Opioids in renal failure. J Pain Symptom Manage 2004;28:497–504.

[15] Eisenberg E, McNicol ED, Carr DB. Efficacy and safety of opioid agonists in the treatment of neuropathic pain of non-malignant origin. Systematic review and mat-analysis of randomized controlled trials. JAMA 2005;293:3043–52.

[16] Furlan AD, Sandoval JA, Mailis-Gagnon A, Tunks E. Opioids for chronic noncancer pain: a meta-analysis of effectiveness and side effects. CMAJ 2006;174:1589–94.

[17] Gasche Y, Daali Y, Fathi M, Chiappe A, Cottini S, Dayer P, Desmeules J. Codeine intoxication associated with ultrarapid CYP2D6 metabolism. N Engl J Med 2004;351:2827–31.

[18] Gourlay GK. Sustained pain relief of chronic pain: pharmacokinetics of SR morphine. Clin Pharmacokin 1998;35:173–90.

[19] Gourlay GK. Treatment of cancer pain with transdermal fentanyl. Lancet Oncol 2001;2:165–72.

[20] Hanks GW, Conno F, Cherny N, Hanna M, Kalso E, McQuay HJ, Mercadante S, Meynadier J, Poulain P, Ripamonti C, Radbruch L, Casas JR, Sawe J, Twycross RG, Ventafridda V; Expert Working Group of the Research Network of the European Association for Palliative Care. Morphine and alternative opioids in cancer pain: the EAPC recommendations. Br J Cancer 2001;84:587–93.

[21] Hassan HE, Myers AL, Lee IJ, Coop A, Eddington ND. Oxycodone induces overexpression of P-glycoprotein (ABCB1) and affects paclitaxel's tissue distribution in Sprague Dawley rats. J Pharm Sci 2007;96:2494–506.

[22] Heiskanen T, Olkkola KT, Kalso E. Effects of blocking the CYP2D6 enzyme on the pharmacokinetics and pharmacodynamics of oxycodone. Clin Pharmacol Ther 1998;64:603–11.

[23] Heiskanen T, Mätzke S, Haakana S, Gergov M, Vuori E, Kalso E. Pharmacokinetics of transdermal fentanyl in normal and cachectic patients with cancer related pain. Pain 2009;144:218–22.

[24] Herrlin K, Segerdahl M, Gustafsson LL, Kalso E. Methadone, ciprofloxacin, and adverse drug reactions. The Lancet 2000;356:2069–70.

[25] Kalso E, Smith L, McQuay HJ, Moore RA. No pain, no gain: clinical excellence and scientific rigour: lessons learned from IA morphine. Pain 2002;98:269–75.

[26] Kalso E, Allan L, Dellemijn PLI, Faura CC, Ilias WK, Jensen TS et al. Recommendations for using opioids in chronic non-cancer pain. Eur J Pain 2003;7:381–6.

[27] Kalso E, Edwards J, Moore RA, McQuay HJ. Opioids in chronic non-cancer pain. A systematic review. Pain 2004;112:372–80.

[28] Katz N, Mazer NA. The impact of opioids on the endocrine system. Clin J Pain 2009;25:170–5.

[29] Kharasch ED, Hoffer C, Whittington D. The effect of quinidine, used as a probe for the involvement of P-glycoprotein, on the intestinal absorption and pharmacodynamics of methadone. Br J Clin Pharmacol 2004;57:600–10.

[30] Kharasch ED, Hoffer C, Altuntas TG, Whittington D. Quinidine as a probe for the role of P-glycoprotein in the intestinal absorption and clinical effects of fentanyl. J Clin Pharmacol 2004;44:224–33.

[31] Kieffer BL, Gavériaux-Ruff C. Exploring the opioid system by gene knock-out. Prog Neurobiol 2002;66:285–306.

[32] Kirchheiner J, Schmidt H, Tzvetkov M, Keulen J-THA, Lötsch J, Roots I, Brockmöller J. Pharmacokinetics of codeine and its metabolite morphine in ultra-rapid metabolizers due to CYP2D6 duplication. Pharmacogenomics J 2007;7:257–65.

[33] Kress HG. Clinical update on the pharmacology, efficacy and safety of transdermal buprenorphine. Eur J Pain 2009;13:219–30.

[34] Kroenke K, Krebs EE, Bair MJ. Pharmacotherapy of chronic pain: a synthesis of recommendations from systematic reviews. Gen Hosp Psychiatry 2009;31:206–19.

[35] Lalovic B, Kharasch E, Hoffer C, Risler L, Liu-Chen L-Y, Shen DD. Pharmacokinetics and pharmacodynamics of oral oxycodone in healthy human subjects: Role of circulating active metabolites. Clin Pharmacol Ther 2006;79:461–79.

[36] Laugesen S, Enggaard TP, Pedersen RS, Sindrup SH, Brosen K. Paroxetine, a cytochrome P450 2D6 inhibitor, diminishes the stereoselective O-demethylation and reduces the hypoalgesic effect of tramadol. Clin Pharmacol Ther 2005;77:312–23.

[37] Lemberg K, Kontinen VK, Siiskonen A, Viljakka K, Yli-Kauhaluoma J, Korpi E, Kalso E. Antinociceptive properties of oxycodone and its metabolites oxymorphone and noroxycodone in rats. Anesthesiology 2006;105:801–12.

[38] Lemberg KK, Siiskonen AO, Kontinen VK, Yli-Kauhaluoma JT, Kalso EA. Noroxymorphone: a novel opioid for spinal analgesia: Synthesis and pharmacological characterization. Anesth Analg 2008;106:463–70.

[39] Lötsch J, Dudziak R, Freynhagen R, Marschner J, Geisslinger G. Fatal respiratory depression after multiple intravenous morphine injections. Clin Pharmacokinet 2006;45:1051–60.

[40] Lötsch J, Geisslinger G. Current evidence for a genetic modulation of the response to analgesics. Pain 2006;121:1–5.

[41] Lötsch J, Skarke C, Wieting J, Oertel B, Schmidt H, Brockmöller J, Geisslinger G. Modulation of the central nervous effects of levomethadone by genetic polymorphism potentially affecting its metabolism, distribution, and drug action. Clin Pharmacol Ther 2006;79:72–89.

[42] Mahlberg R, Kunz D, Sasse J, Kirchheiner J. Serotonin syndrome with tramadol and citalopram. Am J Psychiatry 2004;161:1129.

[43] Martell BA, O'Connor PG, Kerns RD, Becker WC, Morales KH, Kosten TR, Flellin DA. Systematic review: Opioid treatment for chronic back pain: prevalence, efficacy, and association with addiction. Ann Intern Med 2007;146:116–27.

[44] McCance-Katz EF, Rainey P, Friedland G, Jatlow P. The protease inhibitor lopinavir/ritonavir may produce opiate withdrawal in methadone-maintained patients. Clin Infect Dis 2003;37:476–82.

[45] McCance-Katz EF, Moody DE, Morse GD, Ma Q, DiFrancesco R, Friedland G, Pade P, Rainey PM. Interaction between buprenorphine and atazanavir or atazanavir/ritonavir. Drug Alcohol Depend 2007;91:269–78.

[46] McNicol E, Boyce DB, Schumann R, Carr D. Efficacy and safety of mu-opioid antagonists in the treatment of opioid-induced bowel dysfunction: systematic review and meta-analysis of randomized controlled trials. Pain Med 2008;9:634–59.

[47] Mercadante S, Radbruch L, Davies A, Poulain P, Sitte T, Perkins P, Colberg T, Camba MA. A comparison of intranasal fentanyl spray with oral transmucosal fentanyl citrate for the treatment of breakthrough cancer pain: an open-label, randomized, crossover trial. Curr Med Res Opin 2009;25:2805–15.

[48] Nieminen TH, Hagelberg NM, Saari TI, Pertovaara A, Neuvonen M, Laine K, Neuvonen PJ, Olkkola KT. Rifampin greatly reduces the plasma concentrations of intravenous and oral oxycodone. Anesthesiology 2009;110:1371–8.

[49] Nieminen TH, Hagelberg NM, Saari TI, Neuvonen M, Neuvonen PJ, Laine K, Olkkola KT. Grapefruit juice enhances the exposure to oral oxycodone. Basic Clin Pharmacol Toxicol 2010; Epub Apr 15.

[50] Niscola P, Scaramucci L, Vischini G, Giovannini M, Ferrannini M, Massa P, Tatangelo P, Galletti M, Palumbo R. The use of major analgesics in patients with renal dysfunction. Curr Drug Targets 2010;11:752–8.

[51] Park HJ, Shinn HK, Ryu SH, Lee HS, Park CS, Kang JH. Genetic polymorphisms in the ABCB1 gene and the effects of fentanyl in Koreans. Clin Pharmacol Ther 2007;81:539–46.

[52] Porreca F, Ossipov MH. Nausea and vomiting side effects with opioid analgesics during treatment of chronic pain: mechanism implications and management options. Pain Med 2009;10:654–62.

[53] Poulsen L, Brosen K, Arendt-Nielsen L, Gram LF, Elbaek K, Sindrup SH. Codeine and morphine in extensive and poor metabolizers of sparteine: pharmacokinetics, analgesic effect and side effects. Eur J Clin Pharmacol 1996;51:289–95.

[54] Pöyhiä R, Kalso E. Antinociceptive effects and central nervous system depression caused by oxycodone and morphine in rats. Pharmacol Toxicol 1992;70:125–30.

[55] Rakvåg TT, Klepstad P, Baar C, Kvam TM, Dale O, Kaasa S, Krokan HE, Skorpen F. The Val158Met polymorphism of the human catechol-O-methyl-transferase (COMT) gene may influence morphine requirements in cancer pain patients. Pain 2005;116:73–8.

[56] Romundstad L, Breivik H, Roald H, Skolleborg K, Haugen T, Narum J, Stubhaug A. Methylprednisolone reduces pain, emesis, and fatigue after breast augmentation surgery: a single-dose, randomized, parallel-group study with methylprednisolone 125 mg, parecoxib 40 mg, and placebo. Anesth Analg 2006;102:418–25.

[57] Saari TI, Grönlund J, Hagelberg NM, Neuvonen M, Laine K, Neuvonen PJ, Olkkola KT. Effects of itraconazole on the pharmacokinetics and pharmacodynamics of intravenously and orally administered oxycodone. Eur J Clin Pharmacol 2010;66:387–97.

[58] Saper JR, Lake AE. Continuous opioid therapy (COT) is rarely advisable for refractory chronic daily headache: limited efficacy, risks, and proposed guidelines. Headache 2008;48:838–49.

[59] Skarke C, Jarrar M, Erb K, Schmidt H, Geisslinger G, Lötsch J. Respiratory and miotic effects of morphine in healthy volunteers when P-glycoprotein is blocked by quinidine. Clin Pharmacol Ther 2003;74:303–11.

[60] Skarke C, Darimont J, Schmidt H, Geisslinger G, Lötsch J. Analgesic effects of morphine and morphine-6-glucuronide in a transcutaneous electrical pain model in healthy volunteers. Clin Pharmacol Ther 2003;73:107–21.

[61] Solassol I, Bressolle F, Caumette L, Garcia F, Pujol S, Culine S, Pinguet F. Inter- and intraindividual variabilities in pharmacokinetics of fentanyl after repeated 72-hour transdermal applications in cancer pain. Ther Drug Monit 2005;27:491–8.

[62] Thompson CM, Wojno H, Greiner E, May EL, Rice KC, Selley DE. Activation of G-proteins by morphine and codeine congeners: insights to the relevance of O- and N-demethylated metabolites at μ- and δ-opioid receptors. J Pharmacol Exp Ther 2004;308:547-554.

[63] Thompson SJ, Koszdin K, Bernards CM. Opiate-induced analgesia is increased and prolonged in mice lacking P-glycoprotein. Anesthesiology 2000;92:1392–9.

[64] Tiippana E, Hamunen K, Kontinen VK, Kalso E. Do surgical patients benefit from perioperative gabapentin/pregabalin: a systematic review of efficacy and safety. Anesth Analg 2007;104:1545–56.

[65] Turk DC, Swanson KS, Gatchel RJ. Predicting opioid misuse by chronic pain patients: a systematic review and literature synthesis. Clin J Pain 2008;24:497–508.

[66] Tzschentke TM, Christoph T, Kögel B, Schiene K, Hennies H-H, Englberger W et al. (–)-(1R,2R)-3-(3-dimethylamino-1-ethyl-2-methylpropyl)-phenol hydrochloride (tapentadol HCl): a novel μ-opioid receptor agonist/norepinephrine reuptake inhibitor with broad-spectrum analgesic properties. J Pharmacol Exp Ther 2007;323:266–76.

[67] Vissers D, Stam W, Nolte T, Lenre M, Jansen J. Efficacy of intranasal fentanyl spray versus other opioids for breakthrough pain in cancer. Curr Med Res Opin 2010;26:1037–45.

[68] Wade WE, Spurill WJ. Tapentadol hydrochloride: a centrally acting oral analgesic. Clin Ther 2009;31:2804–18.

[69] Wandel C, Kim R, Wood M, Wood A. Interaction of morphine, fentanyl, sufentanil, alfentanil, and loperamide with the efflux drug transporter P-glycoprotein. Anesthesiology 2002;96:913–20.

[70] Yoburn BC, Shah S, Chan K, Duttaroy A, Davis T. Supersensitivity to opioid analgesics following chronic opioid antagonist treatment: relationship to receptor selectivity. Pharmacol Biochem Behav 1995;51:535–9.

[71] Yu C, Kastin AJ, Tu H, Waters S, Pan W. TNF activates P-glycoprotein in cerebral microvascular endothelial cells. Cell Physiol Biochem 2007;20:853–8.

[72] Zwisler ST, Enggaard TP, Noehr-Jensen L, Pedersen RS, Mikkelsen S, Nielsen F, Brosen K, Sindrup SH. The hypoalgesic effect of oxycodone in human experimental pain models in relation to the CYP2D6 oxidation polymorphism. Basic Clin Pharmacol Ther 2009;104:335–44.

[73] Zwisler ST, Enggaard TP, Mikkelsen S, Nielsen F, Brosen K, Sindrup SH. Impact of the CYP2D6 genotype on post-operative intravenous oxycodone analgesia. Acta Anaesthesiol Scand 2010;54:232–40.

Correspondence to: Eija Kalso, MD, DMedSci, Pain Clinic, Helsinki University Central Hospital, P.O. Box 140, FIN-00029 HUS, Helsinki, Finland. Email: eija.kalso@helsinki.fi.

Clinical Pharmacology of Nonsteroidal Anti-Inflammatory Drugs

Raymond A. Dionne, DDS, PhD,[a] Sharon M. Gordon, DDS, MPH, PhD,[b] and May Hamza, MD[c]

[a]National Institute of Nursing Research; National Institutes of Health, Bethesda, Maryland, USA; [b]University of Maryland, Baltimore, Dental School, Baltimore, Maryland, USA; [c]Department of Pharmacology, Faculty of Medicine, Ain Shams University, Cairo, Egypt

Despite the widespread use of nonopioid drugs such as aspirin (acetylsalicylic acid), acetaminophen (paracetamol), and ibuprofen, and the safety implied by their availability without a prescription, their mechanisms of action and clinical effects are not fully understood. Inflammation and pain are symptoms common to injuries, many therapeutic procedures, and chronic diseases. While pain signaling is important to the survival of the organism, interventions that disrupt this physiological process can be problematic, even deleterious, as illustrated by the cardiovascular toxicity attributed to selective cyclooxygenase-2 (COX-2) inhibitors [6,31,44]. The unifying mechanistic hypothesis of COX-mediated prostaglandin (PG) formation and its peripheral inhibition by aspirin-like drugs was revised when it was recognized that there are two isoforms of COX. The subsequent development of selective COX-2 inhibitors was predicted to enhance efficacy and gastrointestinal (GI) safety, but clinical use revealed unexpected COX-2-mediated cardiovascular toxicity. Similar effects have been identified through epidemiological studies for nonsteroidal anti-inflammatory drugs (NSAIDs) [12,36] and acetaminophen [7], but these effects appear to be related to dose and duration of administration. These unexpected findings, and the application of molecular-genetic methods to the study of the mechanisms and safety of analgesics, is resulting in recognition of a wide spectrum of effects produced by these drugs in humans. These mechanisms not only may form the basis for greater efficacy than a single, highly specific mechanism, but may also convey greater safety due to a more balanced physiological impact than unexpected consequences that may result from totally blocking a receptor or pathway with important effects on homeostasis. We review here the multiple mechanisms of NSAIDs and provide recommendations for their therapeutic use.

Cyclooxygenase Inhibition by NSAIDs

While chemically different, aspirin and NSAIDs have the common property of inhibiting COX, thereby reducing the conversion of arachidonic acid to the PG precursor, PGH_2. Although there are at least two different COX isoenzymes (COX-1 and COX-2), these enzymes catalyze identical reactions and exhibit similar kinetics to produce the unstable PGH_2, which functions as an intermediate substrate for the cell-specific biosynthesis of the final forms of PGs. Prostaglandin E_2 (PGE_2) is produced by PGE synthase from many different cell types including neurons, endothelial cells, and neutrophils. When PGE_2 is released in inflamed tissues it sensitizes afferent nerve fibers at peripheral sensory neurons, but it is now also recognized to evoke hyperalgesia at central sites within the spinal cord and brain [47]. PGE_2 is also a pyrogenic mediator that activates the thermoregulatory center in the anterior hypothalamus; increased PGE_2 in the blood facilitates penetration into the brain, further contributing to triggering fever. This spectrum of PG-mediated activity following release due to tissue injury and COX-mediated synthesis results in the initiation of acute pain, edema, and fever that may be sustained by the development of sensitization, leading to hyperalgesia.

Several recent clinical studies affirm the role of COX inhibition in the mechanism of NSAIDs. Evaluation of the in vivo selectivity of ibuprofen and celecoxib in a clinical model of acute inflammation, the surgical removal of impacted third molars [20], examined levels of PGE_2 as a product of both COX-1 and COX-2 in comparison to levels of thromboxane B_2 (TxB_2) as a biomarker for COX-1 activity. PGE_2 levels increased temporally with the onset of pain and the expression of COX-2 [21]. Celecoxib suppressed PGE_2 at the time points consistent with COX-2 inhibition and had no effect on TxB_2, suggestive of COX-2 specificity. Ibuprofen suppressed both PGE_2 and TxB_2 at all time points over the observation period, indicative of dual COX-1 and COX-2 inhibition (see Fig. 1). COX-2 is primarily responsible for the increase in levels of PGE_2 at later time points after tissue injury, but with continued production of PGE_2 by COX-1. Whereas both drugs were analgesic in comparison to placebo, ibuprofen resulted in less pain at virtually all time points compared with celecoxib, suggesting that suppression of *both* COX-1 and COX-2 is needed for maximal NSAID analgesia. Similarly, other studies [22,23] also suggest a functional relationship between PGE_2 levels, pain, and NSAID analgesia, but they do not permit differentiation between a peripheral effect and distribution to the central nervous system with an additional central mechanism of NSAID action [38,57].

Changes over time in expression of the genes responsible for COX-1 and COX-2, along with wide interindividual variability in response to COX-inhibitory drugs, may also affect the efficacy of analgesics [22]. Gene expression in surgical tissue samples shows increased COX-2 gene expression with a slight decrease in COX-1 gene expression [22]. The interindividual variation in COX-2 gene expression at 2–4 hours postsurgery ranged from approximately 2-fold decreases to >16-fold increases in some subjects and was related to a genetic variant in the COX-2 promoter region. Subjects with a genetic variant that resulted in significantly elevated COX-2 expression following

surgery were more sensitive to the COX-2-inhibitory drug, rofecoxib, while those without the genetic variant showed lower COX-2 expression and were more sensitive to the nonselective COX inhibitor, ibuprofen. While COX-1 gene expression was not affected by administration of ibuprofen or rofecoxib, COX-2 gene expression was significantly increased from presurgical levels following 48 hours of repeated administration of both of these COX-inhibitory drugs. These dynamic but variable changes in COX-2 expression in the presence of relatively stable (and overall greater) COX-1 expression suggest that dual COX-1 and COX-

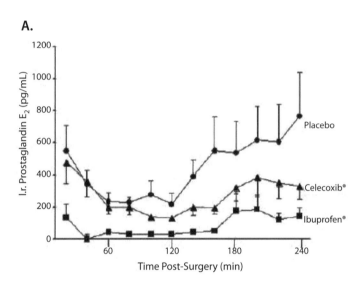

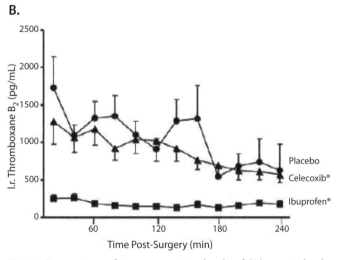

Fig. 1. Comparison of immunoreactive levels of (A) prostaglandin E_2 (PGE_2) and (B) thromboxane B_2 (TXB_2) at the surgical site after extraction of impacted third molars. (A) Ibuprofen suppressed levels of PGE_2 at all time points during the postoperative period. Celecoxib had no effect on levels of PGE_2 at the earlier time points (<60 minutes) but suppressed levels of PGE_2 at the later time points (80 to 240 minutes). (B) Ibuprofen suppressed levels of TXB_2 at all time points, but the effect of celecoxib on levels of TXB_2 did not differ from that of placebo.

2 inhibition is often needed to antagonize tissue injury-mediated synthesis of prostanoids that contribute peripherally to pain and inflammation.

Beyond Cyclooxygenase Inhibition: Multiple Mechanisms of NSAID Analgesia

While COX inhibition is well documented and widely accepted as the mechanism of action of NSAID analgesia, a diverse array of physiological pathways are altered in humans by administration of NSAIDs. Emerging evidence indicates that multiple COX-independent targets exist for both traditional NSAIDs and coxibs.

NSAID Interactions with Endogenous Pain Inhibitory Systems

Pain activates the pituitary-adrenal axis with subsequent pituitary secretion of β-endorphin, leading to elevated circulating β-endorphin levels as part of the endogenous pain inhibitory system. Clinical studies of acute pain demonstrate that β-endorphin is released in response to surgical stress and during postoperative pain. The functional significance of plasma β-endorphin as a component of an endogenous pain inhibitory system is supported by increased clinical pain when β-endorphin levels are decreased by a subtherapeutic dose of dexamethasone [17], and by reduced pain following increased plasma β-endorphin levels due to corticotropin-releasing factor [16]. Ibuprofen affects the release of β-endorphin during both surgical stress [15,50] and postoperative pain [15–17]. For example, administration of 600 mg ibuprofen before minor surgery increases release of β-endorphin intraoperatively in comparison to placebo [50]. Parallel in vivo and in vitro studies indicate that ibuprofen's potentiation of endorphin release is mediated at the level of the pituitary corticotroph cell, possibly by interfering with ultra-short feedback inhibition modulated by PGs [50]. The interaction demonstrated between ibuprofen and β-endorphin release during surgery in conscious patients can probably be attributed to potentiation of stress-induced release. Higher circulating β-endorphin levels following surgery were inversely related to the level of postoperative pain on the day after surgery and resulted in less morphine use [29]. Administration of ketoprofen-lysine to osteoarthritis patients significantly increased circulating β-endorphin levels and lowered substance P, interpreted as a biomarker for the inflammatory response, coincident with the analgesic effect of the ketoprofen [49]. Animal and in vitro studies demonstrate an inhibitory effect of PGE_2 at the level of the pituitary on corticotropin-releasing hormone (CRH)-mediated β-endorphin release [43,52], consistent with increased levels of circulating β-endorphin following NSAID administration. Taken together, these findings support a functional relationship between NSAID administration, increased circulating β-endorphin, and clinical pain that may be contributing to NSAID analgesia.

Ibuprofen Modulation of Multiple Gene Expression Pathways During Inflammation

New insights into the biological properties of COX-2 and its response pathways indicate a complex role, as multiple pathways in the inflammatory cascade are also activated by COX-2 inhibition [53,54]. The function of COX-2 is not limited to inflammation; it has been implicated in other homeostatic functions such as angiogenesis, cell proliferation, and remodeling of extracellular matrix—properties that are associated with wound healing, the development of chronic inflammation, and its resolution [10]. Inhibition of COX-2 derived PGs may cause persistence of inflammation and delays in healing.

COX-2 inhibition, resulting in decreased production of PGs, is also associated with increased risk of cardiovascular diseases and neurodegenerative disorders. Inflammation is common to the processes of wound healing, rheumatoid arthritis, atherogenesis, and neurodegenerative disorders, suggesting a link between COX-2 function and the adverse effects of COX-2 inhibitors across these disorders. For example, administration of ibuprofen over 48 hours in the setting of acute inflammation results in increased expression of the genes for matrix metalloproteinases (MMPs)-1 and -3, along with the genes encoding tissue plasminogen activator (tPA) and interleukin (IL)-8 [53]. Plasminogen is converted to plasmin by tPA, changing the MMPs into their active forms. MMPs play an essential role in the development of inflammation and its resolution. The overexpression of MMP-1 and MMP-3 following ibuprofen treatment is probably a result of the removal of the inhibitory effects of COX-2-dependent PGE_2 on MMP-1 and MMP-3 expression, as similar effects were seen for rofecoxib in this same study [54]. MMP-1 and MMP-3 have been reported in both clinical and experimental studies to be detectable in inflammatory lesions [5], in the synovium of patients with rheumatoid arthritis [37] and in athero-sclerotic plaques [30]. Inhibition of COX-2-derived PG synthesis induces gene expression changes associated with MMP signaling pathways in humans that may impair inflammatory resolution via degradation and remodeling of the extracellular matrix.

Examination of the spectrum of genes and pathways affected by COX inhibition following tissue injury using microarray analysis revealed both significant increases and decreases in comparison to inflammation alone (see Fig. 2) [54]. These changes in gene expression are likely to be interactions between inflammation and COX inhibition. Based on their biological processes and molecular function, the up- or downregulation of the well-characterized genes can be classified into five categories: the arachidonic acid pathway, other biological pathways related to inflammation and pain, angiogenesis and apoptosis pathways, pathways associated with cell adhesion and proteolysis, and signal transduction pathways [54].

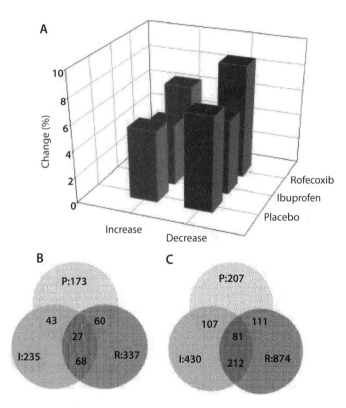

Fig. 2. Gene expression profile induced by acute inflammation and inhibition of cyclooxygenase in a clinical model of tissue injury. (A) Change in percentage of transcripts with significant up- or downregulation following acute inflammation (placebo) and treatments by ibuprofen or rofecoxib. (B) Distribution and intersection of upregulated transcripts (over threefold, $P < 0.05$, $n = 6$ per treatment) following tissue injury in each treatment group. (C) Distribution and intersection of downregulated transcripts (over threefold, $P < 0.05$, $n = 6$ per treatment) following tissue injury in each treatment group [54].

The results of the these studies provide evidence from a clinical model of inflammation and pain that administration of a traditional NSAID, or a selective COX-2 inhibitor, modulates multiple pathways at the gene expression level in addition to the direct effects of COX inhibition. In addition to expected effects on the arachidonic acid pathway during inflammation, both ibuprofen and rofecoxib modulated other cytokine signaling pathways during inflammation. However, rofecoxib was less "selective" than ibuprofen in terms of the number of genes affected and the magnitude of the changes when quantified by reverse transcription polymerase chain reaction [54]. These findings demonstrate that inhibition of COX-2 during inflammation modulates gene expression of both proinflammatory and anti-inflammatory mediators, suggesting a more complex role for COX-2 in the inflammatory cascade than was previously suspected, and it may contribute to the differential toxicity of selective versus nonselective COX-2 inhibitors.

NSAID Modulation of the Endocannabinoid System

Cannabinoids influence a large number of behavioral processes, including pain and inflammation. The endocannabinoids were first recognized two decades ago with demonstration of cannabinoid (CB) binding sites in the rat brain, now described as the CB_1 and CB_2 receptors. The recognition of CB receptors predicted the existence of an endogenous ligand, which resulted in the identification of anandamide and other endogenous cannabinoids. Endocannabinoids are involved in pain and inflammation; they are metabolized by COX to produce a number of products and may contribute to the pharmacological effects of NSAIDs. Evidence from in vitro and in vivo studies suggests a shift in arachidonic acid metabolism toward endocannabinoid formation in response to COX inhibition [4,13,41]. While the precise mechanism for this "endocannabinoid shift" has not been identified, the net effect is inhibition of the release of inflammatory mediators such as calcitonin gene-related peptide in the spinal cord, thereby decreasing nociceptive signaling due to tissue injury.

Fatty acid amide hydrolase (FAAH) is also involved in the inactivation of anandamide, and reduction in its activity is antinociceptive in models of pain [19,25]. An association between cold pain sensitivity in humans and genetic variants in the FAAH gene suggests a functional relationship between FAAH activity and pain in humans [22]. Nonopioids including ibuprofen inhibit the activity of FAAH, particularly at the low pH that is found at sites of inflammation. Synergistic antinociceptive effects have been demonstrated with ibuprofen and anandamide, with increased levels of endocannabinoids in inflamed tissues [14]. These data suggest that ibuprofen's analgesic effects may also be partially mediated through effects on FAAH that enhance the activity of the endocannabinoid system, but this hypothesis awaits confirmation in clinical models of pain and inflammation.

Interactions with Monoaminergic Pathways

Several studies suggest that the antinociceptive effects of nonopioids may be related to their effects on monoaminergic pathways, both serotonergic (5-HT-ergic) and noradrenergic systems. The analgesic activity of aspirin in primates, for example, is antagonized by $5-HT_{2A}$-receptor blockade or depletion of central 5-HT, and enhanced by central administration of 5-HT or its precursor [42]. Similarly, depletion of central 5-HT blocks the antinociceptive effects of aspirin in the first phase of the formalin test [51], rofecoxib in the hotplate test [39], and NSAIDs in the writhing and tail-flick tests in mice [28]. Acetaminophen-induced antinociception is inhibited in animal models by administration of $5-HT_{1B}$-, $5-HT_{2A}$-, and $5-HT_{2C}$-receptor antagonists [9,40] and by a $5-HT_3$-receptor antagonist in a model of mechanical hyperalgesia [2,3]. Acetaminophen analgesia is reversed in humans by $5-HT_3$-receptor antagonists for pain due to electrical stimulation of the median nerve [32]. Increased concentrations of 5-HT in the central nervous system (CNS) following administration of aspirin [51], acetaminophen [9], or coxibs [39], accompanied by downregulation of postsynaptic 5-HT receptors and upregulation of 5-HT transporter [45,46], suggests supraspinal changes in 5-HT release and reuptake [9] that activate descending inhibitory 5-HT-ergic pathways.

The noradrenergic system is involved in pain at spinal and supraspinal levels through activation of α-adrenoceptors and the action of descending inhibitory pathways. Under conditions of persistent noxious input, the descending noradrenergic input to the dorsal horn plays a major role in the modulation of pain [27,56]. Administration of the nonselective α-adrenoceptor antagonist, phentolamine, prevents the effects of the NSAID indomethacin on nociceptive thresholds in rodent models of acute pain, while destruction of spinal noradrenergic neurons blocks indomethacin's effects [48]. Similarly,

pretreatment with an α_2-adrenoceptor antagonist blocks the antinociceptive effects of NSAIDs in a rodent model, whereas an α_1-adrenoceptor antagonist inhibits the effects of acetaminophen [34]. These and similar findings for other NSAIDs and antagonists indicate the involvement of the adrenergic system in their antinociceptive effects by activating supraspinal mechanisms that cause descending inhibitory effects on the spinal transmission of nociceptive inputs [26,34,48].

Cholinergic System Interactions with Nonopioid Analgesia

Acetylcholine in the dorsal horn of the spinal cord mediates antinociceptive effects through both nicotinic and muscarinic receptors to activate descending inhibition and inhibitory interneurons [58]. Administration of the muscarinic antagonist, atropine, inhibits the effect of NSAIDs and acetaminophen, whereas cholinergic depletion prevents the antinociceptive effects of these drugs [35]. Both aspirin and acetaminophen increase intraspinal acetylcholine release, suggesting that intraspinal acetylcholine release could be involved in noninflammatory pain suppression by nonopioids [1]. The possible role of central cholinergic modulation of the antinociceptive effect of nonopioids needs further investigation to identify the mechanism of this modulation.

Considerations for the Clinical Management of Pain and Inflammation

NSAIDs remain one of most widely used drug classes for pain in ambulatory patients, along with aspirin, acetaminophen, and codeine. They are usually more efficacious than these standard drugs in most clinical studies, presumably due to the inflammatory etiology of acute pain. A single dose of 400–600 mg of ibuprofen is generally more effective than combinations of aspirin or acetaminophen and opioids (usually codeine or oxycodone), with fewer side effects, making it preferable for ambulatory patients who generally experience a higher incidence of side effects following an opioid. NSAIDs also exert a modest suppression of swelling following surgical procedures, providing additional therapeutic benefit but without the potential liabilities of administering a steroid. Although selective COX-2 inhibitors were developed to minimize the adverse effects associated with chronic NSAID administration, belated recognition of their cardiovascular effects limits the use of this class until we have greater understanding of the physiological consequences of inhibiting the COX-2 pathway.

While acetaminophen is often recommended as an alternative to aspirin and NSAIDs, an increased recognition of liver toxicity associated with chronic acetaminophen administration, and additive effects when this drug is ingested with ethanol, has resulted in additional warnings regarding its use in the package insert. Many patients previously administered coxibs that were withdrawn from the market are now taking acetaminophen as a safer alternative under the assumption that it does not affect COX-2. Recently published studies in humans comparing the COX selectivity of acetaminophen warrants re-examination of this assumption [18,24]. Acetaminophen was similar to placebo and rofecoxib in its effects on levels of the COX-1 biomarker, thromboxane B_2, as measured by microdialysis and enzyme immunoassay over the first 3 hours postoperatively. Acetaminophen exhibited the same profile as rofecoxib in suppressing PGE_2 from 100 to 180 minutes after surgery, consistent with increasing expression of the COX-2 gene [24]. Continued administration of acetaminophen demonstrated that the COX-2 was significantly upregulated in comparison to placebo, similar to the ketorolac group and consistent with previous findings at 48 hours for rofecoxib [21,33]. These findings suggest that acetaminophen inhibits COX-2 function in vivo and that its analgesic effect, at least in part, may be attributed to peripheral effects in addition to centrally mediated effects [2,8,33]. While it is generally accepted that single or repeated doses of acetaminophen do not have any cardiovascular effects, the similarity between acetaminophen and rofecoxib in a clinical model of inflammation warrants further investigation.

The vast experience gained through nearly 40 years of clinical use of NSAIDs since the introduction of ibuprofen, and recognition of the limitation of coxibs and acetaminophen when administered chronically, suggest that NSAIDs should remain the drugs of choice for the management of pain and inflammation in patients who do not have contraindications to their use. Dual COX-1 and COX-2 inhibition may result in greater suppression of PGE_2-mediated pain than just suppressing the transient increase due to COX-2 expression while avoiding the more widespread effects of coxibs on the inflammatory cascade. A shorter duration of action may also permit the normal physiological effects of COX on

homeostasis and allow for individualization of the dose and dosing interval in response to the wide variability across patients, diseases, and temporal patterns of gene expression. The history of therapeutic innovation has often demonstrated that newer is not always better, that greater potency often translates into greater toxicity, and that drugs with multiple effects are often more effective than highly selective drugs [55]. Management of pain with dual COX-1 and COX-2 inhibition may represent the physiological balance between benefit and risk if prescribed and used correctly.

References

[1] Abelson KS, Kommalge M, Hoglund AU. Spinal cholinergic involvement after treatment with aspirin and paracetamol in rats. Neurosci Lett 2004;368:116–20.

[2] Alloui A, Chassing C, Schmidt J, Ardid D, Dubray C, Cloarec A, Eschalier A. Paracetamol exerts a spinal, tropisetron-reversible, antinociceptive effect in an inflammatory pain model in rats. Eur J Pharmacol 2002;443:71–7.

[3] Alloui A, Pelissier T, Dubray C, Lavarenne J, Eschalier A. Tropisetron inhibits the antinociceptive effects of intrathecally administered paracetamol and serotonin. Fundam Clin Pharmacol 1996;10:406–7.

[4] Ates M, Hamza M, Seidel K, Kotalla CE, Ledent C, Guhring H. Intrathecally applied flurbiprofen produces an endocannabinoid-dependent antinociception in the rat formalin test. Eur J Neurosci 2003;17:597–604.

[5] Baum CL, Arpey CJ. Normal cutaneous wound healing: clinical correlation with cellular and molecular events. Dermatol Surg 2005;31:674–86.

[6] Bresalier RS, Sandler RS, Quan H, Bolognese JA, Oxenius B, Horgan K, Lines C, Riddell R, Morton D, Lanas A, Konstam MA, Baron JA; Adenomatous Polyp Prevention on Vioxx (APPROVe) Trial Investigators. Cardiovascular events associated with rofecoxib in a colorectal adenoma chemoprevention trial. N Engl J Med 2005;352:1092–102.

[7] Chan AT, Manson JE, Albert CM, Chae CU, Rexrode KM, Curhan GC, Rimm EB, Willett WC, Fuchs CS. Nonsteroidal anti-inflammatory drugs, acetaminophen, and the risk of cardiovascular events. Circulation 2006;113:1578–87.

[8] Chen C, Bazan NG. Acetaminophen modifies hippocampal synaptic plasticity via a presynaptic 5-HT$_2$ receptor. Neuroreport 2003;14:743–7.

[9] Courade JP, Caussade F, Martin K, Besse D, Delchambre C, Hanoun N, Hamon M, Eschalier A, Coarec A. Effects of acetaminophen on monoaminergic systems in rat central nervous system. Naunyn Schmiedebergs Arch Pharmacol 2001;364:534–7.

[10] Futugami A, Ishizaki M, Fukuda Y, Kawana S, Yamanaka N. Wound healing involves induction of cyclooxygenase-2 expression in rat skin. Lab Invest 2002;82:1503–13.

[11] Gordon SM, Brahim JS, Rowan R, Kent A, Dionne RA. Peripheral prostanoid levels and nonsteroidal anti-inflammatory drug analgesia: replicate clinical trials in a tissue injury model. Clin Pharmacol Therap 2002;72:175–83.

[12] Graham DJ, Campen D, Hui R, Spence M, Cheetham C, Levy G, Shoor S, Ray WA. Risk of acute myocardial infarction and sudden cardiac death in patients treated with cyclo-oxygenase 2 selective and non-selective non-steroidal anti-inflammatory drugs: nested case-control study. Lancet 2005;365:475–81.

[13] Guhring H, Hamza M, Sergejeva M, Ates M, Kotalla CE, Ledent C, Brune K. A role for endocannabinoids in indomethacin-induced spinal antinociception. Eur J Pharmacol 2002;454:153–63.

[14] Guindon J, DeLean A, Beaulieu P. Local interactions between anandamide, an endocannabinoid, and ibuprofen, a non-steroidal anti-inflammatory drug, in acute and inflammatory pain. Pain 2006;121:85–93.

[15] Hargreaves KM, Dionne RA, Mueller GP, Goldstein DS, Dubner R. Naloxone, fentanyl and diazepam modify plasma beta-endorphin levels during surgery. Clin Pharmacol Ther 1986;40:165–71.

[16] Hargreaves KM, Mueller GP, Dubner R, Goldstein DS, Dionne RA. Corticotrophin-releasing factor (CRF) produces analgesia in humans and rats. Brain Res 1987;422:154–7.

[17] Hargreaves KM, Schmidt E, Mueller GP, Dionne RA. Dexamethasone alters plasma levels of β-endorphin and postoperative pain. Clin Pharmacol Ther 1987;42:601–7.

[18] Hinz B, Cheremina O, Brune K. Acetaminophen (paracetamol) is a selective cyclooxygenase-2 inhibitor in man. FASEB J 2008;22:383–90.

[19] Holt S, Comelli F, Costa B, Fowler CJ. Inhibitors of fatty acid amide hydrolase reduce carrageenan-induced hind paw inflammation in pentobarbital-treated mice: comparison with indomethacin and possible involvement of cannabinoid receptors. Br J Pharmacol 2005;146:467–76.

[20] Khan AA, Brahim JS, Rowan JS, Dionne RA. In vivo selectivity of a selective cyclooxygenase 2 inhibitor in the oral surgery model. Clin Pharmacol Ther 2002;72:44–9.

[21] Khan AA, Iadarola M, Yang H-ST, Dionne RA. Expression of COX-1 and COX-2 in a clinical model of inflammation. J Pain 2007;8:349–54.

[22] Kim H, Mittal DP, Iadarola MJ, Dionne RA. Genetic predictors for acute experimental cold and heat pain sensitivity in humans. J Med Genet 2006;43,e40.

[23] Lee Y-S, Kim H, Wu T-X, Wang X-M, Dionne RA. Genetically mediated interindividual variation in analgesic responses to cyclooxygenase inhibitory drugs. Clin Pharmacol Ther 2006;79:407–18.

[24] Lee Y-S, Kim H, Brahim JS, Rowan J, Lee G, Dionne RA. Acetaminophen selectively suppresses peripheral prostaglandin E2 release and increases COX-2 gene expression in a clinical model of acute inflammation. Pain 2007;129:279–86.

[25] Lichtman AH, Shelton CC, Advani T, Cravatt BF. Mice lacking fatty acid amide hydrolase exhibit a cannabinoid receptor-mediated phenotypic hypoalgesia. Pain 2004;109:319–27.

[26] Lizarraga I, Chambers JP. Involvement of opioidergic and alpha2-adrenergic mechanisms in the central analgesic effects of non-steroidal anti-inflammatory drugs in sheep. Res Vet Sci 2006;80:194–200.

[27] Millan MJ. The role of descending noradrenergic and serotonergic pathways in the modulation of nociception: focus on receptor multiplicity. In: Dickenson A, Besson JM, editors. The pharmacology of pain. Handbook of experimental pharmacology, Vol. 130. Berlin: Springer; 1997. p. 385–446.

[28] Miranda HF, Lemus I, Pinardi G. Effect of the inhibition of serotonin biosynthesis on the antinociception induced by nonsteroidal anti-inflammatory drugs. Brain Res Bull 2003;61:417–25.

[29] Nader-Djalal N, Leon-Casasola OA, Peer GL, Vladutiu AO, Lema MJ. The influence of preoperative concentrations of β-endorphin and met-enkephalin on the duration of analgesia after transurethral resection of the prostate. Anesh Analg 1995;81:591–5.

[30] Newby AC. Dual role of matrix metalloproteinases (Matrixins) in intimal thickening and atherosclerotic plaque rupture. Physiol Rev 2005;85:1–31.

[31] Nussmeier NA, Whelton AA, Brown MT, Langford RM, Hoeft A, Parlow JL, Boyce SW, Verburg KM. Complications of the COX-2 inhibitors parecoxib and valdecoxib after cardiac surgery. N Engl J Med 2005;352:1081–91.

[32] Pickering G, Loriot MA, Libert F, Eschalier A, Beaune P, Dubray C. Analtgesic effect of acetaminophen in humans: first evidence of a central serotonergic mechanism. Clin Pharmacol Ther 2006;79:371–8.

[33] Pelissier T, Alloui A, Caussade F, Dubray C, Cloarec A, Lavarenne J, Eschalier A. Paracetamol exerts a spinal antinociceptive effect involving an indirect interaction with 5-hydroxytryptamine3 receptors: in vivo and in vitro evidence. J Pharmacol Exp Ther 1996;278:8–14.

[34] Pinardi G, Sierralta F, Miranda HF. Adrenergic mechanisms in antinociceptive effects of non-steroidal anti-inflammatory drugs in acute thermal nociception in mice. Inflamm Res 2002;51:219–22.

[35] Pinardi G, Sierralta F, Miranda HF. Atropine reverses the antinociception of nonsteroidal anti-inflammatory drugs in the tail-flick test of mice. Pharmacol Biochem Behav 2003;74:603–8.

[36] Ray WA, Stein CM, Hall K, Daugherty JR, Griffin MR. Non-steroidal anti-inflammatory drugs and risk of serious coronary heart disease: an observational cohort study. Lancet 2002;359:118–23.

[37] Ritchlin CT. Pathogenesis of psoriatic arthritis. Curr Opin Rheumatol 2005;17:406–12.

[38] Samad TA, Moore KA, Sapirstein A, Billet S, Allchorne A, Poole S, Bonventre JV, Woolf CJ. Interleukin-1β-mediated induction of Cox-2 in the CNS contributes to inflammatory hypersensitivity. Nature 2001;410:471–5.

[39] Sandrini M, Vitale G, Pini LA. Effect of rofecoxib on nociception and the serotonin system in the rat brain. Inflamm Res 2002;51:154–9.

[40] Sandrini M, Pini LA, Vitale G. Differential involvement of central 5-HT1B and 5-HT3 receptor subtypes in the antinociceptive effect of paracetamol. Inflamm Res 2003;52:347–52.

[41] Seidel K, Hamza M, Ates M, Guhring H. Flurbiprofen inhibits capsaicin induced calcitonin gene related peptide release from rat spinal cord via an endocannabinoid dependent mechanism. Neurosci Lett 2003;338:99–102.

[42] Skyu KW, Lin MT, Wu TC. Possible role of central serotonergic neurons in the development of dental pain and aspirin-induced analgesia in the monkey. Exp Neurol 1984;84:179–87.

[43] Sobel DO. Characterization of PGE2 inhibition of corticotropin releasing factor-mediated ACTH release. Brain Res 1987;411:102–7.

[44] Solomon SD, McMurray JJ, Pfeffer MA, Wittes J, Fowler R, Finn P, Anderson WF, Zauber A, Hawk E, Bertagnolli M; Adenoma Prevention with Celecoxib (APC) Study Investigators. Cardiovascular risk associated with celecoxib in a clinical trial for colorectal adenoma prevention. J Engl J Med 2005;352:1071–80.

[45] Srikiatkhachorn A, Tarasub N, Govitrapong P. Acetaminophen-induced antinociception via central 5-HT$_{2A}$ receptors. Neurochem Int 1999;34:491–8.

[46] Srikiatkhachorn A, Tarasub N, Govitrapong P. Effect of chronic analgesic exposure on the central serotonin system: a possible mechanism of analgesic abuse headache. Headache 2000;40:343–50.

[47] Svensson CI, Yaksh TL. The spinal phospholipase-cyclooxygenase-prostanoid cascade in nociceptive processing. Annu Rev Pharmacol Toxicol 2002;42:553–83.

[48] Taiwo YO, Levine JD. Prostaglandins inhibit endogenous pain control mechanisms by blocking transmission at spinal noradrenergic synapses. J Neurosci 1988;8:1346–9.

[49] Torri G, Cecchettin M, Bellometti S, Galzigna L. Analgesic effect and plasma beta-endorphin and substance P levels in plasma after short-term administration of a ketoprofen-lysine salt or acetylsalicylic acid in patients with osteoarthrosis. Curr Ther Res 1995;56:62–9.

[50] Troullos E, Hargreaves KM, Dionne RA. Ibuprofen elevates β-endorphin levels in humans during surgical stress. Clin Pharmacol Ther 1997;62:74–81.

[51] Vitale G, Pini LA, Ottani A, Sandrini M. Effect of acetylsalicylic acid on formalin test and on serotonin system in the rat brain. Gen Pharmacol 1998;31:753–8.

[52] Vlaskovska M, Hertting G, Knepel W. Adrenocorticotropin and β-endorphin release from rat adenophyphysis in vitro: Inhibition by prostaglandin E2 formed locally in response to vasopressin and corticotropin-releasing factor. Endocrinol 1984;115:895–903.

[53] Wang X-M, Wu T-X, Lee Y-S, Dionne RA. Rofecoxib regulates the expression of genes related to the matrix metalloproteinase pathway in humans: Implications for the adverse effects of cyclooxygenase-2 inhibitors. Clin Pharmacol Ther 2006;79:303–15.

[54] Wang X-M, Wu T-X, Mamza M, Ramsay ES, Wahl SM, Dionne RA. Rofecoxib modulates multiple gene expression pathways in a clinical model of acute inflammatory pain. Pain 2007;128:136–47.

[55] Woodcock JW, Witter JW, Dionne RA. Individualizing the development of mechanism-based pain therapeutics. Nat Rev Drug Discov 2007;6:703–10.

[56] Xu M, Kontinen VK, Kalso E. Endogenous noradrenergic tone controls symptoms of allodynia in the spinal nerve ligation model of neuropathic pain. Eur J Pharmacol 1999;366:41–5.

[57] Yaksh TL, Dirig DM, Conway CM, Svensson C, Luo ZD, Isakson PC. The acute antihyperalgesic action of nonsteroidal, anti-inflammatory drugs and release of spinal prostaglandin E2 is mediated by inhibition of constitutive spinal cyclooxygenase-2 (COX-2) but not COX-1. J Neurosci 2001;21:5847–53.

[58] Yaksh TL. Central pharmacology of nociceptive transmission. In: McMahon SB, Koltzenburg M, editors. Wall and Melzack's textbook of pain. Elsevier Churchill Livingstone; 2006. p. 371–414.

Correspondence to: Dr. Raymond Dionne, National Institute of Nursing Research, National Institutes of Health, 10 Center Drive, Room 2-1339, Bethesda, MD 20892, USA. Email: dionner@mail.noh.gov.

Part 11

Pain Genes for Unraveling Pain:
A Course for Non-Geneticists

What Are "Pain Genes," and Why Are They Interesting?

23

Marshall Devor, PhD

Department of Cell and Developmental Biology, Institute of Life Sciences and Center for Research on Pain,
The Hebrew University of Jerusalem, Jerusalem, Israel

There is considerable variability in pain reported by different people, regarding both acute pain in response to noxious stimuli and chronic pain associated with injury or disease—even when the provoking stimulus or disorder is essentially identical. A dramatic example is phantom limb pain in amputees. Some amputees report no pain while others have severely disabling pain that lasts a lifetime, even when the level of the amputation is identical [26]. The fact that reamputation usually fails to relieve phantom limb pain points to factors associated with the patient, rather than the surgery, as the underlying cause. Variability is also the rule with pain in day-to-day life. A slap in the face that provokes sobs in one person will be laughed off by another. We each have a different "pain threshold."

Variability in pain expression has traditionally been attributed to psychosocial and cultural factors, personality, personal inclination, and upbringing. It is also irrevocably entangled with the question of how much the outward expression of pain actually reflects the pain felt by the individual, inside. In some societies, for example, people do not hesitate to express their pain, while in others, children are taught to be stoical. Even for a given individual, and with a stimulus of fixed intensity, pain expression may vary wildly with the circumstances. Did that slap in the face indicate a challenge or an insult, or did the tears come just because it hurt? In most cultures there is a marked sex difference in the degree to which pain expression is sanctioned. Boys are taught not to be "crybabies," while for girls tears are expected. Does the resulting difference in outward "pain behavior" only reflect social norms, or is there also a real gender-linked difference in the amount of pain felt by boys and girls in response to identical noxious stimuli? A large body of evidence indicates that women are less tolerant than men of noxious stimuli in laboratory tests, and much more likely to suffer from a variety of chronic pain conditions [2]. Does this finding reflect an inherent, biologically based sex difference in pain *experience*, or just a carryover of patterns of pain *expression* learned in childhood? Is it possible that early socialization alters the amount of pain experienced later in life?

Because of the obvious effect of early socialization, the observation that pain expression tends to run in families and societies has traditionally been interpreted in terms of shared upbringing and environment. New evidence, however, suggests that genetic factors also contribute importantly to pain response and individual variability. In general, traits that run in families (appearance, height, and predispositions) do so for a combination of genetic and environmental reasons. Nonetheless, the concept of genetic influences on pain response is relatively new.

Why Does Pain Genetics Matter?

Why should a pain professional be interested to know that pain experience is affected by genes? First, research on pain genetics has already begun to contribute to the understanding of pain mechanisms and will probably continue to do so. Past experience indicates that this research on mechanisms will ultimately lead to improved diagnostic, prognostic, and treatment options. Indeed, for reasons explained below, pain genetics has a special potential to uncover novel and unexpected insights about pain—insights that might not be achieved by step-by-step pursuit of our current pain physiology. If done right, the genetic approach permits a broad scan for novel pain mechanisms that is unbiased and does not depend on prior knowledge about the physiology of pain.

Second, the study of genetic differences in pain response to analgesic drugs, "pharmacogenetics," promises a new era of individualized pain medicine where the prescription of drug treatments will be tailored to the specific patient, providing increased efficacy with decreased unwanted side effects. In addition, genetic study of drug responses is expected to lead to gene-based diagnostics and prognostics, and perhaps even to gene-based therapy [15].

Finally, people who report having severe pain in the absence of easily observed signs of injury and disease are often stigmatized as complainers and malingerers. Sometimes they are even suspected of being outright liars, trying to cheat "the system" and obtain undeserved sympathy and benefits from caring family members, employers, insurance companies, and the government. Knowledge that pain is variable, and that one person may have much more pain than another for genetic reasons, through no fault of his or her own, may provide some comfort to both patient and therapist. Of course, the fact that pain genes exist does not mean that malingerers and cheats do not.

Heritability of Pain

Most biological traits are affected by genes, environment, and interactions between genes and environment. Why should we be surprised to learn that pain susceptibility is affected by nature as well as by nurture? The short answer is that we shouldn't. Nonetheless, because of the overwhelming influence of environment on both the clinical manifestations of pain response in patients, and in our day-to-day experience of pain, the emergence of an important genetic component took many people by surprise. The first solid indications that pain may be determined by our genes in addition to our socialization came from rare familial disorders inherited by certain family members but not by others. In these individuals pain might be absent, such as in congenital insensitivity to pain with anhidrosis (CIPA), or it may be excessive, such as in Fabry's disease and familial hemiplegic migraine (FHM). As discussed in more detail in the chapter by Gosso and coauthors in this volume, such conditions can usually be traced to disease-causing mutations in specific genes using the method of "positional cloning."

Evidence for pain heritability in humans is also available from epidemiological research, including the study of twins. Pain as a normal trait (e.g., in response to noxious heat and cold in healthy individuals), along with pain in common painful conditions such as backache and sciatica, is more concordant in identical (monozygotic) twins than fraternal (dizygotic) twins [1]. The idea here is that identical twins share all of their gene variants, while fraternal twins share only half. Caveats to this approach remain, however. For example, environment may be more similar for identical twins than for fraternal twins. Information can also be obtained from twins separated at birth and raised apart, in different environments. But this situation is rare. Once heritability has been documented, investigators can undertake more advanced studies, using methods derived from molecular biology, to identify the specific genes that control pain sensitivity. Such genes have come to be called "pain genes."

Twin studies can identify the presence of a heritable component in painful conditions that are genetically complex (e.g., dependent on more than one gene) and hence do not obviously run in families like CIPA or FHM. Unfortunately, however, this approach is not practical for identifying the actual genes involved. More recently a genetic approach termed "genetic association" has gained popularity as a means of determining whether a pain-related trait or condition has a significant heritable component, and also for identifying the underlying gene(s) [10]. In association studies, genetic characteristics are compared in groups of unrelated people, affected individuals and controls. This approach, and current outcomes, are discussed in detail in the chapter by Diatchenko and coauthors in this volume.

The use of animal models of pain provides additional routes for identifying the genetic underpinnings of pain traits. Indeed, such studies to a large extent jump-started the current interest in pain genetics in humans, and they continue to play a role in the discovery of pain genes, as explained below. Two main lines of evidence based on observations of behavioral phenotype in experimental animals point to the conclusion that heritable factors render some individuals predisposed to increased pain response. First is the observation that different inbred strains of rodents, which harbor consistent differences in their genetic makeup, frequently show differences in pain phenotype under identical environmental conditions. Interestingly, a strain that is particularly sensitive in one pain measure, say heat nociception, need not necessarily be sensitive in a second measure. The empirical observation that mouse strains high on one measure of nociception are also high on another is a powerful method for identifying phenotypes that have genetic determinants in common. Measures of nociception that consistently covary across animal strains identify fundamental "types" of pain [17,18]. Inbred strains with different pain sensitivities can be crossed and intercrossed in order to reveal details about the pattern of inheritance, and using advanced methods, to identify the gene(s) that account for the strain differences.

The second line of evidence is based on genetic selection. It has been shown that a single (outbred) rat strain can be separated into distinct phenotypically high and phenotypically low lines by repeated cycles of selective breeding. Selection lines begin with a parental strain with variable phenotype and subsequently diverge as a result of targeted selection pressure. For example, in the study of Devor and Raber [5], rats were selected for breeding based on high (HA) or low (LA) expression of pain phenotype in the neuroma model of neuropathic pain (autotomy behavior). After only a few generations of selection, all offspring of HA parents were high for the trait, and all offspring of LA parents were low. Once the selection lines had been established, intercrossing and backcrossing revealed the pattern of heritability and aided in pinpointing the chromosomal location of relevant genes [20].

Pain Genes

What is a "pain gene"? Genes are parts of DNA molecules that contain the information used by cells to construct protein molecules. They "code" for proteins. Proteins are "products" of gene transcription and translation, the two cellular processes that exploit the information encoded in the sequence of base-pairs in the DNA molecule to manufacture proteins. It is these proteins that carry out the work of the cell, such as enzymatic action, motility, electrical impulse generation, and so on. An essential take-home message is that genes code for protein molecules, *not* for sensory and emotional experiences such as pain. Likewise, when we read in the popular (and in the scientific) press about "genes for generosity," "genes for risk-taking," "genes for social awkwardness," and "genes for empathy" [7, 11, 23], nobody is really proposing that these high-order cognitive phenomena result from the action of individual gene products, i.e., protein molecules. Generosity, risk-taking, and empathy are all complex downstream effects of basic cellular processes. No doubt predisposition to pain is too, at least in many instances.

Only a conscious brain can experience pain or feel empathy for someone else who is in pain. But this does not mean that all of the 25,000 or so genes that are required to make a human body and brain are pain genes. The action or inaction of a certain protein species makes a difference in how pain is perceived by a conscious brain, while actions of other proteins do not. *A pain gene is a gene for which there are one or more polymorphisms (i.e., variations in the sequence of DNA base-pairs) that affect the expression or the functioning of its protein product in a way that affects pain response.*

DNA polymorphisms may include significant portions of the base-pair sequence of A's, T's, C's, and G's that make up the gene. But more commonly the difference is small, often amounting to a change in a single nucleotide base, say from A to C. This kind of variability is called a "single nucleotide polymorphism" or "SNP" (pronounced "snip"). Even such minor changes can have important functional effects. We all have the same complement of genes. Genetic polymorphism means that these genes come with minor variants in different people. A gene that occurs with sequence variations in a population of people is said to have several "alleles." Each variant in an allele of that gene. Think of a Chevrolet Malibu with different engine and trim options.

Sometimes variations in the base-pair sequence, major or minor, are present in the sequence of DNA base-pairs that actually encode for the protein (i.e., in exons). Depending on the details, such variations may alter the amino acid sequence of the protein, changing its shape or charge configuration and hence its functioning. The change might destroy protein function completely, or alter it in more subtle ways, including enhancing its function! Sequence polymorphisms that affect pain response can also occur in nearby regions of the DNA molecule that regulate the "expression" of a pain gene; that is, they affect *how much* of the gene product is synthesized. Such changes generally have no effect on the structure or functioning of the protein product itself. Sequence polymorphisms that affect expression are probably more common than those that affect protein structure and function [29]. A DNA sequence polymorphism can also affect the "bar code" address of a gene's protein product, the part of the sequence that tells the cell where specifically to send this particular protein molecule. The affected protein may work normally and be made in normal amounts. But if it is not sent to the part of the cell where it needs to be sent to do its job (a "trafficking error"), pain processing may not work properly.

At present, we have no idea how many genes there are in which allelic variation affects pain response. The question "How many pain genes are there?" is not even well defined. For example, several hundred genes have been identified so far that, if artificially altered or deleted ("knocked out" in a mouse mutant) affect pain phenotype. There are probably many more. Some (many?) genes, however, are essentially identical among individuals. Genes that are not polymorphic in natural populations do not contribute to pain variability. Therefore, while these genes may play an important role in the machinery of pain processing, if they do not contribute to trait variability, they do not count as "pain genes" as the term is used here. The same is true for genes modified with various molecular technologies for use as tools for studying pain processes and for tracing pain pathways.

Pathology and disease states cannot change the base-pair sequence of genes, although they can change the structure of their protein products (through "alternative gene splicing"). More importantly, pathology and disease can, and do, affect gene expression. For example, in the commonly used rodent neuropathic pain models, the expression of >2,000 genes in sensory neurons may be altered following axotomy [21]. In many of these genes, the degree of altered expression varies from strain to strain, and in quite a few (more than 100) genes, the variation correlates with strain-specific pain behavior. Base-pair variations responsible for the differences in gene expression across strains might qualify as pain genes. Finally, it is likely that sequence polymorphisms also affect protein trafficking, although

this possibility has yet to be explored within the context of pain.

It is estimated that in the human genome, at least 99.9% of the base-pair sequence is identical from one person to the next. However, the remaining 0.1% represents about 3,000,000 base-pairs which might differ among individuals. These base-pairs are distributed across the genome, and therefore there is a good chance that for each of our approximately 25,000 genes, there are one or a few differences in sequences than code for proteins or that regulate gene expression at baseline or in the event of disease. That is, for the large majority of genes there are one or more alleles. Many of these allelic differences have no effect on function, expression, or trafficking. But some do. When sequence variants are rare, occurring in <1% of the population, they are called "mutations." More common variants are called "polymorphisms." For most genes in which there are functionally relevant variations among people, there are only a few common alleles. What makes us genetically different from one another is the mix-and-match combination of the alleles we carry. New mutations are quite rare. The mix-and-match allele combinations that make us unique were determined for each of us at the moment of conception.

Pain response is "polygenic," meaning that many alleles, mixed-and-matched, determine our overall pain sensitivity. But not all alleles are born equal. Alleles of certain genes may have a much stronger effect on our individual pattern of pain response than alleles of others, and an allele with a strong effect on one pain phenotype may have a weak affect on another [18]. Moreover, the effect of alleles may not be additive. Polymorphisms in some genes affect pain only in the presence of the polymorphisms in others. Pain sensitivity is therefore determined not by a simple sum of the various allelic effects present, but by a more complex calculus dependent on the specific combinations of alleles inherited. Finally, in addition to such gene-gene interactions, there are gene-environment interactions [15]. Thus, a genetic polymorphism may have no effect on pain response except under unusual environmental circumstances (e.g., at high altitudes), or if your kids have made you particularly exasperated. Exacerbating this complexity is the fact that most genetic polymorphisms probably have no effect or barely detectable effects. This realization has recently been the source of considerable frustration, and even gloominess about the value of pain genetics [9,16]. Pain genes are of interest to the extent that allelic variants have a reasonably strong effect on pain response and to the extent that they are common in the population. Perhaps strategies can be adopted to enhance the likelihood of finding functionally significant polymorphisms.

Pain Genes and Pain Mechanisms

An essential distinction needs to be made between alleles that cause (or predispose to) diseases that may be painful, and alleles that are (at least partly) responsible for the fact that two different individuals with identical injuries or diseases may report very different levels of pain. Some gene variants (alleles) cause painful disease. An example of such "disease susceptibility genes" are genes that increase the likelihood of developing type 2 diabetes mellitus [28]. This metabolic condition sometimes leads to pain-provoking nerve injury (painful diabetic neuropathy), although usually it leads to nonpainful diabetic neuropathy or no neuropathy at all. The connection between genes, disease, and pain in type 2 diabetes is complex and obscure, and it will probably remain so until we have a better understanding of neuropathic pain mechanisms. So let us first consider the simpler case of point mutations that cause painful disease.

Quite a few mutations have been identified that cause various types of inherited peripheral neuropathies [12]. Some of these conditions are associated with pain. A prominent example is the Thr124Met base-pair substitution that causes painful Charcot-Marie-Tooth (CMT-2) neuropathy in some families. This point mutation in the gene alters the chain of amino acids that make up a key protein in the nerve's myelin sheath (the myelin-associated protein Po). The mutation places a Met (methionine) amino acid in place of the normal Thr (threonine) at position 124 of the protein's amino acid sequence. The resulting protein functions abnormally, causing myelin damage. CMT-2 in other families derives from mutations of different genes that code for different nerve proteins, although the end result is a clinically similar type of neuropathy and functional deficit. Other mutations cause familial neuropathies with different clinical features (and different names), also due to some kind of damage to nerve fibers in affected patients. Overall, pain is present in only a few of the various hereditary neuropathies. And even when it is present and due to a particular point mutation, such as in the Thr124Met form of CMT-2, the degree of pain may vary considerably from individual to individual. The simple fact that the nerve has been damaged does *not* in itself explain the pain.

Why then are some peripheral neuropathies painful while others are not? To answer this question, a deeper understanding of the factors that control the electrical excitability of neurons is required. Only in a few cases are we in a position to take a good guess. For example, when myelin is stripped from some sensory axons, excess numbers of Na^+ channel proteins are inserted into the axonal membrane, which can render the axon more likely to generate abnormal impulse discharge and hence more likely to cause pain [4]. But we lack understanding of why particular forms of neuropathy cause this abnormality and not others. We have the gene but not the mechanism; the glass is half empty. Looked at from the opposite perspective, however, knowledge that particular mutation-induced forms of pathology in fact cause pain while others do not can provide useful experimental leads toward unraveling the pain mechanism (the glass is half full). Indeed, such revelations may ultimately be the most important contribution of pain genetics. Notable examples are migraine headache and temporomandibular joint disorder. In both of these conditions, the root cause of the pain remains uncertain. But discovery of precipitating genetic mutations and polymorphisms may aid in discovering the cause [6].

Although the process of moving from disease-related gene to pain mechanism is a possibility, it is at best uncertain. Indeed, identification of a disease susceptibility gene may even be misleading in the effort to discover pain mechanisms, especially if the connection between the gene and the pain phenotype is indirect. For example, genes that predispose to pain-causing tumors and to painful disk herniations are likely to be very different from one another. Nonetheless, in both cases the cause of pain may be the same, and in both cases only remotely related to the disease susceptibility gene(s). Specifically, both diseases lead to the application of mechanical pressure to nerves. This pressure triggers traumatic neuropathy. The cause of the pain is the nerve compression and consequent myelin damage and axonopathy. It makes little difference what caused the nerve compression in the first place: tumor, disk herniation, or shoes that fit too tightly. For this reason, discovery of the genes responsible for the tumor, or for the disk weakness that led to herniation, are unlikely to hasten understanding of pain in traumatic neuropathy. Indeed, research based on the presumption that the action of the gene is an integral part of the pain mechanism may be wasted work.

Gene alleles may tip a person toward the experience of pain in even more indirect ways than a tumor compressing a nerve. Consider alleles associated with risk-taking behavior [13]. As for pain, there are no genes that encode for risk taking. But there are genes that participate in a chain of causality that leads from gene to protein to behavior to pain. Here is an imaginary, but not unrealistic, scenario. Imagine an allele that encodes for a muscle protein that tends to make a young man more muscular. Being more muscular, he is likely to be more athletic and perhaps more attractive to young women. A probable outcome is that he will be more popular, more self-confident, and perhaps more likely to engage in risky sports. As such, he will be more likely to compete in ski jumping, and hence more likely to suffer injury and pain. After all, the more risks you take, the greater are your chances of being hurt. The gene allele that codes for the muscle protein *is*, by definition, a risk-taking gene. It is also a pain-promoting gene; its presence led to an enhanced likelihood of pain, however indirectly. Moreover, there is a good chance that it will come up in an appropriately large association study of risk taking or of pain. But due to the very indirect link between gene and pain process, identification of the allele affecting the muscle protein is unlikely to lead to better understanding of pain or to the development of novel analgesic drugs. It provides little or no insight into pain mechanisms.

On the other hand, the connection between gene and pain mechanism may be direct and informative. A recent example of particular interest is erythromelalgia, an inherited condition associated with red, warm hands and/or feet and severe burning pain. Like CMT-2 and FHM, causative mutations have been found in affected individuals in affected families. But in this case, the mutated gene pointed directly to a likely pain mechanism. The erythromelalgia gene codes for the $Na_v1.7$ Na^+ channel (gene symbol *SCN9A*), a protein with direct relevance to the excitability of sensory neurons. Specifically, experiments in mice revealed that mutations that cause erythromelalgia pain in patients render sensory neurons hyperexcitable. They are gain-of-function mutations. A fascinating (although certainly not unique) feature of the gene responsible for erythromelalgia is that different mutations in the same gene, found in different families, lead to clinically different pain conditions. Thus, while some mutations

cause erythromelalgia, others cause paroxysmal extreme pain disorder. Moreover, still other mutations, in yet other families, lead to the complete *absence* of pain. When these latter mutations were duplicated in mice, it was found that they cause sensory neurons to be *hypo*excitable (*loss*-of-function mutations) [8]. This is a superb, and unusual, example in which identification of the mutation led directly and rapidly to a better understanding of the pain phenotype. Even here, however, there remain inconsistencies and knowledge gaps. (1) Why does the erythromelalgia mutation cause pain in only certain parts of the body when the gene affects all $Na_v1.7$ proteins? (2) Why do different gain-of-function mutations in the same gene cause quite different painful conditions (erythromelalgia vs. paroxysmal extreme pain disorder)? (3) Why does the loss of $Na_v1.7$ function lead to pain insensitivity in humans but does not cause decreased pain response in $Na_v1.7$ mutant mice [19]?

Tentative evidence is already available indicating that genetic variations can predispose to quite a few different conditions with a pain signature. These include herpes zoster infection and postherpetic neuralgia (PHN), temporomandibular joint (TMJ) disorder, rheumatoid arthritis, various headaches, trigeminal neuralgia, low back pain and sciatica, fibromyalgia, and others. In each case, identification of the mutation or polymorphism that affects disease susceptibility may or may not contribute to an understanding of the underlying pain process. It is difficult to know in advance. In general, identification of disease susceptibility genes may be of considerable medical interest for disease diagnosis and prevention, but a priori, such genes are not likely to be directly related to pain mechanisms. Therefore, if the aim is to understand pain rather than disease, a more likely approach is to identify genes in which sequence variants cause one person to develop pain while another does not, in the presence of the same disease or injury. These are "pain susceptibility genes."

"Disease Susceptibility Genes" versus "Pain Susceptibility Genes"

Genes that facilitate painful disease, or behaviors that lead to pain, can be of considerable interest. But as in the examples of cancer-induced, disk-herniation-induced, or footwear-induced peripheral neuropathy and the risk-taking ski jumper, it is far from certain that they will teach us much about pain processing. The discovery of pain susceptibility genes is a more likely route to a better understanding of pain per se. Finding genes that predispose toward more or less pain in response to experimentally applied stimuli is relatively straightforward. Finding genes that predispose to pain due to disease or injury is more challenging. To find them, it is not sufficient to compare allelic differences in groups of individuals with more pain and less pain. It is also necessary to ensure that the groups being compared have the same pain-inducing pathology. The likelihood of developing type 2 diabetes, for example, is affected by genes (as well as by nutrition). But some people who have diabetes develop painful diabetic neuropathy while others do not. Does this mean that diabetes susceptibility genes directly affect pain processing? Not necessarily. For while it is true that the individuals who develop pain may be inherently pain-prone, an alternative possibility is that these individuals have developed a more severe neuropathy. In principle, this problem might be solved by matching the comparison groups for the extent of diabetic neuropathy present using criteria that are independent of diabetic pain. However, such a procedure would leave considerable uncertainty as we do not yet know with much confidence which criteria to choose. We do not yet know well enough what it is about neuropathy that causes pain. A similar caveat holds for many other painful conditions, among them low back pain, PHN, and TMJ disorder.

There are a few conditions, however, where matching groups for equal pathology is feasible. Examples are neuropathic pains that develop (or do not develop) following standard surgical procedures such as thoracotomy or the harvesting of calf nerves for grafting [3], and osteoarthritic pain, where the groups compared can be balanced for the degree of cartilage erosion (assessed radiologically). Limb amputation presents a particularly interesting potential opportunity. As noted above, some amputees develop severe phantom limb pain while others, with the same amputation level (i.e., the same disease) have none. Such observations provide confidence that pain susceptibility, and not just disease susceptibility, is heritable.

Finding Pain Genes

How do you find pain genes? The search for pain genes, like the search for genes that control any other inherited trait, begins by comparing the genetic makeup of individuals or groups with a contrasting pain phenotype.

There are two basic strategies: (1) The study of large families (lineages, pedigrees) in which some individuals develop the painful condition and others do not. The method is *linkage analysis.* (2) The study large cohorts of matched but unrelated individuals with and without the condition. The method is *association analysis.*

Family studies are advantageous when there is a single gene mutation of major effect (a "Mendelian gene"). As noted above, this approach has yielded a number of important susceptibility genes for painful diseases including CMT-2, FHM, and erythromelalgia. But such conditions are rare, presumably because they have been weeded out over the course of evolution. Moreover, lessons learned from studying them often do not generalize to more common, complex polygenic conditions. In addition, linkage analysis in families is limited to diseases that arise spontaneously. It is not well suited to painful conditions that arise following injury or disease such as low back pain, diabetic neuropathy, or phantom limb pain. It is exceedingly unlikely, for example, that we will ever find large families all of whose members have had a below-the-knee amputation or suffer from a uniform degree of diabetic neuropathy. This is a precondition for finding pain susceptibility genes.

Association studies have the advantage that they are open-ended in terms of the strength of the genetic influence and the pain phenotype that can be tackled. However, due to the intrinsic genetic variability of people who are not related, very large cohorts need to be compared, with commensurate costs. The strengths of association studies and their difficulties are discussed in detail in the chapter by Diatchenko and colleagues in this volume. Here I will provide a general introduction and discuss the special problems involved in identifying pain susceptibility (vs. disease susceptibility) genes using this approach.

In association studies one compares the genomes of large cohorts that differ in the trait of interest but are as similar as possible with regards to other parameters, such as environment and ethnic background (a factor known as "stratification"). The specific size of cohorts required depends on how much variability is present (in genetic background, disease/injury status, and pain phenotype), on how strong an effect the gene in question has in determining the trait, and the strategy used to search for genetic differences. For a Mendelian gene a handful of affected individuals may be enough. However, in the more common situation, in which a given gene makes only a small contribution toward determining the trait, the underlying injury or disease is not uniform across individuals, and the definition of the pain phenotype in question is variable and subjective, very large cohorts need to be compared, numbering in the thousands. Due to practical constraints, often budgetary, association studies are frequently conducted with much smaller sample sizes than necessary. That is, they tend to be "underpowered."

The choice of genetic search strategy is also a critical parameter in association studies. Two alternative strategies are currently available: (1) Testing for allelic differences in a small number of "candidate genes" selected on the basis of prior hypotheses on where differences might lie, and (2) searching for potential differences in all genes and regulatory regions in a hypothesis-free manner ("genome-wide association studies"; GWAS). We are probably only a few years away from the practical implementation of a third strategy, an extension of GWAS that involves comparing the actual base-pair sequence of cohorts with and without pain, rather than just comparing polymorphic SNPs. The latter two strategies have the tremendous theoretical advantage of enabling discovery of entirely novel pathways and mechanisms, independent of preconceptions on how the pain system works. This is because *all* genes would be explored for relevant differences, not just pet candidates, "the usual suspects." Such research can be expected to lead us to proteins that nobody ever imagined to be related to pain, opening new and unexpected chapters in pain physiology. The cost of properly powered whole genome studies, however, is high, and the application of these strategies to the search for pain (as opposed to disease) susceptibility genes forces the price even higher, as explained below. Full-scale GWAS aimed at discovering pain genes have not yet been undertaken.

So how have we been doing so far in the discovery of pain genes using the association approach? Although there is plenty of room for optimism, results so far have been a bit disappointing in terms of reliability, especially considering the fact that the conservative candidate gene-based strategy has been used in most studies [16]. The first study "successful" at finding an association between pain and a particular gene allele is usually published with great fanfare. Initial failures tend not to be published at all, a problem called "publication bias." But then come failures to replicate, or worse, concealment of failures to replicate. An example is the early report that the Val158Met polymorphism,

a simple base-pair substitution in the *COMT* gene, increases pain susceptibility [30]. *COMT* encodes an enzyme (catechol-*O*-methyl transferase) involved in catecholamine degradation. The Val158Met polymorphism reduces the efficiency of the enzyme affecting synaptic catecholamine levels, a change that could well affect pain processing. Unfortunately, a number of attempts to follow up this finding obtained a much weaker signal, or none at all. Equally worrisome with respect to the importance of this gene for *pain* is that the same polymorphism has been implicated, also through association studies, in a wide variety of other "disorders" including anxiety, anorexia nervosa, cocaine addiction, academic achievement, schizophrenia, autism, and attention deficit hyperactivity disorder. In most of these disorders, too, the signal is weak and hard to replicate [14]. It is probably not coincidental if the case of *COMT* sounds to you like the muscle protein gene in the ski jumper that affects popularity with girls, risk taking, and pain. The more indirect an affect, the less informative it is likely to be.

Even more disappointing is the 118G allele of the gene that codes for the mu-opioid receptor (*OPRM1*). The presence of this SNP polymorphism was reported to predict the response of pain patients to opiate analgesics and hence was expected to provide an important step forward in pain pharmacogenetics. And what could be more logical, and more believable, than a morphine-receptor variant affecting analgesic response to morphine? And yet, when looked at in the light of accumulating research experience (meta-analysis), it turns out that this pharmacogenetic effect is at best very weak and may not exist at all [27]. Association studies, mostly underpowered, have reported SNPs for many pain-related medical conditions. One cannot know a priori how many of these reports will ultimately prove reliable.

Along with these examples in which early optimism has changed to uncertainty are some notable successes. Several reliable SNPs have been identified that predispose toward headache and migraine, as well as a variety of inflammatory and immune diseases (e.g. ref. [24]). Effect sizes of a given SNP are typically small, however, and the associations reflect a predisposition to developing a named disease rather than to developing more or less pain. This is to be expected, of course, of work promoted and carried out within classical, disease-oriented medical disciplines. Success in allied disciplines is cause for celebration and optimism.

However, it is likely that the search for pain susceptibility genes, within and across specific disease diagnoses, will ultimately rest on the shoulders of researchers who have a particular interest in pain as a biomedical problem in its own right. A fascinating example has been published recently.

The effects of rare mutations in the *SCN9A* gene that codes for $Na_v1.7$ (erythromelalgia, etc.) were noted above. Interestingly, other sequence variations in this same gene may have much subtler effects on pain sensation. One such SNP was found to associate with pain scores in patients with a variety of conditions including osteoarthritis and pancreatitis, and even to predict pain threshold in healthy individuals [22]. Since its effects are much less debilitating that the mutations discussed above, this SNP is quite common in the general population, qualifying it as a polymorphism rather than a mutation. $Na_v1.7$ (*SCN9A*) is therefore a noteworthy example of a pain gene, initially identified as a rare disease susceptibility mutation in affected families, that was adopted as a promising candidate gene and went on qualify as a likely pain susceptibility gene. This success ought to encourage further attempts at adopting this strategy, perhaps using as candidate genes the peripheral neuropathy mutations noted above (e.g., CMT-2).

Finding Pain Susceptibility Genes by Association

Compared to disease susceptibility genes, alleles that determine whether a particular pathology will be painful or nonpainful are more likely to have a relatively direct relation to the neurobiological processes that are responsible for the pain itself. For example, among the various possibilities, a pain susceptibility gene might determine to what extent sensory neurons that have been damaged generate spontaneous abnormal electrical impulse discharges. Alternatively, the critical genetic polymorphism may affect amplification mechanisms within the spinal cord or brain, differences in neurotransmitter expression, or differences in signal processing in the individual's brain. Knowing the gene or genes involved could lead to deeper understanding and perhaps ultimately to more effective pain management. But how to find pain susceptibility genes?

Association Studies

Family (and twin) studies are not well suited to this aim because of the demand for uniform pathology in all individuals tested. This condition can, however, be met in association studies when the precipitating pathology is known. As noted, limb amputation, postsurgical scar pain, and osteoarthritis are special cases particularly favorable for such analysis. In these conditions, the observable pathology is directly related to the pain (in those individuals who have pain). More difficult, but still possible, are conditions such as sciatica due to compression radiculopathy (lateral stenosis), or cases of trigeminal neuralgia in which there is at least some confidence that pain is caused by a definable pathology (disk herniation or microvascular compression). Subjects with pain would undergo appropriate radiological imaging to confirm the diagnosis, just as in an association study aimed at finding disease susceptibility genes. But the comparison group would be different. Rather than matched controls without sciatica or trigeminal neuralgia, the comparison group would be individuals with the same (radiologically confirmed) pathology but with no pain. The extra screening involved in finding such asymptomatic subjects who have "the disease," but no pain, would add considerably to the cost, of course. Painful conditions in which the relation of pathology to pain (when present) is uncertain, or entirely obscure, are poor targets for a search for pain susceptibility genes.

Hybrid Animal-Human Analysis

The search for pain susceptibility genes might be considerably facilitated by adopting a hybrid approach using animal models in coordination with human cohorts. In this strategy, the animals are first subjected to a uniform pathology that tends to induce a painful condition. Many rodent models are available for provoking subacute and chronic neuropathic or inflammatory pain states. Use of an inbred strain of rats or mice, in which each individual carries an identical set of alleles, is not appropriate. Since the aim is to find genetic variants that contribute to diversity in phenotype (pain), the pathology needs to be applied to populations of animals with at least some genetic diversity. Outbred animals might be suitable, but a better choice is a recombinant population based on breeding two inbred parental strains, one high and one low for the pain trait. Examples of recombinant populations are backcross animals (F_1 × the recessive parental strain), an F_2 generation (F_1 × F_1), or a set of recombinant inbred strains. Comparison of patterns of polymorphisms (haplotypes) across standard inbred strains is another option. Since the animals are genetically heterogeneous, they are expected to be variable in their pain phenotype, some individuals scoring high and some low. Gene hunting tools are now applied to locate allelic differences that distinguish the high- and the low-scoring animals.

As in human studies, finding the allele(s) responsible for a complex trait is not trivial. The task is made easier, however, by the fact that in recombinant populations all of the alleles in the animals tested derived from the two original parental strains. Therefore, rather than searching for all possible genetic differences, or complex haplotypes, the search can be limited to those genes in which the parental strains differ. If the parental strains were chosen wisely in the first place, genetic markers (e.g., SNPs) that distinguish the two strains and that can be used to pinpoint the pain gene(s) will be available in publicly accessible databases. Indeed, the exact base-pair sequence of several inbred mouse strains is currently available online. Using these "informative" markers DNA of the animals that are high and low in the pain phenotype can be compared. Alleles that consistently differ between the two groups indicate genes with a high probability of being responsible for the difference in pain phenotype. These genes—and there are likely to be only a few of them—are promising candidate genes. The human homologues of these candidate genes are then used in an association study of human cohorts with a painful condition similar to that imposed on the animals.

The hybrid strategy has two major advantages. The first is that using animals one can impose any injury or pathology of interest on all individuals, in an almost completely uniform manner, and then easily identify the ones which go on to develop pain. The second is that the search for pain susceptibility genes in recombinant animal populations is a genome-wide search strategy that, like GWAS, is largely free of prior physiological hypotheses and biases. However, it is much simpler and less expensive than a human GWAS because genetic background and environmental factors are much easier to control and because a list of informative markers is at hand. The hypothesis-free nature of the search that yielded the gene candidates carries over to the follow-up human association study. But since only a small number of candidate genes need to be tested in the human cohorts, the association study can be done using a much smaller number of subjects than are required in a straight GWAS of human cohorts. This strategy also sidesteps the need to find cohorts of humans who have

the pathology (which may be hard to diagnose) but no resulting pain.

An example of the animal-human hybrid approach is recent work by Ze'ev Seltzer and colleagues who used recombinant inbred mouse strains and the neuroma model of neuropathic pain to find gene candidates responsible for anesthesia dolorosa or phantom limb pain. This analysis identified a region in the midpart of mouse chromosome 15 that apparently harbors a gene of major effect for this pain trait [25]. The investigators were then able to focus their attention and resources on candidate genes located in the corresponding region of the human genome, chromosome 22. These candidate genes were examined using DNA samples from relatively small cohorts of limb amputees and women who had undergone mastectomy. The strategy has yielded a small number of genes in which minor allelic variations distinguish between the individuals who have chronic pain and those who do not. Further steps of verification are still needed. These steps include replication in independent cohorts, examination of the role of ethnic background and environment, and exploration of genetic association to related painful conditions. In addition, to determine *how* the allele affects predisposition to pain, experimental studies need to examine the effects of gene knockout, potential effects of the allelic polymorphism on the structure and function of the gene product, and the effect of the allele on up- and downregulation and trafficking. Ultimately one wants to show that rescue ("repair") of the suspect pain-related allele returns the pain phenotype to that associated with the alternative allele.

Perspective

Pain genetics is still in its infancy. The basis for expecting substantial payoffs in terms of new understanding and medical applications is firm—even though the results so far have not met early, perhaps unrealistically optimistic, expectations, in terms of ease of replication and magnitude of effects. The reason is that methods used to date have not been optimal, including the underpowered scope of many trials undertaken, and the focus on candidate genes selected on the basis of preconceptions rather than on unbiased GWAS or guidance from animal genetic models. The fact that a gene product is important for pain physiology does not necessarily mean that its alleles are important determinants of variability in natural populations. Finally, the genes that predispose to developing a disease that tends to be painful may be only distantly related to the neural mechanisms of pain processing, which makes for weak genetic association. It is reasonable to predict that pain susceptibility genes, when found in the course of a systematic search, will show stronger association and bear a closer relationship to pain mechanisms. At present we should celebrate the success stories that can be told, and hope that in time these will increase in number. In the meanwhile, knowledge that heritable factors can control the amount of pain felt in the presence of injury or disease ought to reduce the stigma often attached unfairly to individuals whose suffering appears to be excessive.

References

[1]   Battie MC, Videman T, Parent E. Lumbar disc degeneration: epidemiology and genetic influences. Spine 2004;29:2679–90.

[2]   Craft RM, Mogil JS, Aloisi AM. Sex differences in pain and analgesia: the role of gonadal hormones. Eur J Pain 2004;8:397–411.

[3]   Devor M. Evidence for heritability of pain in patients with traumatic neuropathy. Pain 2004;108:200–1.

[4]   Devor M. Pathophysiology of nerve injury. In: Cervero F, Jensen TS, editors. Pain. Handbook of clinical neurology, 3rd series, vol. 81. Edinburgh: Elsevier; 2006. p. 261–76.

[5]   Devor M, Raber P. Heritability of symptoms in an experimental model of neuropathic pain. Pain 1990;42:51–67.

[6]   De Vries B, Frants RR, Ferrari MD, Van Den Maagdenberg AM. Molecular genetics of migraine. Hum Genet 2009;126:115–32.

[7]   Ebstein RP, Israel S, Chew SH, Zhong S, Knafo A. Genetics of human social behavior. Neuron 2010;65:831–44.

[8]   Fischer TZ, Waxman SG. Familial pain syndromes from mutations of the $Na_v1.7$ sodium channel. Ann NY Acad Sci 2010;1184:196–207.

[9]   Goldstein DB. Common genetic variation and human traits. N Engl J Med 2009;360:1696–8.

[10] Hirschhorn JN. Genomewide association studies: illuminating biologic pathways. N Engl J Med 2009;360:1699–701.

[11] Israel S, Lerer E, Shalev I, Uzefovsky F, Reibold M, Bachner-Melman R, Granot R, Bornstein G, Knafo A, Yirmiya N, Ebstein RP. Molecular genetic studies of the arginine vasopressin 1a receptor (AVPR1a) and the oxytocin receptor (OXTR) in human behaviour: from autism to altruism with some notes in between. Prog Brain Res 2008;170:435–49.

[12] Kelley WN, Scherrer SS. Hereditary neuropathies. In: Schmidt RF, Willis WD, editors. Encyclopedia of pain, vol. 2. Berlin: Springer; 2007. p. 885–90.

[13] Knafo A, Israel S, Darvasi A, Bachner-Melman R, Uzefovsky F, Cohen L, Feldman E, Lerer E, Laiba E, Raz Y, Nemanov L, Gritsenko I, Dina C, Agam G, Dean B, Bornstein G, Ebstein RP. Individual differences in allocation of funds in the dictator game associated with length of the arginine vasopressin 1a receptor RS3 promoter region and correlation between RS3 length and hippocampal mRNA. Genes Brain Behav 2008;7:266–75.

[14] Lachman HM. Does COMT val158met affect behavioral phenotypes: yes, no, maybe? Neuropsychopharmacology 2008;33:3027–9.

[15] Mogil JS, editor. The genetics of pain. Progress in pain research and management, vol. 28. Seattle: IASP Press; 2004.

[16] Mogil J. Are we getting anywhere in human pain genetics ? Pain 2009;146:231–2.

[17] Mogil JS, Wilson SG, Bon K, Lee SE, Chung K, Raber P, Pieper JO, Hain HS, Belknap JK, Hubert L, Elmer GI, Chung JM, Devor M. Heritability of nociception I. Responses of 11 inbred mouse strains on 12 measures of nociception. Pain 1999;80:67–82.

[18] Mogil JS, Wilson SG, Bon K, Pieper JO, Lee SE, Chung K, Raber P, Hain HS, Belknap JK, Hubert L, Elmer GI, Chung JM, Devor M. Heritability of nociception. II. "Types" of nociception revealed by genetic correlation analysis. Pain 1999;80:83–93.

[19] Nassar MA, Levato A, Stirling LC, Wood JN. Neuropathic pain develops normally in mice lacking both $Na_v1.7$ and $Na_v1.8$. Mol Pain 2005;1:24.

[20] Nissenbaum J, Shpigler H, Pisante A, Del Canho S, Minert A, Seltzer Z, Devor M, Darvasi A. pain2: a neuropathic pain QTL identified on rat chromosome 2. Pain 2008;135:92–7.

[21] Persson AK, Gebauer M, Jordan S, Metz-Weidmann C, Schulte AM, Schneider HC, Ding-Pfennigdorff D, Thun J, Xu XJ, Wiesenfeld-Hallin Z, Darvasi A, Fried K, Devor M. Correlational analysis for identifying genes whose regulation contributes to chronic neuropathic pain. Mol Pain 2009;5:7.

[22] Reimann F, Cox JJ, Belfer I, Diatchenko L, Zaykin DV, McHale DP, Drenth JP, Dai F, Wheeler J, Sanders F, Wood L, Wu TX, Karppinen J, Nikolajsen L, Männikkö M, Max MB, Kiselycznyk C, Poddar M, Te Morsche RH, Smith S, Gibson D, Kelempisioti A, Maixner W, Gribble FM, Woods CG. Pain perception is altered by a nucleotide polymorphism in SCN9A. Proc Natl Acad Sci USA 2010;107:5148–53.

[23] Rodrigues SM, Saslow LR, Garcia N, John OP, Keltner D. Oxytocin receptor genetic variation relates to empathy and stress reactivity in humans. Proc Natl Acad Sci USA 2009;106:21437–41.

[24] Schurks M, Rist PM, Kurth T. MTHFR 677C>T and ACE D/I polymorphisms in migraine: a systematic review and meta-analysis. Headache 2010;50:588–99.

[25] Seltzer Z, Wu T, Max MB, Diehl SR. Mapping a gene for neuropathic pain-related behavior following peripheral neurectomy in the mouse. Pain 2001;93:101–6.

[26] Sherman R, Devor M, Casey Jones DE, Katz J, Marbach JJ. Phantom pain. New York: Plenum; 1996. p. 1–264.

[27] Walter C, Lotsch J. Meta-analysis of the relevance of the OPRM1 118A>G genetic variant for pain treatment. Pain 2009;146:270–5.

[28] Wolfs MG, Hofker MH, Wijmenga C, Van Haeften TW. Type 2 diabetes mellitus: new genetic insights will lead to new therapeutics. Curr Genomics 2009;10:110–8.

[29] Yan H, Yuan W, Velculescu VE, Vogelstein B, Kinzler KW. Allelic variation in human gene expression. Science 2002;297:1143.

[30] Zubieta JK, Heitzeg MM, Smith YR, Bueller JA, Xu K, Xu Y, Koeppe RA, Stohler CS, Goldman D. COMT val158met genotype affects mu-opioid neurotransmitter responses to a pain stressor. Science 2003;299:1240–3.

Correspondence to: Marshall Devor, PhD, Department of Cell & Developmental Biology, Institute of Life Sciences and Center for Research on Pain, The Hebrew University of Jerusalem, Jerusalem 91904, Israel. Email: marshlu@vms.huji.ac.il.

Pain-Related Mutations in the Human Genome

M. Florencia Gosso, PhD,[a] Curtis F. Barrett, PhD,[a,b] Arn M.J.M. van den Maagdenberg, PhD,[a,b] and Michel D. Ferrari, MD, PhD[b]

[a]Department of Human Genetics and [b]Department of Neurology, Leiden University Medical Centre, Leiden, The Netherlands
M.F.G and C.F.B contributed equally

Pain perception in mammals is mediated by neurons in the pain pathway. Specialized sensory receptors located throughout the peripheral nervous system (the so-called "nociceptors") are responsible for first detecting noxious or aversive thermal, chemical, and mechanical stimuli, and then reporting those stimuli to the central nervous system. Nociceptors carry signals to cell bodies in both the dorsal root ganglion (DRG) and trigeminal ganglion (TG); the cell bodies in turn send out two processes, one to the periphery and another into the brainstem in the upper spinal cord.

Pain results from a specific spatiotemporal pattern of neurological activity in the cerebral cortex; thus, nociceptive neurons express a vast repertoire of proteins involved in the activation and propagation of pain signals [117,144,145]. Consequently, the relationship between stimulus and transduction pathway is a complex process, and as a result, perception of a single stimulus often requires several transduction mechanisms working in concert [84]. In this chapter we will discuss the basics of pain perception and processing, as well as the role played by genetics in modulating sensitivity to painful stimuli.

Nociceptors

Nociceptors are essential for maintaining the body's integrity, by sensing noxious or harmful stimuli and initiating the necessary steps to terminate the encounter with the stimulus (e.g., rapid withdrawal from an intensely unpleasant or painful sensation). The sensory specificity of each nociceptor type is conferred by expression of ion channels tuned to respond to selective mechanical, thermal, or chemical stimuli, usually with high fidelity. Nociceptors are generally comprised of two groups based on their type of afferent fibers (slow or fast conducting), the location of the fiber's target in the dorsal horn, and the transmitter secreted (glutamate or substance P). C fibers have small-diameter cell bodies and slowly conducting, unmyelinated axons, whereas Aδ fibers have medium-diameter cell bodies and fast-conducting, lightly myelinated axons [89]. The terminals of nociceptive axons do not possess specialized end-organ structures; this absence of any encapsulation renders them highly vulnerable to both intrinsic and extrinsic chemical agents. Moreover, in addition to signaling acute pain, nociceptors can also signal persistent and pathological pain occurring in the setting of injury, either after occurrence of slightly painful input (hyperalgesia) or following innocuous stimuli (allodynia) (for review see [113]).

Molecular Mechanisms of Nociceptive Signal Transduction

Upon tissue injury a myriad of ions, nucleotides, lipids, peptides, amino acid derivatives, and proteins are released. These compounds are then capable of activating nociceptors or augmenting nociceptor responses to chemical, mechanical, or thermal stimuli. Certain agents (e.g., protons and capsaicin) directly depolarize nociceptors by activating (opening) select ion channels permeable to sodium and/or calcium; other agents, including bradykinin and nerve growth factor, act on G-protein-coupled receptors and receptor tyrosine kinases, respectively, to initiate intracellular signaling cascades that in turn sensitize depolarizing cation channels. In contrast, other agents (e.g., glutamate, acetylcholine, and adenosine triphosphate) can activate both ion channels and G-protein-coupled receptors, producing a spectrum of direct and indirect effects on nociceptor membrane potential (for review see [104]).

Importantly, nociceptors typically express multiple members of an ion channel family, with certain members being expressed at much higher levels in a given population of neurons than in others. Taken together, this specialized heterogeneity confers nociceptors with finely tuned, kinetically controlled responsiveness. Thus, it is difficult to understand the full effect of individual ion channel mutations simply by studying the mutation in vitro.

Pain Heritability

To justify investments in genetic studies of a trait, one must initially demonstrate that a significant proportion of that trait's variability is heritable. The contribution of genetic influences on traits and diseases in the population can be measured in quantitative terms by estimating heritability, a measure of the extent to which the variance of a trait that is observed in the population might be accounted for by genetic variance [102]. Historically, twin studies have been used to assess most, if not all, human heritable traits. Monozygotic (MZ) twins are genetically identical, whereas dizygotic (DZ) twins share on average half their genetic material. Under certain conditions (e.g., similar shared cultural and familial environments), demonstrating greater

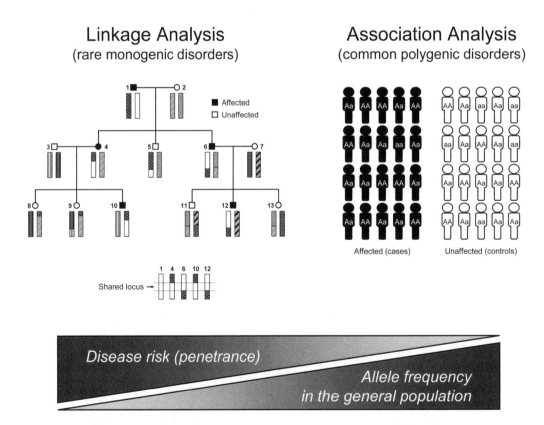

Fig. 1. Overview of whole-genome linkage and association studies. Left: In linkage analysis, large informative families with both affected and unaffected individuals are studied. Shown is a hypothetical family exhibiting a Mendelian disease trait. For each individual, two chromosomal alleles are depicted. Bottom inset: All affected family members have a shared locus with borders defined by recombinations shown as dashed lines (arrow); in contrast, the disease locus is not present in any of the unaffected members. Linkage analysis reveals genetic variants with a high probability of developing the disease (that is, they are highly penetrant); however, these variants are extremely rare in the general population. Squares, male; circles, female. Right: Association analysis examines large groups of unrelated cases and control individuals. In this type of analysis, the frequency of common allele variants is tested for whether they differ significantly between the groups. In the example, the A allele is more frequent in the cases and therefore likely confers an increased relative risk for developing the disease.

phenotypic correlation in MZ than DZ pairs can provide evidence of genetic influence.

From Pain Syndromes to Gene Mutation and Function: How to Study the Genetics of Pain-Related Syndromes

Pain arises from a complex interaction of various transmission, amplification, and suppression systems involving hundreds of molecules. The past successes of pain-related gene hunting owe much to the fact that the first genetic studies of human pain syndromes were of relatively rare, monogenic, highly penetrant disorders that follow the rules of Mendelian inheritance (for review see [46,27]). Pain-related gene variants can be identified by complementary strategies (illustrated in Fig. 1): whole-genome linkage studies, which search for shared genomic regions among affected family members harboring a gene mutation (for review see [81]), and candidate gene association studies and genome-wide association studies (GWAS), which are based on identifying an increased occurrence of specific alleles in cases versus controls. Candidate gene studies are *hypothesis-driven* (with prior knowledge on the tested gene) and generally test one or only a few DNA variants, whereas GWAS are *hypothesis-free* and test hundreds of thousands of DNA variants. Associations can be direct (i.e., the causal allele is the DNA variant studied) or indirect, when the causal allele is linked—that is, in linkage disequilibrium (LD)—with the studied DNA variant (for review see [3,48,60]). Linkage analysis is particularly powerful for studying allelic heterogeneity (different causal mutations in a gene that are sufficient to cause disease are found in different families), as is often observed in channelopathies such as primary erythromelalgia (PE) and familial hemiplegic migraine (FHM).

Although linkage studies are the method of choice when searching for Mendelian diseases influenced by rare, highly penetrant alleles, linkage analysis lacks the power to detect relatively minor genetic effects exerted by multiple loci in polygenic disorders. This limitation stems from the fact that a prohibitive number of informative families are required to map genes of minor to moderate effect that may underlie complex (common) traits [108]. Contrary to linkage studies, association analysis relies on large (clinic- or population-based) samples consisting of unrelated individuals. With linkage analysis,

haplotypes are identified that are inherited intact over several generations (as illustrated by the region indicated with an arrow in Fig. 1, left panel). These haplotypes typically span tens to only a few centimorgans of the genome.[1] In the human genome, 1 cM is on average $\sim10^6$ base pairs. In contrast, association analysis relies on the retention of DNA variants (alleles) at loci located so close that they have not been separated by recombination events.

Combined linkage and mutation detection studies have played a major role in identifying genes and mutations causing disease. Subsequent functional studies unraveling the consequences of these mutations have increased our insight into how these genes are involved in the pathophysiology of pain.

Ion Channels and Pain

Ion channels are membrane-spanning proteins with the principal task of selectively transporting ions into or out of the cell [150]; some ion channels also facilitate ion movement between the cytoplasm and organelles (e.g., the mitochondria and endoplasmic reticulum). Ion channels can be divided into two general categories, voltage-gated and ligand-gated (this distinction is not absolute, however, as the activity of some channels can be regulated by both voltage and ligand binding); a third category of ion channels is the stretch-activated or mechanosensitive channels (these channels will not be discussed further here). From a functional perspective, voltage-gated ion channels sense changes in membrane voltage and respond by opening to allow ions to flux across the membrane. Conversely, ligand-gated channels open upon binding their cognate ligand molecule(s) and permit ions to cross the membrane.

Voltage-gated sodium and potassium channels (and, to a lesser extent, calcium channels) drive action potential propagation and help modulate resting membrane potential and excitability. Voltage-gated calcium channels couple excitation with a variety of downstream cellular responses, including muscle contraction, transcription, and (of particular relevance) neurotransmission [21]. On the other hand, ligand-gated ion channels

---

[1] The centimorgan (also called a map unit) is a measure of recombination frequency, with 1 cM being the distance along a chromosome with a 1% probability that 2 markers (loci) will be separated by a single-generation chromosomal crossing (recombination) event. Thus, the centimorgan can be used to approximate distance along a chromosome.

couple transmitter release to depolarization; this depolarization can in turn activate voltage-gated channels, driving signaling to the nucleus and/or initiating an action potential.

The human genome contains over 400 channel genes, thus representing 1–2% of our genetic endowment [143]. The voltage-gated ion channels are among the most ancient and conserved gene families (at the protein level, more than 50% sequence identity exists between the transmembrane domains of human sodium channel α subunits and those of the simplest multicellular eukaryotes). Importantly, this large, diverse group of channels does not simply reflect redundancy; rather, many channel genes are expressed in a remarkably tissue-specific fashion, whereas others, more broadly expressed, play a prominent role in the physiology of only a few tissue types. Moreover, combinatorial subunit assembly coupled with alternative splicing allows one channel gene to produce a wide range of functionally distinct protein products.

Voltage-Gated Channels

Voltage-gated sodium and calcium channels are closely related members of the ion channel superfamily [150] (voltage-gated potassium channels are also members of this superfamily, but they will not be discussed here). Because of their crucial functions and complex structures, these two ion channel families fall prey to numerous mutations that cause diseases of excitability in the context of pain-related syndromes.

Voltage-Gated Sodium Channels

The human genome contains genes that code for nine functional voltage-gated sodium channel α subunits (named $Na_V1.1$ through $Na_V1.9$) and that differ in both their pattern of tissue expression and their biophysical properties (for review see [149]). The α subunit contains four internally repeated domains (DI–DIV), which each consists of six alpha-helical transmembrane segments (S1–S6) and a pore loop connecting S5 and S6 (Fig. 2C). The α subunit houses the voltage sensor and the ion-conducting pore, and it also serves as the binding site for pharmacological compounds that affect the channel's properties [17]. The association with auxiliary β subunits modifies the kinetics and voltage dependence of gating; in addition, β subunits can serve as cell adhesion molecules interacting with the extracellular matrix, other cell adhesion molecules, and the cytoskeleton [63].

The $Na_V1.1$, $Na_V1.2$, $Na_V1.3$, and $Na_V1.6$ sodium channels, encoded respectively by the *SCN1A*, *SCN2A*, *SCN3A*, and *SCN8A* genes, are the primary sodium channels expressed in the central nervous system [17,131]. $Na_V1.1$ and $Na_V1.3$ channels are primarily localized to cell bodies [146], whereas $Na_V1.2$ channels are located in unmyelinated or premyelinated axons and dendrites [146]; $Na_V1.6$ channels are localized in myelinated axons and in dendrites [13,78]. These channels participate in the generation and propagation of both somatodendritic and axonal action potentials [71,103]. In the peripheral nervous system, $Na_V1.7$ channels (encoded by the *SCN9A* gene) are expressed in sympathetic (superior cervical ganglion [SCG]) neurons, sensory (DRG) neurons, and their axons, whereas $Na_V1.8$ and $Na_V1.9$ (encoded by the *SCN10A* and *SCN11A* genes, respectively) are exclusively expressed in sensory neurons, including peripheral terminal axons and cell bodies [18]. Recent linkage studies have identified several mutations in genes encoding voltage-gated sodium channels as the causal link for human pain-related diseases (for review see [38,27]).

Voltage-Gated Calcium Channels

Calcium (Ca^{2+}) ions initiate or regulate a multitude of physiological processes, from membrane depolarization, neurotransmitter release, and muscle contraction to ion transport, phosphorylation and transcription [7,21]. Voltage-gated calcium channels are structurally quite similar to sodium channels, with the pore-forming $α_1$ subunit being comprised of four repeating units containing six membrane-spanning helices (see Fig. 2A). As with sodium channels, the function (and expression) of calcium channels is modified by auxiliary subunits: β, $α_2δ$, and (in some cases) γ. Adding to the diversity of calcium channels, the auxiliary subunits are encoded by multiple genes (for example, the *CACNB1* through *CACNB4* genes encode the β1 through β4 subunits, respectively) that are themselves subject to alternative splicing.

The $α_1$ subunit of the $Ca_V2.1$ (P/Q–type) voltage-gated calcium channel (encoded by the *CACNA1A* gene) plays a major role in mediating excitation–secretion coupling at the presynaptic terminal, translating membrane depolarization into synaptic release of neurotransmitters [16]. Mutations in voltage-gated calcium channels give rise to a wide variety of diseases (for review see [99,49]). Of note, human mutations in *CACNA1A* have been linked to hemiplegic migraine (sometimes including

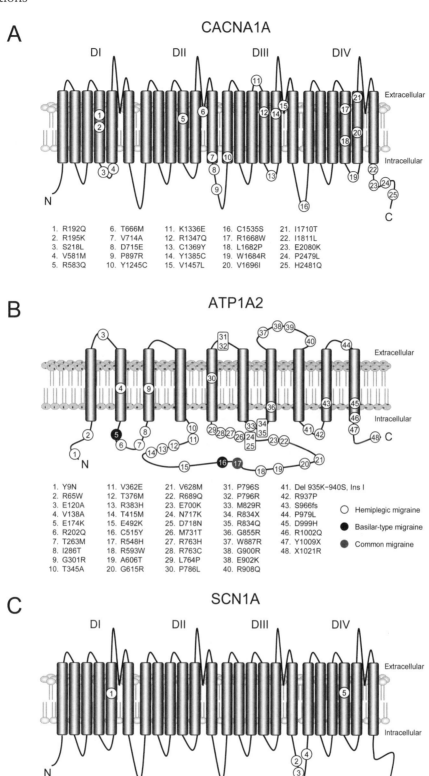

Fig. 2. Schematic representation of sporadic hemiplegic migraine (SHM) and familial hemiplegic migraine (FHM) mutations in FHM gene-encoded proteins. The diagrams show the approximate locations of the mutations. (A) Mutations in the α_{1A} subunit of the $Ca_V 2.1$ (P/Q-type) voltage-gated Ca^{2+} channel encoded by the FHM1 *CACNA1A* gene (Genbank accession number X99897). The protein is located in the plasma membrane and contains four repeat domains (DI–DIV), each containing six transmembrane segments. (B) Mutations in the α_2 subunit of the Na^+,K^+-ATPase encoded by the FHM2 *ATP1A2* gene (Genbank accession number NM_000702). The protein is located in the plasma membrane and contains 10 transmembrane segments. (C) Mutations in the α_1 subunit of the $Na_V 1.1$ voltage-gated Na^+ channel encoded by the FHM3 *SCN1A* gene (Genbank accession number NM_006920). The protein is located in the plasma membrane and has a topography similar to that of $Ca_V 2.1$.

associated symptoms such as seizures, cerebellar ataxia, and head-trauma-induced cerebral edema), episodic ataxia, and spinocerebellar ataxia [137].

Neuronal Ionopathies: Migraine Genes

Migraine is a common, disabling episodic neurovascular disorder [45,51]. Migraine can be broadly classified into migraine with aura and migraine without aura [118]. There are up to four distinct clinical phases of a typical migraine attack [9]. These phases consist of (i) the premonitory phase [50,69], (ii) the aura phase [110], (iii) the headache phase, and (iv) the recovery or resolution phase [70]. Migraine is considered a truly multifactorial complex disorder, and identification of causal genes has proven to be a daunting task. Our current molecular genetic insight into the pathophysiology of migraine predominantly comes from linkage studies among families suffering from a rare monogenic subtype of migraine with aura called familial hemiplegic migraine (FHM).

FHM can be considered a model for the common forms of migraine with aura because the headache and aura features, apart from the hemiparesis, are nearly identical [126]. Furthermore, certain mutations in all identified FHM genes can also produce seizures, suggesting that migraine and epilepsy probably have disease mechanisms and pathways in common. To date, three genes have been linked to FHM, and the functional consequences of many FHM mutations have been studied. In general, these mutations lead to increased excitability in the brain. As a result, the brain of an FHM patient is more susceptible to neuronal input.

FHM1: CACNA1A Gene

The FHM1 CACNA1A gene, located on chromosome 19p13, encodes the ion-conducting, pore-forming α_{1A} subunit of $Ca_V 2.1$ (P/Q-type) voltage-gated neuronal calcium channels [96]. These channels are expressed both at central synapses and in motor nerve terminals, as well as in the cell bodies and dendrites of many neurons (in particular cerebellar Purkinje neurons, for which P-type channels are named). Their principal function upon activation is to mediate Ca^{2+} entry at the nerve terminal, triggering the release of neurotransmitters (see Fig. 4A) [16].

To date, more than 50 CACNA1A mutations have been associated with a wide range of clinical phenotypes, including disorders not associated with FHM (for review see [1,99,137]). Of these, 25 missense mutations have been reported in patients exhibiting a range of hemiplegic migraine phenotypes including pure hemiplegic migraine [39], as well as FHM with associated cerebellar ataxia [2,76] and epilepsy, both during severe FHM attacks [132], or independent of FHM attacks [77,132] (see Fig. 2A).

Functionally, FHM mutations manifest as a gain of function by shifting voltage dependence toward more negative membrane potentials (for review see [101,137]). Consequently, mutant channels can open upon relatively mild depolarization. This shift would lead to increased Ca^{2+} flux and increased neurotransmission, predictions borne true by examining transgenic mice carrying pathogenic FHM1 missense mutations in the orthologous Cacna1a gene [66,130,135,136]. Moreover, consistent with increased central excitability, these mice are highly susceptible to induction of cortical spreading depression [40,41,130,135,136], a propagating wave of neuronal and glial depolarization that plays a prominent role in migraine pathogenesis [10,54].

FHM2: ATP1A2 Gene

The FHM2 ATP1A2 gene, located on chromosome 1q23, encodes the α_2 subunit of a sodium-potassium ATPase exchange pump [26]. During development, ATP1A2 is predominantly expressed in neurons, but expression shifts to glial cells by adulthood [87]. More than 45 ATP1A2 mutations have been reported (see Fig. 2B), with most occurring in individual families (private mutations). Almost all ATP1A2 mutations are amino acid missense mutations, but small deletions [107] and a mutation affecting the stop codon [64] have also been reported. ATP1A2 mutations have been associated mainly with pure FHM [26,64,67,107,100]. However, other clinical manifestations of FHM2 have been reported, including cerebellar ataxia [119], alternating hemiplegia of childhood [5,121], benign focal infantile convulsions [139], and permanent mental retardation [64,140]. Mutations in ATP1A2 have also been associated with other types of migraine, including basilar-type migraine and common migraine [129,141]. Interestingly, and consistent with FHM being a disease of central excitability, the R689Q mutation has also been associated with benign familial infantile convulsions [139].

The functional effect of FHM2 mutations has been investigated, and all mutations studied lead to decreased protein function, in which the pump is less effective at transporting Na^+ and K^+ ions across the cell membrane [14,25,61,75,114,115]. The consequence of such a loss of function is predicted to be impaired K⁺ uptake and, indirectly, reduced removal of glutamate from the synaptic cleft.

FHM3: SCN1A Gene

The FHM3 *SCN1A* gene is located on chromosome 2q24 and encodes the pore-forming α subunit of Na$_V$1.1, a neuronal voltage-gated sodium channel [35]. More than 150 mutations in the *SCN1A* gene have been linked to epilepsy and febrile seizures (for review see [88]). Studies of knockout mice have suggested that Na$_V$1.1 channels are expressed primarily in inhibitory interneurons [151,95]; thus, functional perturbations of this protein will likely lead to a disruption in the balance between excitation and inhibition, giving rise to general hyperexcitability. To date, five FHM3 mutations have been identified [15,35,133,138] (Fig. 2C).

Because of the critical role voltage-gated sodium channels play in action potential firing, it was originally believed that FHM3 mutations increase excitability by exerting a gain-of-function effect on channel function. This belief was based on the observation that, when the Q1489K mutation was introduced into the homologous *SCN5A* cDNA (Na$_V$1.5), there was a significant increase in the channel's ability to recover from inactivation [34]. However, recently this mutation (as well as two additional FHM3 mutations) was introduced into the FHM3 *SCN1A* cDNA. In the context of the Na$_V$1.1 channel, the Q1489K mutation conferred qualitatively opposite effects than in Na$_V$1.5; notably, the channels exhibited *decreased* recovery from inactivation [65]. Na$_V$1.1 channels bearing a second FHM3 mutation, L1649Q, expressed at wild-type levels but were drastically impaired in trafficking to the cell membrane [65], again indicating a loss-of-function effect. Given that *SCN1A* is expressed primarily in inhibitory neurons, these effects would lead to a net increase in central excitability. It is important to note that a third FHM3 mutation, L263V, was also studied in Na$_V$1.1, and it was found to exert a net gain-of-function effect [65]; interestingly, the majority of patients with this mutation also have epilepsy [15]. Based on these results it is therefore difficult to characterize all FHM3 mutations as either gain or loss of function.

The FHM4 Gene and Sporadic Hemiplegic Migraine

The fact that not all FHM families are linked to one of the three known FHM loci implies that there are additional FHM genes yet to be discovered. Recently, a novel FHM locus on chromosome 14q32 was proposed in a Spanish migraine family [23]. In addition, not all hemiplegic migraine patients are part of FHM families. So-called sporadic hemiplegic migraine (SHM) patients exhibit clinical symptoms that are similar to those of hemiplegic migraine patients [128], including attacks of common (nonparetic) migraine. Moreover, the prevalence of familial and sporadic hemiplegic migraine in the general population is similar—both are rare, with an occurrence of approximately 0.01% [128]. Several studies have tried to identify mutations in FHM genes in SHM patients [28,124,127]. Whereas about 15% of SHM patients in a Dutch clinic-based study had gene mutations (predominantly in the *ATP1A2* gene) [28], very few mutations were identified in 100 patients from a Danish population-based study [127].

TREX1 Mutations Associated with Migraine

TREX1 (also called DNAseIII) is a 3-prime repair exonuclease and is a component of the SET complex, acting to rapidly degrade 3' ends of nicked DNA during granzyme A-mediated cell death [68,85,86]. Mutations in the *TREX1* gene have been linked to several disorders (for review see [68]), including Aicardi-Goutieres syndrome 1 (AGS1), retinal vasculopathy with cerebral leukodystrophy (RVCL), familial chilblain lupus (FCL), and systemic lupus erythematosus (SLE). Although the TREX1 protein is not an ion channel, it is interesting to note that mutations in the *TREX1* gene are associated with increased susceptibility to migraine or migraine-like symptoms [29,62,125]. How functional perturbations in a repair exonuclease can cause such a diverse range of conditions is still unknown.

Peripheral Channelopathies

SCN9A Gene

The Na$_V$1.7 sodium channel subtype, encoded by the *SCN9A* gene on chromosome 2q24, is mainly expressed in the peripheral nervous system, in both sympathetic neurons and sensory neurons of the DRG [8,111]. Na$_V$1.7 produces a fast-activating and inactivating inward sodium current and is blocked by nanomolar concentrations of tetrodotoxin (TTX) [74,111]. Recent linkage studies in human patients have directly linked the *SCN9A* gene to three pain disorders: primary erythromelalgia (PE) [147], paroxysmal extreme pain disorder (PEPD) [46], and Na$_V$1.7-associated congenital insensitivity to pain (CIP) [22].

Primary Erythromelalgia

Primary erythromelalgia (PE), also called erythermalgia or inherited erythromelalgia (IEM), is an autosomal dominant disorder with symptoms typically including episodes of burning pain triggered by heat or exercise, together with erythema and mild swelling, primarily in the hands and feet [36]. It is noteworthy to distinguish inherited erythromelalgia from secondary forms of erythromelalgia, which are usually attributed to vascular disorders such as thrombocythemia caused by abnormal platelet-mediated arteriolar inflammation and thrombosis [90]. The onset of PE symptoms may occur within the first decade of life, and both the frequency and severity of pain episodes increase with age, with each episode lasting minutes to hours. PE patients do not report autonomic abnormalities (e.g., orthostatic hypotension or gastrointestinal symptoms). Partial relief of symptoms comes from cooling the affected extremities.

To date, a total of 14 SCN9A mutations have been linked to PE (Fig. 3). All mutations are in highly conserved residues and have been characterized as gain-of-function mutations [33,37,80,147]. Penetrance for these mutations appears to be complete; however, de novo mutations (e.g., I848T, A863P) have

been also reported [59,147], and the L858F mutation was found to show paternal mosaicism [58]. Functionally, all but the F1449V mutation confer slowed deactivation kinetics and larger window currents [20,24,33,43,58,59,79,80,116]. Interestingly, the A1632E mutation causes both PE and PEPD; the functional consequences of the mutation have features common to both PE and PEPD mutations [43].

Despite the direct link between SCN9A mutations and early-onset PE symptoms, no link has been found for the recently reported familial adult-onset PE [12]. Rather, it has been hypothesized that mutations in noncoding regions (e.g., promoter and enhancer regions) of the SCN9A gene may underlie adult-onset forms of PE.

Paroxysmal Extreme Pain Disorder

Paroxysmal extreme pain disorder (PEPD), also known as familial rectal pain, is caused by mutations in the SCN9A gene. Symptoms have an early onset (developing immediately after birth) and are characterized by lifelong pain episodes associated with tonic posturing followed by flushing of the lower limbs that can be either unilateral or bilateral. Unlike PE, which is usually refractory to pharmacological treatment, PEPD patients respond satisfactory to treatment with carbamazepine [6].

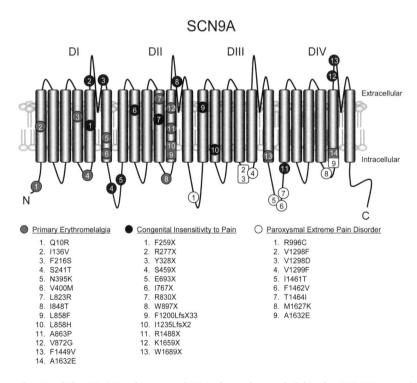

Fig. 3. Mutations in the α_1 subunit of the Na$_v$1.7 voltage-gated Na$^+$ channel encoded by the SCN9A gene (Genbank accession number NP_002968). The diagram shows the approximate locations of the mutations. The protein is located in the plasma membrane and has a topography similar to that of Na$_v$1.1. Mutations linked to primary erythromelalgia (PE), congenital insensitivity to pain (CIP), and paroxysmal extreme pain disorder (PEPD) are indicated.

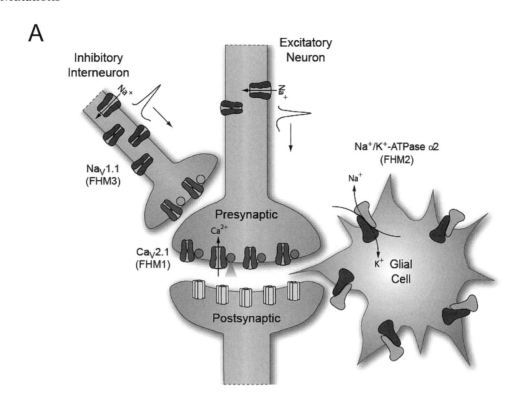

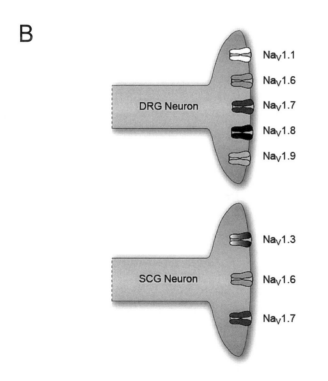

Fig. 4. (A) Cartoon depicting a glutamatergic synapse in the central nervous system and the functional roles of proteins encoded by the FHM1, FHM2, and FHM3 genes. Ca$_V$2.1 calcium channels are located in the presynaptic terminal of excitatory and inhibitory neurons. In response to an invading action potential, these channels gate, allowing Ca^{2+} to enter and triggering vesicle fusion and glutamate release into the synaptic cleft. K$^+$ in the synaptic cleft is removed in part by the action of the Na$^+$/K$^+$-ATPase located at the surface of glial cells (astrocytes). Removing extracellular K$^+$ serves to dampen neuronal excitability and maintains a Na$^+$ gradient, which drives uptake of glutamate from the cleft by transporters (e.g., EAAT1). Lastly, the Na$_V$1.1 voltage-gated sodium channel is expressed in inhibitory interneurons, where it serves to initiate and propagate action potentials. Gain-of-function mutations in Ca$_V$2.1 and loss-of-function mutations in *ATP1A2* and Na$_V$1.1 will each lead to a net effect of increased general excitability (reproduced from [4]). (B) Representation of the cell membrane of dorsal root ganglion (DRG) and superior cervical ganglion (SCG) nerve terminals showing the respective complements of voltage-gated sodium channels that are present in these neurons. The Na$_V$1.8 and Na$_V$1.9 sodium channels require stronger depolarization to activate relative to Na$_V$1.1, Na$_V$1.3, Na$_V$1.6, and Na$_V$1.7. In addition, Na$_V$1.8 and Na$_V$1.9 channels contribute to persistent and slowly inactivating currents, respectively.

Nine *SCN9A* mutations have been linked to PEPD (Fig. 3) [80], most of which have an autosomal dominant pattern of inheritance with complete penetrance, although de novo mutations have been also reported [46].

Channelopathy-Associated Congenital Insensitivity to Pain

Although CIP patients exhibit varying degrees of deficits in terms of sensing pain and their response to painful stimuli (e.g., burns, bone fracture, finger and toe mutilation, and visceral pain), other sensory (non-nociceptive) modalities remain intact [22]. Unlike PE and PEPD, CIP is autosomal recessive and extremely rare [22,52]. To date, 13 CIP alleles have been reported (Fig. 3), all leading to loss-of-function mutations occurring in coding regions of the gene [22,80].

Functional Studies and Molecular Pathophysiology of *SCN9A* Mutations

The role of $Na_V1.7$ in inflammatory pain signaling is supported by knockdown and knockout studies in mice: in vivo knockdown of $Na_V1.7$ with antisense oligonucleotides prevented thermal hyperalgesia [148], and knockout of $Na_V1.7$ in DRG neurons abrogated inflammation-induced mechanical and thermal hyperalgesia [94]. Taken together, such studies indicate that $Na_V1.7$ channels play a key and nonredundant role in nociception. For example, the complete knockout of $Na_V1.7$ by null mutations does not appear to impair other sensory modalities. This finding also suggests that loss-of-function mutations in $Na_V1.7$ channel proteins do not interfere with the function of the other sodium channel isoforms that might be expressed within the same neuron (see Fig. 4B). Finally, persistent lack of pain sensibility observed in adulthood suggests that the role of $Na_V1.7$ channels in nociception is not redundant, and their function cannot be adequately compensated by other channels, such as the sensory-neuron-specific $Na_V1.8$ and $Na_V1.9$ channels [52]. Given the widespread distribution of $Na_V1.7$ channels throughout the sensory nervous system, it is remarkable that PE and PEPD present with pain in such different tissues. PEPD mutations that impair fast inactivation of $Na_V1.7$ would be expected to increase repetitive firing, leading to hyperexcitability of DRG neurons housing the mutant channels [19]. In contrast, the expression of mutant $Na_V1.7$ channels in sympathetic SCG neurons, which normally express several sodium channel classes (including $Na_V1.7$), would decrease excitability [109]. Such opposing cell-specific effects might be explained by two somewhat related factors: (1) TTX-resistant $Na_V1.8$

sodium channels are expressed in sensory but not sympathetic neurons [109]; (2) coexpression of $Na_V1.8$ within DRG neurons permits these cells to generate action potentials and sustain repetitive firing when depolarized [106], so that depolarization would not be expected to abolish action potential firing in DRG neurons expressing $Na_V1.7$ channels bearing PE mutations (Fig. 4B).

Lastly, although functional studies showed a temperature-sensitive shift that brings the activation threshold of PE mutant channels close to that of wild-type $Na_V1.7$ channels, possibly explaining why cooling alleviates pain in PE patients [57], the paroxysmal nature of the painful attacks in PE and PEPD is not fully understood.

SNPs Associated with Altered Pain Perception

Catecholamines (e.g., norepinephrine, epinephrine, and dopamine) have multiple functions in the brain, including processing and modulation of pain (for review see [98]). In recent years, several allelic variants (called single nucleotide polymorphisms or SNPs) have been identified among genes involved in catecholamine metabolism, whose proteins play a role in pain perception [11,93,120,152]. Haplotypes composed of SNPs conferring increased and/or decreased sensitivity to pain have been identified in several genes and are summarized in Table I. Interestingly, several studies of both patients and animal models reported gender differences in pain perception [32,92,93]; experimentally, the threshold for pain from both pressure and electrical stimulation (but not thermal pain stimuli) is lower for females than for males [91,93].

MC1R Gene

The melanocortin-1 receptor (MC1R), encoded by the *MCR1* gene, is a receptor known to play an important role in skin and hair pigmentation [134]. Recently, this receptor has also been studied for its role in relation to pain sensitivity [92,93]. Specifically, both human and animal studies have implicated select gene variants as altering pain sensation (either increasing or decreasing sensitivity) and opioid-mediated analgesia. These SNPs have been previously associated with MC1R loss of function (for review see [112]). Given that this receptor is primarily expressed in melanocytes (and to a lesser extent in keratinocytes, fibroblasts, epithelial cells, and antigen-presenting cells), the connection between decreased MC1R function and altered skin/hair pigmentation is logical. However, how these variants affect pain sensitivity is still unclear, but a key clue comes from a recent paper in which individuals carrying these variants exhibited an increased response to the mu-opioid compound morphine-6-glucuronide (M6G) [92].

COMT Gene

The catechol-*O*-methyltransferase (COMT) enzyme catalyzes the degradation of catecholamines, including the neurotransmitters dopamine, epinephrine, and norepinephrine. Reduced COMT enzymatic activity appears to result in increased pain sensitivity. Although the precise mechanism by which this process occurs remains to be elucidated, decreased COMT activity seems to affect both neurotransmitters and their receptors. Decreased catecholamine metabolism—due to reduced COMT activity—may increase sensitivity to noxious stimuli by decreasing enkephalin levels, leading to an upregulation of mu-opioid receptors, as well as activation of $\beta_{2/3}$ adrenergic receptors [152]. It is interesting to note that pain-altering SNPs have been identified in the *OPRM1* and *OPRD1* genes, which encode the opioid receptors mu-1 and delta-1, respectively (see Table I).

A nonsynonymous SNP on the *COMT* gene that results in a substitution of valine with methionine at position 158 (V158M; SNP rs4680), which reduces thermostability of the enzyme, has been the most-studied functional polymorphism within the gene [83], suggesting that this variant may account for the phenotype. However, a broader study of the haplotype structure of the *COMT* gene was recently conducted [32]. Using both human and in vitro transfection studies, the authors demonstrated that the V158M polymorphism alone is not sufficient to account for the observed variation in pain perception; indeed, an interaction between this polymorphism and other allelic variants determines the final functional outcome. This event subsequently may not affect RNA stability, but rather influences secondary mRNA structure, thereby altering the efficacy of protein synthesis. In this regard it is interesting to note that two SNPs in the haplotype are in coding sequences but are same-sense substitutions, resulting in no change in the protein sequence.

Finally, genetic variation in the *COMT* gene has also been associated with variation in perception of multiple experimental pain stimuli [32,152] and variable susceptibility to common pain conditions such as fibromyalgia [53,142], migraine [42], and temporomandibular disorder [32]. No association was found in other studies with similar phenotypes [31,55,56].

Table I
Haplotypes associated with altered pain perception and/or sensitivity

Gene (Chromosomal Locus)	Protein	SNP(s)* (Location/ Amino Acid Change)	Phenotype	Reference(s)
COMT (22q11.2)	Catechol-*O*-methyltransferase	rs6269 (intronic) rs4633 (H62H) rs4818 (L136L) rs4680 (V158M)	Increased/decreased pain sensitivity	30,32,72,152
GCH1 (14q22.1–q22.2)	GTP cyclohydrolase	rs10483639 (5' UTR) rs3783641 (intronic) rs8007267 (intronic)	Partial analgesia	122,123
MC1R (16q24.3)	Melanocortin 1 receptor	rs1805007 (R151C) rs1805008 (R160W) rs1805009 (D294H)	Increased/decreased pain sensitivity; increased kappa- and mu-opioid-mediated analgesia (see text)	92,93
OPRD1 (1p36.1–p34.3)	Opioid receptor delta-1	rs1042114 (F27C) rs2234918 (G307G)	Increased/decreased acute pain sensitivity	73
OPRM1 (6q24–q25)	Opioid receptor mu-1	rs1799972 (V6A) rs1799971 (N40D)	Decreased pain sensitivity, decreased opioid analgesia	47,82
SCN9A (2q24)	Na$_V$1.7 voltage-gated sodium channel	rs6746030 (R1150W)	Increased pain sensitivity	44,105
TRPV1 (17p13)	Transient receptor potential cation channel V1	rs222747 (M315I) rs8065080 (I585V)	Decreased pain sensitivity	73,97

* NCBI dbSNP126, Build 36.1 (www.ncbi.nlm.nih.gov/projects/SNP/).

GCH1 Gene

Tetrahydrobiopterin (BH4, a cofactor in nitric oxide, serotonin, and catecholamine production), as well as its synthesizing enzyme guanosine triphosphate (GTP) cyclohydrolase (GCH1), has been recently described as playing a role in pain sensitivity. For example, excess BH4 levels are thought to increase pain by increasing nitric oxide production. A pain-protective CGH1 haplotype consisting of three SNPs (rs10483639, rs3783641, and rs8007267) in a regulatory region of the GCH1 gene was identified in about 15% of the population studied, and has been shown to decrease both persistent postsurgical and acute mechanical experimental pain [122,123]. Individuals who are either heterozygous or homozygous for this pain-protective haplotype were also found to show reduced cyclic adenosine monophosphate (cAMP)-mediated GCH1 transcription, resulting in decreased BH4 levels, suggesting that altered GCH1 transcriptional modulation underlies the decreased pain sensitivity observed in these individuals [123].

SCN9A Gene

Recently, the minor A allele of SNP rs6746030 (causing an R1150W substitution in the $Na_v1.7$ protein) was associated with increased pain sensitivity [105]. This SNP was previously identified in a PE family [44]. The effects of the substitution on channel properties were investigated and found to be subtle: in one study a slight positive shift in the voltage dependence of activation was observed in 1150W-containing channels [44], whereas in another study a slight increase in the slope factor of slow (steady-state) inactivation was found [105]. Nevertheless, when expressed in DRG neurons, the 1150W-containing channels led to increased excitability [44], which in humans would increase sensitivity to pain.

Conclusions

The perception of pain provides important information about the health status of the organism. Being able to appropriately detect painful stimuli confers protection, allowing one to take necessary steps to terminate the stimulus. However, being oversensitive to stimuli can be just as dangerous as being undersensitive. Increased (or inappropriate) sensitivity to pain can profoundly affect productivity and quality of life. Thus, a sophisticated system relying on the concerted activity of multiple neuronal networks and molecular pathways has evolved to allow us to correctly identify and avoid potentially harmful situations.

Acknowledgments

Support came from a VICI grant (918.56.602) of the Netherlands Organization for Scientific Research, from a grant from the Centre for Medical Systems Biology within the framework of the Netherlands Genomics Initiative (NGI)/Netherlands Organisation for Scientific Research (NWO), and from TREND (Trauma RElated Neuronal Dysfunction), a Dutch Consortium that is supported by a government grant (BSIK03016).

References

[1] Adams PJ, Snutch TP. Calcium channelopathies: voltage-gated calcium channels. Subcell Biochem 2007;45:215–51.

[2] Alonso I, Barros J, Tuna A, Seixas A, Coutinho P, Sequeiros J, Silveira I. A novel R1347Q mutation in the predicted voltage sensor segment of the P/Q-type calcium-channel alpha-subunit in a family with progressive cerebellar ataxia and hemiplegic migraine. Clin Genet 2004;65:70–2.

[3] Ardlie KG, Kruglyak L, Seielstad M. Patterns of linkage disequilibrium in the human genome. Nat Rev Genet 2002;3:299–309.

[4] Barrett CF, van den Maagdenberg AMJM, Frants RR, Ferrari MD. Familial hemiplegic migraine. Adv Genet 2008;63:57–83.

[5] Bassi MT, Bresolin N, Tonelli A, Nazos K, Crippa F, Baschirotto C, Zucca C, Bersano A, Dolcetta D, Boneschi FM, Barone V, Casari G. A novel mutation in the ATP1A2 gene causes alternating hemiplegia of childhood. J Med Genet 2004;41:621–8.

[6] Bednarek N, Arbues AS, Motte J, Sabouraud P, Plouin P, Morville P. Familial rectal pain: a familial autonomic disorder as a cause of paroxysmal attacks in the newborn baby. Epileptic Disord 2005;7:360–2.

[7] Berridge MJ. Neuronal calcium signaling. Neuron 1998;21:13–26.

[8] Black JA, Dib-Hajj S, McNabola K, Jeste S, Rizzo MA, Kocsis JD, Waxman SG. Spinal sensory neurons express multiple sodium channel alpha-subunit mRNAs. Brain Res Mol Brain Res 1996;43:117–31.

[9] Blau JN. Migraine: theories of pathogenesis. Lancet 1992;339:1202–7.

[10] Bolay H, Moskowitz MA. The emerging importance of cortical spreading depression in migraine headache. Rev Neurol (Paris) 2005;161:655–7.

[11] Bond C, LaForge KS, Tian M, Melia D, Zhang S, Borg L, Gong J, Schluger J, Strong JA, Leal SM, Tischfield JA, Kreek MJ, Yu L. Single-nucleotide polymorphism in the human mu opioid receptor gene alters beta-endorphin binding and activity: possible implications for opiate addiction. Proc Natl Acad Sci USA 1998;95:9608–13.

[12] Burns TM, Te Morsche RH, Jansen JB, Drenth JP. Genetic heterogeneity and exclusion of a modifying locus at 2q in a family with autosomal dominant primary erythermalgia. Br J Dermatol 2005;153:174–7.

[13] Caldwell JH, Schaller KL, Lasher RS, Peles E, Levinson SR. Sodium channel $Na_v1.6$ is localized at nodes of Ranvier, dendrites, and synapses. Proc Natl Acad Sci USA 2000;97:5616–20.

[14] Capendeguy O, Horisberger JD. Functional effects of Na+,K+ATPase gene mutations linked to familial hemiplegic migraine. Neuromolecular Med 2004;6:105–16.

[15] Castro MJ, Stam AH, Lemos C, de Vries B, Vanmolkot KR, Barros J, Terwindt GM, Frants RR, Sequeiros J, Ferrari MD, Pereira-Monteiro JM, van den Maagdenberg AM. First mutation in the voltage-gated $Na_v1.1$ subunit gene SCN1A with co-occurring familial hemiplegic migraine and epilepsy. Cephalalgia 2009;29:308–13.

[16] Catterall WA. Structure and function of neuronal Ca^{2+} channels and their role in neurotransmitter release. Cell Calcium 1998;24:307–23.

[17] Catterall WA. From ionic currents to molecular mechanisms: the structure and function of voltage-gated sodium channels. Neuron 2000;26:13–25.

[18] Catterall WA, Goldin AL, Waxman SG. International Union of Pharmacology. XLVII. Nomenclature and structure-function relationships of voltage-gated sodium channels. Pharmacol Rev 2005;57:397–409.

[19] Catterall WA, Yu FH. Painful channels. Neuron 2006;52:743–4.

[20] Choi JS, Dib-Hajj SD, Waxman SG. Inherited erythermalgia: limb pain from an S4 charge-neutral Na channelopathy. Neurology 2006;67:1563–7.

[21] Clapham DE. Calcium signaling. Cell 2007;131:1047–58.

[22] Cox JJ, Reimann F, Nicholas AK, Thornton G, Roberts E, Springell K, Karbani G, Jafri H, Mannan J, Raashid Y, et al. An SCN9A channelopathy causes congenital inability to experience pain. Nature 2006;444:894–8.

[23] Cuenca-León E, Corominas R, Montfort M, Artigas J, Roig M, Bayes M, Cormand B, Macaya A. Familial hemiplegic migraine: linkage to chromosome 14q32 in a Spanish kindred. Neurogenetics 2009;10:191–8.

[24] Cummins TR, Dib-Hajj SD, Waxman SG. Electrophysiological properties of mutant Na$_v$1.7 sodium channels in a painful inherited neuropathy. J Neurosci 2004;24:8232–6.

[25] De Fusco M, Marconi R, Silvestri L, Atorino L, Rampoldi L, Morgante L, Ballabio A, Aridon P, Casari G. Haploinsufficiency of ATP1A2 encoding the Na$^+$/K$^+$ pump α_2 subunit associated with familial hemiplegic migraine type 2. Nat Genet 2003;33:192–6.

[26] De Fusco M, Marconi R, Silvestri L, Atorino L, Rampoldi L, Morgante L, Ballabio A, Aridon P, Casari G. Haploinsufficiency of ATP1A2 encoding the Na$^+$/K$^+$ pump alpha2 subunit associated with familial hemiplegic migraine type 2. Nat Genet 2003;33:192–6.

[27] de Vries B, Frants RR, Ferrari MD, van den Maagdenberg AMJM. Molecular genetics of migraine. Hum Genet 2009;126:115–32.

[28] de Vries B, Freilinger T, Vanmolkot KR, Koenderink JB, Stam AH, Terwindt GM, Babini E, van den Boogerd EH, van den Heuvel JJ, Frants RR, et al. Systematic analysis of three FHM genes in 39 sporadic patients with hemiplegic migraine. Neurology 2007;69:2170–6.

[29] de Vries B, Steup-Beekman G, Haan J, Bollen E, Luyendijk J, Frants R, Terwindt G, van Buchem M, Huizinga T, van den Maagdenberg AMJM, Ferrari M. TREX1 gene variant in neuropsychiatric systemic lupus erythematosus. Ann Rheum Dis 2010; Epub Apr 13.

[30] Diatchenko L, Nackley AG, Slade GD, Bhalang K, Belfer I, Max MB, Goldman D, Maixner W. Catechol-O-methyltransferase gene polymorphisms are associated with multiple pain-evoking stimuli. Pain 2006;125:216–24.

[31] Diatchenko L, Nackley AG, Tchivileva IE, Shabalina SA, Maixner W. Genetic architecture of human pain perception. Trends Genet 2007;23:605–13.

[32] Diatchenko L, Slade GD, Nackley AG, Bhalang K, Sigurdsson A, Belfer I, Goldman D, Xu K, Shabalina SA, Shagin D, et al. Genetic basis for individual variations in pain perception and the development of a chronic pain condition. Hum Mol Genet 2005;14:135–43.

[33] Dib-Hajj SD, Rush AM, Cummins TR, Hisama FM, Novella S, Tyrrell L, Marshall L, Waxman SG. Gain-of-function mutation in Na$_v$1.7 in familial erythromelalgia induces bursting of sensory neurons. Brain 2005;128:1847–54.

[34] Dichgans M, Freilinger T, Eckstein G, Babini E, Lorenz-Depiereux B, Biskup S, Ferrari MD, Herzog J, van den Maagdenberg AMJM, Pusch M, Strom TM. Mutation in the neuronal voltage-gated sodium channel SCN1A causes familial hemiplegic migraine. Lancet 2005;366:371–7.

[35] Dichgans M, Freilinger T, Eckstein G, Babini E, Lorenz-Depiereux B, Biskup S, Ferrari MD, Herzog J, van den Maagdenberg AMJM, Pusch M, Strom TM. Mutation in the neuronal voltage-gated sodium channel SCN1A in familial hemiplegic migraine. Lancet 2005;366:371–7.

[36] Drenth JP, Michiels JJ. Clinical characteristics and pathophysiology of erythromelalgia and erythermalgia. Am J Med 1992;93:111–4.

[37] Drenth JP, te Morsche RH, Guillet G, Taieb A, Kirby RL, Jansen JB. SCN9A mutations define primary erythermalgia as a neuropathic disorder of voltage gated sodium channels. J Invest Dermatol 2005;124:1333–8.

[38] Drenth JP, Waxman SG. Mutations in sodium-channel gene SCN9A cause a spectrum of human genetic pain disorders. J Clin Invest 2007;117:3603–9.

[39] Ducros A, Denier C, Joutel A, Cecillon M, Lescoat C, Vahedi K, Darcel F, Vicaut E, Bousser MG, Tournier-Lasserve E. The clinical spectrum of familial hemiplegic migraine associated with mutations in a neuronal calcium channel. N Engl J Med 2001;345:17–24.

[40] Eikermann-Haerter K, Baum MJ, Ferrari MD, van den Maagdenberg AMJM, Moskowitz MA, Ayata C. Androgenic suppression of spreading depression in familial hemiplegic migraine type 1 mutant mice. Ann Neurol 2009;66:564–8.

[41] Eikermann-Haerter K, Dilekoz E, Kudo C, Savitz SI, Waeber C, Baum MJ, Ferrari MD, van den Maagdenberg AMJM, Moskowitz MA, Ayata C. Genetic and hormonal factors modulate spreading depression and transient hemiparesis in mouse models of familial hemiplegic migraine type 1. J Clin Invest 2009;119:99–109.

[42] Emin Erdal M, Herken H, Yilmaz M, Bayazit YA. Significance of the catechol-O-methyltransferase gene polymorphism in migraine. Brain Res Mol Brain Res 2001;94:193–6.

[43] Estacion M, Dib-Hajj SD, Benke PJ, Te Morsche RH, Eastman EM, Macala LJ, Drenth JP, Waxman SG. Na$_v$1.7 gain-of-function mutations as a continuum: A1632E displays physiological changes associated with erythromelalgia and paroxysmal extreme pain disorder mutations and produces symptoms of both disorders. J Neurosci 2008;28:11079–88.

[44] Estacion M, Harty TP, Choi JS, Tyrrell L, Dib-Hajj SD, Waxman SG. A sodium channel gene SCN9A polymorphism that increases nociceptor excitability. Ann Neurol 2009;66:862–6.

[45] Ferrari MD. Migraine. Lancet 1998;351:1043–51.

[46] Fertleman CR, Baker MD, Parker KA, Moffatt S, Elmslie FV, Abrahamsen B, Ostman J, Klugbauer N, Wood JN, Gardiner RM, Rees M. SCN9A mutations in paroxysmal extreme pain disorder: allelic variants underlie distinct channel defects and phenotypes. Neuron 2006;52:767–74.

[47] Fillingim RB, Kaplan L, Staud R, Ness TJ, Glover TL, Campbell CM, Mogil JS, Wallace MR. The A118G single nucleotide polymorphism of the mu-opioid receptor gene (OPRM1) is associated with pressure pain sensitivity in humans. J Pain 2005;6:159–67.

[48] Gabriel SB, Schaffner SF, Nguyen H, Moore JM, Roy J, Blumenstiel B, Higgins J, DeFelice M, Lochner A, Faggart M, et al. The structure of haplotype blocks in the human genome. Science 2002;296:2225–9.

[49] Gargus JJ. Genetic calcium signaling abnormalities in the central nervous system: seizures, migraine, and autism. Ann NY Acad Sci 2009;1151:133–56.

[50] Giffin NJ, Ruggiero L, Lipton RB, Silberstein SD, Tvedskov JF, Olesen J, Altman J, Goadsby PJ, Macrae A. Premonitory symptoms in migraine: an electronic diary study. Neurology 2003;60:935–40.

[51] Goadsby PJ, Lipton RB, Ferrari MD. Migraine: current understanding and treatment. N Engl J Med 2002;346:257–70.

[52] Goldberg YP, MacFarlane J, MacDonald ML, Thompson J, Dube MP, Mattice M, Fraser R, Young C, Hossain S, Pape T, et al. Loss-of-function mutations in the Na$_v$1.7 gene underlie congenital indifference to pain in multiple human populations. Clin Genet 2007;71:311–9.

[53] Gursoy S, Erdal E, Herken H, Madenci E, Alasehirli B, Erdal N. Significance of catechol-O-methyltransferase gene polymorphism in fibromyalgia syndrome. Rheumatol Int 2003;23:104–7.

[54] Haerter K, Ayata C, Moskowitz MA. Cortical spreading depression: a model for understanding migraine biology and future drug targets. Headache Currents 2005;2:97–103.

[55] Hagen K, Pettersen E, Stovner LJ, Skorpen F, Zwart JA. The association between headache and Val158Met polymorphism in the catechol-O-methyltransferase gene: the HUNT Study. J Headache Pain 2006;7:70–4.

[56] Hagen K, Pettersen E, Stovner LJ, Skorpen F, Zwart JA. No association between chronic musculoskeletal complaints and Val158Met polymorphism in the catechol-O-methyltransferase gene. The HUNT study. BMC Musculoskelet Disord 2006;7:40.

[57] Han C, Lampert A, Rush AM, Dib-Hajj SD, Wang X, Yang Y, Waxman SG. Temperature dependence of erythromelalgia mutation L858F in sodium channel Na$_v$1.7. Mol Pain 2007;3:3.

[58] Han C, Rush AM, Dib-Hajj SD, Li S, Xu Z, Wang Y, Tyrrell L, Wang X, Yang Y, Waxman SG. Sporadic onset of erythermalgia: a gain-of-function mutation in Na$_v$1.7. Ann Neurol 2006;59:553–8.

[59] Harty TP, Dib-Hajj SD, Tyrrell L, Blackman R, Hisama FM, Rose JB, Waxman SG. Na$_v$1.7 mutant A863P in erythromelalgia: effects of altered activation and steady-state inactivation on excitability of nociceptive dorsal root ganglion neurons. J Neurosci 2006;26:12566–75.

[60] Hirschhorn JN, Daly MJ. Genome-wide association studies for common diseases and complex traits. Nat Rev Genet 2005;6:95–108.

[61] Horisberger JD, Kharoubi-Hess S, Guennoun S, Michielin O. The fourth transmembrane segment of the Na,K-ATPase alpha subunit: a systematic mutagenesis study. J Biol Chem 2004;279:29542–50.

[62] Hottenga JJ, Vanmolkot KR, Kors EE, Kheradmand Kia S, de Jong PT, Haan J, Terwindt GM, Frants RR, Ferrari MD, van den Maagdenberg AMJM. The 3p21.1–p21.3 hereditary vascular retinopathy locus increases the risk for Raynaud's phenomenon and migraine. Cephalalgia 2005;25:1168–72.

[63] Isom LL. The role of sodium channels in cell adhesion. Front Biosci 2002;7:12–23.

[64] Jurkat-Rott K, Freilinger T, Dreier JP, Herzog J, Gobel H, Petzold GC, Montagna P, Gasser T, Lehmann-Horn F, Dichgans M. Variability of familial hemiplegic migraine with novel A1A2 Na$^+$/K$^+$-ATPase variants. Neurology 2004;62:1857–61.

[65] Kahlig KM, Rhodes TH, Pusch M, Freilinger T, Pereira-Monteiro JM, Ferrari MD, van den Maagdenberg AMJM, Dichgans M, George AL Jr. Divergent sodium channel defects in familial hemiplegic migraine. Proc Natl Acad Sci USA 2008;105:9799–804.

[66] Kaja S, van de Ven RC, Broos LA, Veldman H, van Dijk JG, Verschuuren JJ, Frants RR, Ferrari MD, van den Maagdenberg AMJM, Plomp JJ. Gene dosage-dependent transmitter release changes at neuromuscular synapses of *CACNA1A R192Q* knockin mice are non-progressive and do not lead to morphological changes or muscle weakness. Neuroscience 2005;135:81–95.

[67] Kaunisto MA, Harno H, Vanmolkot KR, Gargus JJ, Sun G, Hamalainen E, Liukkonen E, Kallela M, van den Maagdenberg AMJM, Frants RR, et al. A novel missense *ATP1A2* mutation in a Finnish family with familial hemiplegic migraine type 2. Neurogenetics 2004;5:141–6.

[68] Kavanagh D, Spitzer D, Kothari PH, Shaikh A, Liszewski MK, Richards A, Atkinson JP. New roles for the major human 3'-5' exonuclease TREX1 in human disease. Cell Cycle 2008;7:1718–25.

[69] Kelman L. The premonitory symptoms (prodrome): a tertiary care study of 893 migraineurs. Headache 2004;44:865–72.

[70] Kelman L. The postdrome of the acute migraine attack. Cephalalgia 2006;26:214–20.

[71] Khaliq ZM, Raman IM. Relative contributions of axonal and somatic Na channels to action potential initiation in cerebellar Purkinje neurons. J Neurosci 2006;26:1935–44.

[72] Kim H, Mittal DP, Iadarola MJ, Dionne RA. Genetic predictors for acute experimental cold and heat pain sensitivity in humans. J Med Genet 2006;43:e40.

[73] Kim H, Neubert JK, San Miguel A, Xu K, Krishnaraju RK, Iadarola MJ, Goldman D, Dionne RA. Genetic influence on variability in human acute experimental pain sensitivity associated with gender, ethnicity and psychological temperament. Pain 2004;109:488–96.

[74] Klugbauer N, Lacinova L, Flockerzi V, Hofmann F. Structure and functional expression of a new member of the tetrodotoxin-sensitive voltage-activated sodium channel family from human neuroendocrine cells. EMBO J 1995;14:1084–90.

[75] Koenderink JB, Zifarelli G, Qiu LY, Schwarz W, De Pont JJ, Bamberg E, Friedrich T. Na,K-ATPase mutations in familial hemiplegic migraine lead to functional inactivation. Biochim Biophys Acta 2005;1669:61–8.

[76] Kors EE, Haan J, Giffin NJ, Pazdera L, Schnittger C, Lennox GG, Terwindt GM, Vermeulen FL, Van den Maagdenberg AMJM, Frants RR, Ferrari MD. Expanding the phenotypic spectrum of the *CACNA1A* gene T666M mutation: a description of 5 families with familial hemiplegic migraine. Arch Neurol 2003;60:684–8.

[77] Kors EE, Melberg A, Vanmolkot KR, Kumlien E, Haan J, Raininko R, Flink R, Ginjaar HB, Frants RR, Ferrari MD, van den Maagdenberg AMJM. Childhood epilepsy, familial hemiplegic migraine, cerebellar ataxia, and a new *CACNA1A* mutation. Neurology 2004;63:1136–7.

[78] Krzemien DM, Schaller KL, Levinson SR, Caldwell JH. Immunolocalization of sodium channel isoform NaCh6 in the nervous system. J Comp Neurol 2000;420:70–83.

[79] Lampert A, Dib-Hajj SD, Tyrrell L, Waxman SG. Size matters: Erythromelalgia mutation S241T in Na$_v$1.7 alters channel gating. J Biol Chem 2006;281:36029–35.

[80] Lampert A, O'Reilly AO, Reeh P, Leffler A. Sodium channelopathies and pain. Pflugers Arch 2010; Epub Jan 26.

[81] Lander ES, Schork NJ. Genetic dissection of complex traits. Science 1994;265:2037–48.

[82] Lotsch J, Geisslinger G. Relevance of frequent mu-opioid receptor polymorphisms for opioid activity in healthy volunteers. Pharmacogenomics J 2006;6:200–10.

[83] Lotta T, Vidgren J, Tilgmann C, Ulmanen I, Melen K, Julkunen I, Taskinen J. Kinetics of human soluble and membrane-bound catechol-O-methyltransferase: a revised mechanism and description of the thermolabile variant of the enzyme. Biochemistry 1995;34:4202–10.

[84] Lumpkin EA, Caterina MJ. Mechanisms of sensory transduction in the skin. Nature 2007;445:858–65.

[85] Mazur DJ, Perrino FW. Identification and expression of the *TREX1* and *TREX2* cDNA sequences encoding mammalian 3'→5' exonucleases. J Biol Chem 1999;274:19655–60.

[86] Mazur DJ, Perrino FW. Structure and expression of the TREX1 and TREX2 3'→5' exonuclease genes. J Biol Chem 2001;276:14718–27.

[87] McGrail KM, Phillips JM, Sweadner KJ. Immunofluorescent localization of three Na,K-ATPase isozymes in the rat central nervous system: both neurons and glia can express more than one Na,K-ATPase. J Neurosci 1991;11:381–91.

[88] Meisler MH, Kearney JA. Sodium channel mutations in epilepsy and other neurological disorders. J Clin Invest 2005;115:2010–7.

[89] Meyer RA, Campbell JN, Raja SN. Peripheral neural mechanisms of nociception. In: Wall PD, Melzack R, editors. Textbook of pain. Edinburgh: Churchill Livingstone; 1994. p. 13–44.

[90] Michiels JJ, ten Kate FW, Vuzevski VD, Abels J. Histopathology of erythromelalgia in thrombocythaemia. Histopathology 1984;8:669–78.

[91] Mogil JS. The genetic mediation of individual differences in sensitivity to pain and its inhibition. Proc Natl Acad Sci USA 1999;96:7744–51.

[92] Mogil JS, Ritchie J, Smith SB, Strasburg K, Kaplan L, Wallace MR, Romberg RR, Bijl H, Sarton EY, Fillingim RB, Dahan A. Melanocortin-1 receptor gene variants affect pain and mu-opioid analgesia in mice and humans. J Med Genet 2005;42:583–7.

[93] Mogil JS, Wilson SG, Chesler EJ, Rankin AL, Nemmani KV, Lariviere WR, Groce MK, Wallace MR, Kaplan L, Staud R, et al. The melanocortin-1 receptor gene mediates female-specific mechanisms of analgesia in mice and humans. Proc Natl Acad Sci USA 2003;100:4867–72.

[94] Nassar MA, Stirling LC, Forlani G, Baker MD, Matthews EA, Dickenson AH, Wood JN. Nociceptor-specific gene deletion reveals a major role for Na$_v$1.7 (PN1) in acute and inflammatory pain. Proc Natl Acad Sci USA 2004;101:12706–11.

[95] Ogiwara I, Miyamoto H, Morita N, Atapour N, Mazaki E, Inoue I, Takeuchi T, Itohara S, Yanagawa Y, Obata K, et al. Na$_v$1.1 localizes to axons of parvalbumin-positive inhibitory interneurons: a circuit basis for epileptic seizures in mice carrying an Scn1a gene mutation. J Neurosci 2007;27:5903–14.

[96] Ophoff RA, Terwindt GM, Vergouwe MN, van Eijk R, Oefner PJ, Hoffman SM, Lamerdin JE, Mohrenweiser HW, Bulman DE, Ferrari M, et al. Familial hemiplegic migraine and episodic ataxia type-2 are caused by mutations in the Ca^{2+} channel gene *CACNL1A4*. Cell 1996;87:543–52.

[97] Park JJ, Lee J, Kim MA, Back SK, Hong SK, Na HS. Induction of total insensitivity to capsaicin and hypersensitivity to garlic extract in human by decreased expression of TRPV1. Neurosci Lett 2007;411:87–91.

[98] Pertovaara A. Noradrenergic pain modulation. Prog Neurobiol 2006;80:53–83.

[99] Piedras-Rentería ES, Barrett CF, Cao YQ, Tsien RW. Voltage-gated calcium channels, calcium signaling, and channelopathies. In: Krebs J, Michalek M, editors. Calcium: a matter of life or death. New York: Elsevier; 2007. p. 127–66.

[100] Pierelli F, Grieco GS, Pauri F, Pirro C, Fiermonte G, Ambrosini A, Costa A, Buzzi MG, Valoppi M, Caltagirone C, et al. A novel *ATP1A2* mutation in a family with FHM type II. Cephalalgia 2006;26:324–8.

[101] Pietrobon D. Familial hemiplegic migraine. Neurotherapeutics 2007;4:274–84.

[102] Plomin R, Defries JC, McClearn GE. Behavioral genetics: a primer, 2nd ed. Freeman; 1989.

[103] Raman IM, Bean BP. Properties of sodium currents and action potential firing in isolated cerebellar Purkinje neurons. Ann NY Acad Sci 1999;868:93–6.

[104] Ramsey IS, Delling M, Clapham DE. An introduction to TRP channels. Annu Rev Physiol 2006;68:619–47.

[105] Reimann F, Cox JJ, Belfer I, Diatchenko L, Zaykin DV, McHale DP, Drenth JP, Dai F, Wheeler J, Sanders F, et al. Pain perception is altered by a nucleotide polymorphism in SCN9A. Proc Natl Acad Sci USA 2010;107:5148–53.

[106] Renganathan M, Cummins TR, Waxman SG. Contribution of Na$_v$1.8 sodium channels to action potential electrogenesis in DRG neurons. J Neurophysiol 2001;86:629–40.

[107] Riant F, De Fusco M, Aridon P, Ducros A, Ploton C, Marchelli F, Maciazek J, Bousser MG, Casari G, Tournier-Lasserve E. ATP1A2 mutations in 11 families with familial hemiplegic migraine. Hum Mutat 2005;26:281.

[108] Risch N, Merikangas K. The future of genetic studies of complex human diseases. Science 1996;273:1516–7.

[109] Rush AM, Dib-Hajj SD, Liu S, Cummins TR, Black JA, Waxman SG. A single sodium channel mutation produces hyper- or hypoexcitability in different types of neurons. Proc Natl Acad Sci USA 2006;103:8245–50.

[110] Russell MB, Olesen J. A nosographic analysis of the migraine aura in a general population. Brain 1996;119(Pt 2):355–61.

[111] Sangameswaran L, Fish LM, Koch BD, Rabert DK, Delgado SG, Ilnicka M, Jakeman LB, Novakovic S, Wong K, Sze P, et al. A novel tetrodotoxin-insensitive, voltage-gated sodium channel expressed in rat and human dorsal root ganglia. J Biol Chem 1997;272:14805–9.

[112] Schaffer JV, Bolognia JL. The melanocortin-1 receptor: red hair and beyond. Arch Dermatol 2001;137:1477–85.

[113] Schmelz M. Translating nociceptive processing into human pain models. Exp Brain Res 2009;196:173–8.

[114] Segall L, Mezzetti A, Scanzano R, Gargus JJ, Purisima E, Blostein R. Alterations in the alpha2 isoform of Na,K-ATPase associated with familial hemiplegic migraine type 2. Proc Natl Acad Sci USA 2005;102:11106–11.

[115] Segall L, Scanzano R, Kaunisto MA, Wessman M, Palotie A, Gargus JJ, Blostein R. Kinetic alterations due to a missense mutation in the Na,K-ATPase alpha2 subunit cause familial hemiplegic migraine type 2. J Biol Chem 2004;279:43692–6.

[116] Sheets PL, Jackson JO 2nd, Waxman SG, Dib-Hajj SD, Cummins TR. A $Na_v1.7$ channel mutation associated with hereditary erythromelalgia contributes to neuronal hyperexcitability and displays reduced lidocaine sensitivity. J Physiol 2007;581:1019–31.

[117] Shu XQ, Mendell LM. Neurotrophins and hyperalgesia. Proc Natl Acad Sci USA 1999;96:7693–6.

[118] Silberstein SD, Lipton RB, Goadsby PJ. Headache in clinical practice. London: Martin Dunitz; 2002.

[119] Spadaro M, Ursu S, Lehmann-Horn F, Veneziano L, Antonini G, Giunti P, Frontali M, Jurkat-Rott K. A G301R Na^+/K^+-ATPase mutation causes familial hemiplegic migraine type 2 with cerebellar signs. Neurogenetics 2004;5:177–85.

[120] Stamer UM, Stuber F. The pharmacogenetics of analgesia. Expert Opin Pharmacother 2007;8:2235–45.

[121] Swoboda KJ, Kanavakis E, Xaidara A, Johnson JE, Leppert MF, Schlesinger-Massart MB, Ptacek LJ, Silver K, Youroukos S. Alternating hemiplegia of childhood or familial hemiplegic migraine? A novel ATP1A2 mutation. Ann Neurol 2004;55:884–7.

[122] Tegeder I, Adolph J, Schmidt H, Woolf CJ, Geisslinger G, Lotsch J. Reduced hyperalgesia in homozygous carriers of a GTP cyclohydrolase 1 haplotype. Eur J Pain 2008;12:1069–77.

[123] Tegeder I, Costigan M, Griffin RS, Abele A, Belfer I, Schmidt H, Ehnert C, Nejim J, Marian C, Scholz J, et al. GTP cyclohydrolase and tetrahydrobiopterin regulate pain sensitivity and persistence. Nat Med 2006;12:1269–77.

[124] Terwindt G, Kors E, Haan J, Vermeulen F, Van den Maagdenberg AMJM, Frants R, Ferrari M. Mutation analysis of the CACNA1A calcium channel subunit gene in 27 patients with sporadic hemiplegic migraine. Arch Neurol 2002;59:1016–18.

[125] Terwindt GM, Haan J, Ophoff RA, Groenen SM, Storimans CW, Lanser JB, Roos RA, Bleeker-Wagemakers EM, Frants RR, Ferrari MD. Clinical and genetic analysis of a large Dutch family with autosomal dominant vascular retinopathy, migraine and Raynaud's phenomenon. Brain 1998;121(Pt 2):303–16.

[126] Thomsen LL, Eriksen MK, Roemer SF, Andersen I, Olesen J, Russell MB. A population-based study of familial hemiplegic migraine suggests revised diagnostic criteria. Brain 2002;125:1379–91.

[127] Thomsen LL, Oestergaard E, Bjornsson A, Stefansson H, Fasquel AC, Gulcher J, Stefansson K, Olesen J. Screen for CACNA1A and ATP1A2 mutations in sporadic hemiplegic migraine patients. Cephalalgia 2008;28:914–21.

[128] Thomsen LL, Olesen J. Sporadic hemiplegic migraine. Cephalalgia 2004;24:1016–23.

[129] Todt U, Dichgans M, Jurkat-Rott K, Heinze A, Zifarelli G, Koenderink JB, Goebel I, Zumbroich V, Stiller A, Ramirez A, et al. Rare missense variants in ATP1A2 in families with clustering of common forms of migraine. Hum Mutat 2005;26:315–21.

[130] Tottene A, Conti R, Fabbro A, Vecchia D, Shapovalova M, Santello M, van den Maagdenberg AMJM, Ferrari MD, Pietrobon D. Enhanced excitatory transmission at cortical synapses as the basis for facilitated spreading depression in $Ca_v2.1$ knockin migraine mice. Neuron 2009;61:762–73.

[131] Trimmer JS, Rhodes KJ. Localization of voltage-gated ion channels in mammalian brain. Annu Rev Physiol 2004;66:477–519.

[132] Vahedi K, Denier C, Ducros A, Bousson V, Levy C, Chabriat H, Haguenau M, Tournier-Lasserve E, Bousser MG. CACNA1A gene de novo mutation causing hemiplegic migraine, coma, and cerebellar atrophy. Neurology 2000;55:1040–2.

[133] Vahedi K, Depienne C, Le Fort D, Riant F, Chaine P, Trouillard O, Gaudric A, Morris MA, Leguern E, Tournier-Lasserve E, Bousser MG. Elicited repetitive daily blindness: a new phenotype associated with hemiplegic migraine and SCN1A mutations. Neurology 2009;72:1178–83.

[134] Valverde P, Healy E, Jackson I, Rees JL, Thody AJ. Variants of the melanocyte-stimulating hormone receptor gene are associated with red hair and fair skin in humans. Nat Genet 1995;11:328–30.

[135] van den Maagdenberg AM, Pietrobon D, Pizzorusso T, Kaja S, Broos LA, Cesetti T, van de Ven RC, Tottene A, van der Kaa J, Plomp JJ, et al. A Cacna1a knockin migraine mouse model with increased susceptibility to cortical spreading depression. Neuron 2004;41:701–10.

[136] van den Maagdenberg AM, Pizzorusso T, Kaja S, Terpolilli N, Shapovalova M, Hoebeek FE, Barrett CF, Gherardini L, van de Ven RC, Todorov B, et al. High cortical spreading depression susceptibility and migraine-associated symptoms in $Ca_v2.1$ S218L mice. Ann Neurol 2010;67:85–98.

[137] van den Maagdenberg AMJM, Haan J, Terwindt GM, Ferrari MD. Migraine: gene mutations and functional consequences. Curr Opin Neurol 2007;20:299–305.

[138] Vanmolkot KR, Babini E, de Vries B, Stam AH, Freilinger T, Terwindt GM, Norris L, Haan J, Frants RR, Ramadan NM, et al. The novel p.L1649Q mutation in the SCN1A epilepsy gene is associated with familial hemiplegic migraine: genetic and functional studies. Hum Mutat 2007;28:522.

[139] Vanmolkot KR, Kors EE, Hottenga JJ, Terwindt GM, Haan J, Hoefnagels WA, Black DF, Sandkuijl LA, Frants RR, Ferrari MD, van den Maagdenberg AMJM. Novel mutations in the Na^+, K^+-ATPase pump gene ATP1A2 associated with familial hemiplegic migraine and benign familial infantile convulsions. Ann Neurol 2003;54:360–6.

[140] Vanmolkot KR, Stroink H, Koenderink JB, Kors EE, van den Heuvel JJ, van den Boogerd EH, Stam AH, Haan J, De Vries BB, Terwindt GM, et al. Severe episodic neurological deficits and permanent mental retardation in a child with a novel FHM2 ATP1A2 mutation. Ann Neurol 2006;59:310–4.

[141] Vanmolkot KR, van den Maagdenberg AMJM, Haan J, Ferrari MD. New discoveries about the second gene for familial hemiplegic migraine, ATP1A2. Lancet Neurol 2003;2:721.

[142] Vargas-Alarcon G, Fragoso JM, Cruz-Robles D, Vargas A, Lao-Villadoniga JI, Garcia-Fructuoso F, Ramos-Kuri M, Hernandez F, Springall R, Bojalil R, et al. Catechol-O-methyltransferase gene haplotypes in Mexican and Spanish patients with fibromyalgia. Arthritis Res Ther 2007;9:R110.

[143] Venter JC, Adams MD, Myers EW, Li PW, Mural RJ, Sutton GG, Smith HO, Yandell M, Evans CA, Holt RA, et al. The sequence of the human genome. Science 2001;291:1304–51.

[144] Waldmann R, Champigny G, Lingueglia E, De Weille JR, Heurteaux C, Lazdunski M. H^+-gated cation channels. Ann NY Acad Sci 1999;868:67–76.

[145] Waxman SG, Dib-Hajj S, Cummins TR, Black JA. Sodium channels and pain. Proc Natl Acad Sci USA 1999;96:7635–9.

[146] Westenbroek RE, Merrick DK, Catterall WA. Differential subcellular localization of the RI and RII Na^+ channel subtypes in central neurons. Neuron 1989;3:695–704.

[147] Yang Y, Wang Y, Li S, Xu Z, Li H, Ma L, Fan J, Bu D, Liu B, Fan Z, et al. Mutations in SCN9A, encoding a sodium channel alpha subunit, in patients with primary erythermalgia. J Med Genet 2004;41:171–4.

[148] Yeomans DC, Levinson SR, Peters MC, Koszowski AG, Tzabazis AZ, Gilly WF, Wilson SP. Decrease in inflammatory hyperalgesia by herpes vector-mediated knockdown of $Na_v1.7$ sodium channels in primary afferents. Hum Gene Ther 2005;16:271–7.

[149] Yu FH, Catterall WA. Overview of the voltage-gated sodium channel family. Genome Biol 2003;4:207.

[150] Yu FH, Catterall WA. The VGL-chanome: a protein superfamily specialized for electrical signaling and ionic homeostasis. Sci STKE 2004;2004:re15.

[151] Yu FH, Mantegazza M, Westenbroek RE, Robbins CA, Kalume F, Burton KA, Spain WJ, McKnight GS, Scheuer T, Catterall WA. Reduced sodium current in GABAergic interneurons in a mouse model of severe myoclonic epilepsy in infancy. Nat Neurosci 2006;9:1142–9.

[152] Zubieta JK, Heitzeg MM, Smith YR, Bueller JA, Xu K, Xu Y, Koeppe RA, Stohler CS, Goldman D. COMT val158met genotype affects mu-opioid neurotransmitter responses to a pain stressor. Science 2003;299:1240–3.

Correspondence to: Professor Michel D. Ferrari, MD, PhD, Department of Neurology, Leiden University Medical Center, Albinusdreef 2, PO Box 9600, 2300 RC Leiden, The Netherlands. Email: M.D.Ferrari@lumc.nl.

The Search for Human Pain Genes Using Whole-Genome Approaches: Achievements, Failures, and Promises

Shad B. Smith, PhD, Inna E. Tchivileva, MD, William Maixner, DDS, PhD,
and Luda Diatchenko, MD, PhD

Center for Neurosensory Disorders, University of North Carolina, Chapel Hill, North Carolina, USA

Pain perception is one of the most complicated measurable traits because it is an aggregate of several phenotypes associated with peripheral and central nervous system dynamics, stress responsiveness, and inflammatory state. Human persistent pain conditions are very common, with worldwide prevalence ranging from 15% to 20% for adults [4]. As a complex trait, pain is polygenic and is shaped by environmental pressures. There is general agreement that in both humans and rodents the genetic contribution to pain perception is about 50% [38,42,52,53]. A comprehensive catalogue of genes implicated in pain and analgesia in mouse models has recently been consolidated in a pain genes database [37] (http://paingeneticslab.ca/4105/06_02_pain_genetics_database. asp). This database, which continues to grow, catalogues over 300 genes implicated in pain sensitivity using mouse knockout studies. The number of genes contributing to pain perception is probably similar between rodents and humans; however, it is unlikely that each gene contributing to pain perception has genetic variants in the human population that substantially affect the function of its corresponding gene and pain perception. Thus, the number of genes and associated genetic variants that contribute to human pain perception and persistent pain conditions remains an open question. Currently, there is evidence for several genetic variants (i.e., a couple of dozen) that contribute to human pain conditions, human pain perception, and/or

responses to pain therapeutics [15,33,41,58,65]. Essentially all of these variants have been identified through a candidate gene approach. This approach is effective in identifying hypothesis-driven genetic effects in relatively small cohorts or population samples.

Genome-Wide Approaches to Pain

Although significant discoveries have been made using the candidate gene approach, it is now possible to query the entire genome for causal relationships between pain phenotypes and genetic markers. Such genome-wide association studies (GWAS) are facilitated by the recent advent of commercially available, high-throughput genotyping arrays that permit the simultaneous interrogation of over a million single-nucleotide polymorphism (SNP) markers, as well as other genetic features such as copy-number variants (CNVs). The GWAS approach has identified hundreds of novel associations for a wide variety of traits and medical conditions. These include many diseases with a prominent pain component, such as cancer [9] and autoimmune and inflammatory diseases (e.g., rheumatoid arthritis [57,70], lupus [25], Crohn's disease [59,70], celiac disease [67], osteoarthritis [47,72], and sickle-cell anemia [63]). However, the assessed endpoint of all these studies has been disease status, rather than pain per se; to date, no published GWAS has tested associations with pain presence or severity as a dependent variable. There is a single report in a small cohort of oral surgery patients that ketorolac analgesic onset is associated with a DNA-binding protein, *ZNF429*, but significant associations with maximum postoperative pain and postoperative pain onset were not observed [34]. GWAS is currently the most comprehensive method available to researchers to investigate the relationship between genetic factors and disease, and it has considerable potential to advance pain genetics research.

Why Genome-Wide Association Studies?

Twin and family studies have established that the genetic component of interindividual variability, or heritability, of most pain phenotypes is substantial [42,52,53], but to date few genetic variants of large effect have been found (notwithstanding a number of rare Mendelian pain disorders). One mechanistic explanation accounting for the observed variability presumes that there is a large number of genes that contribute to a given phenotype, each contributing a small but measurable effect (the "common disease, common variant" hypothesis [8,15,39]). Because these variants exert small effects, they do not appreciably undergo selection and may appear frequently in a population. These common variants could conceivably be discovered anywhere in the genome, not just within genes with known biological relevance to nociceptive processing, but they are likely to be difficult to detect due to their low penetrance. The GWAS approach offers considerable advantages over other methods (e.g., linkage mapping or candidate gene association) to detect common genetic determinants of pain with limited penetrance [27].

Although the so-called "common disease, common variant" hypothesis needs to hold true for GWAS studies in pain to prove useful, no other hypothesis regarding the specific etiology of a trait or disease is required. The GWAS approach is "hypothesis neutral," meaning no a priori knowledge of phenotype biology is necessary; the spectrum of genomic variation is assessed comprehensively [2,40], either directly or indirectly due to the phenomenon of linkage disequilibrium [32]. Because there are only a few crossover events per generation [46], SNPs in close physical proximity are usually inherited in groups, called "haploblocks" [21]. Genotyping a single representative SNP marker, or "tag SNP," is usually sufficient to characterize multiple

co-inherited SNPs [31]. Even if a disease-causing SNP is not genotyped in the study, its effects will be proxied by genotyped SNPs in linkage disequilibrium (LD) with the causal SNP (Fig.1). In this manner, the hundreds of thousands of SNPs on a GWAS chip provide almost complete coverage of genetic variation, alleviating the need to preselect candidate genes.

The GWAS approach has the potential to uncover disease genes not previously known; in fact, genuinely novel disease genes are as readily detectable as biological candidates. The record for published GWAS shows that while about 20% of associations represent identifiable candidate genes [28,49], the majority are located either in genes without a known biological connection to the trait, or even in regions with no recognized functional consequence (such as introns and intergenic regions). Such discoveries hold great promise for elucidating novel mechanisms of disease as well as new targets for therapeutic interventions [26]. GWAS findings may therefore be especially valuable for pain diseases with poorly understood etiology, such as fibromyalgia and complex regional pain syndrome.

Study Design Issues

Unlike most conditions and traits that previously have been investigated by GWAS, pain is by definition subjective, and diagnosis of painful disease states historically has been contentious. There are numerous study design issues that investigators necessarily will have to resolve before real progress can be made in pain genomics—some common to all GWAS studies, but others unique to the domain of pain research.

The major difference between candidate gene and GWAS studies is simply scale—the ability to examine practically the entire genome for disease-associated variation. Given the size of the full genome (3 billion base pairs, featuring over 10 million SNPs with a minor allele frequency >1% [35]), a large number of markers (500,000–1,000,000) are assessed simultaneously. GWAS look for common variants with necessarily low penetrance, and therefore must be sensitive to odds ratios in the range of 1.3–1.5 [3]. Maintaining sufficient power to be able to detect such a proverbial "needle in a haystack" requires very large study populations, usually thousands each of cases and controls [60]. However, the difficulties of recruiting large numbers of subjects, especially for uncommon diseases, does not give license to disregard considerations of potential bias in study

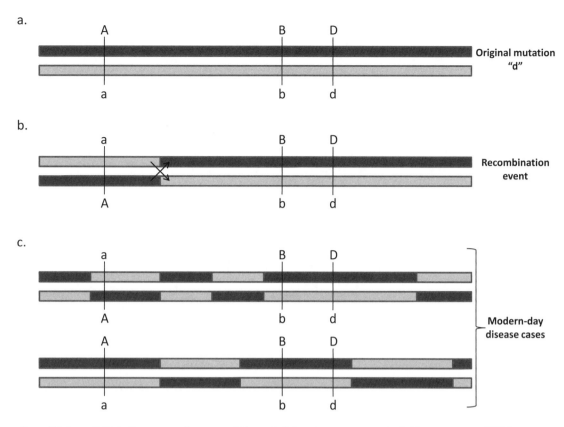

Fig. 1. Linkage disequilibrium (LD) is the nonrandom association of alleles at two or more loci. The presence of LD between nearby single-nucleotide polymorphisms (SNPs) explains why tag SNPs can be used as proxy markers for disease-causing genetic variation. (a) Two copies of an ancestral chromosome bear different alleles at three sites. A novel mutation "d" in one chromosome increases risk for a disease over the other version "D." The alleles "a" and "b" are collinear with d at two SNPs located nearby on the same chromosome. (b) Recombination events result in a "crossover" of genetic material between chromosomes. (c) Over many generations, successive crossover events disrupt the relationship between the causative mutation d and distant allele a, such that no correlation is observed between them. No crossovers have separated the nearby allele b from the disease allele d. The b allele may be considered a marker for d, as the two SNPs are in linkage disequilibrium.

design. In fact, GWAS studies are prone to Type 1 errors from a number of sources, both methodological [10,54,68] and technical [1,20,62].

Successful association studies of disease require a concrete case definition with a basis in biological dysfunction and underlying genetic modulation. In the pain field, demarcations between painful syndromes are frequently imprecise, and symptoms overlap significantly, especially for idiopathic conditions. Individuals with similar symptoms and given the same diagnosis may vary widely in the pathophysiology responsible for the pain. One method to reduce phenotypic heterogeneity is to use as experimental endpoints intermediate or "endophenotypes," presumably with a stronger causal relationship to the underlying biology [5,6]. Alternatively, thorough phenotyping of disease characteristics might facilitate a clustering strategy, whereby groups of subjects with similar presentations are analyzed separately [71].

Similarly, the choice of a suitable control population should be carefully undertaken. Many large published GWAS have used "convenience" population-based controls taken from blood banks or previously genotyped studies of other conditions, under the assumption that the incidence of the uncommon disease under examination will be negligible. However, misclassification bias due to undetected cases in a population-based control sample can lead to a significant loss of power [29], especially for pain studies of common conditions (e.g., migraine, temporomandibular joint disease, and persistent postsurgical pain).

Even more than in candidate gene studies, best-practice epidemiological methods should be rigorously applied to ensure that controls are sampled from the same population as cases. Differing racial and ethnic composition between study groups, known as population stratification, is a notorious source of bias in association studies [7,43]. If the allele frequency at a particular marker differs between the populations that underlie the case and control groups, this difference can emerge as a spurious association signal. To avoid this confound, GWAS have usually involved racially homogeneous samples, with controls either drawn from the same population or carefully matched to cases from a population-based resource. A number of statistical approaches have been developed to detect and correct for racial substructure [66]. Evidence of inflated test statistics due to population stratification is readily identified in a quantile-quantile (Q-Q) plot, in which the expected test statistics under the null hypothesis (i.e., no associated SNPs) are plotted against the observed test statistics. In a Q-Q plot, population stratification (or any other nonrandom bias towards association) is demonstrated by deviation from the expected distribution over a significant portion of the results. This deviation is frequently quantified by a statistic known as the genomic inflation factor, or lambda (λ); it is calculated as the ratio of median values from the expected and observed distributions [19]. The genomic control approach [13], adjusting all study P values by the λ value, is one way to correct for study-wide systematic bias, although it corrects for the average degree of stratification and may not sufficiently account for substructure at every marker. Alternatively, other methods use principal components analysis on the genotypes, identifying dimensions of variance that correspond to background ethnic features, and which can be used as covariates to control for allele frequency differences between populations [54].

Even if all sources of bias have been carefully eliminated, a relatively large number of SNPs will associate strongly with the phenotype of interest, simply because of the vast number of tests being performed. Such chance associations are frequently indistinguishable from true results, given the small effect sizes typically identified in studies of complex traits. To reduce the number of Type 1 errors, investigators choose strict P-value thresholds, such as a Bonferroni correction for the number of markers interrogated, in order to achieve an acceptable genome-wide α level. However, SNPs in LD blocks are not independent of each other, making a strict Bonferroni correction overly conservative (see [17] and [23] for methods to adjust for the correct number of effectively independent SNPs on major commercial GWAS platforms). Others have used Bayesian methods that take into account estimates of the suspected number of true positive associations [69,70]. This approach may improve the success of GWAS studies in pain, as heritability estimates for a variety of painful conditions ranging from 20–40% suggest a strong genetic component to individual differences.

Obstacles to Genome-Wide Analysis

Though the GWAS approach boasts considerable advantages over candidate gene studies, it is worth considering why it has not yet been widely adopted in the pain community. The technological and statistical obstacles involved in genome-wide association analysis have largely been resolved. However, if the pain field is to make progress in this area, there is a need for transformation in the methodology and organization of large pain studies.

As discussed previously, a large number of meticulously phenotyped subjects, with corresponding controls, are necessary for association studies of disease. The size of the cohorts needed for GWAS are unusual in the pain field, and likely will only be realized by collaborative, multi-site efforts. In fact, the consortium model has been widely adopted in other diseases to successfully assemble tens of thousands of subjects [12,22,56,70]. As noted, careful calibration among recruitment sites is necessary for consistent sampling, diagnosis, and genotyping across cohorts [30]. Association with experimental pain measures, which so far has offered inconsistent findings due to a lack of uniformity in testing procedures among laboratories [33], would also benefit from a standardized battery of nociceptive assays.

The large enrollment numbers for GWAS studies will require a correspondingly large expenditure to recruit, examine, and accurately diagnose conditions of interest to pain researchers. Compounding these expenditures are the per-subject genotyping costs, which are currently in the $300–500 range for the newest commercial platforms. Additional resources for DNA sample preparation and storage, as well as burdensome computational demands involved in genotype quality control and statistical analysis, add substantially to the overall cost of GWAS. The level of funding necessary for a GWAS has historically not been available to individual basic or clinical pain scientists. New models of collaboration, and potentially new mechanisms of funding (from both governmental sources and public-private alliances), will be required to assemble the resources for successful studies in the genomic era [45].

A more collaborative environment is not only necessary to prosecute single GWAS, but also to confirm the findings of these studies across populations in multiple studies of the same disease. As has been observed in candidate gene studies, association results are frequently not replicated between laboratories, often due to lack of power in one or both studies. Conversely, a vast number of true associations may fail to meet a statistical threshold for significance in a single GWAS simply because this benchmark must be set so high. The use of meta-analysis methods [58,73] to combine results across studies of many common diseases (aggregating upwards of 100,000 subjects, in some cases) has resulted in much greater power to detect true disease-associated markers, and vastly accelerated gene discovery.

What Will/Won't GWAS Tell Us?

The sequencing of the human genome and the availability of technology to rapidly assess hundreds of thousands of genetic variants have engendered excitement regarding the possibility of personalized medicine, by which disease risk and optimal therapeutic treatments might be informed by a patient's DNA. GWAS methods have been touted as the key to uncovering the genetic variations that determine everything from postsurgical pain severity to opioid efficacy, perhaps over-enthusiastically. With the primary genetic risk determinants for many other diseases and conditions already elucidated, what can we expect the pursuit of genome-wide association to tell us about pain?

With the exception of a few rare conditions marked by congenital spontaneous pain or insensitivity to pain, it is now clear that the vast majority of pain phenotypes and disorders are complex traits, mediated by multiple genes. Each of these genes will only explain a small percentage of the genetic variance, and even less of the overall trait variance. For some well-studied diseases, the cumulative contribution from all discovered SNPs has ranged as high as 10–20%, but even the most predictive loci have rarely been observed to explain more than 1% of the variance by themselves. Common SNP markers may therefore not be of much use for individual predictions of traits or disease risk for many pain phenotypes. However, common disease variants uncovered by GWAS can have a high population attributable risk [3], if their low penetrance is offset by a high degree of exposure to causal alleles in a community.

Even if an associated variant is not substantially predictive of disease risk, it may still offer much information about pathways of disease development [26]. Extensive GWAS efforts of several diseases and traits to date have identified associations in known candidate genes, but the majority of their findings have been localized to genes not previously suspected of playing a causative role. Many well-substantiated findings have not even been linked to any known gene, indicating there may be undiscovered regulatory mechanisms in the vast stretches of DNA between genes. These truly novel findings will expand our understanding of disease and trait etiology, and they will present new targets for pharmacological and gene therapy interventions.

Deep Sequencing for Rare Causal Variants

Complex pain diseases are by definition attributable to multiple genetic and environmental influences. GWAS methods have proven successful at exploring the relationship between common genetic polymorphisms and common traits and diseases, but as yet they have not accounted for the majority of the genetic component of variance for any studied phenotype. It appears increasingly likely that some of the missing heritability is caused by rare genetic variants, with minor allele frequencies of 1–5% or less. Such rare variants are not readily detectable by usual GWAS methods. The SNP selection for commercial GWAS platforms relies on strong LD between chosen tag SNPs and causative polymorphisms, and rare variants are likely to be recent mutations not in LD with neighboring markers [55]. Another practical consideration is the power of GWAS, which decreases proportionally with allele frequency. For uncommon diseases, acquiring the appropriate sample size required to detect statistical differences in allelic frequency below 5% quickly rises beyond the resources of any study. The "common disease—rare variant" hypothesis [55] asserts that a major component of disease susceptibility arises from multiple rare mutations across many genes with increased relative risk.

One method that has been shown to be capable of detecting rare causal variants is resequencing of candidate genes in affected populations [11,18]. Sequence variants that show both a difference in frequency between disease and control groups, as well as plausible biological function, are identified as presumptive causal mutations. The unit of association is the gene, aggregating the effects of multiple rare variants on the phenotype [36]. These individual variants are likely to have a higher penetrance than more common variants, on the order of a twofold to more than fivefold increase in risk [3], while still below the level of single-gene ("Mendelian") diseases [15]. Recent advances in sequencing technology have made this strategy viable for detecting genetic sources of disease susceptibility, with several "next-generation" applications already in the marketplace [44]. The "1000 Genomes Project" currently underway has the formidable goal of cataloging all variation genome-wide in a large number of volunteers, and it should greatly enhance our understanding of the influence of low-frequency variants on traits and diseases (www.1000genomes.org).

Although the application of deep sequencing to the study of pain remains on the horizon, current-day studies should be designed with this emerging technology in mind. Prioritizing pain candidate genes for resequencing will be important given the great costs associated with the technique, and these efforts will continue to be informed by linkage, candidate gene association studies, and GWAS. Because rare variants are likely to have larger effects on a pain phenotype than common polymorphisms, they may be responsible for more severe manifestations of the pain condition and thus might be more readily identified in extreme cases derived from existing population-based studies [15].

Potential Clinical Applications

Substantial progress in the identification of pain-related genetic variants provides promise for future use of these findings for new drug target identification, pharmacogenetic tests, and gene-based diagnostics and prognostic tests. One of the first examples in the area of pharmacogenomics is based on polymorphisms in *CYP2D6*, which encodes cytochrome P-450, a member of a family of enzymes that catalyzes many reactions involved in drug metabolism. Multiple copies of *CYP2D6* are associated with enhanced response to the analgesic codeine, which can increase its toxicity by increasing the metabolism of codeine to morphine 24]. In contrast, codeine and tramadol (another opioid analgesic) are less effective in patients with genetic variants that result in low or no *CYP2D6* activity [61,64]. Another striking example was the discovery of nonfunctional variants of the melanocortin-1 receptor (*MC1R*) that produce a red hair and fair skin phenotype, and which are associated with increased analgesic responses to κ-opioid receptor mediated analgesia [48].

A recent illustration of how association studies can result in the discovery of a new drug target for treatment of common pain conditions with pharmacogenetic

testing is exemplified by genetic variants of the catechol-*O*-methyltransferase (*COMT*) gene, which codes for an enzyme that metabolizes catecholamines (i.e., epinephrine, norepinephrine, and dopamine). *COMT* has been implicated in the regulation of pain perception. Three major haplotypes of *COMT*, designated as low pain-sensitive (LPS), average pain-sensitive (APS), and high pain-sensitive (HPS) have been identified based on a carrier's response to experimental pain stimuli. These three haplotypes account for 11% of the variability to experimental pain sensitivity in young women and are predictive of the risk of onset of a common musculoskeletal pain disorder (i.e., temporomandibular disorders [TMD]) [14,16]. The LPS haplotype produces higher levels of COMT enzymatic activity than the APS or HPS haplotypes [50]. The pharmacological inhibition of COMT in rats results in mechanical and thermal hypersensitivity that is reversed by the nonselective β-adrenergic antagonist propranolol, or by the combined administration of selective β_2- and β_3-adrenergic antagonists, while administration of β_1-adrenergic, α-adrenergic, or dopaminergic receptor antagonists fails to alter COMT-dependent pain sensitivity. These data provide the first direct evidence that low COMT activity leads to increased pain sensitivity via a $\beta_{2/3}$-adrenergic mechanism, and suggest that pain conditions associated with low COMT activity and/or elevated catecholamine levels can be treated with pharmacological agents that block both β_2- and β_3-adrenergic receptors [51]. This finding led to the hypothesis that propranolol, a nonselective β-adrenergic antagonist that is in wide clinical use for treatment of hypertension, may be effective for pain conditions, plausibly in a manner dependent on the subjects' *COMT* diplotype [65].

To test this hypothesis, a double-blind, placebo-controlled, two-period crossover pilot study of efficacy of propranolol was conducted in 40 female patients with TMD. The outcomes of this study demonstrated that propranolol, independent of *COMT* genotype, significantly reduced only a composite pain index, which was calculated as a product of reported clinical pain intensity by pain duration for the past week, but did not decrease other clinical and experimental pressure and heat pain ratings compared to placebo [65]. When stratified by the *COMT* high-activity haplotype (LPS), a beneficial effect of propranolol on pain perception was noted in subjects not carrying this haplotype, a diminished benefit was observed in the heterozygotes, and no benefit was noted in the homozygotes. These findings corroborate that *COMT* gene polymorphism contributes to the variable pharmacodynamic responses to propranolol in patients with chronic musculoskeletal pain. *COMT* haplotypes may serve as genetic predictors of treatment outcomes and permit the identification of a subgroup of patients who will benefit from propranolol therapy. The results of this study may also explain the variability of treatment responses to β-blockers for a broad spectrum of diseases and conditions.

Conclusions

Association studies designed to search for functional human genetic variants and disease markers have undergone tremendous development during the last several years. GWAS, while having a number of deficiencies, inherent problems, and pitfalls, have identified hundreds of genetic variants associated with complex human diseases and traits, and have provided valuable insights into their genetic architecture. The further development of GWAS approaches, combined with whole-genome resequencing approaches, and the application of GWAS to the field of human pain perception, pain disorders, and pain treatments, carry great promise for identifying new drug targets, the development of new drugs, and pharmacogenetics diagnostics and prognostics.

Acknowledgments

This work was supported in part by NIDCR and NINDS grants RO1-DE16558, UO1-DE017018, NS41670 and PO1 NS045685.

References

[1] Anney RJL, Kenny E, O'Dushlaine CT, Lasky-Su J, Franke B, Morris DW, Neale BM, Asherson P, Faraone SV, Gill M. Non-random error in genotype calling procedures: implications for family-based and case-control genome-wide association studies. Am J Med Genet 2008;147B:1379–86.

[2] Barrett JC, Cardon LR. Evaluating coverage of genome-wide association studies. Nat Genet 2006;38:659–62.

[3] Bodmer W, Bonilla C. Common and rare variants in multifactorial susceptibility to common diseases. Nat Genet 2008;40:695–701.

[4] Brennan F, Carr DB, Cousins M. Pain management: a fundamental human right. Anesth Analg 2007;105:205–21.

[5] Camilleri M, Busciglio I, Carlson P, McKinzie S, Burton D, Baxter K, Ryks M, Zinsmeister AR. Candidate genes and sensory functions in health and irritable bowel syndrome. Am J Physiol Gastrointest Liver Physiol 2008;295:G219–25.

[6] Cannon TD, Keller MC. Endophenotypes in the genetic analyses of mental disorders. Annu Rev Clin Psychol 2006;2:267–90.

[7] Cardon LR, Palmer LJ. Population stratification and spurious allelic association. Lancet 2003;361:598–604.

[8] Chakravarti A. Population genetics: making sense out of sequence. Nature Genet 1999;21:56–60.

[9] Chung CC, Magalhaes WCS, Gonzalez-Bosquet J, Chanock SJ. Genome-wide association studies in cancer: current and future directions. Carcinogenesis 2010;31:111–20.

[10] Clayton DG, Walker NM, Smyth DJ, Pask R, Cooper JD, Maier LM, Smink LJ, Lam AC, Ovington NR, Stevens HE, et al. Population structure, differential bias and genomic control in a large-scale, case-control association study. Nat Genet 2005;37:1243–6.

[11] Cohen JC, Kiss RS, Pertsemlidis A, Marcel YL, McPherson R, Hobbs HH. Multiple rare alleles contribute to low plasma levels of HDL cholesterol. Science 2004;305:869–72.

[12] Cornelis MC, Agrawal A, Cole JW, Hansel NN, Barnes KC, Beaty TH, Bennett SN, Bierut LJ, Boerwinkle E, Doheny KF, et al.; GENEVA. The gene, environment association studies consortium (GENEVA): maximizing the knowledge obtained from GWAS by collaboration across studies of multiple conditions. Genet Epidemiol 2010; in press.

[13] Devlin B, Roeder K. Genomic control for association studies. Biometrics 1999;55:997–1004.

[14] Diatchenko L, Nackley AG, Slade GD, Bhalang K, Belfer I, Max MB, Goldman D, Maixner W. Catechol-*O*-methyltransferase gene polymorphisms are associated with multiple pain-evoking stimuli. Pain 2006;125:216–24.

[15] Diatchenko L, Nackley AG, Tchivileva IE, Shabalina SA, Maixner W. Genetic architecture of human pain perception. Trends Genet 2007;23:605–13.

[16] Diatchenko L, Slade GD, Nackley AG, Bhalang K, Sigurdsson A, Belfer I, Goldman D, Xu K, Shabalina SA, Shagin D, Max MB, Makarov SS, Maixner W. Genetic basis for individual variations in pain perception and the development of a chronic pain condition. Hum Mol Genet 2005;14:135–43.

[17] Duggal P, Gillanders E, Holmes T, Bailey-Wilson J. Establishing an adjusted p-value threshold to control the family-wide type 1 error in genome wide association studies. BMC Genomics 2008;9:516.

[18] Fearnhead NS, Winney B, Bodmer W. Rare variant hypothesis for multifactorial inheritance. Cell Cycle 2005;4:521–5.

[19] Freedman ML, Reich D, Penney KL, McDonald GJ, Mignault AA, Patterson N, Gabriel SB, Topol EJ, Smoller JW, Pato CN, et al. Assessing the impact of population stratification on genetic association studies. Nat Genet 2004;36:388–93.

[20] Fu W, Wang Y, Wang Y, Li R, Lin R, Jin L. Missing call bias in high-throughput genotyping. BMC Genomics 2009;10:106.

[21] Gabriel SB, Schaffner SF, Nguyen H, Moore JM, Roy J, Blumenstiel B, Higgins J, DeFelice M, Lochner A, Faggart M, et al. The structure of haplotype blocks in the human genome. Science 2002;296:2225–9.

[22] GAIN Consortium. New models of collaboration in genome-wide association studies: the Genetic Association Information Network. Nat Genet 2007;39:1045–51.

[23] Gao X, Becker LC, Becker DM, Starmer JD, Province MA. Avoiding the high Bonferroni penalty in genome-wide association studies. Genet Epidemiol 2010;34:100–5.

[24] Gasche Y, Daali Y, Fathi M, Chiappe A, Cottini S, Dayer P, Desmeules J. Codeine intoxication associated with ultrarapid *CYP2D6* metabolism. N Engl J Med 2004;351:2827–31.

[25] Graham RR, Hom G, Ortmann W, Behrens TW. Review of recent genome-wide association scans in lupus. J Int Med 2009;265:680–8.

[26] Hirschhorn JN. Genomewide association studies: illuminating biologic pathways. N Engl J Med 2009;360:1699–701.

[27] Hirschhorn JN, Daly MJ. Genome-wide association studies for common diseases and complex traits. Nat Rev Genet 2005;6:95–108.

[28] Hirschhorn JN, Lettre G. Progress in genome-wide association studies of human height. Horm Res 2009;71(Suppl 2):5–13.

[29] Höfler M. The effect of misclassification on the estimation of association: a review. Int J Methods Psychiatr Res 2005;14:92–101.

[30] Ioannidis JPA, Patsopoulos NA, Evangelou E. Heterogeneity in meta-analyses of genome-wide association investigations. PLoS ONE 2007;2:e841.

[31] Johnson GCL, Esposito L, Barratt BJ, Smith AN, Heward J, Di Genova G, Ueda H, Cordell HJ, Eaves IA, Dudbridge F, et al. Haplotype tagging for the identification of common disease genes. Nat Genet 2001;29:233–7.

[32] Jorde LB. Linkage disequilibrium and the search for complex disease genes. Genome Res 2000;10:1435–44.

[33] Kim H, Clark D, Dionne RA. Genetic contributions to clinical pain and analgesia: avoiding pitfalls in genetic research. J Pain 2009;10:663–93.

[34] Kim H, Ramsay E, Lee H, Wahl S, Dionne RA. Genome-wide association study of acute post-surgical pain in humans. Pharmacogenomics 2009;10:171–9.

[35] Kruglyak L, Nickerson DA. Variation is the spice of life. Nat Genet 2001;27:234–6.

[36] Kryukov GV, Shpunt A, Stamatoyannopoulos JA, Sunyaev SR. Power of deep, all-exon resequencing for discovery of human trait genes. Proc Natl Acad Sci USA 2009;106:3871–6.

[37] LaCroix-Fralish ML, Ledoux JB, Mogil JS. The Pain Genes Database: an interactive web browser of pain-related transgenic knockout studies. Pain 2007;131:3.e1–3.e4.

[38] LaCroix-Fralish ML, Mogil JS. Progress in genetic studies of pain and analgesia. Annu Rev Pharmacol Toxicol 2009;49:97–121.

[39] Lander ES. The New Genomics: global views of biology. Science 1996;274:536–9.

[40] Li M, Li C, Guan W. Evaluation of coverage variation of SNP chips for genome-wide association studies. Eur J Hum Genet 2008;16:635–43.

[41] Lötsch J, Geisslinger G, Tegeder I. Genetic modulation of the pharmacological treatment of pain. Pharmacol Ther 2009;124:168–84.

[42] MacGregor AJ, Andrew T, Sambrook PN, Spector TD. Structural, psychological, and genetic influences on low back and neck pain: a study of adult female twins. Arthritis Rheum 2004;51:160–7.

[43] Marchini J, Cardon LR, Phillips MS, Donnelly P. The effects of human population structure on large genetic association studies. Nat Genet 2004;36:512–7.

[44] Mardis ER. Next-generation DNA sequencing methods. Annu Rev Genomics Hum Genet 2008;9:387–402.

[45] Max MB. Moving pain genetics into the genome-wide association era. In: Castro-Lopes J, editor. Current topics in pain: 12th World Congress on Pain. Seattle: IASP Press, 2009. p. 185–97.

[46] McVean GAT, Myers SR, Hunt S, Deloukas P, Bentley DR, Donnelly P. The fine-scale structure of recombination rate variation in the human genome. Science 2004;304:581–4.

[47] Miyamoto Y, Shi D, Nakajima M, Ozaki K, Sudo A, Kotani A, Uchida A, Tanaka T, Fukui N, Tsunoda T, et al. Common variants in DVWA on chromosome 3p24.3 are associated with susceptibility to knee osteoarthritis. Nat Genet 2008;40:994–8.

[48] Mogil JS, Wilson SG, Chesler EJ, Rankin AL, Nemmani KVS, Lariviere WR, Groce MK, Wallace MR, Kaplan L, Staud R, et al. The melanocortin-1 receptor gene mediates female-specific mechanisms of analgesia in mice and humans. Proc Natl Acad Sci USA 2003;100:4867–72.

[49] Mohlke KL, Boehnke M, Abecasis GR. Metabolic and cardiovascular traits: an abundance of recently identified common genetic variants. Hum Mol Genet 2008;17:R102–8.

[50] Nackley A, Shabalina S, Tchivileva I, Satterfield K, Korchynskyi O, Makarov S, Maixner W, Diatchenko L. Human catechol-O-methyltransferase haplotypes modulate protein expression by altering mRNA secondary structure. Science 2006;314:1930–3.

[51] Nackley A, Tan K, Fecho K, Flood P, Diatchenko L, Maixner W. Catechol-O-methyltransferase inhibition increases pain sensitivity through activation of both beta2- and beta3-adrenergic receptors. Pain 2007;128:199–208.

[52] Nielsen CS, Stubhaug A, Price DD, Vassend O, Czajkowski N, Harris JR. Individual differences in pain sensitivity: genetic and environmental contributions. Pain 2008;136:21–9.

[53] Norbury TA, MacGregor AJ, Urwin J, Spector TD, McMahon SB. Heritability of responses to painful stimuli in women: a classical twin study. Brain 2007;130:3041–9.

[54] Price AL, Patterson NJ, Plenge RM, Weinblatt ME, Shadick NA, Reich D. Principal components analysis corrects for stratification in genome-wide association studies. Nat Genet 2006;38:904–9.

[55] Pritchard JK. Are rare variants responsible for susceptibility to complex diseases? Am J Hum Genet 2001;69:124–37.

[56] Psychiatric Genetics Consortium. A framework for interpreting genome-wide association studies of psychiatric disorders. Mol Psychiatry 2008;14:10–7.

[57] Raychaudhuri S, Thomson BP, Remmers EF, Eyre S, Hinks A, Guiducci C, Catanese JJ, Xie G, Stahl EA, Chen R, et al. Genetic variants at CD28, PRDM1 and CD2/CD58 are associated with rheumatoid arthritis risk. Nat Genet 2009;41:1313–8.

[58] Reimann F, Cox JJ, Belfer I, Diatchenko L, Zaykin DV, McHale DP, Drenth JPH, Dai F, Wheeler J, Sanders F, et al. Pain perception is altered by a nucleotide polymorphism in SCN9A. Proc Natl Acad Sci USA 2010; in press.

[59] Rioux JD, Xavier RJ, Taylor KD, Silverberg MS, Goyette P, Huett A, Green T, Kuballa P, Barmada MM, Datta LW, et al. Genome-wide association study identifies new susceptibility loci for Crohn disease and implicates autophagy in disease pathogenesis. Nat Genet 2007;39:596–604.

[60] Risch N, Merikangas K. The future of genetic studies of complex human diseases. Science 1996;273:1516–7.

[61] Sachse C, Brockmoller J, Bauer S, Roots I. Cytochrome P450 2D6 variants in a Caucasian population: allele frequencies and phenotypic consequences. Am J Hum Genet 1997;60:284–95.

[62] Sampson J, Zhao H. Genotyping and inflated type I error rate in genome-wide association case/control studies. BMC Bioinformatics 2009;10:68.

[63] Sebastiani P, Solovieff N, Hartley SW, Milton JN, Riva A, Dworkis DA, Melista E, Klings ES, Garrett ME, Telen MJ, et al. Genetic modifiers of the severity of sickle cell anemia identified through a genome-wide association study. Am J Hematol 2010;85:29–35.

[64] Stamer UM, Lehnen K, Hothker F, Bayerer B, Wolf S, Hoeft A, Stuber F. Impact of CYP2D6 genotype on postoperative tramadol analgesia. Pain 2003;105:231–8.

[65] Tchivileva IE, Lim PF, Smith SB, Slade GD, Diatchenko L, McLean SA, Maixner W. Effect of catechol-O-methyltransferase polymorphism on response to propranolol therapy in chronic musculoskeletal pain: a randomized, double-blind, placebo-controlled, crossover pilot study. Pharmacogenet Genomics 2010; in press.

[66] Tiwari HK, Barnholtz-Sloan J, Wineinger N, Padilla MA, Vaughan LK, Allison DB. Review and evaluation of methods correcting for population stratification with a focus on underlying statistical principles. Hum Hered 2008;66:67–86.

[67] van Heel DA, Franke L, Hunt KA, Gwilliam R, Zhernakova A, Inouye M, Wapenaar MC, Barnardo MCNM, Bethel G, Holmes GKT, et al. A genome-wide association study for celiac disease identifies risk variants in the region harboring IL2 and IL21. Nat Genet 2007;39:827–9.

[68] Voight BF, Pritchard JK. Confounding from cryptic relatedness in case-control association studies. PLoS Genet 2005;1:e32.

[69] Wacholder S, Chanock S, Garcia-Closas M, El ghormli L, Rothman N. Assessing the probability that a positive report is false: an approach for molecular epidemiology studies. J Natl Cancer Inst 2004;96:434–42.

[70] Wellcome Trust Case Control Consortium. Genome-wide association study of 14,000 cases of seven common diseases and 3,000 shared controls. Nature 2007;447:661–78.

[71] Wessman J, Paunio T, Tuulio-Henriksson A, Koivisto M, Partonen T, Suvisaari J, Turunen JA, Wedenoja J, Hennah W, Pietilainen OPH, et al. Mixture model clustering of phenotype features reveals evidence for association of DTNBP1 to a specific subtype of schizophrenia. Biol Psychiatry 2009;66:990–6.

[72] Zhai G, van Meurs JBJ, Livshits G, Meulenbelt I, Valdes AM, Soranzo N, Hart D, Zhang F, Kato BS, Richards JB, et al. A genome-wide association study suggests that a locus within the ataxin 2 binding protein 1 gene is associated with hand osteoarthritis: the Treat-OA consortium. J Med Genet 2009;46:614–6.

[73] Zintzaras E, Lau J. Trends in meta-analysis of genetic association studies. J Hum Genet 2007;53:1–9.

Correspondence to: Luda Diatchenko, PhD, Center for Neurosensory Disorders, Carolina Center for Genome Sciences, University of North Carolina at Chapel Hill, 2120 Old Dental Building, Columbia and Manning, CB 7455, Chapel Hill, NC 27599, USA. Email: lbdiatch@email.unc.edu.

Part 12

Neuropathic Pain: From Basic Mechanisms to Clinical Management

Clinical Manifestations of Neuropathic Pain and Distinguishing Features from Other Types of Pain

Per Hansson, MD, DMSc, DDS

Pain Center, Department of Anesthesiology and Intensive Care, Karolinska University Hospital, Solna; Clinical Pain Research, Department of Molecular Medicine and Surgery, Karolinska Institute, Stockholm, Sweden

A crude but often-employed classification of pain sufficient for clinical management comprises the following four types of pain: nociceptive/inflammatory, neuropathic (peripheral and central), pain of unknown origin, and psychogenic pain. Not infrequently, a patient will have a mixture of pain types, which may pose differential diagnostic issues.

Recently, a novel definition of neuropathic pain was suggested by a group of experts from the neurological, neurosurgical, and pain communities [28]: "Pain arising as a direct consequence of a lesion or disease affecting the somatosensory system." This suggestion challenges the 1994 International Association for the Study of Pain (IASP) version [23], which is still in effect and defines neuropathic pain as "pain initiated or caused by a primary lesion or dysfunction in the peripheral or central nervous system". The word "dysfunction" has been regarded an ill-defined term [16] that may erroneously be interpreted as including the normal plasticity of the provoked nociceptive system; that is, pain due to secondary changes in the nociceptive system (given its inherent plasticity) resulting from sufficiently strong nociceptive stimulation. The vagueness of the term "dysfunction" may also allow for the inclusion of conditions such as complex regional pain syndrome type I, fibromyalgia, and irritable bowel syndrome. In addition, the IASP definition does not distinguish neuropathic pain from, for example, musculoskeletal pains that arise in the course of neurological disorders; that is, pains that are secondary to a neurological condition.

Neuropathic Pain Is a Direct Consequence of a Lesion or Disease Affecting the Somatosensory System

The novel definition of neuropathic pain [28] underlines the compulsory existence of an underlying lesion or disease that affects the somatosensory part of the nervous system as a prerequisite for the manifestation of any kind of neuropathic pain. It is important to consider the possibility of a latency, more or less extensive, between the time of injury or start of disease and the onset of pain. In central neuropathic pain due to spinal cord injury [26] or stroke [20,21], a latency of up to several years has been reported that may be related to healing processes in the central nervous system (CNS). In spinal cord injury, syringomyelia should be suspected when the onset of pain is delayed for years, and especially if the level of sensory loss is moving in a cranial direction. In peripheral neuropathic pain, the phenomenon of latency has not been studied in detail, but clinical empiricism speaks in favor of this possibility.

A Suggested Diagnostic Work-Up Algorithm of Neuropathic Pain and the Problem of Identifying the Pain Part of the Problem

In parallel with their suggested definition of neuropathic pain [28], Treede et al. also put forth a diagnostic work-up algorithm that builds upon a recent study by Rasmussen and coworkers [25] and offers three levels of diagnostic certainty. Scrutinizing the work-up algorithm makes it plain that it focuses on the identification of a lesion or disease of the nervous system and not on the pain aspect of the problem. The only reference to pain in the algorithm refers to pain being neuroanatomically distributed; that is, experienced within the distribution of a lesioned nerve or diseased part of the nervous system. In the diagnostic work-up of peripheral neuropathic pain it may be difficult, however, to determine if pain in a region with nerve injury is neuropathic, because other pains may also be present in such areas; for example, there may be muscle pain due to altered movement pattern or overuse of atrophic muscles if mixed sensory and motor nerves are involved. It seems likely that the pain is neuropathic in an area with nerve lesion if the pain is experienced in the entire innervation territory of the injured nervous structure. Such a distribution is, however, far from the clinical reality in many patients because partial lesion is the most common type of nerve injury. In partial nerve injury a limited number of fascicles are damaged, and if a neuropathic pain condition emerges, the distribution of symptoms would be limited to the innervation territory of one or several injured fascicles.

The case of central neuropathic pain is even more complex because the distribution of such pain is difficult to anticipate based on the location of the CNS lesion or disease. The distribution of pain in any case of central neuropathic pain is explained by basic neuroanatomy, that is, the somatotopic organization in sensory pathways, nuclei, and cortical regions. Hence, the distribution of pain needs to conform to the somatotopic representation of the body within the CNS [28]. Pain in the entire half of the left or right side of the body after stroke or in the entire area below the level of the lesion in spinal cord injury is probably central neuropathic pain. On the other hand, a pain condition in multiple sclerosis, or after a stroke or spinal cord injury, that is "patchier" in distribution but is located in a region with signs of somatosensory dysfunction poses a differential diagnostic problem. Importantly, no gold standard exists on how to identify neuropathic pain in such instances.

Can Sensory Descriptors Assist in Identifying Neuropathic Pain?

Several independent research groups have published a variety of questionnaires to be used for diagnosis or assessment of neuropathic pain [5,6,9]. These questionnaires focus on sensory descriptors and their potential usefulness as diagnostic adjuncts. It is clear from such efforts that no pathognomonic descriptors exist, although descriptors such as burning, lancinating, numbness, and electric shocks are more common on a group level in neuropathic pain than in non-neuropathic conditions [9]. The first three descriptors are also among the most commonly used in patients with non-neuropathic pain. Such group-level findings are not helpful in the clinical situation, however, where physicians must work with individual patients [15]. The work-up algorithm by Treede et al. [28], importantly, does not include guidance from pain descriptors because the authors questioned the validity of such an approach. Questionnaires have also been implemented in epidemiological studies of neuropathic pain. A recent study from Canada [27], using the French DN4 questionnaire [9], reported a prevalence of such pain in 17.9% of the population. Such a conspicuous overestimation serves as a solid basis for seriously questioning the usefulness of such questionnaires. The possibility cannot be excluded, however, that if questionnaires are refined they may provide some guidance in the future in identifying neuropathic pain states.

Characteristics of Painful Symptoms and Signs in Neuropathic Pain

Painful neuropathic conditions express themselves with spontaneous and/or abnormal stimulus-evoked pain [13]. Most patients report ongoing spontaneous pain, although a minority suffer from only stimulus-evoked pain. Although no detailed information can be gathered from the literature, it is suggested that most neuropathic pain conditions do not express themselves only intermittently or paroxysmally, but in fact are usually continuous with varying intensities, sometimes with superimposed intermittent or paroxysmal painful or nonpainful symptoms. Important exceptions to this generalization are trigeminal and glossopharyngeal neuralgia, where pain characteristically is paroxysmal with a duration of a few seconds, sometimes repeated hundreds of times a day.

Evoked pain is defined as allodynia when it is caused by normally nonpainful stimuli [23], usually a light moving mechanical stimulus (dynamic mechanical allodynia), a light static mechanical stimulus (static mechanical allodynia) or a cold object. Importantly, the phenomenon of pain caused by usually nonpainful stimuli is not peculiar to neuropathic pain but may occur also in non-neuropathic conditions such as skin injury (due to sunburn or surgery, for example) and joint inflammation, as well as in psychogenic pain conditions. Neuropathic pain states are also often associated with nonpainful, abnormal spontaneous and evoked sensory phenomena such as paresthesia and dysesthesia [13]. To what extent such phenomena are expressed in non-neuropathic conditions is not known.

The distribution of pain in long-term neuropathic pain states is usually stable over time, and this characteristic distinctly defines such pain from referred components in nociceptive pain states [7]. An example of the latter is variable referred sensory components to the extremities, including pain, in patients with focal pain in the region of the cervical or lumbar spine [7].

A recent study [3] that used the NPSI (Neuropathic Pain Symptom Inventory) to examine the association of positive symptoms across different etiologies of neuropathic pain demonstrated that there are more similarities than differences in such symptoms associated with a large variety of peripheral and central lesions. Hence, condition-specific manifestations are not to be expected.

Characteristics of Sensory Abnormalities in Neuropathic and Non-Neuropathic Pain Conditions

In neuropathic pain states the distribution of sensory loss usually matches the innervation territory of the damaged nervous structure. Sensory alterations were originally described in the context of neuropathic pain, but recent findings have indicated that subgroups of patients with nociceptive pain (e.g., musculoskeletal pain) may report similar but transitory and variable sensory

disturbances in the focal pain area and/or in areas of referred symptoms with a distribution lacking distinct borders [12,18,19]. Given that such phenomena do not rely on nerve lesions or diseases of the nervous system, distinct neuroanatomical boundaries related to a level of a lesion or disease of the nervous system do not apply. Therefore, the mapping of the distribution of sensory abnormalities is important in the diagnostic work-up. Cases with qualitative aberrations such as dynamic mechanical allodynia may demonstrate evoked pain spreading beyond the anticipated neuroanatomical borders. Extraterritorial spread of pain and sensory dysfunction should be accepted only after careful consideration and differential diagnostic reasoning regarding non-neurological conditions [16]. This phenomenon occurs occasionally and may develop after a period of proper distribution of symptom and signs. In some cases it can also be interpreted as variations in the innervation territories of nerves or roots.

No common somatosensory denominator has been identified in peripheral neuropathic pain states. From detailed studies in patients with central neuropathic pain due to stroke [2,8] or multiple sclerosis [24], the common denominator regarding signs at somatosensory examination seems to be involvement of the spino-(trigemino-)thalamo-cortical system resulting in altered sensibility to temperature and/or pain stimuli. The painful condition seems to be unrelated to alterations in other somatosensory channels or in the motor system. Nonsymptomatic trigeminal neuralgia is usually not paralleled by sensory abnormalities at bedside examination, and hence it does not qualify as a definite neuropathic pain according to the recently published diagnostic work-up algorithm [28].

Importantly, again, signs of sensory aberrations in a pain condition are not equivalent to neuropathic pain. Regarding the outcome of somatosensory examination, specific characteristics apply to true neuropathic conditions; that is, modality profile and distinct borders of abnormalities are reproducible at least during one examination. The physiological basis for the abnormal somatosensory findings in nociceptive/inflammatory pain states are unknown, but such findings indicate an interaction between different somatosensory channels due to activity in the nociceptive system [14]. Increased sensitivity in such pains may of course be due to peripheral sensitization. In addition, patients with psychogenic pain conditions (e.g., conversion hysteria) sometimes report sensory abnormalities, indicating prominent interactions between the psyche and the soma. As alluded to previously, a crucial part of the sensory examination is to carefully map the distribution of the sensory abnormalities using bedside tools, trying to link the distribution to a suspected neuroanatomical level extracted from the history. Given that sensory alterations are not confined to neuropathic pain states, the outcome of sensory examinations, especially in the hands of clinicians lacking experience in detailed sensory examination, could be a source of confusion and possible diagnostic errors.

Response to Treatment Gives Little Guidance as to Pain Type

It has become increasingly clear that nociceptive/inflammatory and neuropathic pain conditions may respond to similar drugs, which indicates shared pathophysiological mechanisms between nociceptive and neuropathic pain conditions or shared, unspecific targets that, when activated, may lower excitability in the nociceptive system regardless of pain type. In addition, different neuropathic pain conditions may be relieved by the same drugs for the same reasons [17]. Gabapentin reduces neuropathic pain [4] as well as postoperative pain [22] in humans, and the same holds true for N-methyl-D-aspartate (NMDA) receptor-antagonists such as ketamine [10,11]. In addition, accumulating evidence indicates that upregulation of subtypes of sodium channels takes place in both neuropathic and inflammatory models of pain [1], pointing to possible shared mechanisms of pain and perhaps susceptibility to drugs interacting with such ion channels. Taken together, the evidence suggests that drug effects in individual patients are not sufficient to indicate the nature of the painful condition, and hence cannot be used to solve differential diagnostic issues related to pain.

Summary

(1) Neuropathic pain is always linked to a lesion or disease of the nervous system. (2) The distribution of pain in neuropathic pain states is neuroanatomically correlated to the level of the lesion or disease. (3) The possibility of a latency, more or less extensive, between the time of lesion or onset of disease and pain onset should be considered. (4) No pathognomonic sensory descriptors exist in neuropathic pain, and the overlap with

non-neuropathic conditions is extensive. (5) Sensory abnormalities are usually confined to the innervation territory of the damaged nervous structure. Such findings may be present also in non-neuropathic conditions. If so, they do not obey neuroanatomical rules and regulations. (6) Shared pathophysiological mechanisms have been suggested between nociceptive and neuropathic pain conditions, as well as shared, unspecific targets that when activated may lower excitability in the nociceptive system regardless of pain type. Therefore, the response to different treatment modalities does not indicate the nature of the painful condition and thus cannot be used to solve differential diagnostic issues related to pain.

References

[1]   Amir R, Argoff CE, Bennett GJ, Cummins TR, Durieux ME, Gerner P, Gold MS, Porreca F, Strichartz GR. The role of sodium channels in chronic inflammatory and neuropathic pain. J Pain 2006;7:S1–29.

[2]   Andersen G, Vestergaard K, Ingeman-Nielsen M, Jensen TS. Incidence of central post-stroke pain. Pain 1995;61:187–93.

[3]   Attal N, Fermanian C, Fermanian J, Lanteri-Minet M, Alchaar H, Bouhassira D. Neuropathic pain: are there distinct subtypes depending on the aetiology or anatomical lesion? Pain 2008;138:343–53.

[4]   Backonja M, Beydoun A, Edwards KR, Schwartz SL, Fonseca V, Hes M, LaMoreaux L, Garofalo E. Gabapentin for the symptomatic treatment of painful neuropathy in patients with diabetes mellitus: a randomized controlled trial. JAMA 1998;280:1831–6.

[5]   Bennett MI, Attal N, Backonja MM, Baron R, Bouhassira D, Freynhagen R, Scholz J, Tolle TR, Wittchen HU, Jensen TS. Using screening tools to identify neuropathic pain. Pain 2007;127:199–203.

[6]   Bennett MI, Smith BH, Torrance N, Potter J. The S-LANSS score for identifying pain of predominantly neuropathic origin: validation for use in clinical and postal research. J Pain 2005;6:149–58.

[7]   Bogduk N. On the definitions and physiology of back pain, referred pain, and radicular pain. Pain 2009;147:17–9.

[8]   Boivie J, Leijon G, Johansson I. Central post-stroke pain: a study of the mechanisms through analyses of the sensory abnormalities. Pain 1989;37:173–85.

[9]   Bouhassira D, Attal N, Alchaar H, Boureau F, Brochet B, Bruxelle J, Cunin G, Fermanian J, Ginies P, Grun-Overdyking A, et al. Comparison of pain syndromes associated with nervous or somatic lesions and development of a new neuropathic pain diagnostic questionnaire (DN4). Pain 2005;114:29–36.

[10] De Kock MF, Lavand'homme PM. The clinical role of NMDA receptor antagonists for the treatment of postoperative pain. Best Pract Res Clin Anaesthesiol 2007;21:85–98.

[11] Eide PK, Stubhaug A, Stenehjem AE. Central dysesthesia pain after traumatic spinal cord injury is dependent on N-methyl-D-aspartate receptor activation. Neurosurgery 1995;37:1080–7.

[12] Geber C, Magerl W, Fondel R, Fechir M, Rolke R, Vogt T, Treede RD, Birklein F. Numbness in clinical and experimental pain: a cross-sectional study exploring the mechanisms of reduced tactile function. Pain 2008;139:73–81.

[13] Hansson P. Neuropathic pain: clinical characteristics and diagnostic workup. Eur J Pain 2002;6(Suppl A):47–50.

[14] Hansson P, Backonja M, Bouhassira D. Usefulness and limitations of quantitative sensory testing: clinical and research application in neuropathic pain states. Pain 2007;129:256–9.

[15] Hansson P, Haanpaa M. Diagnostic work-up of neuropathic pain: computing, using questionnaires or examining the patient? Eur J Pain 2007;11:367–9.

[16] Hansson P, Lacerenza M, Marchettini P. Aspects of clinical and experimental neuropathic pain: the clinical perspective. In: Hansson PT, Fields HL, Hill RG, Marchettini P, editors. Neuropathic pain: pathophysiology and treatment. Progress in pain research and management, vol. 21. Seattle: IASP Press; 2001. p. 1–18.

[17] Hansson PT, Dickenson AH. Pharmacological treatment of peripheral neuropathic pain conditions based on shared commonalities despite multiple etiologies. Pain 2005;113:251–4.

[18] Leffler AS, Hansson P, Kosek E. Somatosensory perception in patients suffering from long-term trapezius myalgia at the site overlying the most painful part of the muscle and in an area of pain referral. Eur J Pain 2003;7:267–76.

[19] Leffler AS, Kosek E, Hansson P. The influence of pain intensity on somatosensory perception in patients suffering from subacute/chronic lateral epicondylalgia. Eur J Pain 2000;4:57–71.

[20] Leijon G, Boivie J, Johansson I. Central post-stroke pain: neurological symptoms and pain characteristics. Pain 1989;36:13–25.

[21] MacGowan DJ, Janal MN, Clark WC, Wharton RN, Lazar RM, Sacco RL, Mohr JP. Central poststroke pain and Wallenberg's lateral medullary infarction: frequency, character, and determinants in 63 patients. Neurology 1997;49:120–5.

[22] Mathiesen O, Moiniche S, Dahl JB. Gabapentin and postoperative pain: a qualitative and quantitative systematic review, with focus on procedure. BMC Anesthesiol 2007;7:6.

[23] Merskey H, Bogduk N. Classification of chronic pain: descriptions of chronic pain syndromes and definitions of pain terms. Seattle: IASP Press; 1994.

[24] Osterberg A, Boivie J, Thuomas KA. Central pain in multiple sclerosis: prevalence and clinical characteristics. Eur J Pain 2005;9:531–42.

[25] Rasmussen PV, Sindrup SH, Jensen TS, Bach FW. Symptoms and signs in patients with suspected neuropathic pain. Pain 2004;110:461–9.

[26] Siddall PJ, McClelland JM, Rutkowski SB, Cousins MJ. A longitudinal study of the prevalence and characteristics of pain in the first 5 years following spinal cord injury. Pain 2003;103:249–57.

[27] Toth C, Lander J, Wiebe S. The prevalence and impact of chronic pain with neuropathic pain symptoms in the general population. Pain Med 2009;10:918–29.

[28] Treede RD, Jensen TS, Campbell JN, Cruccu G, Dostrovsky JO, Griffin JW, Hansson P, Hughes R, Nurmikko T, Serra J. Neuropathic pain: redefinition and a grading system for clinical and research purposes. Neurology 2008;70:1630–5.

Correspondence to: Per Hansson, MD, DMSc, DDS, Department of Molecular Medicine and Surgery, Karolinska Institute, 17176 Stockholm, Sweden. Email: per.hansson@ki.se.

Neurobiological Mechanisms of Neuropathic Pain and Its Treatment

27

Anthony H. Dickenson BSc, PhD, FMedSci, and Lucy A. Bee, PhD

Department of Neuroscience, Physiology, and Pharmacology, University College London, London, United Kingdom

In 1994, the International Association for the Study of Pain (IASP) Taxonomy Subcommittee defined neuropathic pain as "pain initiated or caused by a primary lesion or dysfunction of the nervous system," yet there have since been calls for a revised definition [73]. In particular, it has been suggested that "dysfunction" in the original definition should be removed. This is because some dysfunctions of the nervous system, such as allodynia (pain due to a stimulus that does not usually provoke pain) and hyperalgesia (an increased response to an already painful stimulus) are not forms of neuropathic pain, nor are they exclusive symptoms of neuropathic pain (these phenomena may also result from inflammatory pain as a normal and reversible consequence of functional plasticity). Indeed, animal models of nerve *and* tissue damage both lead to hypersensitivity to previously innocuous and noxious mechanical stimuli. An advantage of animal models of neuropathic pain is that they all involve damage to peripheral nerves, yet we agree with the premise that animals cannot inform on allodynia and hyperalgesia and so the term "hypersensitivity" is more apt. Animal models are critical for revealing the mechanisms behind the pain state and showing how and where drugs work, yet they are limited in their ability to inform about side effects elicited in patients that may preclude clinical usefulness.

Animal Models of Neuropathic Pain

There is a need for basic science and surrogate animal models to complement, and in some cases guide, clinical and human research. The key advantage of animal models that approximate human neuropathic pain conditions is that they enable access to the full spectrum of pathophysiologies in both the peripheral nervous system (PNS) and the central nervous system (CNS) and allow the molecular and cellular events underlying abnormal sensory processing and disproportionate pain to be explored [37]. Additionally, they can be used to assess the pharmacology of the pain state, which can explain the actions of existing analgesic drugs, provide information about efficacy, and identify rational therapeutic targets for future drugs.

These models, which must adhere to guidelines set by IASP for the care and use of laboratory animals to minimize suffering [57,84], can be broadly divided into peripheral mononeuropathy, peripheral polyneuropathy, and central neuropathic pain, in line with the human situation (see Table I). There are in particular several models of peripheral mononeuropathy, yet the spinal nerve ligation (SNL) model, in which the L5 and L6 spinal nerves are unilaterally ligated close to their respective ganglia to produce a restricted partial denervation of the hind limb, is

Table I

Mechanisms of neuropathic pain with corresponding drug targets
and pharmacotherapies (current and potential)

Mechanism	Target	Drug
Peripheral sensitization	TRPV1 receptors	Capsaicin: low and high doses
Altered expression, distribution, and function of ion channels	Voltage-gated K+ channels	–
	Voltage-gated Na+ channels	Local anesthetics, e.g., lidocaine; antiepileptics, e.g., carbamazepine, lacosamide, lamotrigine; anti-arrhythmic agents, e.g., mexiletine
	HCN channels	–
	P2X-receptor-gated channels	–
	Voltage-gated Ca²⁺ channels	Ziconotide, gabapentin, pregabalin
Increased central excitation	NMDA receptors	Ketamine, ifenprodil
	NK1 receptors	–
Reduced spinal inhibition	Opioid receptors	Morphine, oxycodone, tramadol, tapentadol
	GABA receptors	Baclofen
	Glycine receptors	–
Deregulated supraspinal control	Monoamines	Tricyclic antidepressants, e.g., amitryptiline; serotonin and norepinephrine reuptake inhibitors, e.g., duloxetine, tramadol, tapentadol
Immune system involvement	Cytokines	NSAIDs
	TNF-α	–
	Microglia	–
Schwann cell dedifferentiation	Growth factors	–

Abbreviations: HCN channels, hyperpolarization-activated cyclic nucleotide-gated channels; NMDA, *N*-methyl D-aspartate; NSAIDs, nonsteroidal anti-inflammatory drugs; TNF-α, tumor necrosis factor alpha; TRPV1, transient receptor potential vanilloid 1.

favored by many for various reasons. One reason is the stereotypical injury that is induced, which gives rise to consistent and reproducible sensory abnormalities over a sustained postoperative period and fits with reports that the pain that persists postoperatively in humans after surgical trauma is a form of neuropathic pain. The sensory abnormalities in the animal models manifest as evoked (and arguably ongoing) behavioral responses that can be evaluated by sensory testing using mechanical, heat, and cooling stimuli. In head-to-head comparisons of different animal models of experimental neuropathic pain carried out by single laboratories using a standardized testing procedure, the SNL model showed the largest and most stable magnitudes of behavioral hypersensitivities to applied peripheral stimuli [17,33].

One apparent puzzle is why only a minority of patients with nerve injury have pain symptoms, yet almost all animals with an induced nerve injury display behavioral hypersensitivities. This discrepancy is explicable in terms of the consistent genetic background of the inbred rodents selected for the model, the reproducibility and severity of the nerve injury, and possibly the animals' lack of prior pain experience. Obviously, animals will not be subject to certain confounding issues such as complex societal, socioeconomic, and higher cognitive functions that are unique to humans.

Contribution of Schwann Cells, Growth Factors, and Phenotypic Switches to Neuropathic Pain

The degree of primary afferent fiber myelination, which confers fiber conduction velocity, depends on the integrity of enveloping Schwann cells that control sensory neuron development and function. Nerve injury can result in Schwann cell de-differentiation and a consequent switch from normal myelin production to the dysregulated synthesis of neurotrophic factors. Prolonged exposure of the neuronal environment to excess growth factors can have adverse effects on neighboring intact and injured neurons, contributing to the pain phenomenon [50,81].

The constitutive availability of growth factors in the peripheral targets of large- and small-diameter sensory neurons maintains normal neuronal phenotype. Nerve growth factor (NGF), for example, is taken up from its source by free sensory nerve endings and is transported retrogradely to the cell body, where it controls the expression of genes that are crucial for smooth sensory function. These genes include those that encode neurotransmitters, receptors, and ion channels. Traumatic nerve injury can disrupt the delivery of NGF along the axon, which necessarily leads to miscommunication between the cell body and its neuronal targets. One consequence is a downregulation of substance P and calcitonin gene-related polypeptide (CGRP) in peptidergic fibers, with a concomitant upregulation of the usually quiescent substance P in Aβ fibers [77]. Tissue NGF can additionally drive peripheral and central sensitization by upregulating neuronal content of brain-derived neurotrophic factor (BDNF). Experimental evidence duly confirms the proalgesic actions of BDNF, since antagonizing it, or sequestering its TrkB receptor in vivo, can greatly attenuate behavioral measures of chronic pain [31]. In terms of treatment, surrogate sources of glial-derived neurotrophic factor (GDNF) have potent neuroprotective effects on axotomized sensory neurons, can prevent mechanical sensitivities that develop after SNL surgery, and can reverse some of the changes in Na^+ channel expression that are consequent to Schwann cell disorganization and neuropathic pain [9].

Ion Channels Underlying Neuropathic Pain and Their Therapeutic Potential

Ion channel plasticity is known to be intimately linked with neuropathic pain, and many analgesic drugs have been designed (sometimes serendipitously) to modulate these channels. In particular, channels that are voltage-gated for Na^+, K^+, and Ca^{2+} ions (as well as the N-methyl-D-aspartate [NMDA] receptor complex) underlie the processing of sensory information and are key targeting candidates.

Voltage-Gated Na^+ Channels

Voltage-gated Na^+ channels propagate action potentials along neurons and spur hyperexcitability after nerve injury. Different voltage-gated Na^+ channel isoforms, with different kinetic and pharmacological properties, have been delineated in sensory neurons. The $Na_V1.8$ and $Na_V1.9\alpha$ subunits are expressed exclusively in small, unmyelinated fibers and are resistant to block by tetrodotoxin (TTX), whereas the $Na_V1.7\alpha$ subunit, which is susceptible to block by TTX, is expressed in sensory and sympathetic neurons. Tissue and nerve damage can lead to a change in the expression and function of α subunits, with a resultant change in neuronal excitability to the detriment of the sensory system [54,63]. Tellingly, inherited "gain-of-function" mutations in the $Na_V1.7\alpha$ subunit in humans result in erythromelalgia, a painful condition characterized by intolerable burning sensations in the extremities [83], while other mutations in this channel result in paroxysmal extreme pain disorder.

Peripheral nerve damage leads to a downregulation of 1.8 and 1.9 transcripts in the dorsal root ganglia (DRG) (despite the translocation, insertion and clustering of Na^+ channels containing these subunits at injury and neuroma sites) [32]. The newly dense distribution of Na^+ channels along the sensory neuron after nerve injury supports ectopic firing, whereby action potentials propagate along the neuron in the absence of a stimulus. Such spontaneous discharges, which result partly from Schwann cell de-differentiation as mentioned above, can be replicated experimentally by the addition of a demyelinating agent (the detergent lysolecithin) to Aδ fibers [78], and are known to promote cross-talk between damaged and uninjured fibers by means of ephaptic communication.

Ion channel modulators compromise ion flow under specific (patho)physiological conditions by virtue of state-dependence. This principle underlies the analgesic capacity of antiepileptic drugs such as carbamazepine and the structurally related oxcarbazepine. These agents slow the recovery of rapidly firing voltage-gated Na^+ channels in a frequency-dependent manner, and have been shown to be effective in the treatment of trigeminal neuralgia, diabetic neuropathy, and postherpetic neuralgia [7]. Lamotrigine, another antiepileptic agent, works in a similar way, while the antiarrhythmic mexiletine, as well as the local anesthetic lidocaine, nonselectively block voltage-gated Na^+ channels to ease neuropathic symptoms (the latter usually applied as a 5% topical patch), regardless of the channel's location in the body. Several of these drugs have shown a degree of efficacy in patients with pain due to Na$_V$1.7 mutations, yet they have side effects that relate to their lack of selectivity within the sodium channel family. The recent development of a selective Na$_V$1.8 blocker, shown to be effective in preclinical models of neuropathy, may be key in improving the therapeutic index of drugs acting on sodium channels [29]. Additional compounds have also been identified that have varying blocking potentials when tested on the Na$_V$1.8 channel in different species [35]. The development of a selective blocker for Na$_V$1.7 channels will undoubtedly prove an important milestone in the development of analgesic agents for neuropathic pain; phlotoxin 1, a peptide isolated from the venom of a tarantula, is reported to be a potent blocker of Na$_V$1.7, blocking selectively at concentrations below 2 µm [18], and so further work needs to establish whether this agent has analgesic potential. In addition to their regulation by nerve injury, transgenic mice lacking Na$_V$1.7 or Na$_V$1.8 channel subunits have marked deficits in neuronal coding of acute mechanical stimuli, indicating that these channels may be key contributors to transmission of this important modality [48].

Voltage-Gated K$^+$ Channels

In contrast to voltage-gated Na$^+$ channels, voltage-gated K$^+$ channels act as brakes in the system, repolarizing active neurons to restore baseline membrane potentials. K$_V$7 (KCNQ) channels operate at low thresholds in the CNS and are responsible for the inhibitory M current in DRG neurons. Retigabine is an agent that facilitates the M current through the opening of K$_V$7 channels, and it has accordingly been shown to inhibit electrically evoked dorsal horn neuronal responses in vivo in a dose-dependent manner. Moreover, retigabine's actions are retained, if not enhanced, after nerve injury (despite alterations in K$^+$ channel expression), hence there is interest in the development of this opener as an analgesic that can be used in the mainline treatment of neuropathic pain, in addition to openers that operate at other potassium channels, for example those belonging to the SK family of small-conductance calcium-activated potassium channels [1].

HCN Channels

Bearing significant structural homology to K$^+$ channels are the hyperpolarization-activated cyclic nucleotide-gated (HCN) channels, which are permeable to both K$^+$ and Na$^+$ ions. These channels prevail in cardiac tissue and DRG neurons, where they modulate the rhythm and waveform of action potentials and contribute to resting membrane potentials [58]. Accumulating evidence points toward an important role of HCN channels in A-fiber-mediated mechanical allodynia and spontaneous neuronal discharges associated with peripheral nerve injury; a specific blocker has been shown to dose-dependently suppress behavioral hypersensitivities in SNL rats and reduce spontaneous A-fiber discharge in the absence of adverse effects (i.e., cardiotoxicity and death), yet it leaves normal sensory transduction intact [41].

Voltage-Gated Ca^{2+} Channels

Voltage-gated Ca^{2+} channels conduct Ca^{2+} ions into the neuron during depolarization, and therefore they play a role in synaptic transmitter release, membrane excitability, and intracellular signaling events that can alter gene expression and lay the foundations for long-term potentiation (LTP). Different voltage-gated Ca^{2+} channels subserve different functional roles relative to their cellular locations. L channels are key determinants of membrane excitability, whereas N and P/Q channels are involved with transmitter release at synaptic junctions. Supporting this release are the R channels, which are particularly prevalent in nociceptive spinal cord pathways. T channels are low-voltage-activated channels that permit Ca^{2+} flux at resting membrane potentials, hence their role in pacemaking, neuronal bursting, and synaptic signal boosting. Various experiments point to an altered role of voltage-gated Ca^{2+} channels after neuropathy, and specific blockers have been shown to differentially attenuate the behavioral hypersensitivities and altered dorsal horn neuronal responses that accompany experimental neuropathic pain [45–47].

Gabapentin, a drug used in neuropathic pain, is now known to modulate voltage-gated Ca^{2+} channel (VGCC) function [24]. At first it was assumed that gabapentin had γ-aminobutyric acid (GABA)-mimetic properties, but this assumption was contraindicated by findings that gabapentin (and pregabalin) did not bind to GABA receptors or change GABA levels [4,36,72]. A gabapentin binding site was eventually isolated and identified as the α$_2$δ subunit of VGCCs [24], and evidence followed regarding the drug's ability to reduce Ca^{2+} currents in excitable neurons [62]. Since this discovery, other agents modeled on gabapentin, including pregabalin, have been shown to have analgesic potencies in sensitized states that correlate with their binding affinity and stereospecificity at the $\alpha_2\delta$ subunit [16,19]. Furthermore, the $\alpha_2\delta$ subunit is upregulated after nerve injury [42], forming a potential basis for the ability of the drug to selectively reduce transmission after nerve damage [12,61,65]. It has recently been shown that the antiallodynic effect of pregabalin in vivo is associated with impaired anterograde trafficking of $\alpha_2\delta_1$ subunits, resulting in a decreased density of these subunits on presynaptic terminals, which in turn results in reduced neurotransmitter release and spinal sensitization (factors that are otherwise important for the maintenance of neuropathic pain) [3]. It should be mentioned, however, that both gabapentin and pregabalin have actions that are regulated by brainstem mechanisms.

Primary Afferent Fiber Reorganization

Erroneous sprouting of primary afferent fibers may also underlie symptoms of neuropathic pain; the PNS has regenerative capacity such that following nerve transection, Schwann cells accrue and promote neuronal redevelopment, resulting in de-afferentation of injured and uninjured fibers. Such collateral branching can lead to misdirected targeting of fibers, and inappropriate peripheral innervation, such that cutaneous areas once occupied by the lesioned nerve become hyperinnervated by low- and high-threshold fibers. The behavioral manifestation of this sprouting, which has been demonstrated in skin samples from neuropathic patients, includes touch-evoked pain.

Whether or not peripheral reorganization of the nervous system after nerve injury is matched by central reorganization in the spinal cord has been the subject of considerable debate. This follows seminal work suggesting that central terminals of myelinated afferents redistribute after nerve injury into dorsal horn laminae, which in the normal state are exclusively occupied by the central terminals of unmyelinated neurons [82]. This purported shift in fiber termination would enable low-threshold sensory fibers to access nociceptive-specific relay neurons, meaning that innocuous stimuli would be inappropriately translated and painfully perceived. Subsequent observations that the bulk-labeling procedure indiscriminately labels the terminals of both myelinated *and* unmyelinated fibers (and not just myelinated fibers, as originally thought) casts doubt on this concept, and it is now agreed that

any potential dorsal horn reorganization following nerve injury is markedly less significant than was once thought [26].

If allodynia is not a consequence of low-threshold Aβ fibers tapping into an altered CNS after nerve injury, it may alternatively be caused by central changes. Central sensitization not only can lead to increased responsivity of neurons but additionally can result in an expansion of the sensory neuron's peripheral receptive field [64]. The barrage of peripheral activity that follows nerve injury can increase neuronal transmitter release and unleash NMDA receptors in the dorsal horn of the spinal cord, triggering central sensitization [14].

Immune System Involvement in Neuropathic Pain

Immune system products such as tumor necrosis factor (TNF) α may trigger caspase-signaling pathways, resulting in cell death. The immune system plays an obvious role in inflammatory pain [49], yet its previously underestimated role in neuropathic pain is being increasingly recognized [43]. In the periphery, newly expressed cytokines are released from injured nerves, and chemoattractant signals are released from Schwann cells, resulting in sequential macrophage infiltration in the damaged area if the neuropathy has inflammatory components. The Schwann cells themselves release proinflammatory agents, resulting in further macrophage recruitment, sustaining the cycle of nociceptor sensitization. Microglia are the resident immune cells in the CNS (functionally equivalent to peripheral macrophages), and together with astrocytes, they constitute the glial population. Glia entangle with central neurons and play a key role in pathophysiological pain [23].

Fractalkine is a neuron-to-glia signal [11] that can trigger release of neurostimulating agents such as nitric oxide (NO), adenosine triphosphate (ATP), excitatory amino acids (EAAs), and classical immune mediators, inducing spinal nociceptive facilitation [52]. Fluorocitrate and compounds that inhibit microglia activation reduce the development of nerve-injury-induced hypersensitivities, yet do not reverse established pain behaviors [71]. Given that glial cells are not involved in normal pain processing and only become activated during excessive nervous system activity, agents targeting these cells, or their neuroactive products, may hold increased analgesic hope for the future.

The Spinal Cord and Spinal Neurons

The central terminals of primary afferent fibers show highly organized, topographic termination patterns in the dorsal horn of the spinal cord. Afferent neurons arriving from the periphery enter the spinal cord via dorsal root entry zones, and terminate in specific laminae in keeping with their neuronal type and sensory signal.

Lamina I is a thin "marginal" layer that receives synaptic input from small-diameter unmyelinated C fibers and finely myelinated Aδ fibers. It comprises small neurons that are largely nociceptive-specific (NS), with a smaller number of neurons being thermoreceptive or sensitive to itch stimuli. Many lamina I neurons project long-distance axons to the brain along designated tracts (for example the spinoparabrachial tract), while other neurons send dendrites to local neurons within the same lamina, or dorsally to distal neurons in other laminae. Lamina I neurons can modulate the excitability of neurons in deeper laminae directly via intraspinal pathways, or indirectly in loop form via pathways that descend from brainstem areas [65].

Lamina II, known as the "substantia gelatinosa," is where nociceptive interneurons involved in the processing of noxious input are principally located. Accordingly, fibers conveying noxious input from the periphery terminate here; the outer aspect of lamina II (II_o) receives input from Aδ fibers and isolectin B4-positive nonpeptidergic C fibers, whilst the more basal, inner aspect (II_i) receives the terminals of TrkA-positive peptidergic C fibers. Like lamina I cells, neurons within the substantia gelatinosa can send projections beyond their segmental area to modulate neuronal activity in other laminae (i.e., I and IV).

Laminae III and IV are collectively known as the "nucleus proprius." They contain cells that respond to innocuous input such as that arriving along Aβ fibers.

Lamina V, which is set deep in the dorsal horn, receives convergent input from low- and high-threshold sensory fibers. The ability of neurons in lamina V to amalgamate sensory input ranging from the innocuous to the noxious affords the prefix "wide-dynamic-range" (WDR). WDR neurons have large receptive fields and a high propensity for wind-up, so that upon repeated stimulation they temporally summate incoming action potentials and react to given stimuli with exaggerated response [51]. This phenomenon is frequency-dependent and depends on NMDA receptors. These complexes, which

gate Ca^{2+} entry into the neuron, require dual activation by the excitatory transmitter glutamate and depolarizing membrane potentials. This reliance on coincident pre- and postsynaptic activity (which affords them the term "coincidence detectors") ensures that the receptors are activated, and the Ca^{2+} channel is opened, only during intense synaptic activity. NMDA receptors are thus involved in central sensitization [13,15], and their expression and docking at synaptic sites increases after nerve injury. However, the multiple roles of NMDA receptors in normal and abnormal nervous system function (memory and learning vs. pathological pain processing) impose important constraints on therapeutics that block or modulate their conductance, with benefits offset by side effects that include dizziness and sedation [25]. Pharmacological properties of channel modulators can, however, be refined so that agents preferentially bind to open channels, conferring a pathologically activated state that has superior tolerability. This is the mechanism of action of memantine and nitromemantine.

In contrast to WDR neurons, NS neurons in superficial laminae have small receptive fields and undergo minimal wind-up in response to repetitive stimulation. Following nerve injury, NS neurons may take on characteristics of WDR neurons and therefore become responsive to a more spatially and sensory diverse range of stimuli [64]. WDR neurons can project in the spinothalamic tract and relay to cortical areas of the brain, whereupon they are decoded into sensory-discriminative and affective-motivational components. Indeed, the ability of the WDR neurons to wind-up and code innocuous and noxious mechanical and thermal stimuli makes them ideal candidates for driving the sensory components of pain, as well as generating abnormal signals that lead to allodynia and hyperalgesia.

Laminae V–VI receive input from the afferents of specialized muscle structures, which may also penetrate and make synaptic contact in the ventral horn of the spinal cord. Simple synaptic contact between incoming sensory neurons and motor neurons can effect reflex responses via skeletal muscles, including the nocifensive withdrawal reflex that serves to unconsciously protect an organism from impending injury, and it forms a basis for many of the behavioral measures used in preclinical studies.

Lamina I Projections

Two main pathways connect lamina I nociceptive projection neurons with the brain. The first of these is the spinoparabrachial pathway [6]. The parabrachial area collects and integrates far-ranging nociceptive signals, before processing them and distributing them onwards [8]. Its key output areas are the amygdala, hypothalamus, and periaqueductal gray (PAG). The amygdala triggers emotional affect, including aversion, anxiety, and fear-induced avoidance learning [44], while the hypothalamus aligns homeostatic processes (e.g., blood pressure and heart rate) to the painful input [75]. In turn, the PAG triggers emotional behaviors that include passive and active coping strategies (withdrawal from the environment versus engagement) [40], as well as opioid and nonopioid endogenous analgesia [38]. Thus, this pathway serves the affective-motivational dimension of pain [59]. The other main pathway from lamina I (which is less dense than the spinoparabrachial pathway) projects to caudal parts of the thalamus, which itself projects to the insular and somatosensory cortices for sensory discrimination and interoception [5].

Lamina V Projections

Like lamina I projection neurons, neurons from the deep dorsal horn project to one of two major sites, namely the thalamus (hence the spinothalamic pathway) and the caudal reticular formation. The thalamus projects to the prefrontal cortex, which is involved with attention and motivational aspects of pain (and therefore would play an important role in people who overly attend to, and catastrophize, their pain) [79]. The caudal reticular formation, on the other hand, underlies the motor response to pain, while its intrinsic subnucleus reticularis dorsalis processes the quality, modality, and intensity of the incoming stimulus [76]. Lamina V neurons additionally project to the striatum and globus pallidus.

Thus, deep laminae projection neurons play a large role in somatic responses and sensory decoding and, via thalamocortical projections, a lesser role in the emotional coupling of the painful stimulus.

Supraspinal Control of Spinal Sensory Processing

Complex networks of pathways from various sites in the brain integrate together to modulate the spinal processing of sensory information in a top-down fashion. Higher-order cognitive and emotional processes such as anxiety, mood, and attention can influence the perception of pain through the convergence of somatic and limbic systems into a so-called descending modulatory system, providing a neural substrate through which the brain can control pain. This network enables significant feedback regulation of the nociceptive signal via a spinobulbospinal loop, which first projects up from the spinal cord to the brain as described, before descending back down to the spinal cord via brainstem structures to alter the level of sensory gain within the spinal cord [65]. One consequence of this system in the context of neuropathic pain is that nociceptive information can precipitate supraspinal neuroplastic changes to further facilitate incoming spinal inputs, resulting in an enhanced pain state.

The pharmacology of the descending systems is complex, but broadly speaking the two major defined transmitters in the pathways from brain to spinal cord are the monoamines, norepinephrine (NE) and 5-hydroxytryptamine (5-HT).

The PAG and rostral ventromedial medulla (RVM), which lie in the midbrain and brainstem respectively, are key structures in the descending modulatory repertoire [20]. The PAG collects, processes, and integrates ascending nociceptive inputs with descending information from the diencephalon and limbic forebrain, and then projects via the RVM to the dorsal horn. In turn, the RVM, a crucial junction and relay site in this descending control, receives information from autonomic, homeostatic, affective, and sensory systems and projects directly to the spinal cord via the dorsolateral funiculus. The source of other projections to the spinal cord include the dorsal reticular formation and the locus ceruleus (LC). This latter area contains the source of spinal NE pathways, whereas spinal 5-HT appears to originate from the RVM. Within the dorsal horn, descending projections may alter the tone of sensory signals in the spinal cord via direct presynaptic actions on the dorsal horn terminals of primary afferent fibers, via postsynaptic actions on second-order projection neurons, and also via actions on intrinsic interneurons within the spinal cord [22].

The brainstem can facilitate or inhibit spinal cord activity via RVM "ON" and "OFF" cells, respectively [21]. The net output of the descending facilitatory and inhibitory pathways determines whether neuronal activity in the spinal cord is enhanced or suppressed. Opioid agents can modulate this output because they (directly) inhibit excitatory ON cells and (indirectly) activate inhibitory OFF cells [2]. Thus, opioids exert their analgesic actions at the supraspinal level, in addition to the spinal level.

There are no intrinsic NE or 5-HT neurons within the spinal cord, and so the overriding control of the role of the spinal monoamine systems derives from activity in brain structures, with the final descending pathways running from the LC and RVM. It is well established that the major spinal receptor for NE is the inhibitory α_2-adrenoceptor. Agonists at this receptor, such as clonidine and dexmedetomidine, are analgesic, but they have sedative and hypotensive actions that limit their use. There are multiple 5-HT receptors at spinal levels, with the 5-HT$_1$ receptor likely to serve an inhibitory function, whereas the 5-HT$_3$ receptor is a powerful excitatory receptor. The function and potential of the 5-HT$_{1B/D}$ receptor appears to be restricted to cranial pain mechanisms, and accordingly triptans act here for the relief of headache and migraine.

In addition, the terminals that release the two monoamines in the spinal cord are likely targets for antidepressant drugs used in neuropathic pain. The analgesic capacity of the old drugs such as amitriptyline and newer agents such as the selective serotonin reuptake inhibitor (SSRI) fluoxetine, and the balanced NE/5-HT reuptake blockers such as duloxetine, varies with actions that involve increased synaptic levels of NE and 5-HT—mechanisms common to amitriptyline and duloxetine—drugs that have better efficacy than the SSRIs, which themselves have no direct effects of NE-mediated controls. Thus, it appears that the increased synaptic levels of NE may promote more α_2-adrenoceptor mediated inhibition at spinal levels via actions at receptors that are located both pre- and postsynaptically. Furthermore, amitriptyline is reported to have additional actions that may include Na$^+$ channel block and at extreme doses, NMDA-receptor actions, which may explain the high efficacy yet confounding side effects of this drug.

The ability of the antidepressants to be effective in neuropathic pain comes from their actions on the monoamine systems, yet until recently it was not known whether NE and 5-HT transmission was altered by nerve injury, or whether drugs simply enhanced normal monoamine function. The former appears to be the case because preclinical studies show that the role of the inhibitory adrenoceptor function is *decreased* whereas the facilitatory function of the 5-HT$_3$ receptor is *increased* following nerve injury [53,56,66]. Agents are beginning to emerge that target both the monoamine and opioid systems to analgesic effect; tramadol, for example, is a weak opioid that can block the reuptake of NE and 5-HT, and tapentadol is a next-generation, centrally acting analgesic that combines mu-opioid agonist action with NE reuptake inhibition within a single molecule [74]. This elimination of any 5-HT modulatory action (relative to tramadol) would be expected to remove the potential pronociceptive effect of increased 5-HT turnover, and also reduce any gastrointestinal and emetic actions. Moreover, it has recently been shown that activity at spinal 5-HT receptors is permissive for the inhibitory efficacy of gabapentin [67].

There are various hypotheses relating to the "non-$\alpha_2\delta$" inhibitory actions of gabapentin and pregabalin. Most of these consider the drugs' spinal actions, which have been demonstrated in various studies [27,30,60], yet these agents are additionally thought to exert supraspinal antinociceptive effects [69]. Indeed, pharmacological functional magnetic resonance imaging (fMRI) studies, which reliably detect the central effects of analgesic drugs [80], have shown that gabapentin significantly reduces brainstem activity during central sensitization in humans [28]. This brainstem site of action is supported by reports that systemic administration of gabapentin reduces descending influences from the reticular formation onto trigeminal sensory neurons [34]. These effects may not be due to direct actions of gabapentin on the brainstem; they may instead be secondary to spinal or peripheral actions (since a reduced spinal drive results in decreased spinobulbospinal activity) [65], yet despite clear preclinical demonstrations of gabapentin's spinal actions, an additional (independent or linked) supraspinal mechanism has been agreed upon by others [39,55,70].

The mechanisms underlying the proposed supraspinal actions of gabapentin involve activation of the descending noradrenergic system [68]. Specifically, gabapentin is thought to presynaptically reduce GABAergic transmission in the LC following nerve injury, which consequently releases (via disinhibition) descending neurons that terminate on inhibitory α_2-adrenoceptors in the dorsal horn. These studies are not, however, the only references to gabapentin's dependency on the supraspinal monoamine system, since the injury-dependent interaction of an ascending lamina I projection-brainstem descending serotonergic system with spinal 5-HT$_3$ receptors is also important for the analgesic actions of gabapentin in neuropathic animals [67]. In particular, a central permissive role exerted by excitatory serotonergic influences from the brainstem on gabapentin's inhibitory efficacy has been demonstrated, with a hypothesized interplay between presynaptic VGCCs and 5-HT$_3$ receptors in primary afferent fibers [67]. In particular, the increased descending input to spinal 5-HT$_3$ receptors after nerve injury [66] may depolarize the terminals of primary afferent fibers to the extent that the opening of VGCCs is prolonged, possibly giving gabapentin increased access to the $\alpha_2\delta$ subunit. With interruption of this pathway in SNL rats, behavioral hypersensitivities are reduced and gabapentin has no effect on neuronal responses [67]. Importantly, gabapentin's inhibitory efficacy in neuropathic animals could be blocked by antagonizing spinal 5-HT$_3$ receptors with ondansetron, or induced in normal animals by 5-HT$_3$-receptor activation [67].

Gabapentin's requirement for enhanced activity at spinal 5-HT$_3$ receptors following nerve injury ultimately means that the same brainstem-reaching circuits that influence nociception and perceived pain also influence treatment outcome. Those midbrain areas involved in the processing of fear, stress, and anxiety are contacted by spinobulbospinal circuits, and activity in the anterior cingulate cortex directly affects descending modulatory structures [10]. These circuits may therefore represent an anatomical link between the sensory and emotional components of pain, and thus the neural substrate through which depression, anxiety, and sleep disorders (for example) can influence pain.

Conclusions

Neuropathic pain arises from initiating changes in the damaged nerve, which in turn alter processing in the spinal cord and the brain and also cause plasticity in areas adjacent to those directly influenced by the neuropathy. The loss of peripheral function appears to drive central compensations so that the mechanisms involved in the pain are likely to be multiple and located at a number of sites. Thus, marked central changes are likely to occur, even when a neuropathy arises from purely peripheral origins. The fact that aberrant processing of sensory information leads to hyperalgesia and allodynia suggests central compensations, as does the simple consideration that damage to a nerve would be expected to cause sensory loss, and not increased pain. Possibly, increased central hyperexcitability is a maladaptive compensation for the marked loss

of peripheral input that occurs after nerve injury. The cascade of changes start to occur within the peripheral nerve, mainly involving ion channels and growth factors. The central terminals of these afferent fibers are altered, as are transmitter release and function; these changes then increase spinal sensory neuron excitability and induce facets of central sensitization. Finally, descending controls alter and shift toward facilitatory effects. The presently used clinical drugs and also potential new drugs interact with these multiple mechanisms at different sites in the nervous system, and the multiplicity of these mechanisms is a rational basis for combination therapy: different drugs acting through different targets can modulate more than one mechanism at more than one site.

Acknowledgments

The London Pain Consortium and The Wellcome Trust supported this work.

References

[1] Bahia PK, Suzuki R, Benton DC, Jowett AJ, Chen MX, Trezise DJ, Dickenson AH, Moss GW. A functional role for small-conductance calcium-activated potassium channels in sensory pathways including nociceptive processes. J Neurosci 2005;25:3489–98.

[2] Barbaro NM, Heinricher MM, Fields HL. Putative pain modulating neurons in the rostral ventral medulla: reflex-related activity predicts effects of morphine. Brain Res 1986;366:203–10.

[3] Bauer CS, Nieto-Rostro M, Rahman W, Tran-Van-Minh A, Ferron L, Douglas L, Kadurin I, Sri Ranjan Y, Fernandez-Alacid L, Millar NS, et al. The increased trafficking of the calcium channel subunit alpha2delta-1 to presynaptic terminals in neuropathic pain is inhibited by the alpha2delta ligand pregabalin. J Neurosci 2009;29:4076–88.

[4] Ben-Menachem E. Pregabalin pharmacology and its relevance to clinical practice. Epilepsia 2004;45(Suppl 6):13–8.

[5] Bester H, Chapman V, Besson JM, Bernard JF. Physiological properties of the lamina I spinoparabrachial neurons in the rat. J Neurophysiol 2000;83:2239–59.

[6] Bester H, Matsumoto N, Besson JM, Bernard JF. Further evidence for the involvement of the spinoparabrachial pathway in nociceptive processes: a c-Fos study in the rat. J Comp Neurol 1997;383:439–58.

[7] Beydoun S, Alarcon F, Mangat S, Wan Y. Long-term safety and tolerability of oxcarbazepine in painful diabetic neuropathy. Acta Neurol Scand 2007;115:284–8.

[8] Blomqvist A, Ma W, Berkley KJ. Spinal input to the parabrachial nucleus in the cat. Brain Res 1989;480:29–36.

[9] Boucher TJ, Okuse K, Bennett DL, Munson JB, Wood JN, McMahon SB. Potent analgesic effects of GDNF in neuropathic pain states. Science 2000;290:124–7.

[10] Calejesan AA, Kim SJ, Zhuo M. Descending facilitatory modulation of a behavioral nociceptive response by stimulation in the adult rat anterior cingulate cortex. Eur J Pain 2000;4:83–96.

[11] Chapman GA, Moores K, Harrison D, Campbell CA, Stewart BR, Strijbos PJ. Fractalkine cleavage from neuronal membranes represents an acute event in the inflammatory response to excitotoxic brain damage. J Neurosci 2000;20:RC87.

[12] Chapman V, Suzuki R, Dickenson AH. Electrophysiological characterization of spinal neuronal response properties in anaesthetized rats after ligation of spinal nerves L5–L6. J Physiol 1998;507(Pt 3):881–94.

[13] Dickenson AH. A cure for wind up: NMDA receptor antagonists as potential analgesics. Trends Pharmacol Sci 1990;11:307–9.

[14] Dickenson AH. Spinal cord pharmacology of pain. Br J Anaesth 1995;75:193–200.

[15] Dickenson AH, Sullivan AF. Evidence for a role of the NMDA receptor in the frequency dependent potentiation of deep rat dorsal horn nociceptive neurones following C fibre stimulation. Neuropharmacology 1987;26:1235–8.

[16] Dissanayake VU, Gee NS, Brown JP, Woodruff GN. Spermine modulation of specific [3H]-gabapentin binding to the detergent-solubilized porcine cerebral cortex alpha 2 delta calcium channel subunit. Br J Pharmacol 1997;120:833–40.

[17] Dowdall T, Robinson I, Meert TF. Comparison of five different rat models of peripheral nerve injury. Pharmacol Biochem Behav 2005;80:93–108.

[18] Escoubas P, Rash L. Tarantulas: eight-legged pharmacists and combinatorial chemists. Toxicon 2004;43:555–74.

[19] Field MJ, McCleary S, Hughes J, Singh L. Gabapentin and pregabalin, but not morphine and amitriptyline, block both static and dynamic components of mechanical allodynia induced by streptozocin in the rat. Pain 1999;80:391–8.

[20] Fields HL, Basbaum AI. Brainstem control of spinal pain-transmission neurons. Annu Rev Physiol 1978;40:217–48.

[21] Fields HL, Bry J, Hentall I, Zorman G. The activity of neurons in the rostral medulla of the rat during withdrawal from noxious heat. J Neurosci 1983;3:2545–52.

[22] Fields HL, Heinricher MM, Mason P. Neurotransmitters in nociceptive modulatory circuits. Annu Rev Neurosci 1991;14:219–45.

[23] Garrison CJ, Dougherty PM, Kajander KC, Carlton SM. Staining of glial fibrillary acidic protein (GFAP) in lumbar spinal cord increases following a sciatic nerve constriction injury. Brain Res 1991;565:1–7.

[24] Gee NS, Brown JP, Dissanayake VU, Offord J, Thurlow R, Woodruff GN. The novel anticonvulsant drug, gabapentin (Neurontin), binds to the alpha2delta subunit of a calcium channel. J Biol Chem 1996;271:5768–76.

[25] Haines DR, Gaines SP. N of 1 randomised controlled trials of oral ketamine in patients with chronic pain. Pain 1999;83:283–7.

[26] Hughes DI, Scott DT, Todd AJ, Riddell JS. Lack of evidence for sprouting of Abeta afferents into the superficial laminas of the spinal cord dorsal horn after nerve section. J Neurosci 2003;23:9491–9.

[27] Hwang JH, Yaksh TL. Effect of subarachnoid gabapentin on tactile-evoked allodynia in a surgically induced neuropathic pain model in the rat. Reg Anesth 1997;22:249–56.

[28] Iannetti GD, Zambreanu L, Wise RG, Buchanan TJ, Huggins JP, Smart TS, Vennart W, Tracey I. Pharmacological modulation of pain-related brain activity during normal and central sensitization states in humans. Proc Natl Acad Sci USA 2005;102:18195–200.

[29] Jarvis MF, Honore P, Shieh CC, Chapman M, Joshi S, Zhang XF, Kort M, Carroll W, Marron B, Atkinson R, et al. A-803467, a potent and selective $Na_V1.8$ sodium channel blocker, attenuates neuropathic and inflammatory pain in the rat. Proc Natl Acad Sci USA 2007;104:8520–5.

[30] Kaneko M, Mestre C, Sanchez EH, Hammond DL. Intrathecally administered gabapentin inhibits formalin-evoked nociception and the expression of Fos-like immunoreactivity in the spinal cord of the rat. J Pharmacol Exp Ther 2000;292:743–51.

[31] Kerr BJ, Bradbury EJ, Bennett DL, Trivedi PM, Dassan P, French J, Shelton DB, McMahon SB, Thompson SW. Brain-derived neurotrophic factor modulates nociceptive sensory inputs and NMDA-evoked responses in the rat spinal cord. J Neurosci 1999;19:5138–48.

[32] Kim CH, Oh Y, Chung JM, Chung K. The changes in expression of three subtypes of TTX sensitive sodium channels in sensory neurons after spinal nerve ligation. Brain Res Mol Brain Res 2001;95:153–61.

[33] Kim KJ, Yoon YW, Chung JM. Comparison of three rodent neuropathic pain models. Exp Brain Res 1997;113:200–6.

[34] Kondo T, Fromm GH, Schmidt B. Comparison of gabapentin with other antiepileptic and GABAergic drugs. Epilepsy Res 1991;8:226–31.

[35] Krafte DS, Chapman M, Marron B, Atkinson R, Liu Y, Ye F, Curran M, Kort M, Jarvis MF. Block of $Na_V1.8$ by small molecules. Channels (Austin) 2007;1:152–3.

[36] Lanneau C, Green A, Hirst WD, Wise A, Brown JT, Donnier E, Charles KJ, Wood M, Davies CH, Pangalos MN. Gabapentin is not a GABAB receptor agonist. Neuropharmacology 2001;41:965–75.

[37] Le Bars D, Gozariu M, Cadden SW. Animal models of nociception. Pharmacol Rev 2001;53:597–652.

[38] Lewis VA, Gebhart GF. Evaluation of the periaqueductal central gray (PAG) as a morphine-specific locus of action and examination of morphine-induced and stimulation-produced analgesia at coincident PAG loci. Brain Res 1977;124:283–303.

[39] Loscher W, Honack D, Taylor CP. Gabapentin increases aminooxyacetic acid-induced GABA accumulation in several regions of rat brain. Neurosci Lett 1991;128:150–4.

[40] Lovick TA. Ventrolateral medullary lesions block the antinociceptive and cardiovascular responses elicited by stimulating the dorsal periaqueductal grey matter in rats. Pain 1985;21:241–52.

[41] Luo L, Chang L, Brown SM, Ao H, Lee DH, Higuera ES, Dubin AE, Chaplan SR. Role of peripheral hyperpolarization-activated cyclic nucleotide-modulated channel pacemaker channels in acute and chronic pain models in the rat. Neuroscience 2007;144:1477–85.

[42] Luo ZD, Chaplan SR, Higuera ES, Sorkin LS, Stauderman KA, Williams ME, Yaksh TL. Upregulation of dorsal root ganglion $\alpha_2\delta$ calcium channel subunit and its correlation with allodynia in spinal nerve-injured rats. J Neurosci 2001;21:1868–75.

[43] Marchand F, Perretti M, McMahon SB. Role of the immune system in chronic pain. Nat Rev Neurosci 2005;6:521–32.

[44] Maren S. Neuroscience. The threatened brain. Science 2007;317:1043–4.

[45] Matthews EA, Bee LA, Stephens GJ, Dickenson AH. The Cav2.3 calcium channel antagonist SNX-482 reduces dorsal horn neuronal responses in a rat model of chronic neuropathic pain. Eur J Neurosci 2007;25:3561–9.

[46] Matthews EA, Dickenson AH. Effects of ethosuximide, a T-type Ca^{2+} channel blocker, on dorsal horn neuronal responses in rats. Eur J Pharmacol 2001;415:141–9.

[47] Matthews EA, Dickenson AH. Effects of spinally delivered N- and P-type voltage-dependent calcium channel antagonists on dorsal horn neuronal responses in a rat model of neuropathy. Pain 2001;92:235–46.

[48] Matthews EA, Wood JN, Dickenson AH. $Na_V1.8$-null mice show stimulus-dependent deficits in spinal neuronal activity. Mol Pain 2006;2:5.

[49] McMahon SB, Cafferty WB, Marchand F. Immune and glial cell factors as pain mediators and modulators. Exp Neurol 2005;192:444–62.

[50] McMahon SB, Jones NG. Plasticity of pain signaling: role of neurotrophic factors exemplified by acid-induced pain. J Neurobiol 2004;61:72–87.

[51] Mendell LM, Wall PD. Responses of single dorsal cord cells to peripheral cutaneous unmyelinated fibres. Nature 1965;206:97–9.

[52] Milligan E, Zapata V, Schoeniger D, Chacur M, Green P, Poole S, Martin D, Maier SF, Watkins LR. An initial investigation of spinal mechanisms underlying pain enhancement induced by fractalkine, a neuronally released chemokine. Eur J Neurosci 2005;22:2775–82.

[53] Oatway MA, Chen Y, Weaver LC. The 5-HT3 receptor facilitates at-level mechanical allodynia following spinal cord injury. Pain 2004;110:259–68.

[54] Okuse K, Chaplan SR, McMahon SB, Luo ZD, Calcutt NA, Scott BP, Akopian AN, Wood JN. Regulation of expression of the sensory neuron-specific sodium channel SNS in inflammatory and neuropathic pain. Mol Cell Neurosci 1997;10:196–207.

[55] Petroff OA, Rothman DL, Behar KL, Lamoureux D, Mattson RH. The effect of gabapentin on brain gamma-aminobutyric acid in patients with epilepsy. Ann Neurol 1996;39:95–9.

[56] Rahman W, Suzuki R, Rygh LJ, Dickenson AH. Descending serotonergic facilitation mediated through rat spinal 5HT3 receptors is unaltered following carrageenan inflammation. Neurosci Lett 2004;361:229–31.

[57] Ren K, Dubner R. Inflammatory models of pain and hyperalgesia. ILAR J 1999;40(3):111–8.

[58] Robinson RB, Siegelbaum SA. Hyperpolarization-activated cation currents: from molecules to physiological function. Annu Rev Physiol 2003;65:453–80.

[59] Saper CB. The spinoparabrachial pathway: shedding new light on an old path. J Comp Neurol 1995;353:477–9.

[60] Shimoyama N, Shimoyama M, Davis AM, Inturrisi CE, Elliott KJ. Spinal gabapentin is antinociceptive in the rat formalin test. Neurosci Lett 1997;222:65–7.

[61] Stanfa LC, Singh L, Williams RG, Dickenson AH. Gabapentin, ineffective in normal rats, markedly reduces C-fibre evoked responses after inflammation. Neuroreport 1997;8:587–90.

[62] Stefani A, Spadoni F, Bernardi G. Gabapentin inhibits calcium currents in isolated rat brain neurons. Neuropharmacology 1998;37:83–91.

[63] Strichartz GR, Zhou Z, Sinnott C, Khodorova A. Therapeutic concentrations of local anaesthetics unveil the potential role of sodium channels in neuropathic pain. Novartis Found Symp 2002;241:189–201.

[64] Suzuki R, Kontinen VK, Matthews E, Williams E, Dickenson AH. Enlargement of the receptive field size to low intensity mechanical stimulation in the rat spinal nerve ligation model of neuropathy. Exp Neurol 2000;163:408–13.

[65] Suzuki R, Morcuende S, Webber M, Hunt SP, Dickenson AH. Superficial NK1-expressing neurons control spinal excitability through activation of descending pathways. Nat Neurosci 2002;5:1319–26.

[66] Suzuki R, Rahman W, Hunt SP, Dickenson AH. Descending facilitatory control of mechanically evoked responses is enhanced in deep dorsal horn neurones following peripheral nerve injury. Brain Res 2004;1019:68–76.

[67] Suzuki R, Rahman W, Rygh LJ, Webber M, Hunt SP, Dickenson AH. Spinal-supraspinal serotonergic circuits regulating neuropathic pain and its treatment with gabapentin. Pain 2005;117:292–303.

[68] Takasu K, Honda M, Ono H, Tanabe M. Spinal alpha$_2$-adrenergic and muscarinic receptors and the NO release cascade mediate supraspinally produced effectiveness of gabapentin at decreasing mechanical hypersensitivity in mice after partial nerve injury. Br J Pharmacol 2006;148:233–44.

[69] Takeuchi Y, Takasu K, Honda M, Ono H, Tanabe M. Neurochemical evidence that supraspinally administered gabapentin activates the descending noradrenergic system after peripheral nerve injury. Eur J Pharmacol 2007;556:69–74.

[70] Tanabe M, Takasu K, Kasuya N, Shimizu S, Honda M, Ono H. Role of descending noradrenergic system and spinal alpha$_2$-adrenergic receptors in the effects of gabapentin on thermal and mechanical nociception after partial nerve injury in the mouse. Br J Pharmacol 2005;144:703–14.

[71] Tawfik VL, Nutile-McMenemy N, Lacroix-Fralish ML, DeLeo JA. Efficacy of propentofylline, a glial modulating agent, on existing mechanical allodynia following peripheral nerve injury. Brain Behav Immun 2007;21:238–46.

[72] Taylor CP, Gee NS, Su TZ, Kocsis JD, Welty DF, Brown JP, Dooley DJ, Boden P, Singh L. A summary of mechanistic hypotheses of gabapentin pharmacology. Epilepsy Res 1998;29:233–49.

[73] Treede RD, Jensen TS, Campbell JN, Cruccu G, Dostrovsky JO, Griffin JW, Hansson P, Hughes R, Nurmikko T, Serra J. Neuropathic pain: redefinition and a grading system for clinical and research purposes. Neurology 2008;70:1630–5.

[74] Tzschentke TM, Christoph T, Kogel B, Schiene K, Hennies HH, Englberger W, Haurand M, Jahnel U, Cremers TI, Friderichs E, De Vry J. (-)-(1R,2R)-3-(3-dimethylamino-1-ethyl-2-methyl-propyl)-phenol hydrochloride (tapentadol HCl): a novel mu-opioid receptor agonist/norepinephrine reuptake inhibitor with broad-spectrum analgesic properties. J Pharmacol Exp Ther 2007;323:265–76.

[75] Vidal C, Suaudeau C, Jacob J. Regulation of body temperature and nociception induced by non-noxious stress in rat. Brain Res 1984;297:1–10.

[76] Villanueva L, de Pommery J, Menetrey D, Le Bars D. Spinal afferent projections to subnucleus reticularis dorsalis in the rat. Neurosci Lett 1991;134:98–102.

[77] Villar MJ, Cortes R, Theodorsson E, Wiesenfeld-Hallin Z, Schalling M, Fahrenkrug J, Emson PC, Hokfelt T. Neuropeptide expression in rat dorsal root ganglion cells and spinal cord after peripheral nerve injury with special reference to galanin. Neuroscience 1989;33:587–604.

[78] Wallace VC, Cottrell DF, Brophy PJ, Fleetwood-Walker SM. Focal lysolecithin-induced demyelination of peripheral afferents results in neuropathic pain behavior that is attenuated by cannabinoids. J Neurosci 2003;23:3221–33.

[79] Wiech K, Seymour B, Kalisch R, Stephan KE, Koltzenburg M, Driver J, Dolan RJ. Modulation of pain processing in hyperalgesia by cognitive demand. Neuroimage 2005;27:59–69.

[80] Wise RG, Rogers R, Painter D, Bantick S, Ploghaus A, Williams P, Rapeport G, Tracey I. Combining fMRI with a pharmacokinetic model to determine which brain areas activated by painful stimulation are specifically modulated by remifentanil. Neuroimage 2002;16:999–1014.

[81] Woolf CJ, Salter MW. Neuronal plasticity: increasing the gain in pain. Science 2000;288:1765–9.

[82] Woolf CJ, Shortland P, Coggeshall RE. Peripheral nerve injury triggers central sprouting of myelinated afferents. Nature 1992;355:75–8.

[83] Yang Y, Wang Y, Li S, Xu Z, Li H, Ma L, Fan J, Bu D, Liu B, Fan Z, Wu G, Jin J, Ding B, Zhu X, Shen Y. Mutations in SCN9A, encoding a sodium channel alpha subunit, in patients with primary erythermalgia. J Med Genet 2004;41:171–4.

[84] Zimmermann M. Ethical guidelines for investigations of experimental pain in conscious animals. Pain 1983;16:109–10.

Correspondence to: Anthony H. Dickenson, PhD, FMedSci, Department of Neuroscience, Physiology, Pharmacology, University College London, Gower Street, London WC1E 6BT, United Kingdom. Email: anthony.dickenson@ucl.ac.uk.

Management of Neuropathic Pain

Troels Staehelin Jensen, MD, DMSc, and Nanna Brix Finnerup, MD, DMSc

Department of Neurology and Danish Pain Research Center, Aarhus University Hospital, Aarhus, Denmark

Damage to the somatosensory nervous system represents a potential risk for the development of neuropathic pain. Neuropathic pain is defined by the International Association for the Study of Pain (IASP) as "pain initiated or caused by a primary lesion, dysfunction or transitory perturbation in the peripheral or central nervous system" [21]. Recently, a group of neurologists has proposed a sharpening of this definition by excluding the word "dysfunction" to eliminate conditions for which there are no objective signs of nervous system pathology. According to this novel proposal, neuropathic pain is defined as "pain arising as a direct consequence of a lesion or disease affecting the somatosensory system" [37].

Neuropathic pains consist of a variety of different diseases and conditions including nerve compression, neuropathies, and diseases of the central nervous system, such as stroke and multiple sclerosis. In addition to the long list of different etiologies causing neuropathic pain, these pains also differ in anatomical location and can be localized anywhere from the peripheral nociceptor to the highest centers in the brain [3,5,11,16–19,41].

The consequences of injury to the nervous system include an array of neurobiological events resulting in degeneration and regeneration phenomena, with sensitization as the main factor for the development of pain. A cascade of pain-generating events occurs, with changes at the injury site, in dorsal root ganglion cells, in the spinal cord, and at synaptic relays upstream in the nervous system. These multiple sites in the nervous system where neuronal hyperexcitability develops not only are foci for pain development but also represent potential targets for pain modulation by reducing neuronal hyperexcitability. Our understanding of neuropathic pain has improved dramatically following the discovery of multiple signaling systems in pain [3,5,18,36,41]. This novel information has also resulted in an improvement in treating neuropathic pain, but there is still an unmet need for better treatment, as evidenced by the fact that two-thirds of patients with neuropathic pain do not get sufficient pain relief from the current treatments [1,10]. In chronic pain conditions, elimination of the causative agent is rarely possible, and symptomatic treatment of pain is often the best that can be achieved. It is still unclear how such symptomatic treatment should be carried out, and various algorithms have been proposed [1,7,8,10,12]. This review will outline the current therapy of neuropathic pain, emphasizing recent advancements in pharmacological treatment and neurostimulation techniques.

Efficacy Measures in Neuropathic Pain

The assessment of neuropathic pain is essential in the evaluation of different types of treatment options, and it is equally important to find adequate efficacy measures.

Despite their heterogeneity, neuropathic pains share a range of characteristics [3,5,17,19], including:

- Pain located in a neuroanatomical area with partial or complete sensory loss
- Ongoing pain (stimulus-independent)
- Evoked types of pain (stimulus-dependent)
- Hyperexcitability
- Aftersensations
- Abnormal summation of pain
- Sympathetic involvement

These elements are, therefore, worth measuring as efficacy endpoints, either alone or together. The problem here is that these symptoms or phenomena may occur in various combinations; they are not necessarily all present at the same time, and there may also be differences in symptom presentation over time in individual patients. To reduce the variation in efficacy, measures of treatment success need to be standardized. Pharmacological trials usually assess efficacy based on stable dosing and average scoring of pain within a specified period, such as average daily pain ratings over the last week of treatment. Some symptoms are more bothersome than others, and at present, we do not know how each subcomponent contributes to the entire picture of pain. As for other chronic pain conditions, we know that neuropathic pain is influenced not only by biological but also by psychological and sociological factors.

Targets for Treatment

If pathophysiological mechanisms contributing to the pain can be identified, and if such mechanisms translate into specific symptoms and signs, then it is assumed that the result will be an improved treatment of neuropathic pain [3–5,18]. The problem is that we are rarely in a situation where such translation can be documented, and for that reason most treatments of neuropathic pain are limited to the general management of peripheral and central neuronal hyperexcitability; most of the existing treatments are directed nonspecifically toward such increased neuronal excitability. However, as shown below, there are now data indicating that by targeting either specific sites or certain molecular aspects of neuronal hyperexcitability, we can demonstrate clinical pain relief of certain neuropathic pain states.

For space reasons, we will only consider treatments for which Class 1 or Class 2 evidence has been provided. Class 1 evidence indicates an adequately powered prospective, randomized, controlled clinical trial fulfilling specific quality requirements or an adequately powered systematic review of prospective randomized, controlled clinical trials. Class 2 evidence indicates a prospective matched-group cohort study, which may lack one of the requirements for sufficient quality. These parameters limit the review to pharmacological treatment and neurostimulation techniques. It is important, however, to emphasize that other sorts of treatment are also beneficial. For example, coping strategies, reduction of anxiety, improvement of sleep, treatment of depression, physical therapy, and psychosocial support are often used in the treatment of chronic pain.

Principles of Pharmacological Treatment

Improvement in pain by a treatment is generally assessed by measuring the change in pain intensity on a visual analogue scale, or on an 11-point numerical rating scale anchored with no pain at one end and the worst possible pain at the other end. These measures are often supplemented by a measurement of degree of pain relief on similar scales and by various measures of life quality and the patient's or assessor's impression of change.

The following subsections will briefly summarize the drugs for which randomized, controlled clinical trials have shown efficacy.

Antidepressants

Antidepressants have a well-established beneficial effect in various neuropathic pain states. Antidepressants used in neuropathic pain treatment include tricyclic antidepressants (TCAs), the selective serotonin-norepinephrine reuptake inhibitors (SNRIs), and the selective serotonin reuptake inhibitors (SSRIs) [27,32–34]. TCAs are characterized by their multiple modes of action, with a particular ability to inhibit reuptake of the monoamines, serotonin and norepinephrine, from presynaptic terminals. But they also have cholinergic, adrenergic, and histaminergic blocking properties, and can block ion channels (including Na^+ channels). Antidepressants relieve pain independently of their antidepressant effects. However, because of their dual effect, they may be the first drug choice in patients with coexisting depression. TCAs, of which there are several (including amitriptyline, imipramine, clomipramine, and nortriptyline), have been widely used for the treatment of various types of neuropathic pain. A large number of randomized, double-blind, placebo-controlled trials of TCAs have been performed. Efficacy has been documented for painful diabetic neuropathy, other polyneuropathies, nerve injury pain, postherpetic neuralgia, central poststroke pain (for review see [1,8,10]), and more recently also in spinal cord injury pain [25]. TCAs have several side effects; the most important ones are cardiac conduction disturbances, dry mouth, urine retention, sedation, dizziness, and orthostatic hypotension. An electrocardiogram is mandatory before start of treatment. Specific serotonergic reuptake inhibitors such as citalopram and paroxetine have limited effect on neuropathic pain, but a recent study with the SSRI escitalopram confirmed that SSRIs do have a weak analgesic effect [23]. SNRIs are effective in reducing pain in painful neuropathy. Five of seven controlled clinical trials showed effects of duloxetine and venlafaxine [1,7,8,10]. Data from one of these studies comparing TCAs with SNRIs suggest that the pain-relieving effect of TCAs might be related to monoamine reuptake inhibition rather than to Na^+ channel-blocking effects [32].

Anticonvulsants

Anticonvulsants have several pharmacological actions that may interfere with processes involved in neuronal hyperexcitability by either decreasing excitatory or increasing inhibitory neuronal transmission. The main compounds are gabapentin, pregabalin, lamotrigine, valproate, levetiracetam, topiramate, oxcarbazepine, and carbamazepine.

Gabapentin and Pregabalin

Gabapentin and pregabalin, which are structural analogues to γ-aminobutyric acid (GABA), have no effect at GABAergic receptors but bind to the $\alpha_2\delta$ subunit of voltage-dependent Ca^{2+} channels and reduce Ca^{2+} influx into cells. Because of the wide distribution of Ca^{2+} channels in the central nervous system, these drugs are likely to influence the neuronal function at many sites. Gabapentin and pregabalin have documented efficacy in painful diabetic neuropathy, postherpetic neuralgia, mixed neuropathic pain conditions, and phantom limb pain (for reviews see [1,7,8,10]). More recently, the evidence has been extended to include other conditions such as central pain and HIV neuropathy [29,31,40]. The evidence for a pain-relieving effect in these conditions is generally based on a large number of parallel-designed studies. Gabapentin and pregabalin are generally well tolerated, with no major drug interactions, but sedation, dizziness, and peripheral edema are common side effects.

Lamotrigine

Lamotrigine blocks voltage-dependent Na^+ channels and inhibits Na^+-influx-mediated release of excitatory amino acids from presynaptic neurons. In small (usually crossover) trials, lamotrigine has shown efficacy in trigeminal neuralgia, HIV neuropathy, painful diabetic neuropathy, and central poststroke pain at doses greater than 200 mg/day [10]. However, more recent large, parallel, double-blind, placebo-controlled studies in painful diabetic neuropathy and HIV neuropathy were not able to find a pain-relieving effect of lamotrigine [1,39]. So at present, the effect of lamotrigine seems to be limited to central poststroke pain.

Valproate

The role of valproate in treating neuropathic pain is unclear. There are six published studies [10] with valproate in painful neuropathy, spinal cord injury pain, and postherpetic neuralgia showing either no effect or a surprisingly large effect in painful neuropathy and postherpetic neuralgia.

Topiramate

The anticonvulsant topiramate was initially thought to have an effect in neuropathic pain, but three large studies in painful diabetic neuropathy were all negative [35], and topiramate is currently not recommended for the treatment of this type of pain.

Levetiracetam

Levetiracetam, which is thought to act by inhibiting presynaptic neurotransmitter release by binding to the synaptic vesicle protein SV2A in the brain and spinal cord, has been used for treating partial seizures and has also recently been tried in neuropathic pain. Two recently conducted trials failed to find an effect in postmastectomy neuropathic pain and spinal cord injury pain [13,38].

Lacosamide

Lacosamide is a functionalized amino acid with neuronal antihyperexcitability properties. It has been shown to increase the inactivation of voltage-gated ion channels. Its role in neuropathic pain is unclear. One study showed an effect in painful diabetic neuropathy, while other studies failed to do so [28,42,44].

Phenytoin

Phenytoin, an old antiepileptic with sodium-channel-blocking properties, is useful for the acute termination of bouts of trigeminal neuralgia, but otherwise this drug does not have any place in chronic neuropathic pain therapy.

Carbamazepine and Oxcarbazepine

Carbamazepine and oxcarbazepine are the treatment of choice for trigeminal neuralgia, despite surprisingly weak documentation with small and old placebo-controlled trials.

Opioids

The three types of opioid receptors—mu, kappa, and delta—are widely distributed in the nervous system. Opioids inhibit noxious transmission via multiple mechanisms including peripheral, presynaptic, and postsynaptic opioid receptors located in the dorsal horn and at sites in the brain. Several randomized, controlled trials have convincingly shown opioids to be effective in relieving pain in postherpetic neuralgia, painful diabetic neuropathy, mixed neuropathic pain, spinal cord injury, and postamputation pain [1,7,8,9,10,26]. The most common side effects are constipation, cognitive side effects, and nausea. The risk of drug abuse and immunological side effects is a limiting factor for using these drugs in nonmalignant pain. There is no general agreement regarding how opioids should be dosed, but usually these drugs are given as short-acting opioids every 4–6 hours followed by a switch to long-acting opioids after 1–2 weeks.

Tramadol is a compound that has both opioid analgesic properties and a weak monoaminergic reuptake-inhibiting action. Several trials have documented the effectiveness of tramadol for painful polyneuropathies, in particular those caused by diabetes [1,7,8,10]. The abuse potential of tramadol is less than for the strong opioid analgesics. Side effects are sedation, dizziness, and nausea. In a recent study, tramadol up to 400 mg daily was found to be significantly better than placebo in spinal cord injury patients with at- or below-level neuropathic pain [1,7].

NMDA Antagonists

NMDA (N-methyl-D-aspartic acid) blockers including dextromethorphan, memantine, and riluzole have provided mixed results, with, for example, an effect of dextromethorphan in diabetic neuropathy, but no effect in postherpetic neuralgia. Memantine, another NMDA antagonist, has generally been ineffective (for review see [1]).

Cannabinoids

Cannabinoids have been used in five trials for the relief of pain in multiple sclerosis, plexus avulsion, and mixed neuropathic pain. In a recent trial, Nurmikko et al. [22] used tetrahydrocannabinol in 125 patients with neuropathic pain of peripheral origin in a randomized, double-blind, parallel, placebo-controlled study. There was significant pain reduction and improvement of a number of secondary outcome parameters. Sedation and gastrointestinal side effects were limitations in this and other studies.

Topical Agents

Lidocaine

Lidocaine blocks voltage-gated sodium channels, and its topical application is thought to silence ectopic discharges on small afferent fibers by blocking sodium channels nonspecifically. Lidocaine was introduced a long time ago, and lidocaine patches are now increasingly used in the treatment of postherpetic neuralgia and focal peripheral neuropathic pain [1]. Randomized trials have shown efficacy of lidocaine patches in postherpetic neuralgia and mixed peripheral focal neuropathy and also in post-traumatic neuralgia [1]. So far, only patients with concomitant allodynia have been studied in randomized trials, but lidocaine relieves nonallodynic symptoms as well. Lack of systemic side effects makes topical lidocaine suitable for focal peripheral neuropathic pain with allodynia or hyperalgesia.

Capsaicin

Topically applied capsaicin (usually in a weak concentration of 0.075%) has had limited or no effect in painful diabetic neuropathy, postherpetic neuralgia, HIV-related neuropathic pain, and postsurgical neuropathic pain. Recent studies using high concentrations of capsaicin (8%) applied topically have, however, produced long-lasting pain relief in HIV-related neuropathic pain [30] and postherpetic neuralgia [2].

Combination Therapies

There have been only limited studies of combination therapies in neuropathic pain. In a crossover study of 41 patients with painful diabetic neuropathy and postherpetic neuralgia, Gilron and colleagues determined daily pain intensity in patients receiving maximal tolerated

Table I
Number needed to treat using various analgesics for different neuropathies

Drug	No. Trials/ No. Positive Trials	Number Needed to Treat (95% CI)				
		Central Pain	Painful Poly-neuropathy	Post-herpetic Neuralgia	Peripheral Nerve Injury	Mixed Neuropathic Pain
Tricyclic antidepressants	23/20	2.7 (1.7–6.1)	2.1 (1.9–2.6)	2.8 (2.2–3.8)	2.5 (1.4–11)	NA
SNRIs	7/5	ND	5.0 (3.9–6.8)	ND	NA	ND
SSRIs	4/3	ND	6.8 (3.9–27)	ND	ND	ND
Gabapentin	14/8	NA	6.4 (4.3–12)	4.3 (3.3–6.1)	NA	8.0 (5.9–32)
Pregabalin	14/13	5.6 (3.5–14)	4.5 (3.6–5.9)	4.2 (3.4–5.4)	ns	3.8 (2.6–7.3)
Opioids	9/8	ND	2.6 (1.7–6.0)	2.6 (2.0–3.8)	5.1 (2.7–3.6)	2.1 (1.5–3.3)
Tramadol	6/6	ns	4.9 (2.1–9.0)	4.8 (2.6–27)	NA	ND
NMDA antagonists	13/2	ND	3.4 (1.8–6.6)	ns	ns	ns
Lidocaine patch	3/2	ND	ND	NA	NA	4.4 (2.5–17)
Cannabinoids	6/5	3.4 (1.8–23)	ns	ND	ns	ns
Capsaicin	11/6	ND	11 (5.5–316)	3.2 (2.2–5.9)	ns	NA
NGX capsaicin	3/3	ND	ND	ns	ND	ND
Botulinum toxin A	2/2	2.3 (1.5–4.7)	ND	ND	ND	3.0 (1.6–22)
Nitrate spray	3/3	NA	ND	ND	ND	ND

Source: N.B. Finnerup et al., unpublished observations.
Abbreviations: NA, dichotomized data are not available for calculating number needed to treat (NNT); ND, studies not done; NMDA, N-methyl-D-aspartate; ns, absolute risk difference not significant; SNRIs, serotonin norepinephrine reuptake inhibitors; SSRIs, selective serotonin reuptake inhibitors.

doses of morphine and gabapentin. They showed a higher pain reduction with gabapentin and morphine at lower doses than when either compound was given alone [14]. In a recent study, a similar beneficial effect was shown for the combination of gabapentin and a tricyclic antidepressant [15].

Novel Therapeutic Approaches

Botulinum toxin, which has been shown to inhibit vanilloid receptors and to inhibit release of glutamate and substance P, has also been shown to have a pain-relieving effect in patients with focal peripheral neuropathic pain and allodynia [34] and in diabetic neuropathic pain [43]. Other substances such as glycine antagonists, cyclooxygenase-2 inhibitors, acetylcarnitine, and neurotrophic factors have failed in clinical trials [10].

Practical Guidelines for Pharmacological Therapy

Before choosing a neuropathic pain treatment, clinicians need to consider the benefits and hazards of a specific treatment. Table I presents a list of the number-needed-to-treat (NNT) values for various drug classes against different groups of neuropathic pain conditions. In general, the simpler and less harmful treatments should be chosen, and the efficacy of one compound should always be compared with its adverse effects. It is mandatory that clinicians be familiar with contraindications; this is particularly important in the elderly. Cardiac conduction abnormalities (e.g., AV block), congestive heart failure, and convulsive disorders are contraindications for treatment with TCAs. For anticonvulsants the contraindications are fewer, but side effects such as sedation, dizziness, tremor, and skin rashes are not uncommon.

Adverse effects are important in the decision of any treatment for pain. The calculation of adverse effects, usually as the number needed to harm (NNH), is rarely done in a systematic way that permits an analysis of the specific harm caused by one agent. In most cases, the only harmful effect that can be calculated in a systematic fashion is the number of patients who drop out of a trial [10], and in these cases it is assumed that dropouts are due to side effects.

Before starting a pharmacological treatment, the clinician must consider the patient's age, concomitant medical conditions, depression, sleep disturbances, and other psychosocial factors. Realistic expectations for the outcome of a given treatment should be discussed with the patient, and it should be explained that often only partial pain relief can be expected.

Table II
Pharmacological agents with documented effect in neuropathic pain

Drug	Start Dose and Maximum Dose	Documented Effect	Side Effects
Gabapentin	Start: 300 mg/day; Max: 3600 mg/day	PHN, PDN, mixed neuropathic pain	Sedation, dizziness, edema
Pregabalin	Start: 25 mg/day; Max: 600 mg/day	PHN, PDN, mixed neuropathic pain, central pain	Sedation, dizziness, edema
Tricyclic antidepressants	Start: 25 mg/day; Max: 75–150 mg/day	PHN, PDN, central pain, mixed neuropathic pain	Cardiac conduction disturbances, anticholinergic side effects, sedation
SNRIs	Venlafaxine: Start: 37.5 mg; Max: 225–375 mg/day; Duloxetine: Start: 60 mg	Painful neuropathy	Sedation
Carbamazepine (oxcarbazepine)	Start: 300 mg/day; Max: 1200–1800 mg (1/3 higher dose for oxcarbazepine)	Trigeminal neuralgia	Sedation, dizziness, ataxia
Tramadol	Start: 50 mg/day; Max: 400 mg/day	Painful neuropathy	Sedation, dizziness, constipation
Lamotrigine	Start: 25 mg/day, titrate slowly; Max: 400–600 mg/day	Trigeminal neuralgia, poststroke central pain	Sedation, tremor, rash
Opioids	Start: 5–10 mg/day, titrate; substitute long-acting opioids; Max: variable	PHN, PDN, postamputation pain	Sedation, dizziness, tolerance, drug abuse
Lidocaine medicated patch	5%	PHN, traumatic nerve injury	Allergic reaction
Capsaicin cream	0.075% and 8%	PHN, PDN, HIV	

Abbreviations: HIV, human immunodeficiency virus-related; PDN, painful diabetic neuropathy; PHN, postherpetic neuralgia; SNRIs, serotonin norepinephrine reuptake inhibitors.

The treatment effect is not always predictable, and patients with the same disease or symptom may respond differently to treatment. There is little evidence for specific symptoms to be treated with specific drugs [10]. Although sodium channel blockers, such as carbamazepine, are the drug of choice for treating paroxysmal pain in trigeminal neuralgia, there is little evidence for choosing sodium channel blockers for pain dominated by paroxysmal pain and antidepressants for burning, pricking, and ongoing pain. Based on current evidence, the European Federation of Neurological Societies (EFNS) has provided guidelines for the pharmacological treatment of neuropathic pain [10]. Table II presents a list of drugs for the treatment of neuropathic pain, with recommended doses for different conditions and major side effects.

Stimulation Therapy

There has been increasing interest in using electrical and magnetic neurostimulation techniques for treating neuropathic pain. Based on published guidelines [6], there is no documentation that peripheral nerve or nerve root stimulation has any effect in neuropathic pain. Spinal cord stimulation has been used for some neuropathic pain conditions. For so-called failed back surgery syndrome and complex regional pain syndrome type I, there is level B evidence (established as probably effective from at least one convincing Class 2 study or overwhelming evidence from Class 2 studies, i.e., other controlled trials) that spinal cord stimulation has an effect.

The effect of deep brain stimulation in central poststroke pain is still unclear, but there seems to be an effect in postamputation pain (level D evidence; expert opinion without critical appraisal). Motor cortex stimulation and transcranial magnetic stimulation are other options for the treatment of neuropathic pain. There is level C evidence (probably effective from at least two convincing Class 3 studies) that motor cortex stimulation is effective in patients with poststroke pain and in facial pains of neuropathic origin. Transcranial magnetic stimulation is a technique in which analgesia is obtained by noninvasive cortical stimulation. There is level B evidence that this technique provides slight pain relief in patients with central poststroke pain and certain other types of neuropathic pain [6]. While transcutaneous nerve stimulation and repetitive transcranial magnetic stimulations are practically harmless and without risk, spinal cord, deep brain, and motor cortex stimulation have adverse effects such as lead migration and infections, and some of these may be serious. Another disadvantage is the cost associated with the invasive procedures; therefore, in general, these techniques should only be used when other types of treatment have failed.

Conclusion

Before choosing a neuropathic pain treatment, clinicians need to consider the benefits and hazards of a particular treatment. There are no exact data that permit the presentation of a treatment algorithm for all types of neuropathic pain. In practice, treatments are often combined. In the future we will see more studies of combined treatments, which makes sense given the multiple mechanisms contributing to neuropathic pain in individual patients. However, side effects will be a limiting factor for any type of systemic therapy applied.

References

[1] Attal N, Cruccu G, Haanpaa M, Hansson P, Jensen TS, Nurmikko T. EFNS guidelines on pharmacological treatment of neuropathic pain: 2009 revision. Eur J Neurol 2010;13:1153–69.

[2] Backonja M, Wallace MS, Blonsky ER, Cutler BJ, Malan P, Jr., Rauck R, Tobias J. NGX-4010, a high-concentration capsaicin patch, for the treatment of postherpetic neuralgia: a randomised, double-blind study. Lancet Neurol 2008;7:1106–12.

[3] Baron R. Mechanisms of disease: neuropathic pain: a clinical perspective. Nat Clin Pract Neurol 2006;2:95–106.

[4] Besson JM. The neurobiology of pain. Lancet 1999;353:1610–5.

[5] Costigan M, Scholz J, Woolf CJ. Neuropathic pain: a maladaptive response of the nervous system to damage. Annu Rev Neurosci 2009;32:1–32.

[6] Cruccu G, Aziz TZ, Garcia-Larrea L Hansson P, Jensen TS, Lefaucheur JP, Simpson BA, Taylor RS. EFNS guidelines on neurostimulation therapy for neuropathic pain. Eur J Neurol 2007;14:952–70.

[7] Dworkin RH, O'Connor AB, Backonja M, Farrar JT, Finnerup NB, Jensen TS, Kalso EA, Loeser JD, Miaskowski C, Nurmikko TJ, et al. Pharmacologic management of neuropathic pain: evidence-based recommendations. Pain 2007;132:237–51.

[8] Dworkin RH, O'Connor AB, Audette J, Baron R, Gourlay GK, Haanpaa ML, Kent JL, Krane EJ, Lebel AA, Levy RM, et al. Recommendations for the pharmacological management of neuropathic pain: an overview and literature update. Mayo Clin Proc 2010;85:S3–14.

[9] Eisenberg E, McNicol E, Carr DB. Opioids for neuropathic pain. Cochrane Database Syst Rev 2006;3:CD006146.

[10] Finnerup NB, Otto M, McQuay HJ, Jensen TS, Sindrup SH. Algorithm for neuropathic pain treatment: an evidence-based proposal. Pain 2005;118:289–305.

[11] Finnerup NB, Jensen TS. Mechanisms of disease: mechanism-based classification of neuropathic pain: a critical analysis. Nat Clin Pract Neurol 2006;2:107–15.

[12] Finnerup NB, Sindrup SH, Jensen TS. An evidence based algorithm for the treatment of neuropathic pain. Med Gen Med 2007;9:36.

[13] Finnerup NB, Grydehoj J, Bing J, Johannesen IL, Biering-Sorensen F, Sindrup SH, Jensen TS. Levetiracetam in spinal cord injury pain: a randomized controlled trial. Spinal Cord 2009;47:861–7.

[14] Gilron I, Bailey JM, Tu D, Holden RR, Weaver DF, Houlden RL. Morphine, gabapentin, or their combination for neuropathic pain. N Engl J Med 2005;352:1324–34.

[15] Gilron I, Bailey JM, Tu D, Holden RR, Jackson AC, Houlden RL. Nortriptyline and gabapentin, alone and in combination for neuropathic pain: a double-blind, randomised controlled crossover trial. Lancet 2009;374:1252–61.

[16] Hansson PT, Dickenson AH. Pharmacological treatment of peripheral neuropathic pain conditions based on shared commonalities despite multiple etiologies. Pain 2005;113:251–4.

[17] Jensen TS, Gottrup H, Sindrup SH, Bach FW. The clinical picture of neuropathic pain. Eur Pharmacol 2001;429:1–11.

[18] Jensen TS, Baron R. Translation of symptoms and signs into mechanisms in neuropathic pain, Pain 2003;102:1–8.

[19] Jensen TS, Hansson P. Classification of neuropathic pain syndromes based on symptoms and signs. In: Cervero F, Jensen TS, editors. Pain. Handbook of clinical neurology, vol. 81. Amsterdam: Elsevier; 2006. p. 517–26.

[20] Kanai A, Segawa Y, Okamoto T, Koto M, Okamoto H. The analgesic effect of a metered-dose 8% lidocaine pump spray in posttraumatic peripheral neuropathy: a pilot study. Anesth Analg 2009;108:987–91.

[21] Merskey H, Bogduk N. Classification of chronic pain: descriptions of chronic pain syndromes and definitions of pain terms. Seattle: IASP Press; 1994.

[22] Nurmikko TJ, Serpell MG, Hoggart B, Toomey PJ, Morlion BJ, Haines D. Sativex successfully treats neuropathic pain characterised by allodynia: a randomised, double-blind, placebo-controlled clinical trial. Pain 2007;133:210–20.

[23] Otto M, Bach FW, Jensen TS, Brosen K, Sindrup SH. Escitalopram in painful polyneuropathy: a randomized, placebo-controlled, cross-over trial. Pain 2008;139:275–83.

[24] Ranoux D, Attal N, Morain F, Bouhassira D. Botulinum toxin type A induces direct analgesic effects in chronic neuropathic pain. Ann Neurol 2008;64:274–83.

[25] Rintala DH, Holmes SA, Courtade D, Fiess RN, Tastard LV, Loubser PG. Comparison of the effectiveness of amitriptyline and gabapentin on chronic neuropathic pain in persons with spinal cord injury. Arch Phys Med Rehabil 2007;88:1547–60.

[26] Rowbotham MC, Twilling L, Davies PS, Reisner L, Taylor K, Mohr D. Oral opioid therapy for chronic peripheral and central neuropathic pain. N Engl J Med 2003;348:1223–32.

[27] Saarto T, Wiffen PJ. Antidepressants for neuropathic pain. Cochrane Database Syst Rev 2007;CD005454.

[28] Shaibani A, Fares S, Selam JL, Arslanian A, Simpson J, Sen D, Bongardt S. Lacosamide in painful diabetic neuropathy: an 18-week double-blind placebo-controlled trial. J Pain 2009;10:818–28.

[29] Siddall PJ, Cousins MJ, Otte A, Griesing T, Chambers R, Murphy TK. Pregabalin in central neuropathic pain associated with spinal cord injury: a placebo-controlled trial. Neurology 2006;67:1792–800.

[30] Simpson DM, Brown S, Tobias J. Controlled trial of high-concentration capsaicin patch for treatment of painful HIV neuropathy. Neurology 2008;70:2305–13.

[31] Simpson DM, Schifitto G, Clifford DB, Murphy TK, Durso-De CE, Glue P, Whalen E, Emir B, Scott GN, Freeman R. Pregabalin for painful HIV neuropathy: a randomized, double-blind, placebo-controlled trial. Neurology 2010;74:413–20.

[32] Sindrup SH, Bach FW, Madsen C, Gram LF, Jensen TS. Venlafaxine versus imipramine in painful polyneuropathy: a randomized, controlled trial. Neurology 2003;60:1284–9.

[33] Sindrup SH, Otto M, Finnerup NB, Jensen TS. Antidepressants in the treatment of neuropathic pain. Basic Clin Pharmacol Toxicol 2005;96:399–409.

[34] Sindrup SH, Finnerup NB, Otto M, Jensen TS. Principles of pharmacological treatment. In: Cervero F, Jensen TS, editors. Pain. Handbook of clinical neurology, vol. 81. Amsterdam: Elsevier; 2006. p. 843–53.

[35] Thienel U, Neto W, Schwabe SK, Vijapurkar U. Topiramate in painful diabetic polyneuropathy: findings from three double-blind placebo-controlled trials. Acta Neurol Scand 2004;110:221–31.

[36] Tracey I, Mantyh PW. The cerebral signature for pain perception and its modulation. Neuron 2007;55:377–91.

[37] Treede RD, Jensen TS, Campbell JN, Cruccu G, Dostrovsky JO, Griffin JW, Hansson P, Hughes R, Nurmikko T, Serra J. Neuropathic pain: redefinition and a grading system for clinical and research purposes. Neurology 2008;70:1630–5.

[38] Vilholm OJ, Cold S, Rasmussen L, Sindrup SH. Effect of levetiracetam on the postmastectomy pain syndrome. Eur J Neurol 2008;15:851–7.

[39] Vinik AI, Tuchman M, Safirstein B, Corder C, Kirby L, Wilks K, Quessy S, Blum D, Grainger J, White J, Silver M. Lamotrigine for treatment of pain associated with diabetic neuropathy: results of two randomized, double-blind, placebo-controlled studies. Pain 2007;128:169–79.

[40] Vranken JH, Dijkgraaf MG, Kruis RM, van der Vegt MH, Hollmann MW, Heesen M. Pregabalin in patients with central neuropathic pain: a randomized, double-blind, placebo-controlled trial of a flexible-dose regimen. Pain 2007;136:150–7.

[41] Woolf CJ. Pain: moving from symptom control toward mechanism-specific pharmacologic management. Ann Int Med 2004;140:441–51.

[42] Wymer JP, Simpson J, Sen D, Bongardt S; Lacosamide SP742 Study Group. Efficacy and safety of lacosamide in diabetic neuropathic pain: an 18-week double-blind placebo-controlled trial of fixed-dose regimens. Clin J Pain 2009;25:376–85.

[43] Yuan RY, Sheu JJ, Yu JM, Chen WT, Tseng IJ, Chang HH, Hu CJ. Botulinum toxin for diabetic neuropathic pain: a randomized double-blind crossover trial. Neurology 2009;72:1473–8.

[44] Ziegler D, Hidvegi T, Gurieva I, Bongardt S, Freynhagen R, Sen D, Sommerville K. Efficacy and safety of lacosamide in painful diabetic neuropathy. Diabetes Care 2010;33:839–41.

Correspondence to: Professor Troels Staehelin Jensen, MD, DMSc, Danish Pain Research Center, Aarhus University Hospital, Norrebrogade 44, Building 1A, 8000 Aarhus C, Denmark. Email: tsjensen@ki.au.dk.

Part 13
Interventional Therapies for Acute and Chronic Pain

Interventional Therapies for Chronic Pain: Indications and Efficacy

James P. Rathmell, MD[a,b] and Mark Wallace, MD[c,d]

[a]Department of Anaesthesia, Harvard Medical School, and [b]Division of Pain Medicine, Massachusetts General Hospital, Boston, Massachusetts, USA; [c]Division of Pain Medicine, Department of Anesthesiology, University of California San Diego, and [d]UCSD Center for Pain Medicine, La Jolla, California, USA

Minimally Invasive Treatments for Spine-Related Pain

Interventional pain therapy refers to a group of targeted treatments used for specific spine disorders, ranging from epidural injection of steroids to percutaneous intradiskal techniques. Some have been rigorously tested in randomized controlled trials (RCTs), whereas others are in widespread use without critical evaluation. When these treatment techniques are used for the disorders they are most likely to benefit (Table I), they can be highly effective; however, when used haphazardly, they are unlikely to be helpful and, indeed, may cause harm.

Definitions

Low back pain, a nonspecific term, refers to pain centered over the lumbosacral junction. To be precise in our approach to diagnosis and treatment, we differentiate pain primarily over the axis of the spinal column from that which refers primarily to the leg (Fig. 1). Lumbar spinal pain is pain inferior to the tip of the 12th thoracic spinous process and superior to the tip of the first sacral spinous process. Sacral spinal pain is inferior to the first sacral spinous process and superior to the sacrococcygeal joint [47]. Lumbosacral spinal pain is pain in either or both regions and constitutes "low back pain." Other patients present with "sciatica," or pain predominantly localized in the leg. The proper term, however, is "radicular pain" because stimulation of the nerve roots or the dorsal root ganglion of a spinal nerve evokes the pain.

Pathophysiology

The basic functional unit of the spine comprises two adjacent vertebral bodies with two posterior facet joints, an intervertebral disk, and the surrounding ligamentous structures (Fig. 2). The intervertebral disk absorbs energy and distributes weight evenly from one spinal segment to the next while allowing movement of the protective bony elements [57]. Lifting, bending, twisting, or whole-body vibration can damage elements of the spine. With injury and aging, progressive degenerative changes appear in each element of the functional spinal unit, along with the onset of characteristic symptoms (Fig. 2). The earliest change in the lumbar facet joints is synovitis, which progresses to degradation of the articular surfaces, capsular laxity and subluxation, and finally, enlargement of the articular processes (facet hypertrophy). Progressive degeneration also occurs within the intervertebral disks, starting with loss of hydration of the nucleus pulposus, followed by the appearance of circumferential or radial tears within the annulus fibrosis (internal disk disruption).

Lumbosacral pain can arise from the facet joints or the annulus fibrosis [61]. With internal disruption of the annulus, some of the gelatinous central

Table I
Rational sequence for application of medical therapies in treating spinal pain,
along with the level of evidence* supporting each treatment

Pain Type	Initial Pain Therapy	Therapy for Persistent Pain
Acute radicular pain	A 7–10-day course of an oral analgesic (NSAID or acetaminophen, with or without an opioid analgesic) with a muscle relaxant, for those with superimposed muscle spasm (Level I) [21].	Between 2 and 6 weeks following onset of acute radicular pain, consider lumbar epidural steroid injection to speed resolution of radicular symptoms (Level II) [3].
Chronic radicular pain	TCAs (e.g., nortriptyline, desipramine) and newer SNRIs (e.g., venlafaxine, duloxetine) are effective in the treatment of neuropathic pain. Antiepileptic drugs (e.g., gabapentin, pregabalin) also treat neuropathic pain effectively (Level I) [30]. Chronic radicular pain may respond to treatment with chronic opioids, but neuropathic pain is less responsive to opioids than nociceptive pain (Level II) [5,20].	Consider evaluation for a trial of spinal cord stimulation (Level II) [19].
Acute lumbosacral pain	A 7–10-day course of an oral analgesic (NSAID or acetaminophen, with or without an opioid analgesic) with a muscle relaxant, for those with superimposed muscle spasm (Level I) [21].	Between 2 and 6 weeks after onset of chronic radicular pain, consider referral for physical therapy for stretching, strengthening, and aerobic exercise in conjunction with patient education (Level I) [22].
Chronic lumbosacral pain	Consider diagnostic medial branch blocks of the nerves to the facet joints. If there is >50% pain relief with the diagnostic blocks, consider radiofrequency treatment (Level II) [64].	Consider enrollment in a formal multidisciplinary pain program that incorporates medical management, behavioral therapy, and physical therapy (Level I) [36]. Consider cognitive-behavioral therapy (Level I) [68]. If there is no response to diagnostic facet blocks and MRI shows early degenerative disk disease affecting no more than two intervertebral disks, consider diagnostic provocative diskography (Level III) [15]. If diskography is concordant (pain is reproduced at anatomically abnormal levels and there is no pain at an adjacent anatomically normal level), consider IDET at the symptomatic level(s) (Level II) [1].

Abbreviations: IDET, intradiskal electrothermal therapy; MRI, magnetic resonance imaging; NSAID, nonsteroidal anti-inflammatory drug; SNRI, serotonin norepinephrine reuptake inhibitor; TCA, tricyclic antidepressant.
* Level of evidence is based on the Oxford Evidence Based Medicine Levels for Treatment: Level I, high-quality randomized controlled trials (RCTs) or systematic reviews of RCTs; Level II, low-quality RCTs, cohort studies or systematic reviews of cohort studies; Level III, case-control studies or systematic reviews of case-control studies; Level IV, case series; Level V, expert opinion.

nucleus pulposus can extend beyond the disk margin, as a disk herniation (herniated nucleus pulposus; HNP). When HNP extends to the region adjacent to the spinal nerve, it incites an intense inflammatory reaction [52]. Patients with HNP typically present with acute radicular pain. Hypertrophy of the facet joints and calcification of the ligamentous structures can reduce the size of the intervertebral foramina and/or central spinal canal (spinal stenosis), with onset of radicular pain and/or neurogenic claudication.

Patients with prior lumbar surgery and either recurrent or persistent low back pain, often termed "failed back surgery syndrome," need mention [53]. It is essential to know the type of surgery, the indications for and results of the surgery, and the time course and characteristics of any changes in the pattern and severity of postoperative pain. Recurrent pain or progressive symptoms signal the need for further diagnostic evaluation.

Initial Evaluation and Treatment

In the initial evaluation of a patient with low back pain, several features in the history—"red-flag" conditions—require prompt investigation, including new onset or worsening of back pain after trauma, infection, or previous cancer. Patients with progressive neurological deficits (typically worsening numbness or weakness) or bowel or bladder dysfunction also warrant immediate radiologic imaging to rule out a compressive lesion [40].

If no red-flag condition is apparent, diagnosis and treatment rely on location and duration of symptoms, and on determination of whether the pain is acute or chronic and primarily radicular or lumbosacral in nature. Acute low back pain is pain that is present for less than 3 months, while chronic low back pain is defined as being present for a longer period of time [47].

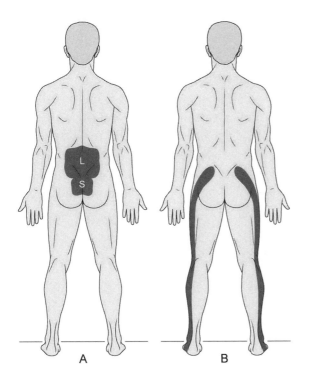

Fig. 1. The definition of low back pain. (A) "Low back pain" is more precisely termed "lumbosacral spinal pain," which encompasses both lumbar spinal pain (L) and sacral spinal pain (S). (B) Radicular pain describes pain that is referred to the lower extremity and is caused by stimulation of a spinal nerve.

Acute Radicular Pain

Herniated nucleus pulposus typically causes acute radicular pain, with or without radiculopathy (signs of dysfunction including numbness, weakness, or loss of deep tendon reflexes referable to a specific spinal nerve). In elderly patients and those with extensive lumbar spondylosis, acute radicular symptoms caused by narrowing of one or more intervertebral foramina can occur [16]. Initial treatment is symptomatic, and symptoms resolve without specific treatment in about 90% of patients [59]. For those with persistent pain after HNP, lumbar diskectomy may be indicated. A controlled trial of surgical versus nonoperative treatment showed significant improvement in both groups over 2 years, but it was inconclusive about the superiority of either approach [72].

Chronic Radicular Pain

Persistent leg pain in the distribution of a spinal nerve may occur in patients with a disk herniation with or without subsequent surgery. In those with persistent pain, a search for a reversible cause of nerve root compression is warranted. In many individuals, scarring around the nerve root at the operative site can be seen with magnetic resonance imaging (MRI) [7], and electrodiagnostic studies show a pattern suggesting

chronic radiculopathy [73]. This patient group has characteristics similar to those with other nerve injuries, and initial management should consist of pharmacological treatment for neuropathic pain [18].

Acute Lumbosacral Pain

Most patients presenting with acute onset of lumbosacral pain without radicular symptoms have no obvious abnormal physical findings [29], and radiologic imaging is unlikely to be helpful [39]. Traumatic sprain of the muscles and ligaments of the lumbar spine or the zygapophyseal joints, and early internal disk disruption, are significant causes of acute lumbosacral pain. Similar to patients with acute radicular pain, this group is best managed symptomatically.

Chronic Lumbosacral Pain

There are many causes of chronic lumbosacral pain, and the anatomical cause cannot be identified with certainty in up to 90% of cases [40]. The structures most

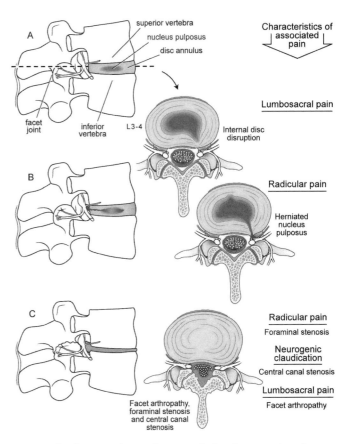

Fig. 2. The functional spinal unit and the degenerative changes that lead to lumbosacral and radicular pain. (A) The normal functional spinal unit. (B) The degenerative changes leading to lumbosacral pain (disk disruption, facet joint arthropathy) and radicular pain (herniated nucleus pulposus). (C) The degenerative changes of lumbar spondylosis leading to lumbosacral (facet joint) pain, radicular (foraminal stenosis) pain, and neurogenic claudication (central canal stenosis).

commonly implicated include the sacroiliac joint, lumbar facets, and lumbar intervertebral disks. In chronic low back pain, the incidence of internal disk disruption has been estimated at 39% (range 29–49%), that of facet joint pain at 15% (10–20%), and that of sacroiliac joint pain at 15% (7–23%) [10]. The gold standard for diagnosing sacroiliac and facet joint pain is injection of local anesthetic at the site [24]. However, the use of uncontrolled local anesthetic blocks for diagnostic purposes is plagued by high placebo response [9]. For patients achieving significant short-term pain relief with diagnostic blocks, radiofrequency treatment offers a simple, minimally invasive intervention that can provide pain reduction for 3–6 months in those with facet-related pain. Degenerating intervertebral disks are also a source of chronic axial back pain [10]. Diagnostic provocative diskography may identify symptomatic disks prior to management with therapies such as intradiskal electrothermal therapy (IDET) or surgical fusion.

Medical Therapies

Numerous pharmacological agents and minimally invasive treatments are beneficial in treating specific types of pain. There is no consensus on how these therapies should be sequenced in treating persistent low back pain; the general approach to using each therapy is shown in Table I.

Treatments of neuropathic pain such as chronic lumbar radicular pain are extrapolated from RCTS examining two common forms of neuropathic pain: painful diabetic neuropathy and postherpetic neuralgia [30,31]. Tricyclic antidepressants (TCAs), such as nortriptyline or desipramine, and newer selective norepinephrine reuptake inhibitors (SNRIs), such as venlafaxine or duloxetine, are effective in the treatment of neuropathic pain [30,31]. Antiepileptic drugs, such as gabapentin or pregabalin, also can effectively treat neuropathic pain [30,31]. Decisions regarding pharmacological treatment of neuropathic pain may be based on an analysis of the number needed-to-treat (NNT); the NNT (with 95% confidence intervals) is 3.1 for TCA (CI 2.7–3.7); 6.8 for SNRIs (CI 3.4–4.41); and 4.7 for gabapentin/pregabalin (CI 4.0–5.6) [31].

Interventional Therapies

Epidural Injection of Steroids

Numerous RCTs have examined the efficacy of epidural corticosteroid injection for acute radicular pain. Such injections into the epidural space are thought to combat the inflammatory response that is associated with acute disk herniation [46]. In acute radicular pain with HNP, the evidence [2,46,74] shows that epidural steroids reduce the severity and duration of leg pain if given between 3 and 6 weeks after onset. Adverse effects, such as injection site pain and transient worsening of radicular pain, occur in less than 1% of treated subjects [2]. Beyond 3 months from treatment, there appear to be no long-term reductions in pain or improvements in function [2]. This therapy has never proven helpful for lumbosacral pain without radicular symptoms.

Facet Blocks and Radiofrequency Treatment

Pain from the lumbar facet joints affects up to 15% of patients with chronic low back pain [26]. Patients are identified based on typical patterns of referred pain, with maximal pain located directly over the facet joints and patient report of pain on palpation over the facets; radiographic findings are variable, but some degree of facet arthropathy is typically present [25]. A few low-quality studies suggest that the intra-articular injection of anesthetics and corticosteroids leads to intermediate-term pain relief (for 1–3 months) in patients with an active inflammatory process [26]. Radiofrequency denervation delivers energy through an insulated, small-diameter needle positioned adjacent to the sensory nerve to the facet joint, creating a small area of tissue coagulation that denervates the facet joint. Two systematic reviews concluded that there is moderate evidence that radiofrequency denervation provides better pain relief than sham intervention [35,64]. The quality of the six available RCTs was deemed adequate, but they were conducted in a technically heterogeneous manner (with varying inclusion criteria and differing treatment protocols), thus limiting analysis of their findings. Approximately 50% of patients treated report at least 50% pain reduction. Pain typically returns within 6 to 12 months after treatment, and denervation can be repeated without lessening of efficacy [60]. Adverse events are uncommon; in 1% of treated patients, pain occurred at the treatment site that lasted 2 weeks or less [41].

Intradiskal Electrothermal Therapy

The intervertebral disk is thought to be involved in 29–49% of patients with chronic low back pain [15]. Provocative diskography is a controversial diagnostic test that employs a series of needles placed in the central portion of the intervertebral disks; a small volume of saline or radiographic contrast is then introduced to try to reproduce the patient's typical pain, to determine the offending disk. This test has been used to select patients for surgical fusion, but its ability to predict outcome is questionable [15].

Diskography has also been used to select patients for a procedure called IDET, which is used to treat diskogenic chronic lumbosacral pain. IDET employs a steerable thermal resistance wire placed along the posterior annulus fibrosus. Thermal energy is applied to destroy penetrating nociceptive fibers and to change the cross-linking of glucosaminoglycans, thereby stiffening the intervertebral disk [33]. Clinical study results are mixed; one high-quality RCT showed that 40% of patients achieved greater than 50% pain relief, while 50% of the patients had no appreciable benefit (NNT to achieve 75% relief of pain = 5) [55]. A second high-quality RCT showed no effect [32]. When all studies are combined, a 50% reduction in pain is suggested, as is improvement in sitting and standing tolerance in 40–50% of patients receiving IDET at a single level, with concordant diskography and well-preserved disk height [1]. Despite ongoing reports of successful use of IDET [4], recent evidence-based guidelines for nonsurgical low back pain interventions found little evidence for use of IDET [19].

Percutaneous Diskectomy: Plasma Disk Decompression and Other Emerging Techniques

The development of minimally invasive, percutaneous techniques to treat lumbar disk herniations and persistent radicular pain has had a long history, starting with chemonucleolysis using chymopapain and evolving through a series of techniques, from laser-assisted disk decompression through radiofrequency-based techniques such as plasma disk decompression (nucleoplasty). Many of these techniques have undergone extensive clinical testing and failed to show efficacy comparable to open diskectomy using an operative microscope. Nonetheless, there is ongoing interest in further developing effective percutaneous interventions to treat small symptomatic disk herniations. Our group has recently published long-term outcomes of an RCT comparing nucleoplasty to transforaminal injection of steroid in a cohort of patients with persistent radicular pain associated with contained disk herniations, demonstrating durable reduction in pain and improvements in functional status 2 years after treatment [34].

Intrathecal Drug Delivery for Chronic Pain

Introduction and Patient Selection

Before considering implantable therapy, the patient should have progressed through the pain treatment continuum or the World Health Organization ladder. This process assures that the patient has been given a fair trial of more conservative therapies before embarking on invasive pain treatment. One area of controversy is understanding when a spinal cord stimulator should be utilized versus a spinal drug delivery system. Spinal cord stimulation is considered a more conservative therapy, because no drugs are involved and there is less use of the health care system for management [66]. As discussed below, with newer spinal agents for neuropathic pain, the decision to use spinal cord stimulation or spinal drug delivery should be based more on pain distribution. With advancements in the technology of spinal cord stimulation, this view may become obsolete. The current recommendation is spinal cord stimulation for axial pain with extremity pain and spinal drug delivery for axial or trunk pain, or for pain unresponsive to spinal cord stimulation.

Nociceptive pain is mediated by an intact and functioning nervous system. Neuropathic pain is elicited by a damaged peripheral or central nervous system. Historically, it was thought that nociceptive pain is more responsive to intrathecal drug therapy, whereas neuropathic pain is more responsive to spinal cord stimulation. However, with the development of nonopioid drugs, this consensus may no longer hold. Preclinical studies have demonstrated that the spinal delivery of agents such as clonidine and sodium or calcium channel blockers are more effective than opioids in treating neuropathic pain [17]. With these better drugs and better technology for spinal cord stimulation, definite lines between spinal cord stimulation and spinal drug delivery are obscured [66].

Another area of controversy is the absence or presence of a known pain generator. Should patients without an identified pain generator be managed with implantable devices? An example is the low back pain patient with normal imaging studies, no physical findings, and negative diagnostic injections. These patients present a dilemma because undiagnosed psychological disorders may be overshadowing the problem. Objective evidence of pathology is more important for nonmalignant pain than for malignant pain because of psychological issues surrounding pain of unknown etiology. It is not to say that patients without objective evidence of pathology should be excluded; rather, they should be evaluated closely for psychological issues (discussed below). If they are declared psychologically stable for implantation, then one should proceed, even in the absence of objective pathology [71].

Historically, it has been a requirement to demonstrate some response to systemically administered opioids. The decision to proceed with spinal drug delivery was usually made if patients experienced a partial, unacceptable response or unacceptable side effects in spite of adequate pain relief. The absence of any appreciable pain relief at reasonable doses of an opioid in a nociceptive pain patient probably precludes the use of intraspinal opioids. However, this criterion is controversial for neuropathic pain. It has been demonstrated in the Chung model of neuropathic pain that intrathecal opioids are ineffective in relieving pain whereas systemic opioids are effective [44]. This study is an example of a situation in which a partial response of a systemically administered opioid in no way predicts the effect of the intrathecal opioid. This situation explains why some patients still require systemic opioids in addition to the spinal nonopioid agents. However, most patients who demonstrate some response to systemic opioids will respond to spinal opioids. A general rule of thumb is that as the injury gets closer to the central nervous system, pharmacological therapy will become less and less effective, whether opioids or nonopioids are used. Demonstration of opioid responsiveness is a strict criterion that will lead to fewer failures. In severe cases, neuropathic pain often cannot be effectively managed with a nonopioid alone. A nonopioid is usually added to an opioid to enhance analgesia.

Psychological Screening

Most experts will agree that psychological screening is mandatory prior to embarking on chronic intraspinal drug therapy. In spite of this consensus, there are few reports on the efficacy of psychological screening in predicting outcome. This lack of research probably reflects the research challenges in this area and the difficulties in predicting long-term success based on psychological screening. However, there are some reports in the literature supporting psychological screening, and in general these studies find that patients with a psychological profile deemed appropriate for implantable therapy have better outcomes than those deemed inappropriate [43]. However, some early reports have questioned the utility of a psychological evaluation in predicting outcome. Several studies state that depression, hysteria, and hypochondriasis are common in pain patients and do not constitute a contraindication to implants [13,14,62]. Burton went as far as to question the need for psychological evaluation per se, while admitting that psychological testing can identify significant problems that may interfere with long-term success [13]. Others have agreed with this point of view [63]; however, specialists with the most experience with implantables for pain relief hold strong to the belief that psychological screening is crucial to the long-term success of implantables for chronic pain management [49].

Most of the literature on psychological screening involves spinal cord stimulation; however, this information can be applied to chronic intraspinal drug delivery. The majority of studies in this area use the Minnesota Multiphasic Personality Inventory (MMPI) as a predictor of outcome with spinal implantables. North et al. [50] reported on the predictive value of psychological testing on the outcome of spinal cord stimulation. He concluded that low scores on two psychological traits—anxiety and problems with authority (as measured by the Derogatis Affects Balance Scale and the Wiggins scales of the MMPI, respectively)—predicted pain relief following a spinal cord stimulation trial but not 3 months after permanent electrode implantation. These authors pointed out that their sample could have been biased, but they still supported psychological screening.

Burchiel et al. [12] studied 40 patients with chronic low back and leg pain who underwent spinal cord stimulation. They used the MMPI, the visual analogue pain rating scale (VAS), the McGill Pain Questionnaire (MPQ), the Oswestry Disability Questionnaire, the Beck Depression Inventory, and the Sickness Impact Profile to predict treatment outcome. Regression analysis revealed that increased patient age and scores on subscale D of the MMPI correlated with poor outcomes. Higher scores on the evaluative subscale of the MPQ correlated with an improved outcome. From this study, the authors developed the following equation, which correctly predicted success or failure at 3 months in 88% of their patients: % delta VAS = 112.57 − 1.98 (D) − 1.68 (Age) + 35.54 (MPQe).

Brandwin and Kewman [11] found that treatment-resistant patients had relatively lower hysteria and hypochondriasis scores than did successful patients. They also concluded that higher elevations of the depression scale were associated with treatment failure. Daniel et al. [27] used a six-point rating scale based on the results of a psychological interview, a pain questionnaire, a health index, the Cornell Medical Index, the MPQ, the Beck Depression Inventory, and the MMPI. They reported a 76.5% accuracy in the psychologists predicting outcome based on this scale.

In a focus article, Nelson et al. [48] summarized certain psychological-behavioral features that would exclude a patient from further consideration for implantable therapy. These include the following:

Active psychosis. Psychotic patients can have very real pain, but their perception of the pain is often distorted. If they are stabilized on neuroleptics, they may be reconsidered for implantation but must be carefully monitored.

Active suicidality. Stabilization of the suicidal thoughts and associated mood disturbances is necessary before further consideration.

Active homicidality. It is difficult to stabilize these individuals, and they are often too unstable to engage in any treatment of this sort.

Major uncontrolled depression or other mood disorders. Patients with severe depression may experience increases in pain. If the depression is treated, then pain may decrease significantly enough to eliminate the need for invasive therapy.

Somatization disorder or other somatoform disorders. These patients are at risk of developing other symptoms in response to the implant. This exclusionary criterion should be used with caution because many chronic pain patients have vague pain complaints with no identifiable etiology.

Alcohol or drug dependency. Patients with major alcohol or drug problems who demonstrate a minimum of 3 months of appropriate control of substance use may be reconsidered.

Compensation or litigation resolution. Although treatment obstacles may occur if a patient has a monetary incentive to remain disabled by pain, most pain experts agree that such patients should be evaluated on a case-by-case basis for implantable therapy.

Lack of appropriate social support. This is not an absolute exclusionary criterion, but it should be considered because the pain treatment team cannot assume all responsibility for the patient's needs.

Neurobehavioral cognitive deficits. Severe cognitive impairments may interfere with the patient's reasoning and judgment, making it difficult for him or her to assume the shared responsibility required for implantable therapy.

In summary, psychological testing serves as a screening tool to identify the appropriateness of invasive therapy for the management of chronic pain. Using the exclusionary criteria of Nelson et al. [48], the psychological evaluation should focus on identifying these problems that may interfere with a successful outcome. As our medical judgment on the treatment of chronic pain is not infallible, neither is psychological screening. However, when the two are used together, better outcomes are more likely.

Screening Trials

Although most clinicians recommend a screening trial prior to pump placement, a screening protocol that accurately predicts a successful outcome has not been established [42,45,69]. In general, screening trials can be divided into the following: (1) single injection, (2) multiple injections, and (3) continuous infusion. There are no studies supporting one over the other, and clinicians should use their own judgment to decide which technique best suits their practice. It is recommended that the initial screening be done as an inpatient in a monitored setting. After 24 hours of observation, patients may have the drug continuously infused in the comfort of their own home. A retrospective review of 429 physicians found that 33.7% used a single intrathecal injection technique, 18.3% used a multiple injection with blinded placebo technique, and 35.3% used a continuous epidural infusion technique [54]. Currently, the most common technique appears to be a continuous intrathecal infusion [51].

The single injection technique involves a single administration of drug intrathecally or epidurally. The morphine dose is usually 0.5–1.0 mg intrathecally or 5–10 mg epidurally. An intrathecal or epidural equivalent of the patient's daily systemic dose may also be used. The single injection technique has the advantages of low cost, low risks, and ease of use. In addition, this technique probably overestimates side effects, so if no adverse effects arise, it is likely that the drug will be tolerated over the long term and at higher doses. Disadvantages are lack of correlation with a continuous infusion and higher placebo response.

With the multiple injection technique, the patient is administered a series of injections, either intrathecally or epidurally. Morphine doses are similar to those used for the single injection technique. Advantages of this technique are that the patients may receive a placebo injection for comparison with actual drug administration. A disadvantage is the lack of correlation with a continuous infusion.

A continuous infusion may be administered intrathecally or epidurally through a temporary catheter connected to an external pump [6,56]. The response to therapy can be determined over days to weeks. The initial morphine dose is 20 µg/hour intrathecally or 200 µg/hour epidurally, or the equivalent to the patient's daily systemic dose. The dose may be increased every 12–48 hours until pain relief or unacceptable side effects are reached. The advantage of this method is that it more closely mimics the implantable system. In addition, response to therapy can be more accurately assessed in the patient's own environment, during normal daily activities. The single injection and multiple injections are performed in the clinic or hospital setting, making it difficult to accurately assess the patient's response.

When performing the screening infusion trial, one would like to mimic long-term delivery as closely as possible. Chronic daily infusion rates may range from as low as 0.1 mL/day (with a SynchroMed pump) to 1.5 mL/day (with constant flow rate pumps). The lower limit of commonly used infusion pumps is 0.1 mL/hour, which equals 2.4 mL/day. It is unclear if there is much difference in analgesic outcome with the same dose delivered at 0.1 mL/day versus 2.4 mL/day. However, preclinical pharmacokinetic studies have demonstrated that drug spread through the cerebrospinal fluid is volume-dependent. Therefore, a larger volume may result in a higher dermatomal spread of the drug, which may affect analgesia. This finding explains why some patients report excellent analgesia during the screening trial when higher volumes are infused, only to find this pain relief disappear when the infusion pump is implanted and the same dose is infused at a lower volume. The best method to mimic chronic infusion therapy is with a microinfusion pump with a lower volume of 20 µL/hour. However, these infusion pumps are expensive, which limits their use.

Drug Selection for Chronic Intrathecal Therapy

Much uncertainty clouds the decision-making process surrounding drug selection and dosing for chronic spinal drug delivery. According to an Internet survey consisting of 413 physicians who represented management of 13,342 patients, the responding physicians chose morphine most often, but they selected many other drugs without clear indications. There was evidence of wide variations in clinical practice among physicians who use this modality [38]. An interdisciplinary panel with extensive clinical experience in intraspinal infusion therapy evaluated the results of the Internet survey, the systematic reviews of the literature, and their own clinical experience. This panel proposed a scheme for the selection of drugs and doses for intraspinal therapy [8]. They developed a hierarchy of therapeutic strategies that can be used during the screening process. Since the first polyanalgesic consensus meeting, the guidelines have been updated twice, in 2003 and 2007 [28,37].

To date, only two agents have U.S. Food and Drug Administration (FDA) approval for chronic spinal drug delivery to treat pain: morphine and ziconotide. Of the currently available drugs used for chronic spinal drug delivery, only ziconotide has been subjected to rigorous RCTs. The positive results of these trials led to FDA approval in 2004 [58,67,70]. Only one RCT has compared intraspinal drug delivery with conventional medical management in cancer pain. The investigators randomized 202 cancer patients to receive intrathecal drug delivery or comprehensive medical management. More patients receiving intrathecal therapy achieved success with significantly lower toxicity scores [65].

Many complicating factors should be weighed when determining the upper daily dose limit, or concentration. If the choice is restricted to commercially available drugs, there are limitations on drug concentrations. If patients require higher doses, there will be frequent refills. The commercially available concentrations include: morphine, 50 mg/mL; ziconotide, 100 µg/mL; hydromorphone, 10 mg/mL; fentanyl and sufentanil, 50 µg/mL; meperidine, 100 mg/mL; bupivacaine, 7.5 mg/mL; clonidine, 500 µg/mL; and baclofen, 2000 µg/mL. The upper dose limit will depend on the availability of drug compounding. The goal is to try and keep the refill intervals between 1 and 3 months. However, there is growing concern over the development of catheter tip inflammatory masses [23]. It has been suggested that the risk of granuloma formation is dependent upon the concentration of the drug delivered [75]. The exact drug concentration that will predispose to granuloma formation is unknown; however, it is recommended that the lowest concentration possible be used.

With the development of the patient hand-held activator for bolus dosing, guidelines for drug selection and dosing may change drastically. However, it is too early to determine the impact of this technology on the selection process.

Intrathecal drug delivery is technically feasible, even for the long-term treatment of noncancer pain. However, patient selection remains empirical, and there are no long-term controlled studies to guide the overall placement of this therapy within the pain treatment armamentarium. Until more data emerge, this therapy will be reserved for that small group of patients whose pain is severe, limiting, and unable to be controlled with more conservative measures.

References

[1] Appleby D, Andersson G, Totta M. Meta-analysis of the efficacy and safety of intradiscal electrothermal therapy (IDET). Pain Med 2006;7:308–16.

[2] Arden NK, Price C, Reading I, Stubbing J, Hazelgrove J, Dunne C, Michel M, Rogers P, Cooper C. A multicentre randomized controlled trial of epidural corticosteroid injections for sciatica: the WEST study. Rheumatology (Oxford) 2005;44:1399–406.

[3] Armon C, Argoff CE, Samuels J, Backonja MM. Assessment: use of epidural steroid injections to treat radicular lumbosacral pain: report of the Therapeutics and Technology Assessment Subcommittee of the American Academy of Neurology. Neurology 2007;68:723–9.

[4] Assietti R, Morosi M, Block JE. Intradiscal electrothermal therapy for symptomatic internal disc disruption: 24-month results and predictors of clinical success. J Neurosurg Spine;12:320–6.

[5] Ballantyne JC, Mao J. Opioid therapy for chronic pain. N Engl J Med 2003;349:1943–53.

[6] Bedder MD. The anesthesiologist's role in neuroaugmentative pain control techniques: spinal cord stimulation and neuraxial narcotics. Prog Anesthesiol 1990;4:226–36.

[7] BenDebba M, Augustus van Alphen H, Long DM. Association between peridural scar and activity-related pain after lumbar discectomy. Neurol Res 1999;21(Suppl 1):S37–42.

[8] Bennett G, Burchiel K, Buchser E, Classen A, Deer T, Du Pen S, Ferrante FM, Hassenbusch SJ, Lou L, Maeyaert J, et al. Clinical guidelines for intraspinal infusion: report of an expert panel. J Pain Symptom Manage 2000;20:S37–S43.

[9] Bogduk N. Diagnostic blocks: a truth serum for malingering. Clin J Pain 2004;20:409–14.

[10] Bogduk N. Role of anesthesiologic blockade in headache management. Curr Pain Headache Rep 2004;8:399–403.

[11] Brandwin MA, Kewman DG. MMPI indicators of treatment response to spinal epidural stimulation in patients with chronic pain and patients with movement disorders. Psychol Rep 1982;51:1059–64.

[12] Burchiel K. Prognostic factors of spinal cord stimulation for chronic back and leg pain. Neurosurgery 1995;36:1101–11.

[13] Burton C. Dorsal column stimulation: optimization of application. Surg Neurol 1975;4:171–6.

[14] Burton C. Session on spinal cord stimulation: safety and clinical efficacy. Neurosurgery 1977;1:214–5.

[15] Carragee EJ, Lincoln T, Parmar VS, Alamin T. A gold standard evaluation of the "discogenic pain" diagnosis as determined by provocative discography. Spine (Phila Pa 1976) 2006;31:2115–23.

[16] Chad DA. Lumbar spinal stenosis. Neurol Clin 2007;25:407–18.

[17] Chaplan S, Pogrel J, Yaksh T. Pharmacology of tactile allodynia in the streptozotocin diabetic rat. J Pharmacol Exp Ther 1994;269:1117–23.

[18] Chen H, Lamer TJ, Rho RH, Marshall KA, Sitzman BT, Ghazi SM, Brewer RP. Contemporary management of neuropathic pain for the primary care physician. Mayo Clin Proc 2004;79:1533–45.

[19] Chou R, Atlas SJ, Stanos SP, Rosenquist RW. Nonsurgical interventional therapies for low back pain: a review of the evidence for an American Pain Society clinical practice guideline. Spine (Phila Pa 1976) 2009;34:1078–93.

[20] Chou R, Fanciullo GJ, Fine PG, Miaskowski C, Passik SD, Portenoy RK. Opioids for chronic noncancer pain: prediction and identification of aberrant drug-related behaviors: a review of the evidence for an American Pain Society and American Academy of Pain Medicine clinical practice guideline. J Pain 2009;10:131–46.

[21] Chou R, Huffman LH. Medications for acute and chronic low back pain: a review of the evidence for an American Pain Society/American College of Physicians clinical practice guideline. Ann Intern Med 2007;147:505–14.

[22] Chou R, Qaseem A, Snow V, Casey D, Cross JT Jr, Shekelle P, Owens DK. Diagnosis and treatment of low back pain: a joint clinical practice guideline from the American College of Physicians and the American Pain Society. Ann Intern Med 2007;147:478–91.

[23] Coffey RJ, Burchiel K. Inflammatory mass lesions associated with intrathecal drug infusion catheters: Report and observations on 41 patients. Neurosurgery 2002;50:78–87.

[24] Cohen SP. Sacroiliac joint pain: a comprehensive review of anatomy, diagnosis, and treatment. Anesth Analg 2005;101:1440–53.

[25] Cohen SP, Hurley RW, Christo PJ, Winkley J, Mohiuddin MM, Stojanovic MP. Clinical predictors of success and failure for lumbar facet radiofrequency denervation. Clin J Pain 2007;23:45–52.

[26] Cohen SP, Raja SN. Pathogenesis, diagnosis, and treatment of lumbar zygapophysial (facet) joint pain. Anesthesiology 2007;106:591–614.

[27] Daniel MS, Long C, Hutcherson WL, Hunter S. Psychological factors and outcome of electrode implantation for chronic pain. Neurosurgery 1985;17:773–7.

[28] Deer T, Krames ES, Hassenbusch SJ, et al. Polyanalgesic consensus conference 2007: Recommendations for the management of pain by intrathecal drug delivery: Report of an interdisciplinary expert panel. Neuromodulation 2007;10:300–28.

[29] Deyo RA, Weinstein JN. Low back pain. N Engl J Med 2001;344:363–70.

[30] Dworkin RH, O'Connor AB, Backonja M, Farrar JT, Finnerup NB, Jensen TS, Kalso EA, Loeser JD, Miaskowski C, Nurmikko TJ, et al. Pharmacologic management of neuropathic pain: evidence-based recommendations. Pain 2007;132:237–51.

[31] Finnerup NB, Otto M, McQuay HJ, Jensen TS, Sindrup SH. Algorithm for neuropathic pain treatment: an evidence based proposal. Pain 2005;118:289–305.

[32] Freeman BJ, Fraser RD, Cain CM, Hall DJ, Chapple DC. A randomized, double-blind, controlled trial: intradiscal electrothermal therapy versus placebo for the treatment of chronic discogenic low back pain. Spine (Phila Pa 1976) 2005;30:2369–77; discussion 2378.

[33] Freeman BJ, Walters RM, Moore RJ, Fraser RD. Does intradiscal electrothermal therapy denervate and repair experimentally induced posterolateral annular tears in an animal model? Spine (Phila Pa 1976) 2003;28:2602–8.

[34] Gerszten PC, Smuck M, Rathmell JP, Simopoulos TT, Bhagia SM, Mocek CK, Crabtree T, Bloch DA. Plasma disc decompression compared with fluoroscopy-guided transforaminal epidural steroid injections for symptomatic contained lumbar disc herniation: a prospective, randomized, controlled trial. J Neurosurg Spine 2010;12:357–71.

[35] Geurts JW, van Wijk RM, Stolker RJ, Groen GJ. Efficacy of radiofrequency procedures for the treatment of spinal pain: a systematic review of randomized clinical trials. Reg Anesth Pain Med 2001;26:394–400.

[36] Guzman J, Esmail R, Karjalainen K, Malmivaara A, Irvin E, Bombardier C. Multidisciplinary rehabilitation for chronic low back pain: systematic review. BMJ 2001;322:1511–16.

[37] Hassenbusch SJ, Portenoy RK, Cousins M, Buchser E, Deer TR, Du Pen SL, Eisenach J, Follett KA, Hildebrand KR, Krames ES, et al. Polyanalgesic Consensus Conference 2003: An update on the management of pain by intraspinal drug delivery: report of an expert panel. J Pain Symptom Manage 2004;27:540–63.

[38] Hassenbusch SJ, Portenoy RK. Current practices in intraspinal therapy: a survey of clinical trends and decision making. J Pain Symptom Manage 2000;20:S4–S11.

[39] Jarvik JG, Deyo RA. Diagnostic evaluation of low back pain with emphasis on imaging. Ann Intern Med 2002;137:586–97.

[40] Koes BW, van Tulder MW, Thomas S. Diagnosis and treatment of low back pain. BMJ 2006;332:1430–4.

[41] Kornick C, Kramarich SS, Lamer TJ, Todd Sitzman B. Complications of lumbar facet radiofrequency denervation. Spine (Phila Pa 1976) 2004;29:1352–4.

[42] Krames ES. Intrathecal infusional therapies for intractable pain: patient management guidelines. J Pain Symptom Manage 1993;8:36–46.

[43] Kupers RC, Van den Oever R. Spinal cord stimulation in Belgium: a nation-wide survey on incidence, indications and therapeutic efficacy by the health insurer. Pain 1994;56:211–6.

[44] Lee YW, Chaplan SR, Yaksh TL. Systemic and supraspinal, but not spinal, opiates suppress allodynia in a rat neuropathic pain model. Neurosci Lett 1995;199:111–4.

[45] Maniker AH, Krieger AJ, Adler RJ. Epidural trial in implantation of intrathecal morphine infusion pumps. N Engl J Med 1991;88:780–97.

[46] McLain RF, Kapural L, Mekhail NA. Epidural steroid therapy for back and leg pain: mechanisms of action and efficacy. Spine J 2005;5:191–201.

[47] Merskey H, Bogduk N, editors. Classification of chronic pain: descriptions of chronic pain syndromes and definitions of pain terms, 3rd ed. Seattle: IASP Press; 1994.

[48] Nelson DV, Kennington M, Novy DM, Squitieri P. Psychological selection criteria for implantable spinal cord stimulators. Pain Forum 1996;5:93–103.

[49] North RA, Kidd DH, Zahurak M, James CS, Long DM. Spinal cord stimulation for chronic intractable pain: experience over two decades. Neurosurgery 1991;32:384–95.

[50] North RB, Kidd DH. Prognostic value of psychological testing in patients undergoing spinal cord stimulation: a prospective study. Neurosurgery 1996;39:301–11.

[51] Oakley J, Staats P. The use of implanted drug delivery systems. In: Raj PP, editor. The practical management of pain, vol. II. St Louis: Mosby; 2000. p. 768–78.

[52] Olmarker K. Radicular pain: recent pathophysiologic concepts and therapeutic implications. Schmerz 2001;15:425–9.

[53] Onesti ST. Failed back syndrome. Neurologist 2004;10:259–64.

[54] Paice JA, Penn RD, Shott S. Intraspinal morphine for chronic pain: a retrospective, multicenter study. J Pain Symptom Manage 1996;11:71–80.

[55] Pauza KJ, Howell S, Dreyfuss P, Peloza JH, Dawson K, Bogduk N. A randomized, placebo-controlled trial of intradiscal electrothermal therapy for the treatment of discogenic low back pain. Spine J 2004;4:27–35.

[56] Penn RD, Paice JA. Chronic intrathecal morphine for intractable pain. J Neurosurg 1987;67:182–7.

[57] Pope MH, DeVocht JW. The clinical relevance of biomechanics. Neurol Clin 1999;17:17–41.

[58] Rauck RL, Wallace MS, Leong MS, Minehart M, Webster LR, Charapata SG, Abraham JE, Buffington DE, Ellis D, Kartzinel R; Ziconotide 301 Study Group. A randomized, double-blind, placebo-controlled study of intrathecal ziconotide in adults with severe chronic pain. J Pain Symptom Manage 2006;31:393–406.

[59] Saal JA, Saal JS. Nonoperative treatment of herniated lumbar intervertebral disc with radiculopathy. An outcome study. Spine (Phila Pa 1976) 1989;14:431–7.

[60] Schofferman J, Kine G. Effectiveness of repeated radiofrequency neurotomy for lumbar facet pain. Spine (Phila Pa 1976) 2004;29:2471–3.

[61] Schwarzer AC, Aprill CN, Derby R, Fortin J, Kine G, Bogduk N. The prevalence and clinical features of internal disc disruption in patients with chronic low back pain. Spine (Phila Pa 1976) 1995;20:1878–83.

[62] Shealy CN. Dorsal column stimulation: optimization of application. Surg Neurol 1975;4:142–5.

[63] Simpson BA. Spinal cord stimulation in 60 cases of intractable pain. J Neurol Neurosurg Psychiatry 1991;554:196–9.

[64] Slipman CW, Bhat AL, Gilchrist RV, Issac Z, Chou L, Lenrow DA. A critical review of the evidence for the use of zygapophysial injections and radiofrequency denervation in the treatment of low back pain. Spine J 2003;3:310–6.

[65] Smith TJ, Staats PS, Deer T, Stearns LJ, Rauck RL, Boortz-Marx RL, Buchser E, Catala E, Bryce DA, Coyne PJ, Pool GE. Randomized clinical trial of an implantable drug delivery system compared with comprehensive medical management for refractory cancer pain: impact on pain, drug-related toxicity, and survival. J Clin Oncol 2002;20:4040–9.

[66] Staats P, Mitchell V. Future directions for intrathecal analgesia. Prog Anesthesiol 1997;19:367–82.

[67] Staats PS, Yearwood T, Charapata SG, Presley RW, Wallace MS, Byas-Smith M, Fisher R, Bryce DA, Mangieri EA, Luther RR, et al. Intrathecal ziconotide in the treatment of refractory pain in patients with cancer or AIDS: a randomized controlled trial. JAMA 2004;291:63–70.

[68] van Tulder MW, Ostelo R, Vlaeyen JW, Linton SJ, Morley SJ, Assendelft WJ. Behavioral treatment for chronic low back pain: a systematic review within the framework of the Cochrane Back Review Group. Spine (Phila Pa 1976) 2001;26(3):270–81.

[69] Waldman SD, Feldstein GS, Alen ML, Turnage G. Selection of patients for implantable intraspinal narcotic delivery systems. Anesth Analg 1986;65:883–5.

[70] Wallace MS, Charapata SG, Fisher R, et al. Intrathecal ziconotide in the treatment of chronic nonmalignant pain: a randomized, double-blind, placebo-controlled clinical trial. Neuromodulation 2006;9:75–86.

[71] Wallace MS, Yaksh TL. Long-term intraspinal drug therapy: a review. Reg Anesth Pain Med 2000;25:117–57.

[72] Weinstein JN, Lurie JD, Tosteson TD, Skinner JS, Hanscom B, Tosteson AN, Herkowitz H, Fischgrund J, Cammisa FP, Albert T, Deyo RA. Surgical vs nonoperative treatment for lumbar disk herniation: the Spine Patient Outcomes Research Trial (SPORT) observational cohort. JAMA 2006;296:2451–9.

[73] Wilbourn AJ, Aminoff MJ. AAEM minimonograph 32: the electrodiagnostic examination in patients with radiculopathies. American Association of Electrodiagnostic Medicine. Muscle Nerve 1998;21:1612–31.

[74] Wilson-MacDonald J, Burt G, Griffin D, Glynn C. Epidural steroid injection for nerve root compression. A randomised, controlled trial. J Bone Joint Surg Br 2005;87:352–5.

[75] Yaksh TL, Hassenbusch SJ, Burchiel K. Inflammatory masses associated with intrathecal drug infusion: a review of preclinical evidence and human data. Pain Med 2002;3:300–12.

Correspondence to: James P. Rathmell, MD, Division of Pain Medicine, Massachusetts General Hospital, 55 Fruit Street, GRB 444, Boston, MA 02116, USA. Email: jrathmell@partners.org. Mark Wallace, MD, Department of Anesthesiology, University of California San Diego, UCSD Center for Pain Medicine, 9300 Campus Point Drive, MC 7651, La Jolla, CA 92037-7651, USA. Email: mwallace@ucsd.edu.

Continuous Peripheral Nerve Blocks for Treating Acute Pain in the Hospital and the Ambulatory Environment

Brian M. Ilfeld, MD, MS

Division of Regional Anesthesia, Department of Anesthesiology, University of California at San Diego, San Diego, California, USA

The last decade has witnessed a renewed interest in continuous peripheral nerve blocks (CPNBs), also called "perineural local anesthetic infusions." This technique involves the percutaneous insertion of a catheter directly adjacent to the peripheral nerve or nerves supplying the surgical site (as opposed to a "wound" catheter placed directly at a surgical site). Infusing local anesthetic via the perineural catheter then provides potent, site-specific analgesia. This method was first described in 1946 using a cork to stabilize a needle placed adjacent to the brachial plexus divisions to provide a "continuous" supraclavicular block [4]. Subsequently, Sarnoff and Sarnoff [100] described the use of an indwelling plastic catheter allowing repeated boluses of local anesthetic along the phrenic nerve to treat intractable hiccups. Additional sporadic techniques and applications of CPNB were reported [22,31,73], but it was not until the 1990s that technological advances in needle technology, placement techniques (e.g., nerve stimulators), catheter design, and infusion pump mechanics brought a plethora of CPNB research activity [8,112]. As a result, a great deal of published information is now available to practitioners.

Indications and Selection Criteria

Surgical Indications

Given the inherent risks with CPNB (see the section below on complications), the majority of series and studies limit this technique to patients expected to have at least *moderate* postoperative pain of a duration greater than 24 hours that is not easily managed with oral opioids [35,93]. However, CPNB may be used following *mildly* painful procedures—defined here as those usually well-managed with oral opioids—to decrease opioid requirements and opioid-related side effects [91,92]. Because not all patients desire, or are capable of accepting, the extra responsibility that comes with the catheter and pump system, appropriate patient selection is crucial for safe CPNB, particularly in the ambulatory environment. Although recommendations exist for the use of various catheter locations for specific surgical procedures [7], there is little published information that specifically describes this issue. In general, axillary, cervical paravertebral, infraclavicular, or supraclavicular infusions are used for surgical procedures involving the hand, wrist, forearm, and elbow; interscalene, cervical paravertebral, and intersternocleidomastoid catheters are used for surgical procedures involving the shoulder or proximal humerus; thoracic paravertebral catheters are used for breast or thorax procedures; psoas compartment catheters are used for hip surgery; fascia iliaca, femoral, and psoas compartment catheters are used for knee or thigh procedures; and popliteal or subgluteal catheters are used for surgical procedures of the leg, ankle, and foot.

Patient Selection

Little published information is available regarding the balancing of potential perineural infusion risks and benefits for patients with significant comorbidities. Investigators often exclude patients with known hepatic or renal insufficiency, in an effort to avoid local anesthetic toxicity [32]. For infusions that may effect the phrenic nerve and ipsilateral diaphragm function (e.g., interscalene or cervical paravertebral catheters), patients with heart or lung disease are often excluded because *continuous* interscalene local anesthetic infusions have been shown to cause frequent ipsilateral diaphragm paralysis [87]. Although the effect on overall pulmonary function may be minimal for relatively healthy patients [15], practitioners must be aware of the possible related risks and be prepared to manage complications (see the section on complications below).

Equipment and Techniques

Stimulating vs. Nonstimulating Catheters

Inaccurate catheter placement occurs in a substantial number of cases—as high as 40% in some reports [95]. Multiple techniques and equipment are available for catheter insertion. One common technique involves giving a bolus of local anesthetic via an insulated needle to provide a surgical block, followed by the introduction of a "nonstimulating" catheter [65]. However, using this technique, it is possible to provide a successful surgical block, but inaccurate catheter placement [56]. For outpatients, this complication becomes more pressing as the inadequate perineural infusion often will not be detected until after surgical block resolution following home discharge [56]. Some investigators first insert the catheter and then administer a bolus of local anesthetic via the catheter in an effort to avoid this problem, with a reported failure rate of 1–8% [10,11]. Alternatively, catheters that deliver current to their tips have been developed, in an attempt to improve initial placement success rates [8]. These catheters provide feedback on the positional relationship of the catheter tip to the target nerve prior to local anesthetic dosing [88]. While there is evidence that passing current via the catheter may improve the accuracy of catheter placement with minor benefits in the lower extremity [21,80,94,97], there are currently no investigations directly comparing stimulating and nonstimulating catheters. Further study is required to identify the optimal placement techniques and equipment for ambulatory perineural infusion. Regardless of the equipment and technique used, a "test dose" of local anesthetic with epinephrine should be administered via the catheter in an effort to identify intrathecal, epidural, or intravascular placement prior to infusion initiation.

Techniques and Approaches

Numerous catheter-placement techniques have been reported—from ultrasound [45,46] and fluoroscopic guidance [89] to nerve-stimulation [44] and listening for a fascial "click" [102]—yet few studies specifically address the question of which technique is optimal for the various catheter locations. Regarding the various approaches, success rates range widely from 50% to 100%, but there are few comparisons between approaches specifically involving perineural catheters (as opposed to single-injection techniques). Although many proponents voice firm opinions based on their experience and/or imaging studies, clinical data are scarce. Therefore, the optimal approach for catheter placement at each anatomic location remains unknown and deserves future study. However, ultrasound guidance is gaining adherents at an astonishing pace and deserves further description below.

Ultrasound-Guided Catheter Insertion

For ultrasound-guided procedures, the term "long axis" is used when the length of a nerve is within the ultrasound beam, compared with "short axis" when viewed in cross-section [45]. A needle inserted with its length within a two-dimensional ultrasound beam is described as "in plane," while a needle inserted across a two-dimensional ultrasound beam is "out of plane" [45].

Needle-in-Plane, Nerve-in-Short-Axis Approach

This approach is the most-frequently published *single*-injection peripheral nerve block orientation, because this view allows for easier identification and differentiation of the target nerve from surrounding structures [45]. When the long axis of the needle is inserted within the ultrasound plane, the needle tip location can be more easily identified relative to the target nerve. Local anesthetic spread may be observed if the initial local anesthetic bolus is placed through the needle, and the needle tip may be adjusted when necessary. However, when the perineural catheter is inserted past the needle tip, it has the tendency to bypass the nerve because of the perpendicular orientation of the block needle and target nerve [33], although there are certain anatomic locations that will often allow a catheter to be passed and remain perineural [76,118]. Some practitioners have advocated either passing the catheter a minimal distance past the needle tip, or advancing the catheter further initially and then, after needle removal, retracting the catheter such that its orifice lies a minimal distance (<2 cm) past the original needle tip position [40] (although yet others have suggested that this procedure may result in a dislodged catheter tip as the needle is withdrawn over the catheter, especially by trainees). Some advocate using an extremely flexible perineural catheter in an attempt to keep the catheter tip in close proximity to the target nerve if the catheter is inserted more than a minimal distance [74,75,98]. Still others describe reorienting the needle from an in-plane to a more parallel trajectory and inserting a stimulating catheter to better monitor catheter tip location [83].

There are multiple benefits of the needle-in-plane, nerve-in-short-axis approach. First, practitioners need to learn only one technique because it may be used for both single-injection and catheter insertion procedures. Furthermore, it may be used for nearly all anatomic catheter locations, even for deeper target nerves [75]. If a 17- or 18-gauge needle is used, the needle tip may be more easily identified and will remain within the ultrasound plane due to its rigidity compared with smaller gauge needles [101]. While some have speculated that the use of a large needle is more painful, seven prospective studies reported a median catheter-insertion pain score of 0–2 on a 0–10 numeric rating scale (10 = the most pain imaginable) when the needle track was first anesthetized with lidocaine using a 25–27-gauge needle [37,40,41,74,75,77,78]. In addition, the potential benefits of using a larger needle gauge (fewer needle passes given the relative ease of keeping a rigid, larger-gauge needle in plane, and less risk of undesired tissue contact due to misinterpretation of the needle shaft for the needle tip) must be weighed against the potential risks (increased patient discomfort, increased tissue trauma, and increased injury if a vessel is punctured).

There are disadvantages of this approach as well. They include new needle entry sites relative to the nerve compared with more traditional nerve stimulation modalities that typically use a parallel needle-to-nerve insertion; challenges in keeping the needle shaft in-plane [110]; difficult needle tip visualization for relatively deep nerves [26,109]; and, as noted above, the fact that the catheter tip may bypass the target nerve, given the perpendicular orientation of the needle and nerve [33]. If an extremely flexible catheter is used in an attempt to minimize this issue, it is sometimes difficult to thread past the tip of the placement needle.

Needle-out-of-Plane, Nerve-in-Short Axis Approach

The potential benefits of this approach include a generally familiar parallel needle-to-nerve trajectory used with traditional nerve stimulation techniques (and also vascular access); and, because the needle is parallel to the target nerve, the catheter theoretically may remain in closer proximity to the nerve, even when threaded more than a centimeter past the needle tip [40,41]. However, a disadvantage of this technique is the relative inability to visualize the advancing needle tip [38,40], which some speculate increases the likelihood of unwanted contact with nerves, vessels, peritoneum, pleura, or even meninges [70]. Practitioners often use a combination of tissue movement and "hydro-location," in which fluid is injected and the resulting expansion infers the needle tip location (either with or without color Doppler flow) [6,38]. It has been suggested that for superficial catheters (e.g., interscalene and femoral), the consequent "longitudinal" orientation of needle with nerve makes precise visualization of the needle tip less critical, because when it is advanced beyond the ultrasound beam, the needle tip tends to remain relatively close to the nerve. However, for deeper nerves, this technique is not as straightforward as guiding the needle tip to a target nerve as in the in-plane technique described above, and it may be more difficult to master (and, at times, nearly impossible) [26,109].

Needle-in-Plane and Nerve-in-Long-Axis Approach

Superficially, this technique appears to have the benefits of both approaches described previously, with few limitations. The nerve can be viewed along with the needle shaft/tip, and the catheter monitored as it exits the needle parallel to the target nerve. The difficulty lies in keeping three structures—the needle, nerve, and catheter—in the ultrasound plane [67]. In addition, to view the nerve in long axis, the nerve itself must be relatively straight, and there can be only one target nerve as opposed to multiple trunks or cords as found within the brachial plexus. Evidence of this technique's difficulties may be found in the scarcity of published reports [67,115].

Limitations on the length of this chapter preclude a discussion of multiple additional ultrasound-related issues, such as transducer selection, the concomitant use of nerve stimulation (an important tool in a subset of patients) [39], and various methods for catheter tip localization [113]. Although many proponents voice firm opinions based on their personal experience, there is a shortage of clinical data comparing aspects of any one placement technique with another.

Infusates

Local Anesthetic

The majority of perineural infusion publications have involved bupivacaine or ropivacaine, although the use of levobupivacaine and shorter-acting agents has been reported. As these local anesthetics have varying durations of action, investigations involving one may not necessarily be applied to another. One trial involving interscalene infusion found that ropivacaine 0.2% and bupivacaine 0.15% provided similar analgesia, but ropivacaine was associated with better preservation of strength in the hand and less paresthesia in the fingers [14]. However, another study of interscalene infusion found ropivacaine 0.2% and levobupivacaine 0.125% to be equivalent following shoulder surgery, with patients receiving levobupivacaine consuming a lower volume of anesthetic [20]. Similarly, a third investigation found no difference between 0.125% bupivacaine and ropivacaine provided as self-administered bolus doses via axillary catheter following mildly painful surgery of the upper extremity [91]. Unfortunately, the precise equipotent local anesthetic concentrations within the peripheral nervous system remain undetermined, making the evaluation of comparisons problematic. Currently, there is insufficient information to determine if there is an optimal local anesthetic for CPNB. When deciding on an infusate, providers should consider the risk of local anesthetic toxicity as the concentration of local anesthetic increases.

Investigators have added clonidine to long-acting local anesthetic (1–2 μg/mL), for *continuous* perineural femoral [16], anterior lumbar plexus [104,106,108], interscalene [107], and popliteal [103] infusions. Unfortunately, while clonidine increases the duration of *single-injection* nerve blocks [61], the only controlled investigations of adding clonidine to a *continuous* ropivacaine infusion (1 or 2 μg/mL) failed to reveal any clinically relevant benefits [52,54]. Additionally, opioids and epinephrine have been added to local anesthetic infusions [119,120], but there are currently insufficient published data to draw any

conclusions regarding the safety of the former [86] or the efficacy of the latter [82,90].

Dosing Strategies

Investigations of interscalene [57,107], infraclavicular [53], axillary [62,79], fascia iliaca [36], extended femoral [106,108], subgluteal [34], and popliteal [58] catheters suggest that the optimal local anesthetic dosing regimen varies with anatomical location. Therefore, data from studies involving one catheter location cannot necessarily be applied to another location. Many variables probably affect the optimal regimen, including surgical procedure, catheter location, physical therapy regimen, and the specific local anesthetic infused. The available published data related to dosing regimen optimization involve surgical procedures producing at least moderate postoperative pain [34,36,53,57,58,62,79,106–108]. It is possible—even probable—that adequate analgesia for procedures inducing *mild* postoperative pain would be adequately treated with a bolus-only dosing regimen [91]. Additionally, there is a theoretical possibility that stimulating catheters may be placed, on average, closer to the target nerve/plexus compared with nonstimulating devices [97]. If this surmise proves accurate, then potentially different dosing regimens, basal rates, and bolus doses would be optimal for different types of catheters.

Available inpatient and outpatient data suggest that following procedures producing moderate-to-severe pain, providing patients with the ability to self-administer local anesthetic doses increases perioperative benefits and decreases local anesthetic consumption. Unfortunately, insufficient information is available to base recommendations on the optimal basal rate, bolus volume, or lockout period accounting for the many variables that may affect these values (e.g., catheter type, location, surgical procedure). Until recommendations based on prospectively collected data are published, practitioners should be aware that investigators have reported successful analgesia using the following with long-acting local anesthetics: a basal rate of 5–10 mL/hour, a bolus volume of 2–5 mL, and a lockout duration of 20–60 minutes. Additionally, the maximum safe doses for the long-acting local anesthetics remain unknown. However, multiple investigations involving patients free of renal or hepatic disease have reported blood concentrations within acceptable limits following up to 5 days of perineural infusion with similar dosing schedules.

Potential Benefits

A plethora of prospective, randomized investigations suggest many benefits of CPNB, but I will focus mainly on double-masked, placebo-controlled studies since they generally provide the highest quality data by minimizing potential bias. Such studies have involved patients scheduled for moderately painful procedures who received an infraclavicular [51], interscalene [56,59], posterior popliteal [55,123], femoral [42,47], or psoas compartment [121] perineural catheter. Overwhelmingly, patients receiving perineural local anesthetic achieved both clinically and statistically significant lower resting and breakthrough pain scores while requiring dramatically less oral analgesic medication. Patients who received perineural local anesthetic also experienced additional benefits related to improved analgesia. Zero to 30% of patients receiving perineural ropivacaine reported insomnia due to pain, compared with 60–70% of patients using only oral opioids [51,55,56]. Patients receiving perineural ropivacaine awoke from sleep because of pain an average of 0.0–0.2 times on the first postoperative night, compared with 2.0–2.3 times for patients receiving perineural saline [51,55,56]. Dramatically lower opioid consumption in patients receiving perineural local anesthetic resulted in fewer opioid-related side effects, including a lower rate of nausea, vomiting, pruritis, and sedation [51,55,56,123]. Furthermore, patients receiving perineural local anesthetic reported satisfaction with their postoperative analgesia (on a scale of 0–10, where 10 = highest satisfaction) of 8.8–9.8 compared with 5.5–7.7 for patients receiving placebo [51,55,56,59,123]. Two unmasked but randomized studies suggest that continuous femoral nerve blocks following total knee arthroplasty result in a more rapid resumption of knee flexion [16,104]. These two studies from Europe also found that following total knee arthroplasty or knee arthrolysis, using a 48- or 72-hour hospital-based continuous femoral block decreased rehabilitation center stays from 21 to 17 days and from 50 to 40 days, respectively [16,104]. However, as previously noted [114], these data did not suggest that hospital length of stay is likely to be reduced in the United States, where the average institutional stay of patients is already less than 1 week. Two additional randomized studies failed to demonstrate a decrease in hospitalization duration using a hospital-based 48-hour continuous femoral block over a single-injection femoral block, although one study was unmasked [96]

and the other possibly underpowered (with no power analysis provided) [47]. Finally, one study reported a decreased time to adequate ambulation and optimization of daily activities using ambulatory CPNB compared with intravenous opioids [18].

Potential Risks/Complications

Although accumulating evidence shows that CPNB provides multiple benefits, complications involving this technique do occur. Unfortunately, the relatively recent widespread use of perineural local anesthetic infusion and the lack of large clinical studies make it difficult to evaluate the incidence of related complications. Two of the largest prospective investigations to date, involving over 2,100 patients combined, suggest that the incidence of related complications is very low—at least as low as, if not lower than, single-injection techniques [11,19]. Smaller prospective studies involving continuous infraclavicular and popliteal perineural infusions suggest a similar incidence of complications [10,12].

Inaccurate Catheter Placement

The reported range of what has been called "secondary block failure" is 0–40% [65,95]. The incidence of this complication is presumably dependent on many factors, including the experience of the practitioner, the equipment and technique used, as well as patient factors such as body shape [27,84]. In an effort to decrease the chances of an unidentified misplacement, investigators have first inserted the catheter, and then injected the initial local anesthetic via the catheter [11,53,57,58,88]. If a surgical block does not develop, the catheter may be replaced.

Vascular Puncture/Hematoma

While puncturing a vessel is certainly a well-known complication of single-injection peripheral nerve blocks, this event may be more significant when placing a perineural catheter, since the needle gauge is often larger to allow for endoluminal catheter insertion. The incidence of this complication is reportedly between 0% and 11%, and it is most likely influenced significantly by such variables as the anatomical location of the block and needle/catheter design [9,12,13,19,53,65]. Prolonged Horner's syndrome due to neck hematoma is a rare complication that has been reported [35]. While a hematoma may require weeks for resolution (months for Horner's syndrome), practitioners and patients should be reassured with the multiple case reports of complete neural recovery following hematoma resolution [13,35,64,122]. If vascular puncture does occur, it is still possible to successfully place a perineural catheter following a period of direct pressure, although a resulting hematoma will conduct electrical current and may decrease the ability to stimulate the target nerve with subsequent attempts [53]. Clinically significant hematoma formation has been reported in patients with a psoas compartment catheter who received low molecular weight heparin for anticoagulation [64,122]. These occurrences have led some practitioners to manage patients with a psoas compartment catheter in much the same way as those having neuraxial block when thromboprophylaxis is ordered [122], although others have questioned this practice [23]. The American Society of Regional Anesthesia consensus statement on neuraxial anesthesia and anticoagulation notes that, "conservatively, the [recommendations] … may be applied to plexus and peripheral techniques. However, this may be more restrictive than necessary" and that "additional information is needed to make definitive recommendations" [49].

Intravascular Local Anesthetic Injection

Even if the bolus of local anesthetic for initial surgical block placement is given via the catheter, intravascular injection with subsequent toxicity is possible. When a bolus is given via the needle, subsequent intravascular catheter placement is still possible [51,117]. Therefore, investigators have recommended injecting a "test dose" containing epinephrine via the catheter prior to local anesthetic infusion initiation [63].

Perineuraxis Injection

When placing a catheter near the neuraxis, as with the psoas compartment and interscalene locations, it is possible to cannulate the epidural [28,30,72] or intrathecal [69] spaces. Injection of local anesthetic is potentially catastrophic and may result in unconsciousness and extreme hypotension, requiring aggressive resuscitation. As with intravascular catheter placement, it is possible to accurately inject the initial bolus of local anesthetic via the needle, followed by cannulation of the epidural [28], intrathecal [69], and even intrapleural spaces with the catheter [111]. When working close to the neuraxis, it is possible to obtain epidural local anesthetic spread even with an accurately placed perineural catheter, resulting in a sympathectomy and possible hypotension.

Nerve Injury

Nerve injury is a recognized complication following placement of both single-injection block and CPNB, presumably related to needle trauma or subsequent local anesthetic/adjuvant neurotoxicity [2]. The prospective clinical evidence from human subjects suggests that the incidence of neural injury from a perineural catheter and ropivacaine (0.2%) infusion is no higher than that following single-injection regional blocks [5,10,11,13]. There are two case reports of interscalene perineural catheters possibly resulting in brachial plexus irritation [93]. In both of these cases, repeated boluses of 0.25% bupivacaine had been injected over a period of days, and patient discomfort ceased upon removal of the catheters [93]. There is also evidence that in diabetes, the risk of local anesthetic-induced nerve injury is increased [48].

Dislodgement

The most common complication during perineural infusion is simply inadvertent catheter dislodgement. The reported incidence of dislodgement varies greatly between 0% and 30%, which is most likely related to the anatomical location, equipment type, and technique used to secure the catheter. Every effort to optimally secure the catheter must be made to maximize patient benefits. Measures have included the use of sterile liquid adhesive (e.g., benzoin), sterile tape (e.g., "Steri-Strips"), securing of the catheter-hub connection with either tape or specifically designed devices (e.g., "Statlock"), subcutaneous tunneling of the catheter, and the use of 2-octyl cyanoacrylate glue [66]. Using a combination of these maneuvers, investigators have reported a catheter retention rate of 95–100% for 6–9 days of infusion [3,60].

Infection

While catheter site bacterial colonization is relatively common [29,43], clinically relevant infection is not [13,19,43]. In prospective investigations of interscalene [11,13], posterior popliteal [10], and multiple-site [19] catheters involving over 2,700 patients combined, infection rates varied from 0–3%, with one psoas compartment abscess forming after femoral CPNB. In these few cases, all infections completely resolved within 10 days [1,19]. Limiting catheter use to 3–4 days may further decrease the incidence of this complication, and practitioners should balance the need for analgesia with the risk of infection [19,43].

Pulmonary Complications

For infusions that may effect the phrenic nerve and ipsilateral diaphragm function (e.g., interscalene or cervical paravertebral catheters), caution is warranted because interscalene CPNBs have been shown to cause frequent ipsilateral diaphragm paralysis [87]. Although the effect on overall pulmonary function may be minimal for relatively healthy patients [15], a case of clinically relevant lower lobe collapse in a patient with an interscalene infusion at home and two cases of acute respiratory failure have occurred [19,99].

Catheter Migration

While there are case reports of initially misplaced catheters, spontaneous migration into adjacent anatomical structures following a documented correct placement has been described in only one patient [19]. Possible complications include intravascular or interpleural migration, resulting in local anesthetic toxicity, and epidural/intrathecal migration when using an interscalene, paravertebral, or psoas compartment catheter. It is possible to accidentally position the catheter tip in the epidural space (and presumably other structures) following partial catheter withdrawal [28].

Delayed Local Anesthetic Toxicity

All practitioners using continuous block techniques should consider systemic local anesthetic toxicity due to CPNB. The maximum safe doses for the long-acting local anesthetics as well as the incidence of systemic toxicity are unknown. There have been cases of patients reporting early symptoms of toxicity, such as perioral numbness, that resolved with termination of the infusion [5,116]. Providing patients with the ability to self-administer bolus doses decreases local anesthetic consumption [24,34,36,50,53,57,58,62,106–108]. Investigators often exclude patients from a long-duration CPNB with known hepatic or renal insufficiency in an effort to avoid local anesthetic toxicity [32,51,55,56].

Catheter Knotting and Retention

Several case reports of catheter retention have been published, although the overall incidence of this complication is unknown [53,71,81,85]. The most common etiology is knot formation below the skin or fascia, which has been reported in fascia iliaca [85], femoral [81], and psoas compartment catheters [71]. Two of these cases required surgical exploration for catheter removal [71,81]. However, removal of a knotted fascia iliaca catheter was achieved without surgical intervention with simple hip flexion [85]. In all of these cases, the catheter had been advanced over 5 cm past the needle tip. Advancing the catheter more than 3–5 cm is often attempted in an effort to decrease the risk of dislodgement, or to "thread" the catheter tip towards the lumbar plexus when using the femoral or fascia iliaca insertion points [17]. However, retention rates of 95–100% have been reported using a maximum distance of 5 cm [51–58], and in the absence of using a catheter-over-wire Seldinger technique [104–106,108], the catheter tip rarely reaches the lumbar plexus following a femoral insertion [17]. Therefore, although there is no consensus regarding the optimal distance of catheter insertion, the available data suggest that insertion greater than 5 cm is unnecessary and may increase the risk of catheter knotting [85].

Catheter Shearing

It is possible to "shear off" a segment of catheter if, after its insertion past the needle tip, the catheter itself is withdrawn back into the needle. Therefore, this maneuver should only be attempted when using needle/catheter combinations that have been specifically designed for catheter withdrawal. When specifically designed needle/catheter combinations are used—such as some stimulating catheters—catheter withdrawal should cease with any resistance, and the needle itself should be retracted until the catheter resistance resolves [25,53,54,57,58]. In one reported case, a 6-cm femoral catheter fragment was sheared off and remained in situ for 1 week, causing persistent pain of the ipsilateral groin, thigh, and knee [68]. Despite an embedded radio-opaque strip, the catheter fragment could not be visualized with plain radiographs. However, a computerized tomographic scan did localize the fragment, and the femoral nerve neuralgia resolved in the week following surgical extraction of the fragment [68]. In an additional case, an axillary catheter fragment was diagnosed with ultrasonography and was surgically extracted [5]. In all of the case reports of retained catheters/fragments, no patient has experienced persistent symptoms following their removal [5,25,53,68].

Conclusions

A large and growing body of evidence shows that continuous peripheral nerve blocks provide a multitude of clinical benefits. However, because of the relatively recent evolution of modern techniques, illuminating data are often unavailable. Future prospective investigation is required to determine the true incidence of complications associated with perineural infusion, as well as the necessary procedures to minimize their incidence and optimize diagnostic evaluation and subsequent management.

References

[1]   Adam F, Jaziri S, Chauvin M. Psoas abscess complicating femoral nerve block catheter. Anesthesiology 2003;99:230–1.

[2]   Al Nasser B, Palacios JL. Femoral nerve injury complicating continuous psoas compartment block. Reg Anesth Pain Med 2004;29:361–3.

[3]   Ang ET, Lassale B, Goldfarb G. Continuous axillary brachial plexus block: a clinical and anatomical study. Anesth Analg 1984;63:680–4.

[4]   Ansbro FP. A method of continuous brachial plexus block. Am J Surg 1946;71:716–22.

[5]   Bergman BD, Hebl JR, Kent J, Horlocker TT. Neurologic complications of 405 consecutive continuous axillary catheters. Anesth Analg 2003;96:247–52.

[6]   Bloc S, Ecoffey C, Dhonneur G. Controlling needle tip progression during ultrasound-guided regional anesthesia using the hydrolocalization technique. Reg Anesth Pain Med 2008;33:382–3.

[7]   Boezaart AP. Perineural infusion of local anesthetics. Anesthesiology 2006;104:872–80.

[8]   Boezaart AP, de Beer JF, du Toit C, van Rooyen K. A new technique of continuous interscalene nerve block. Can J Anaesth 1999;46:275–81.

[9]   Boezaart AP, de Beer JF, Nell ML. Early experience with continuous cervical paravertebral block using a stimulating catheter. Reg Anesth Pain Med 2003;28:406–13.

[10] Borgeat A, Blumenthal S, Karovic D, Delbos A, Vienne P. Clinical evaluation of a modified posterior anatomical approach to performing the popliteal block. Reg Anesth Pain Med 2004;29:290–6.

[11] Borgeat A, Dullenkopf A, Ekatodramis G, Nagy L. Evaluation of the lateral modified approach for continuous interscalene block after shoulder surgery. Anesthesiology 2003;99:436–42.

[12] Borgeat A, Ekatodramis G, Dumont C. An evaluation of the infraclavicular block via a modified approach of the Raj technique. Anesth Analg 2001;93:436–41.

[13] Borgeat A, Ekatodramis G, Kalberer F, Benz C. Acute and nonacute complications associated with interscalene block and shoulder surgery: a prospective study. Anesthesiology 2001;95:875–80.

[14] Borgeat A, Kalberer F, Jacob H, Ruetsch YA, Gerber C. Patient-controlled interscalene analgesia with ropivacaine 0.2% versus bupivacaine 0.15% after major open shoulder surgery: the effects on hand motor function. Anesth Analg 2001;92:218–23.

[15] Borgeat A, Perschak H, Bird P, Hodler J, Gerber C. Patient-controlled interscalene analgesia with ropivacaine 0.2% versus patient-controlled intravenous analgesia after major shoulder surgery: effects on diaphragmatic and respiratory function. Anesthesiology 2000;92:102–8.

[16] Capdevila X, Barthelet Y, Biboulet P, Ryckwaert Y, Rubenovitch J, d'Athis F. Effects of perioperative analgesic technique on the surgical outcome and duration of rehabilitation after major knee surgery. Anesthesiology 1999;91:8–15.

[17] Capdevila X, Biboulet P, Morau D, Bernard N, Deschodt J, Lopez S, d'Athis F. Continuous three-in-one block for postoperative pain after lower limb orthopedic surgery: where do the catheters go?. Anesth Analg 2002;94:1001–6.

[18] Capdevila X, Dadure C, Bringuier S, Bernard N, Biboulet P, Gaertner E, Macaire P. Effect of patient-controlled perineural analgesia on rehabilitation and pain after ambulatory orthopedic surgery: a multicenter randomized trial. Anesthesiology 2006;105:566–73.

[19] Capdevila X, Pirat P, Bringuier S, Gaertner E, Singelyn F, Bernard N, Choquet O, Bouaziz H, Bonnet F. Continuous peripheral nerve blocks in hospital wards after orthopedic surgery: a multicenter prospective analysis of the quality of postoperative analgesia and complications in 1,416 patients. Anesthesiology 2005;103:1035–45.

[20] Casati A, Borghi B, Fanelli G, Montone N, Rotini R, Fraschini G, Vinciguerra F, Torri G, Chelly J. Interscalene brachial plexus anesthesia and analgesia for open shoulder surgery: a randomized, double-blinded comparison between levobupivacaine and ropivacaine. Anesth Analg 2003;96:253–9.

[21] Casati A, Fanelli G, Koscielniak-Nielsen Z, Cappelleri G, Aldegheri G, Danelli G, Fuzier R, Singelyn F. Using stimulating catheters for continuous sciatic nerve block shortens onset time of surgical block and minimizes postoperative consumption of pain medication after halux valgus repair as compared with conventional nonstimulating catheters. Anesth Analg 2005;101:1192–7.

[22] Cheeley LN. Treatment of peripheral embolism by continuous sciatic nerve block. Curr Res Anesth Analg 1952;31:211–2.

[23] Chelly JE, Greger JR, Casati A, Gebhard R, Ben David B. What has happened to evidence-based medicine? Anesthesiology 2003;99:1028–9.

[24] Chelly JE, Greger J, Gebhard R. Ambulatory continuous perineural infusion: are we ready? Anesthesiology 2000;93:581–2.

[25] Chin KJ, Chee V. Perforation of a Pajunk stimulating catheter after traction-induced damage. Reg Anesth Pain Med 2006;31:389–90.

[26] Chin KJ, Perlas A, Chan VW, Brull R. Needle visualization in ultrasound-guided regional anesthesia: challenges and solutions. Reg Anesth Pain Med 2008;33:532–44.

[27] Coleman MM, Chan VW. Continuous interscalene brachial plexus block. Can J Anaesth 1999;46:209–14.

[28] Cook LB. Unsuspected extradural catheterization in an interscalene block. Br J Anaesth 1991;67:473–5.

[29] Cuvillon P, Ripart J, Lalourcey L, Veyrat E, L'Hermite J, Boisson C, Thouabtia E, Eledjam JJ. The continuous femoral nerve block catheter for postoperative analgesia: bacterial colonization, infectious rate and adverse effects. Anesth Analg 2001;93:1045–9.

[30] De Biasi P, Lupescu R, Burgun G, Lascurain P, Gaertner E. Continuous lumbar plexus block: use of radiography to determine catheter tip location. Reg Anesth Pain Med 2003;28:135–9.

[31] DeKrey JA, Schroeder CF, Buechel DR. Continuous brachial plexus block. Anesthesiology 1969;30:332.

[32] Denson DD, Raj PP, Saldahna F, Finnsson RA, Ritschel WA, Joyce TH III, Turner JL. Continuous perineural infusion of bupivacaine for prolonged analgesia: pharmacokinetic considerations. Int J Clin Pharmacol Ther Toxicol 1983;21:591–7.

[33] Dhir S, Ganapathy S. Comparative evaluation of ultrasound-guided continuous infraclavicular brachial plexus block with stimulating catheter and traditional technique: a prospective-randomized trial. Acta Anaesthesiol Scand 2008;52:1158–66.

[34] di Benedetto P, Casati A, Bertini L. Continuous subgluteus sciatic nerve block after orthopedic foot and ankle surgery: comparison of two infusion techniques. Reg Anesth Pain Med 2002;27:168–72.

[35] Ekatodramis G, Macaire P, Borgeat A. Prolonged Horner syndrome due to neck hematoma after continuous interscalene block. Anesthesiology 2001;95:801–3.

[36] Eledjam JJ, Cuvillon P, Capdevila X, Macaire P, Serri S, Gaertner E, Jochum D. Postoperative analgesia by femoral nerve block with ropivacaine 0.2% after major knee surgery: continuous versus patient-controlled techniques. Reg Anesth Pain Med 2002;27:604–11.

[37] Fredrickson MJ. A prospective randomized comparison of ultrasound guidance versus neurostimulation for interscalene catheter placement. Reg Anesth Pain Med 2010; in press.

[38] Fredrickson M. "Oblique" needle-probe alignment to facilitate ultrasound-guided femoral catheter placement. Reg Anesth Pain Med 2008;33:383–4.

[39] Fredrickson MJ. The sensitivity of motor response to needle nerve stimulation during ultrasound guided interscalene catheter placement. Reg Anesth Pain Med 2008;33:291–6.

[40] Fredrickson MJ, Ball CM, Dalgleish AJ, Stewart AW, Short TG. A prospective randomized comparison of ultrasound and neurostimulation as needle end points for interscalene catheter placement. Anesth Analg 2009;108:1695–700.

[41] Fredrickson MJ, Danesh-Clough TK. Ambulatory continuous femoral analgesia for major knee surgery: a randomised study of ultrasound-guided femoral catheter placement. Anaesth Intensive Care 2009;37:758–66.

[42] Ganapathy S, Wasserman RA, Watson JT, Bennett J, Armstrong KP, Stockall CA, Chess DG, MacDonald C. Modified continuous femoral three-in-one block for postoperative pain after total knee arthroplasty. Anesth Analg 1999;89:1197–202.

[43] Gaumann DM, Lennon RL, Wedel DJ. Continuous axillary block for postoperative pain management. Reg Anesth Pain Med 1988;13:77–82.

[44] Grant SA, Nielsen KC, Greengrass RA, Steele SM, Klein SM. Continuous peripheral nerve block for ambulatory surgery. Reg Anesth Pain Med 2001;26:209–14.

[45] Gray AT. Ultrasound-guided regional anesthesia: current state of the art. Anesthesiology 2006;104:368–73.

[46] Guzeldemir ME, Ustunsoz B. Ultrasonographic guidance in placing a catheter for continuous axillary brachial plexus block. Anesth Analg 1995;81:882–3.

[47] Hirst GC, Lang SA, Dust WN, Cassidy JD, Yip RW. Femoral nerve block. Single injection versus continuous infusion for total knee arthroplasty. Reg Anesth 1996;21:292–7.

[48] Horlocker TT, O'Driscoll SW, Dinapoli RP. Recurring brachial plexus neuropathy in a diabetic patient after shoulder surgery and continuous interscalene block. Anesth Analg 2000;91:688–90.

[49] Horlocker TT, Wedel DJ, Benzon H, Brown DL, Enneking FK, Heit JA, Mulroy MF, Rosenquist RW, Rowlingson J, Tryba M, Yuan CS. Regional anesthesia in the anticoagulated patient: defining the risks (the second ASRA Consensus Conference on Neuraxial Anesthesia and Anticoagulation). Reg Anesth Pain Med 2003;28:172–97.

[50] Ilfeld BM, Enneking FK. A portable mechanical pump providing over four days of patient-controlled analgesia by perineural infusion at home. Reg Anesth Pain Med 2002;27:100–4.

[51] Ilfeld BM, Morey TE, Enneking FK. Continuous infraclavicular brachial plexus block for postoperative pain control at home: a randomized, double-blinded, placebo-controlled study. Anesthesiology 2002;96:1297–304.

[52] Ilfeld BM, Morey TE, Enneking FK. Continuous infraclavicular perineural infusion with clonidine and ropivacaine compared with ropivacaine alone: a randomized, double-blinded, controlled study. Anesth Analg 2003;97:706–12.

[53] Ilfeld BM, Morey TE, Enneking FK. Infraclavicular perineural local anesthetic infusion: a comparison of three dosing regimens for postoperative analgesia. Anesthesiology 2004;100:395–402.

[54] Ilfeld BM, Morey TE, Thannikary LJ, Wright TW, Enneking FK. Clonidine added to a continuous interscalene ropivacaine perineural infusion to improve postoperative analgesia: a randomized, double-blind, controlled study. Anesth Analg 2005;100:1172–8.

[55] Ilfeld BM, Morey TE, Wang RD, Enneking FK. Continuous popliteal sciatic nerve block for postoperative pain control at home: a randomized, double-blinded, placebo-controlled study. Anesthesiology 2002;97:959–65.

[56] Ilfeld BM, Morey TE, Wright TW, Chidgey LK, Enneking FK. Continuous interscalene brachial plexus block for postoperative pain control at home: a randomized, double-blinded, placebo-controlled study. Anesth Analg 2003;96:1089–95.

[57] Ilfeld BM, Morey TE, Wright TW, Chidgey LK, Enneking FK. Interscalene perineural ropivacaine infusion: a comparison of two dosing regimens for postoperative analgesia. Reg Anesth Pain Med 2004;29:9–16.

[58] Ilfeld BM, Thannikary LJ, Morey TE, Vander Griend RA, Enneking FK. Popliteal sciatic perineural local anesthetic infusion: a comparison of three dosing regimens for postoperative analgesia. Anesthesiology 2004;101:970–7.

[59] Ilfeld BM, Vandenborne K, Duncan PW, Sessler DI, Enneking FK, Shuster JJ, Theriaque DW, Chmielewski TL, Spadoni EH, Wright TW. Ambulatory continuous interscalene nerve blocks decrease the time to discharge readiness after total shoulder arthroplasty: a randomized, triple-masked, placebo-controlled study. Anesthesiology 2006;105:999–1007.

[60] Ilfeld BM, Wright TW, Enneking FK, Mace JA, Shuster JJ, Spadoni EH, Chmielewski TL, Vandenborne K. Total shoulder arthroplasty as an outpatient procedure using ambulatory perineural local anesthetic infusion: a pilot feasibility study. Anesth Analg 2005;101:1319–22.

[61] Iskandar H, Guillaume E, Dixmerias F, Binje B, Rakotondriamihary S, Thiebaut R, Maurette P. The enhancement of sensory blockade by clonidine selectively added to mepivacaine after midhumeral block. Anesth Analg 2001;93:771–5.

[62] Iskandar H, Rakotondriamihary S, Dixmerias F, Binje B, Maurette P. [Analgesia using continuous axillary block after surgery of severe hand injuries: self-administration versus continuous injection.] Ann Fr Anesth Reanim 1998;17:1099–103.

[63] Klein SM. Beyond the hospital: continuous peripheral nerve blocks at home. Anesthesiology 2002;96:1283–5.

[64] Klein SM, D'Ercole F, Greengrass RA, Warner DS. Enoxaparin associated with psoas hematoma and lumbar plexopathy after lumbar plexus block. Anesthesiology 1997;87:1576–9.

[65] Klein SM, Grant SA, Greengrass RA, Nielsen KC, Speer KP, White W, Warner DS, Steele SM. Interscalene brachial plexus block with a continuous catheter insertion system and a disposable infusion pump. Anesth Analg 2000;91:1473–8.

[66] Klein SM, Nielsen KC, Buckenmaier CC III, Kamal AS, Rubin Y, Steele SM. 2-Octyl cyanoacrylate glue for the fixation of continuous peripheral nerve catheters. Anesthesiology 2003;98:590–1.

[67] Koscielniak-Nielsen ZJ, Rasmussen H, Hesselbjerg L. Long-axis ultrasound imaging of the nerves and advancement of perineural catheters under direct vision: a preliminary report of four cases. Reg Anesth Pain Med 2008;33:477–82.

[68] Lee BH, Goucke CR. Shearing of a peripheral nerve catheter. Anesth Analg 2002;95:760–1.

[69] Litz RJ, Vicent O, Wiessner D, Heller AR. Misplacement of a psoas compartment catheter in the subarachnoid space. Reg Anesth Pain Med 2004;29:60–4.

[70] Luyet C, Eichenberger U, Greif R, Vogt A, Szucs FZ, Moriggl B. Ultrasound-guided paravertebral puncture and placement of catheters in human cadavers: an imaging study. Br J Anaesth 2009;102:534–9.

[71] MacLeod DB, Grant SA, Martin G, Breslin DS. Identification of coracoid process for infraclavicular blocks. Reg Anesth Pain Med 2003;28:485.

[72] Mahoudeau G, Gaertner E, Launoy A, Ocquidant P, Loewenthal A. [Interscalenic block: accidental catheterization of the epidural space.] Ann Fr Anesth Reanim 1995;14:438–41.

[73] Manriquez RG, Pallares V. Continuous brachial plexus block for prolonged sympathectomy and control of pain. Anesth Analg 1978;57:128–30.

[74] Mariano ER, Cheng GS, Choy LP, Loland VJ, Bellars RH, Sandhu NS, Bishop ML, Lee DK, Maldonado RC, Ilfeld BM. Electrical stimulation versus ultrasound guidance for popliteal-sciatic perineural catheter insertion: a randomized, controlled trial. Reg Anesth Pain Med 2009;34:480–5.

[75] Mariano ER, Loland VJ, Bellars RH, Sandhu NS, Bishop ML, Abrams RA, Meunier MJ, Maldonado RC, Ferguson EJ, Ilfeld BM. Ultrasound guidance versus electrical stimulation for infraclavicular brachial plexus perineural catheter insertion. J Ultrasound Med 2009;28:1211–8.

[76] Mariano ER, Loland VJ, Ilfeld BM. Interscalene perineural catheter placement using an ultrasound-guided posterior approach. Reg Anesth Pain Med 2009;34:60–3.

[77] Mariano ER, Loland VJ, Sandhu NS, Bellars RH, Bishop ML, Afra R, Ball ST, Meyer RS, Maldonado RC, Ilfeld BM. Ultrasound guidance versus electrical stimulation for femoral perineural catheter insertion, J Ultrasound Med 2009;28:1453–60.

[78] Mariano ER, Loland VJ, Sandhu NS, Bellars RH, Bishop ML, Meunier MJ, Afra R, Ferguson EJ, Ilfeld BM. A randomized, controlled comparison of two techniques for interscalene perineural catheter insertion involving ultrasound and nerve stimulation. J Ultrasound Med 2010; in press.

[79] Mezzatesta JP, Scott DA, Schweitzer SA, Selander DE. Continuous axillary brachial plexus block for postoperative pain relief. Intermittent bolus versus continuous infusion. Reg Anesth 1997;22:357–62.

[80] Morin AM, Eberhart LH, Behnke HK, Wagner S, Koch T, Wolf U, Nau W, Kill C, Geldner G, Wulf H. Does femoral nerve catheter placement with stimulating catheters improve effective placement? A randomized, controlled, and observer-blinded trial. Anesth Analg 2005;100:1503–10.

[81] Motamed C, Bouaziz H, Mercier FJ, Benhamou D. Knotting of a femoral catheter. Reg Anesth 1997;22:486–7.

[82] Murphy DB, McCartney CJ, Chan VW. Novel analgesic adjuncts for brachial plexus block: a systematic review. Anesth Analg 2000;90:1122–8.

[83] Niazi AU, Prasad A, Ramlogan R, Chan VW. Methods to ease placement of stimulating catheters during in-plane ultrasound-guided femoral nerve block. Reg Anesth Pain Med 2009;34:380–1.

[84] Nielsen KC, Guller U, Steele SM, Klein SM, Greengrass RA, Pietrobon R. Influence of obesity on surgical regional anesthesia in the ambulatory setting: an analysis of 9,038 blocks. Anesthesiology 2005;102:181–7.

[85] Offerdahl MR, Lennon RL, Horlocker TT. Successful removal of a knotted fascia iliaca catheter: principles of patient positioning for peripheral nerve catheter extraction. Anesth Analg 2004;99:1550–2.

[86] Partridge BL. The effects of local anesthetics and epinephrine on rat sciatic nerve blood flow. Anesthesiology 1991;75:243–50.

[87] Pere P. The effect of continuous interscalene brachial plexus block with 0.125% bupivacaine plus fentanyl on diaphragmatic motility and ventilatory function. Reg Anesth 1993;18:93–7.

[88] Pham-Dang C, Kick O, Collet T, Gouin F, Pinaud M. Continuous peripheral nerve blocks with stimulating catheters. Reg Anesth Pain Med 2003;28:83–8.

[89] Pham-Dang C, Meunier JF, Poirier P, Kick O, Bourreli B, Touchais S, Le Corre P, Pinaud M. A new axillary approach for continuous brachial plexus block. A clinical and anatomic study. Anesth Analg 1995;81:686–93.

[90] Picard PR, Tramer MR, McQuay HJ, Moore RA. Analgesic efficacy of peripheral opioids (all except intra-articular): a qualitative systematic review of randomised controlled trials. Pain 1997;72:309–18.

[91] Rawal N, Allvin R, Axelsson K, Hallen J, Ekback G, Ohlsson T, Amilon A. Patient-controlled regional analgesia (PCRA) at home: controlled comparison between bupivacaine and ropivacaine brachial plexus analgesia. Anesthesiology 2002;96:1290–6.

[92] Rawal N, Axelsson K, Hylander J, Allvin R, Amilon A, Lidegran G, Hallen J. Postoperative patient-controlled local anesthetic administration at home. Anesth Analg 1998;86:86–9.

[93] Ribeiro FC, Georgousis H, Bertram R, Scheiber G. Plexus irritation caused by interscalene brachial plexus catheter for shoulder surgery. Anesth Analg 1996;82:870–2.

[94] Rodriguez J, Taboada M, Carceller J, Lagunilla J, Barcena M, Alvarez J. Stimulating popliteal catheters for postoperative analgesia after hallux valgus repair. Anesth Analg 2006;102:258–62.

[95] Salinas FV. Location, location, location: continuous peripheral nerve blocks and stimulating catheters. Reg Anesth Pain Med 2003;28:79–82.

[96] Salinas FV, Liu SS, Mulroy MF. The effect of single-injection femoral nerve block versus continuous femoral nerve block after total knee arthroplasty on hospital length of stay and long-term functional recovery within an established clinical pathway. Anesth Analg 2006;102:1234–9.

[97] Salinas FV, Neal JM, Sueda LA, Kopacz DJ, Liu SS. Prospective comparison of continuous femoral nerve block with nonstimulating catheter placement versus stimulating catheter-guided perineural placement in volunteers. Reg Anesth Pain Med 2004;29:212–20.

[98] Sandhu NS, Capan LM. Ultrasound-guided infraclavicular brachial plexus block. Br J Anaesth 2002;89:254–9.

[99] Sardesai AM, Chakrabarti AJ, Denny NM. Lower lobe collapse during continuous interscalene brachial plexus local anesthesia at home. Reg Anesth Pain Med 2004;29:65–8.

[100] Sarnoff SJ, Sarnoff LC. Prolonged peripheral nerve block by means of indwelling plastic catheter. Treatment of hiccup. Anesthesiology 1951;12:270–5.

[101] Schafhalter-Zoppoth I, McCulloch CE, Gray AT. Ultrasound visibility of needles used for regional nerve block: an in vitro study. Reg Anesth Pain Med 2004;29:480–8.

[102] Selander D. Catheter technique in axillary plexus block. Presentation of a new method. Acta Anaesthesiol Scand 1977;21:324–9.

[103] Singelyn FJ, Aye F, Gouverneur JM. Continuous popliteal sciatic nerve block: an original technique to provide postoperative analgesia after foot surgery. Anesth Analg 1997;84:383–6.

[104] Singelyn FJ, Deyaert M, Joris D, Pendeville E, Gouverneur JM. Effects of intravenous patient-controlled analgesia with morphine, continuous epidural analgesia, and continuous three-in-one block on postoperative pain and knee rehabilitation after unilateral total knee arthroplasty. Anesth Analg 1998;87:88–92.

[105] Singelyn FJ, Gouverneur JM. Postoperative analgesia after total hip arthroplasty: i.v. PCA with morphine, patient-controlled epidural analgesia, or continuous "3-in-1" block?: a prospective evaluation by our acute pain service in more than 1,300 patients. J Clin Anesth 1999;11:550–4.

[106] Singelyn FJ, Gouverneur JM. Extended "three-in-one" block after total knee arthroplasty: continuous versus patient-controlled techniques. Anesth Analg 2000;91:176–80.

[107] Singelyn FJ, Seguy S, Gouverneur JM. Interscalene brachial plexus analgesia after open shoulder surgery: continuous versus patient-controlled infusion. Anesth Analg 89 1999;1216–20.

[108] Singelyn FJ, Vanderelst PE, Gouverneur JM. Extended femoral nerve sheath block after total hip arthroplasty: continuous versus patient-controlled techniques. Anesth Analg 2001;92:455–9.

[109] Sites BD, Brull R, Chan VW, Spence BC, Gallagher J, Beach ML, Sites VR, Abbas S, Hartman GS. Artifacts and pitfall errors associated with ultrasound-guided regional anesthesia. Part II: a pictorial approach to understanding and avoidance. Reg Anesth Pain Med 2007;32:419–33.

[110] Sites BD, Spence BC, Gallagher JD, Wiley CW, Bertrand ML, Blike GT. Characterizing novice behavior associated with learning ultrasound-guided peripheral regional anesthesia. Reg Anesth Pain Med 2007;32:107–15.

[111] Souron V, Reiland Y, De Traverse A, Delaunay L, Lafosse L. Interpleural migration of an interscalene catheter. Anesth Analg 2003;97:1200–1.

[112] Steele SM, Klein SM, D'Ercole FJ, Greengrass RA, Gleason D. A new continuous catheter delivery system. Anesth Analg 1998;87:228.

[113] Swenson JD, Davis JJ, DeCou JA. A novel approach for assessing catheter position after ultrasound-guided placement of continuous interscalene block. Anesth Analg 2008;106:1015–6.

[114] Todd MM, Brown DL. Regional anesthesia and postoperative pain management: long-term benefits from a short-term intervention. Anesthesiology 1999;91:1–2.

[115] Tsui BC, Ozelsel TJ. Ultrasound-guided anterior sciatic nerve block using a longitudinal approach: "expanding the view". Reg Anesth Pain Med 2008;33:275–6.

[116] Tuominen M, Pitkanen M, Rosenberg PH. Postoperative pain relief and bupivacaine plasma levels during continuous interscalene brachial plexus block. Acta Anaesthesiol Scand 1987;31:276–8.

[117] Tuominen MK, Pere P, Rosenberg PH. Unintentional arterial catheterization and bupivacaine toxicity associated with continuous interscalene brachial plexus block. Anesthesiology 1991;75:356–8.

[118] van Geffen GJ, Gielen M. Ultrasound-guided subgluteal sciatic nerve blocks with stimulating catheters in children: a descriptive study. Anesth Analg 2006;103:328–33.

[119] Wajima Z, Nakajima Y, Kim C, Kobayashi N, Kadotani H, Adachi H, Inoue T, Ogawa R. IV compared with brachial plexus infusion of butorphanol for postoperative analgesia. Br J Anaesth 1995;74:392–5.

[120] Wajima Z, Shitara T, Nakajima Y, Kim C, Kobayashi N, Kadotani H, Adachi H, Ishikawa G, Kaneko K, Inoue T. Comparison of continuous brachial plexus infusion of butorphanol, mepivacaine and mepivacaine-butorphanol mixtures for postoperative analgesia. Br J Anaesth 1995;75:548–51.

[121] Watson MW, Mitra D, McLintock TC, Grant SA. Continuous versus single-injection lumbar plexus blocks: comparison of the effects on morphine use and early recovery after total knee arthroplasty. Reg Anesth Pain Med 2005;30:541–7.

[122] Weller RS, Gerancher JC, Crews JC, Wade KL. Extensive retroperitoneal hematoma without neurologic deficit in two patients who underwent lumbar plexus block and were later anticoagulated. Anesthesiology 2003;98:581–5.

[123] White PF, Issioui T, Skrivanek GD, Early JS, Wakefield C. The use of a continuous popliteal sciatic nerve block after surgery involving the foot and ankle: does it improve the quality of recovery? Anesth Analg 2003;97:1303–9.

Correspondence to: Brian M. Ilfeld, MD, MS (Clinical Investigation), Department of Anesthesiology, UCSD Center for Pain Medicine, 9300 Campus Point Dr, MC 7651, La Jolla, CA 92037-7651, USA. Email: bilfeld@ucsd.edu.

Part 14
Pain and Addiction: Optimizing Outcome, Reducing Risk

Pain and Addiction: Prevalence, Neurobiology, Definitions

Roman D. Jovey, MD

Medical Director, CPM Centres for Pain Management and Physician Director, Credit Valley Hospital,
Addiction and Concurrent Disorders Centre, Mississauga, Canada

Physicians, nurses, psychologists, and others frequently report that their training included little formal teaching about pain. There is little doubt that professional education about addiction lags even further behind, and that training on the pain addiction/interface is virtually non-existent. For the good of our patients and our communities, all prescribers of controlled substances need to have at least a fundamental knowledge of addiction medicine.

Chronic pain presents a significant burden to society in terms of lost workforce productivity and significant health care costs. For the individual, chronic pain significantly affects quality of life and overall functioning; comorbidities, particularly depression, are especially prevalent in chronic pain patients, resulting in a doubling of suicide rates compared to the general population. Chronic pain has traditionally been poorly managed, with large population surveys repeatedly demonstrating patient dissatisfaction. In the absence of more readily available interdisciplinary treatment resources, pain clinicians have used long-term opioid therapy for chronic pain management as part of the solution for this silent epidemic of undertreated pain.

The disease of addiction also presents a significant burden of illness to society and has also traditionally been under-recognized and undertreated. Unfortunately, in our well-intentioned desire to provide better pain management for patients with pain, clinicians have contributed, at least to some extent, to the growing problem of prescription analgesic abuse. Are there solutions that balance appropriate treatment for patients in pain against the serious public health implications of drug misuse and diversion?

For the clinical practice of pain management to make real progress, communication between the domains of pain medicine and addiction medicine is essential. It is equally incorrect to state that all patients with pain on long-term opioids are addicted as it is to say that no patient taking opioids for "legitimate" pain can develop an addiction to opioids. We need to replace rhetoric and opinion with science, knowledge, and reason. The pain management community needs to understand that all pain management goes on against a backdrop of our substance-abusing society (which goes far beyond opioids, to nicotine, cannabis, alcohol, and other licit and illicit drugs). Addiction specialists must accept that the use of opioids to treat chronic pain is an evidence-based practice, and must assist pain clinicians with the management of complex patients with both problems.

Meanwhile, the education of pain specialists in principles of addiction medicine is essential in order to optimize outcomes for patients suffering from chronic pain. Training should include techniques for screening and risk stratification of individual patients, along with a range of tailored management strategies to deliver opioid therapy in the safest way possible for each individual. A physician treating a patient who is suffering from intractable noncancer pain is always faced with following the core guiding principles of our profession: cure when possible, give comfort always, but above all, do no harm.

Concerns Regarding Iatrogenic Opioid Addiction: Historical Basis

In deciding whether or not to offer a patient with chronic noncancer pain a trial of long-term opioid therapy, clinicians are concerned about the possibility of contributing to iatrogenic opioid addiction. Is there a scientific basis for this fear?

In a study published in 1925, and another in 1954, between 9% and 27% of white male opioid addicts reported that their addiction started with a prescription from a doctor for an opioid analgesic to treat a painful condition [20,28]. Asking an identified addict population, who often demonstrate significant levels of denial, how they began their addiction is inviting a rationalizing and blaming response. Most importantly, however, the denominator in these studies was missing. The researchers did not ask the following question: How many patients prescribed opioids for a painful condition did *not* develop an addiction to their opioids? In a similar study of 58 patients, the authors warn physicians that: "severe oral opioid dependence occurs more frequently than previously recognized" [7]. Yet this paper did not discuss an estimated incidence or prevalence and therefore also did not address the denominator issue. Millions of patients worldwide are regularly exposed to opioid analgesics for the treatment of pain.

What Is the Estimated Overall Rate of Substance Abuse/Dependence in the Population?

The most recent results from the 2008 National Survey on Drug Use and Health (NSDUH), an annual American population survey of over 67,000 people, estimated that 8.9% of the population aged 12 or older were classified with substance dependence or abuse in the past year based on criteria specified in the American Psychiatric Association's *Diagnostic and Statistical Manual of Mental Disorders,* 4th edition (DSM-IV). The survey further reported an 8% prevalence of any illicit drug use in the past month, a 1.9% prevalence rate for misuse of any prescription opioid in the past month, and a 0.7% prevalence rate for opioid abuse or dependence in the past year [32].

These percentages were stable from 2002 to 2008, and, in fact, the misuse of prescription opioids by people aged 17–25 has declined over this same time period [32].

Previous studies have found that substance use disorders (SUDs) are common among inpatients of general medical hospitals. A study using standardized diagnostic instruments to measure current and lifetime alcohol and other drug abuse or dependence among a sample of 363 inpatients on general medical, general surgical, and orthopedic wards of a university hospital reported a current and lifetime prevalence rate of SUDs of 22% and 50%, respectively. The prevalence rates of current problems with alcohol alone, other drugs alone, and both alcohol and other drugs were 16%, 2.5%, and 3%, respectively. Males in this study had a current SUD rate of almost 30% [6].

Is the Prevalence of Substance Use Disorders Higher in Patients with Chronic Pain?

Older surveys from chronic pain clinics quoted prevalence rates of addiction among their patients from a low of 3% up to a high of 27% [12,15,8]. However many of these older studies used nonstandardized definitions or relied on physiological criteria to diagnose addiction.

In a systematic review of the use of opioids to treat chronic back pain, the authors reported a prevalence of aberrant medication-taking behaviors ranging from 5% to 24% [24]. Only one of the seven studies reviewed had an acceptable quality score, and this study is discussed in more detail below. Studies were not explicit in separating iatrogenic opioid dependence from preexisting substance use disorders and did not account for behaviors related to inadequately treated pain.

The only high-quality prospective study in the above review was conducted in a community family practice clinic, comparing a group of patients with chronic severe low back pain with a control group attending for other reasons. The study used standardized and validated diagnostic instruments and definitions of substance abuse and dependence. The lifetime prevalence for any SUD was 52–54%, the current prevalence of SUD was 23%, and the lifetime prevalence of prescription opioid abuse was 13–15%. The authors found no significant difference in the prevalence rates of SUD among patients with severe chronic back pain versus controls. They concluded that the presence of severe chronic back pain does not appear to be associated with an increased risk for substance abuse in general, or with prescribed opioid abuse in particular [5].

Another study recruited 801 adults receiving daily opioid therapy from 235 primary care practices in six health care systems in Wisconsin. The point prevalence of current substance abuse and/or dependence using DSM-IV criteria in the past 30 days was 9.7%. The prevalence of opioid use disorder in this study was 3.8%. A logistic regression model found that increased risk for opioid abuse was associated with age between 18 and 30 years (odds ratio [OR] = 6.17), severity of lifetime psychiatric disorders (OR = 6.17), a positive toxicology test for cocaine (OR = 5.92) or marijuana (OR = 3.52), and four or more aberrant drug-related behaviors (OR = 11.48). In this study, opioid use disorders were noted to be four-times higher in patients receiving opioid therapy compared with general population samples (3.8% versus 0.9%) [13].

In a 2009 structured evidence-based review of available published studies of patients on chronic opioid agonist therapy (COAT), Fishbain et al. [11] noted that 3.3% of patients on COAT manifested behaviors consistent with substance "abuse" or "addiction." In studies of COAT that excluded patients with a current or past history of a SUD, this rate was only 0.2%. An average of 11.5% of patients demonstrated one or more aberrant drug-related behaviors, but in those without a history of SUD, this rate was only 0.6%. In a subset of five studies using urine drug testing that did not exclude high-risk patients, 20.4% of patients had no detectable prescribed opioid in their urine, whereas 14.5% had an illicit substance detected.

A 2010 Cochrane review of long-term opioid therapy for chronic noncancer pain found that in those studies specifically reporting on this outcome, signs of opioid addiction were found in only 0.3% of study patients. These studies typically excluded patients with a past history of SUD [27].

Is the Prevalence of Chronic Pain Higher in Patients with Addiction Disorders?

A study of 248 patients attending a methadone maintenance treatment program (MMTP) found that 61.3% complained of a chronic pain problem [16]. Compared with patients without pain, those with pain reported significantly more health problems, more psychiatric disturbance, more prescription and nonprescription drug use, and greater belief that they were undertreated. In another study, pain of any type or duration during the past week was reported by 80% of outpatient MMTP patients and by 78% of patients attending inpatient addiction treatment programs. Chronic severe pain was reported by 37% of MMTP patients and by 24% of inpatients. Among those with chronic severe pain, 65% of MMTP patients and 48% of inpatients reported high levels of pain-related interference in physical and psychosocial functioning. Among those with chronic severe pain, inpatients were significantly more likely than MMTP patients to have used illicit drugs, as well as alcohol, to treat their pain complaint but were less likely to have been prescribed pain medications [30].

Where does this conflicting evidence leave the pain clinician? It appears that the overall prevalence of substance abuse or dependence in the population is approximately 10%, with a prevalence of prescription opioid dependence of less than 1%. The few studies available on prevalence of substance abuse/dependence in patients with chronic pain have conflicting results. Patients with chronic pain will at least be similar to the general population and at worst have 2–4 times the risk of opioid use disorders. However, even in the latter case, fewer than one in 10 pain patients will have a concurrent abuse/addiction problem. A patient addicted to one mood-modifying substance is more likely to become cross-addicted to another. Based on the Fishbain [11] and Cochrane [27] reviews, at least in low-risk patients, the risk of developing iatrogenic opioid addiction due to the prescribing of opioids for pain appears to be low.

Therefore, physicians treating patients with chronic noncancer pain with opioid analgesics need to be able to screen patients for addiction risk. This is not necessarily to deny patients with a past history of SUD a trial of opioid therapy, but rather to identify those at higher risk for more careful assessment and closer monitoring. To do so effectively, it is helpful to understand some fundamental concepts of the addictive process.

The Neurochemistry of Addiction

Addiction begins as a disorder of brain reward centers, which exist to ensure survival of the organism and species. Reward centers have evolved to grab our attention, dominate motivation, and compel behavior toward survival even in the presence of danger. Eating, sex, social interaction, and unexpected novel stimuli activate these reward circuits under normal circumstances. All of the usual drugs of abuse have an ability to turn on reward circuits to a much greater extent for a longer period of time than natural stimuli. By activating and dysregulating endogenous reward centers, addictive drugs hijack brain circuits that take over behavior, leading to progressive loss of control over drug intake in spite of medical, emotional, interpersonal, occupational, and legal consequences.

The mesolimbic reward pathway connects the ventral tegmental area (VTA) with the nucleus accumbens, the amygdala, hippocampus, hypothalamus, and prefrontal cortex. Some of these areas are part of the brain's conventional memory-processing system. Increasing evidence suggests that important aspects of the addictive process may involve powerful emotional memories. Dopamine is released in the VTA and nucleus accumbens in response to rewarding drugs, and it appears to influence the motivational state of wanting or expectation. The persistent release of dopamine as a result of chronic drug use eventually results in a reduction in dopamine release in response to drug use (tolerance), requiring higher drug doses for effect, progressively recruits limbic brain regions and the prefrontal cortex, and "programs" drug cues via glutamatergic mechanisms [26]. Another circuit involving the amygdala, anterior cingulate, orbitofrontal cortex, and dorsolateral prefrontal cortex contributes to the obsessive craving for drugs. Persistent dopamine release results in the formation of the protein cyclic adenosine monophosphate (cAMP) response element-binding protein (CREB) which dampens reward circuitry in the nucleus accumbens, and ΔFosB, which causes prolonged sensitization of reward pathways to reexposure to drugs. Thus the abstinent, addicted brain can be triggered to return to compulsive drug use via a single exposure to a drug, contextual drug cues, craving, or stress—each originating in a relatively distinct brain region or neural pathway [1]. The compulsion to use drugs is complemented by deficits in impulse control and decision-making mediated by glutamate-based circuits in the orbitofrontal cortex and anterior cingulate gyrus [21].

Laboratory animals can be bred to exhibit greater and lesser sensitivity in parts of the reward pathway, with a correspondingly greater or lesser propensity to develop addictive behaviors to chemicals of abuse [22,25]. It is therefore equally likely that certain humans are also born with a greater or lesser sensitivity in the reward pathways. Some people are probably genetically "wired" to be at increased risk for developing an addictive disorder.

Based on results from the 2008 NSDUH, regular heroin users make up only 0.2% of the total population. They tend to cluster in the core of larger cities or transportation hubs that serve as importation and distribution sites for illicit drugs. Some researchers believe that these predisposed individuals may be using illicit opioids to fill some type of neurochemical deficit in their brain chemistry. Unfortunately, the repetitive use of a rapidly absorbed, short-acting opioid such as heroin by intermittent, intravenous bolus dosing not only contributes to devastating secondary causes of morbidity and mortality, but also causes disruption in other central nervous system (CNS) neurochemical processes, such as the hypothalamic-pituitary-adrenal axis. Opioid agonist therapy with methadone or buprenorphine is therefore not simply the substitution of one safer addicting drug for another. Rather, it may serve to stabilize some aspect of deficient brain chemistry in these predisposed individuals [23].

Fig. 1 illustrates a suggested simplified model of the contributors to the addictive process. To be sure, an individual requires the presence of an addicting substance or behavior to develop an addictive disorder, but other risk factors are also required. Certain mental health problems such as bipolar disorder, attention deficit hyperactivity disorder, schizophrenia, and antisocial and psychopathic personality disorders are associated with an increased risk of comorbid addictive disorders [29]. Certain psychological traits such as extreme shyness, borderline personality tendencies, an anxiety-prone personality, poor stress-coping capabilities, and alexithymia (difficulty in cognitively evaluating one's emotional state) may increase the risk. Environment can also be important. A past history of physical, sexual, or emotional trauma increases the risk of future substance misuse. Similarly, a child growing up in a family where alcohol or sedative abuse is the main method of coping with life stresses may mimic this behavior as an adult [18]. Environment and personality may play a major role in the recovery process from addiction. However, the basic science and clinical research discussed above is increasingly identifying the altered neurochemistry of biogenetically predisposed individuals as having the primary role in the development of

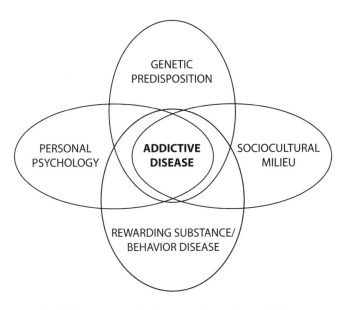

Fig. 1. The etiology of addiction: a biopsychosocial illness.

addictive disorders. As we continue to learn more about brain chemistry, it may turn out, after all, that addicts are born, not made.

The Overlap between Pain and Addiction Neurobiology

Certain regions of the brain, such as the nucleus accumbens and anterior cingulate gyrus, are involved in both pain and addiction. Aversive stimuli, such as noxious thermal stimuli (46°C), produce significant signal changes in reward circuitry as well as in classic pain circuitry, suggesting that there may be a shared neural system for evaluation of both aversive and rewarding stimuli [4]. Both chronic pain and addiction involve sensitization and synaptic plasticity, which alters the response of a nerve circuit to sensory input, including painful stimuli. This process involves glutamate, α-amino-3-hydroxy-5-methyl-4-isoxazolepropionic acid (AMPA) and N-methyl-D-aspartate (NMDA) receptors, similar to the process responsible for long-term memory formation in the hippocampus [17]. Both cocaine- and opioid-addicted people show decreased cold pressor pain tolerance, which may respond to gabapentin [9,10]. In some circumstances, the regular use of opioids can result in opioid hyperalgesia, an increased sensitivity to pain [3]. In acute pain models, some addictive responses to opioids, such as euphoria and physical withdrawal, are reduced [33,35]. Finally, normal and pathological pain circuitry involves various endogenous opioids and cannabinoids, also important in addiction pathways [14].

The initial presentation of patients with addictive disease and those with chronic pain syndromes can be strikingly similar, despite their different focus (compulsive drug use versus experience of pain). Both groups of patients may develop widespread systems dysfunction, including sleep disturbance, mood disturbance, anhedonia, chronic fatigue, pharmacological drug dependence, dysfunction in multiple life roles (work, relationships, and recreation), an increase in life stressors, and inability to cope with stress. When pain and addiction occur together, they may act as mutually reinforcing conditions. Undetected or untreated addiction to prescribed opioids or to street drugs or alcohol may exacerbate the experience of pain and may undermine both compliance with and responses to treatment. Untreated or ineffectively treated pain may make a commitment to recovery from addiction difficult, by perpetuating addictive use of prescribed medications, or street drugs or alcohol, in an attempt to find relief. Thus, the identification and management of a concurrent addictive disorder is important to the safe and effective treatment of pain.

Defining Opioid Addiction in the Patient with Pain

Under the current classification system for psychiatric illness, DSM-IV (TR), the term "substance dependence" continues to be used instead of the term "addiction." When DSM-IIIR was developed, this change in terminology was partly a well-meaning attempt to decrease the stigma attached to the term "addict." However, it has resulted in a less precise definition, especially when referring to substances with a therapeutic use such as opioids. Under DSM-IV, three out of seven of the defining criteria for "opioid dependence" rely on symptoms related to tolerance, physical dependence, and withdrawal [2]. These criteria may be quite appropriate for alcohol abuse or illicit heroin use, but they are not appropriate when the drug in question is prescribed for a therapeutic purpose. It is hoped that this confusion will be corrected with the publication of DSM-V.

In the meantime, the Liaison Committee on Pain and Addiction (LCPA) of the American Academy of Pain Medicine (AAPM), the American Pain Society (APS), and the American Society of Addiction Medicine (ASAM) endorsed and published a consensus document in 2001, which includes a set of more appropriate and clinically useful definitions for assessing the use of opioids in the context of pain treatment [31]:

Physical dependence "is a state of adaptation that often includes tolerance and is manifested by a drug class-specific withdrawal syndrome that can be produced by abrupt cessation, rapid dose reduction, decreasing blood level of the drug, and/or administration of an antagonist." Physical dependence on opioids is an expected physiological response in most individuals in the presence of continuous opioid use for therapeutic or nontherapeutic purposes. It may develop in as short a period as 7–10 days. The area of the brain where physical dependence is thought to occur is anatomically and functionally separate from the brain pathways that are known to be related to reward. Therefore, physical dependence on opioids is not, by itself, diagnostic of addiction.

Tolerance "is a state of adaptation in which exposure to a drug induces changes that result in a diminution of one or more of the drug's effects over time." With steady-state dosing, tolerance to most of the unwanted opioid side effects, such as respiratory depression, sedation, and nausea, occurs readily and is a welcome phenomenon. However, some patients may also develop tolerance to the analgesic effects of opioids, indicated by the need for increasing or more frequent doses of the medication to maintain analgesic effect. The regions of the CNS involved in tolerance to analgesia are also anatomically and functionally separate from the reward pathways. The occurrence of tolerance to opioids, in and of itself, does not imply addiction.

Addiction "is a primary, chronic, neurobiological disease, with genetic, psychosocial, and environmental factors influencing its development and manifestations. It is characterized by behaviors that include one or more of the following (also known as the "4 C's"):

(1) Impaired <u>C</u>ontrol over drug use, (2) <u>C</u>ompulsive use, (3) Continued use despite harm (<u>C</u>onsequences), (4) <u>C</u>raving." *Impaired control* over the use of opioids might be reflected in multiple episodes of requests for early prescription refills, "double doctoring," or using street sources of opioids or other drugs. *Compulsive preoccupation with obtaining opioids*, despite the presence of adequate analgesia, may be reflected in noncompliance with nonopioid components of pain treatment, inability to acknowledge psychosocial contributors to pain, and the perception that no interventions other than opioids have any impact on pain and

suffering. *Consequences* associated with the use of opioids may include persistent oversedation or euphoria, deteriorating levels of function despite relief of pain, or an increase in pain-associated distresses such as anxiety, sleep disturbance, or depressive symptoms. Common and expected medication side effects, such as constipation, should not be interpreted as adverse consequences in this context. *Craving* is an intense desire to use a substance for its psychoactive effect.

These phenomena may be accompanied by distortions in thought, chiefly denial, and a tendency to relapse once in recovery. Physical dependence and/or tolerance may, or may not, be present in addiction. "It should be emphasized that no single event is diagnostic of addictive disorder. Rather, the diagnosis is made in response to a pattern of behavior that usually becomes obvious over time."

Pseudoaddiction is a phenomenon first reported in the cancer pain literature [34]. Individuals with severe, unrelieved pain may become intensely focused on finding relief for that pain. Such patients may appear to be preoccupied with obtaining opioids, but the preoccupation is with finding pain relief, rather than with the use of opioids per se. Such therapeutic preoccupation can be distinguished from true addiction by observing that when effective analgesia is obtained, by whatever means, the previous behaviors, which may have suggested addiction, resolve. Controversy continues over the use of the term "pseudoaddiction" [19]. There is a risk that clinicians can misinterpret true addictive behaviors as pseudoaddiction. If medications are being used appropriately for pain treatment, the patient will not use opioids in a manner that persistently causes sedation or euphoria, level of function is increased rather than decreased, and medications are used as prescribed without loss of control over use.

To summarize, SUDs affect about 10% of the general population. Based on very limited high-quality published data, patients with chronic pain either have the same or a somewhat higher risk of concurrent substance abuse or addiction. The development of addiction requires not only repeated exposure to a potentially addicting substance or behavior, but an individual with a particular biopsychogenetic vulnerability living in a particular social milieu. Without the presence of these risk factors, the risk that a physician can "create" an addict de novo from an opioid-naive patient by prescribing opioids for pain appears to be low. Due to sensitized reward pathways in the brain, there is a high risk of cross-addiction to opioids in patients with previous addiction to other substances. Therefore, physicians can certainly enable the "rekindling" of a previous addictive disorder by failing to screen patients for risk factors, or by ignoring the early symptoms and signs of a developing addiction to prescribed opioids. It is important to use appropriate terminology when discussing patients with pain on therapeutic opioids in order clarify communication among health professionals and reduce stigma for patients.

References

[1] Adinoff B. Neurobiologic processes in drug reward and addiction. Harv Rev Psychiatry 2004;12:305–20.

[2] American Psychiatric Association. Diagnostic and statistical manual of mental disorders, 4th ed. Washington, DC: American Psychiatric Association; 1994.

[3] Bannister K, Dickenson AH. Opioid hyperalgesia. Curr Opin Support Palliat Care 2010;4:1–5.

[4] Becerra L, Breiter HC, Wise R, Gonzalez RG, Borsook D. Reward circuitry activation by noxious thermal stimuli. Neuron 2001;32:927–46.

[5] Brown RL, Fleming MF, Patterson JJ. Chronic opioid analgesic therapy for chronic low back pain. J Am Board Fam Pract 1996;9:191–204.

[6] Brown RL, Leonard T, Saunders LA, Papasouliotis O. The prevalence and detection of substance use disorders among inpatients ages 18 to 49: an opportunity for prevention. Prev Med 1998;27:101–10.

[7] Busto UE, Sproule BA, Knight K, Romach MK, Sellers EM. Severe dependence on oral opioids. Can J Clin Pharmacol 1998; 5: 23–8.

[8] Chabal C, Erjavec MK, Jacobson L, Mariano A, Chaney E. Prescription opiate abuse in chronic pain patients: clinical criteria, incidence, and predictors. Clin J Pain1997;13:150–5.

[9] Compton P, Charuvastra VC, Kintaudi K, Ling W. Pain responses in methadone-maintained opioid abusers. J Pain Symptom Manage 2000;20:237–45.

[10] Compton P, Kehoe P, Sinha K, Torrington MA, Ling W. Gabapentin improves cold-pressor pain responses in methadone-maintained patients. Drug Alcohol Depend 2010; Epub Feb 15.

[11] Fishbain DA, Cole B, Lewis J, Rosomoff HL, Rosomoff RS. What percentage of chronic nonmalignant pain patients exposed to chronic opioid analgesic therapy develop abuse/addiction and/or aberrant drug-related behaviors? A structured evidence-based review. Pain Med 2008;9:444-59.

[12] Fishbain DA, Rosomoff HL, Rosomoff RS. Drug abuse, dependence, and addiction in chronic pain patients. Clin J Pain. 1992;8:77–85.

[13] Fleming MF, Balousek SL, Klessig CL, Mundt MP, Brown DD. Substance use disorders in a primary care sample receiving daily opioid therapy. J Pain 2007;8:573–82.

[14] Gardner EL. Endocannabinoid signaling system and brain reward: emphasis on dopamine. Pharmacol Biochem Behav. 2005;81:263–84.

[15] Hoffman N, Olofsson O. Prevalence of abuse and dependency in chronic pain patients. Int J Addictions 1995;30:919–27.

[16] Jamison RN, Kauffman J, Katz NP. Characteristics of methadone maintenance patients with chronic pain. J Pain Symptom Manage 2000;19:53–62.

[17] Ji RR, Kohno T, Moore KA, Woolf CJ. Central sensitization and LTP: do pain and memory share similar mechanisms? Trends Neurosci 2003;26:696–705.

[18] Johnson B, Muffler J. Sociocultural. In: Lowinson J, Ruiz P, Millman R, Langrod J, editors. Substance abuse, 3rd ed. Philadelphia: Williams and Wilkins; 1997. p. 107–18.

[19] Kirsh KL, Whitcomb LA, Donaghy K, Passik SD. Abuse and addiction issues in medically ill patients with pain: attempts at clarification of terms and empirical study. Clin J Pain. 2002;18(4 Suppl):S52–60.

[20] Kolb L. Types and characteristics of drug addicts. Ment Hyg 1925;9:300.

[21] Koob GF, Volkow ND. Neurocircuitry of addiction. Neuropsychopharmacology 2010;35:217–38.

[22] Koob GF. The neurobiology of addiction: a neuroadaptational review relevant for diagnosis. Addiction 2006;101(Suppl 1):23–30.

[23] Kreek MJ. Opiates, opioids and addiction. Mol Psychiatry 1996;1:232–54.

[24] Martell BA, O'Connor PG, Kerns RD, Becker WC, Morales KH, Kosten TR, Fiellin DA. Systematic review: opioid treatment for chronic back pain: prevalence, efficacy, and association with addiction. Ann Intern Med 2007;146:116–27.

[25] Nestler EJ. Genes and addiction. Nat Genet 2000; 26:277–81.

[26] Nestler EJ. Is there a common molecular pathway for addiction? Nat Neurosci 2006;8:1445–9.

[27] Noble M, Treadwell JR, Tregear SJ, Coates VH, Wiffen PJ, Akafomo C, Schoelles KM. Long-term opioid management for chronic noncancer pain. Cochrane Database Syst Rev 2010;1:CD006605.

[28] Rayport M. Experience in the management of patients medically addicted to narcotics. JAMA 1954;165:684–91.

[29] Regier DA, Myers JK, Kramer M, Robins LN, Blazer DG, Hough RL, Eaton WW, Locke BZ. The NIMH Epidemiologic Catchment Area program. Historical context, major objectives, and study population characteristics. Arch Gen Psychiatry 1984;41:934–41.

[30] Rosenblum A, Joseph H, Fong C, Kipnis S, Cleland C, Portenoy RK. Prevalence and characteristics of chronic pain among chemically dependent patients in methadone maintenance and residential treatment facilities. JAMA. 2003;289:2370–8.

[31] Savage SR, Joranson DE, Covington EC, Schnoll SH, Heit HA, Gilson AM. Definitions related to the medical use of opioids: evolution towards universal agreement. J Pain Symptom Manage 2003;26:655–67.

[32] Substance Abuse and Mental Health Services Administration. Results from the 2008 National Survey on Drug Use and Health: national findings. Office of Applied Studies, NSDUH Series H-36, HHS Publication No. SMA 09-4434. Rockville, MD; 2009. Available at: www.oas.samhsa.gov/nsduh/2k8nsduh/2k8Results.cfm. Accessed Feb 28, 2010.

[33] Vaccarino AL, Marek P, Kest B, Ben-Eliyahu S, Couret LC Jr, Kao B, Liebeskind JC. Morphine fails to produce tolerance when administered in the presence of formalin pain in rats. Brain Res 1993;627:287–90.

[34] Weissman DE, Haddox JD. Opioid pseudoaddiction--an iatrogenic syndrome. Pain 1989;36:363–6.

[35] Zacny JP, McKay MA, Toledano AY, Marks S, Young CJ, Klock PA, Apfelbaum JL. The effects of a cold-water immersion stressor on the reinforcing and subjective effects of fentanyl in healthy volunteers. Drug Alcohol Depend 1996;42:133–42.

Correspondence to: Roman D. Jovey, MD, Medical Director, CPM Centres for Pain Management, 6400 Millcreek Drive, Unit 9, Mississauga, ON L5N 3E7, Canada. Fax: 905-858-2144; email: drjovey@sympatico.ca

Identifying and Addressing Risks for Opioid Misuse in Opioid Therapy of Pain

32

Seddon R. Savage, MD, MS

*Dartmouth Center on Addiction Recovery and Education; Manchester VA Medical Center, Manchester, New Hampshire;
Department of Anesthesiology, Dartmouth Medical School, Hanover, New Hampshire, USA*

Over the past several decades, the use of opioids for the treatment of pain—including acute pain, cancer-related pain, and chronic nonterminal pain—has increased significantly as pain treatment has become a higher priority in society. Expanding therapeutic use of opioids has been paralleled by expanding nonmedical use [22]. The 2006 National Survey on Drug Use and Health (NSDUH) found that 13.6% of Americans reported lifetime nonmedical use of opioids, and 5.1% and 2.1% reported nonmedical use in the past year or past month, respectively [36]. Misuse of opioids has resulted in increasing emergency department visits related to prescription opioids [12] and increased admissions for treatment of prescription opioid addiction (rising between 1992 and 2007 from 0.9% to 5% of addiction treatment requests nationally at federally funded treatment centers and from 1.1% to 20% in West Virginia, a region rife with prescription opioid abuse) [35]. It also has led to increased involvement of opioid medications in overdose drug deaths [21].

To improve the clinical safety and efficacy of prescribed opioids and to prevent diversion and misuse, it is important that clinicians appreciate various subtypes of misuse and be able to identify patients at risk for misuse and apply management strategies that reduce risk.

Types of Opioid Misuse

In order to prevent and address misuse, it is important to consider the diverse motivations that may lead to misuse. There is little epidemiological information on the relative distribution of reasons for misuse [47]; however, among the recognized motivators of misuse are self-medication of symptoms, elective use to produce reward or euphoria, compulsive use due to addiction, and diversion for profit.

Self-Medication of Non-Pain Symptoms

In addition to their indicated clinical uses in the treatment of pain, addiction, cough, and diarrhea, opioids may produce other effects that some individuals may experience as therapeutic: sedation may help to induce sleep or blunt anxiety, euphoria may elevate depressive symptoms [3], and the impact of traumatic memories may be modulated [32]. Therefore, people with access to opioids—either clinically prescribed or through street sources—may use them to self-medicate diverse symptoms. More specific, effective, and longitudinally appropriate treatments are usually preferred; however, when such effects accompany legitimate treatment and are resonant with the goals of therapy, they may be perceived as beneficial side effects. The risks of self-medication include the potential for unsafe dosing and for ignoring more effective treatments. Theoretically, the reinforcing effects of opioids may result in increased symptoms, increased medication use, alternating periods of relief and withdrawal, and enhanced vulnerability to addiction [1,20].

Self-Medication of Pain

Much of the nonmedical use of opioids in the general population may in fact reflect self-medication of pain. A recent Internet survey of more than 3,500 college students found that 13.9% reported lifetime use and 7.2% reported past-year use of opioid medications that were not prescribed for them. Among lifetime users, 42.4% reported use only to relieve pain, 23.9% reported use to get high, and 33.9% reported mixed self-treatment and recreational use [24].

Patients for whom opioids are prescribed for pain may use them in higher doses than prescribed to self-medicate their pain. Patients are usually advised to titrate opioids only with supervision of their prescribing clinician. Repeated episodes of self-initiated titration may indicate an emerging opioid use disorder. However, there are several reasons that patients may require higher-than-anticipated doses of opioids to achieve analgesia, and some patients may auto-titrate doses if clinicians do not recognize and accommodate these circumstances.

Analgesic dose requirements for the same pain generator may vary widely between individuals based on genetic and other influences [30]. Neuropathic pain may shift the opioid dose-response curve such that higher dose of opioids are required to achieve the same level of analgesia than in non-neuropathic pain [10]. Tolerance may occur over time, with some individuals developing tolerance more rapidly than others. Finally, some patients appear to develop increasing generalized pain or painful hypersensitivity (allodynia) that may be caused by opioids. Opioid-induced hyperalgesia is suggested by the observation of increasing nonfocal or more diffuse pain and hypersensitivity with diminishing duration and intensity of analgesic responses, in the absence of apparent progression of pathology [9]. Patients may feel driven to increase their medication doses with the hope of attenuating the increasing pain.

Emerging evidence suggests that hyperalgesia, progressive tolerance, medication use problems, and/or generally diminishing returns are more common with higher-dose opioids, which some experts define as greater than the analgesic equivalent of 200 mg of morphine per day [7]. Therefore, when opioid dose requirements appear to be climbing beyond this level in persons with chronic noncancer pain and stable pathology, some clinicians recommend rotating to a new opioid at somewhat lower equianalgesic doses to avoid or address tolerance or hyperalgesia [33]. As incomplete cross-tolerance usually occurs with a new opioid, better analgesia at lower doses of the new drug may occur.

Using this technique, some patients can be managed by rotating as needed between moderate doses of different opioids [39]. Alternatively, some patients with escalating pain in the context of stable pathology appear to experience improved analgesia by simply tapering opioid doses, possibly due to the reversal of hyperalgesic mechanisms [40].

Despite these concerns, some patients clearly benefit from opioid doses well above 200 mg of morphine equivalents per day, so clinical judgment must be used to determine whether to rotate, taper, maintain, or increase the dose. Stability of pain relief in response to dose increase, the focal versus generalized nature of the pain, and the overall well-being and function of the patient must be considered in decision making. Special care is indicated in monitoring patients who require higher-than-usual doses of opioids.

Use for Reward

Opioids induce euphoria (reward) in some, but not all, individuals, and some who experience reward may use opioids electively to get high. Genetics shapes individual responses to opioids, including analgesic responses, reward, and side effects [19]. It is clear that different opioids (e.g., morphine, oxycodone, methadone, fentanyl, and hydrocodone) variably affect different opioid receptor subtypes and that different individuals vary in their expression of these subtypes and thus may respond differently to different medications [34]. It is conceivable that someday, through genetic profiling, clinicians will be able to match opioids to individual patients based on prospective identification of relative analgesia and reward effects [43].

Diversion

Diversion of opioids from their intended therapeutic track may occur in a variety of ways. Preclinical diversion may occur through theft at manufacturing plants, in transit, or from pharmacies [18]. Pharmacists, physicians, or other healthcare professionals may sell, trade, or misuse medications. Postclinical diversion occurs when patients share, sell, or misuse medications they have been prescribed or when medications are stolen from them. Some diversion may seem relatively innocent (e.g., a patient sharing medication left over from surgery with a spouse for an acute pain problem) or clearly criminal (e.g., a "doctor shopper" feigning pain to obtain opioids to sell for profit); however, all diversion risks harmful consequences.

The 2006 NSDUH study found that among individuals who reported nonmedical use of opioids, 70.5% obtained opioids from friends or relatives, 19.1% had prescriptions from one doctor, 1.6% had prescriptions from more than one doctor, 3.9% obtained them from a dealer or stranger, and 0.1% acquired them via the Internet. Of those who obtained opioids from friends or relatives, 80.7% believed their sources obtained opioids from one doctor, and 3.3% from more than one doctor [36]. This information suggests that about 20% of those who use opioids nonmedically receive them directly themselves as patients, but that patients (with or without their knowledge) are a major source of diverted opioids.

Clinical Presentation of Opioid Misuse

Opioid misuse may present in diverse, aberrant drug-related behaviors such as requests for early renewals, reports of lost or stolen prescriptions, observable intoxication or withdrawal, demanding behaviors, or a failure to respond to treatment. Identified aberrant drug-related behaviors merit careful assessment to identify and appropriately address their cause. With the exception of diversion for profit, misuse most often reflects co-occurring clinical problems that require further clinical attention.

Predictors of Risk for Prescription Opioid Misuse, Abuse, and Addiction

Comorbidity of Chronic Pain, Substance Use Disorders, and Mental Health Conditions

Chronic pain frequently co-occurs with psychological conditions, including anxiety, depression, and posttraumatic stress disorder. In turn, these conditions have a high co-occurrence with substance use disorders (SUDs). The convergence of psychological comorbidities with chronic pain and SUDs suggests a potentially high risk among chronic pain patients for misuse of prescribed opioids directed at self-medication or use for reward or due to addiction. Individuals presenting for substance abuse treatment have a relatively high prevalence of chronic pain. As noted previously, however, the actual prevalence of opioid misuse, abuse, and addiction in individuals prescribed opioids for chronic noncancer pain appears to be relatively low. It may be that clinicians prescribe opioids less frequently to people with substance use or mental health conditions.

Some evidence suggests that opioid reward is reduced in the presence of pain [28,48], which may reduce risks of misuse to some degree. Nonetheless, a subset of chronic pain patients prescribed opioids do misuse opioids, and several recent studies have attempted to characterize who is at risk.

Prescription Opioid Misuse and Mental Health Conditions

A 2009 analysis of the 2002 National Epidemiologic Study of Alcohol and Related Conditions, a survey of more than 40,000 people, found that mood disorders (including a spectrum of depressive and anxiety disorders) were associated with an elevated risk for prescription opioid misuse and supported a self-medication model of misuse [23]. The same study also found that individuals who misused opioids had an increased risk of developing mood disorders in the absence of preexisting comorbidity.

An analysis of the 2003 NSDUH study found that individuals with any co-occurring mental health conditions had twice the risk for initiation of non-medical use of opioids, and those with depressed feelings for two or more weeks had 2.5 times the risk of those with no co-occurring condition [11]. The NSDUH study also found that any lifetime use of marijuana, cocaine, or heroin was associated with increased likelihood of nonmedical use of prescription opioids and that whites had twice the likelihood of African Americans.

A recent study of patients presenting to an emergency department for a renewal of opioids found that trait anxiety and panic disorder, as assessed using five validated self-report instruments and a structured clinical interview, correlated with a positive screen for risk of opioid misuse using a validated instrument [45].

Prescription Opioid Misuse and Co-occurring Substance Use Disorders

Mounting evidence supports history of an SUD as a major risk factor for misuse of prescription opioids. A study of longitudinal administrative data on 15,160 veterans found a history of an SUD to be a strong predictor of opioid misuse, and a co-occurring mental health disorder to be a moderately strong predictor of recognized prescription opioid abuse or dependence. Because mental health disorders were more prevalent (45.3% versus 7.6%), they accounted for greater attributable risk in the population than history of an SUD [13]. A more-controlled study of 127 veterans prescribed opioids in a primary care setting found that patients with a history of an SUD were three to six times more likely to misuse opioid medications than patients without such a history [27].

One study found that younger age, a history of alcohol abuse or current marijuana or cocaine use, and a history of legal problems with alcohol or drugs increased the risk of prescription opioid misuse [17], and another study found that individuals with evidence of cocaine use were much less likely to resolve opioid misuse in a structured prescribing program than other patients [25].

A recent study found that individuals seeking treatment for prescription opioid addiction were more likely to recall reward effects on their first exposure to opioids than a control group of chronic pain patients on long-term opioid treatment who did not develop addiction [4]. Another identified craving for medication as a predictor of prescribed opioid misuse [41]. These studies support a perception that an inherent vulnerability in the limbic reward system may drive prescribed opioid misuse.

Taken in aggregate, these studies support expectations that individuals with some mental health disorders, preexisting SUDs, and/or substance-related legal problems may be at higher risk for prescription opioid misuse. Two recent reviews of evidence related to prediction of opioid misuse risk generally supported these conclusions; however, both noted that available evidence is limited, that studies could not always determine whether SUDs or mental health conditions preceded or were a consequence of chronic pain and opioid treatment, and that more research is needed to confirm the suggested associations [8,37]. In addition, these studies emphasized that risk prediction does not equate to actual misuse, so recognition of variables associated with increased risk must be integrated with other clinical information.

Detection of Risk for Misuse, Abuse, or Addiction in Clinical Settings

Clinical Evaluation

Clinical history, physical examination, and pertinent laboratory review can provide important clinical information for patients being considered for opioid treatment of chronic pain. In addition to comprehensive pain evaluation, history-taking should include personal and family substance use histories, current substance use patterns, any history of legal problems associated with alcohol or drugs, and assessment for co-occurring psychiatric conditions. Physical examination for findings associated with potentially harmful drug or alcohol use (e.g., signs of intravenous injection or alcoholism) or signs of intoxication or withdrawal may be revealing. Laboratory findings such as increased liver function studies; mean corpuscular volume; or positivity for HIV, hepatitis B, or hepatitis C antibodies may suggest a need to further evaluate for alcohol or injection drug use. Urine drug screening may provide objective evidence of recent use of illicit drugs or nonprescribed controlled substances.

Tools to Predict Risk of Misuse

Standard screens for SUDs such as the Alcohol Use Disorders Identification Test (AUDIT), CAGE-AID (CAGE-Adapted to Include Drugs), Short-Michigan Alcohol Screening Test-Adapted to Include Drugs (SMAST-AID), Drug Abuse Screening Test (DAST), and others may help to identify active substance use problems associated with elevated risk of opioid misuse. However, they are not designed to identify individuals without current use problems who may be at risk for misuse of prescribed opioids. Two promising tools in development for this purpose are the Opioid Risk Tool (ORT) and the Revised Screener and Opioid Assessment for Patients with Pain (SOAPP).

The ORT is a 10-item screen with questions related to age, personal and family substance histories, specific mental health diagnoses, and history of child sexual trauma that can be self- or clinician-administered. Scored results stratify respondents into low-, moderate-, and higher-risk groups. Clinical management recommendations were recently suggested for different ORT risk groups, although no outcomes data on the recommendations are currently available [38]. A copy of the ORT questionnaire can be obtained at http://www.emergingsolutionsinpain.com.

The SOAPP is available in a number of iterations, as 24-item, 14-item, and 5-item screens that use a five-point scale for each item. A score above 18 is reported to have a sensitivity of 80% in predicting actual risk behaviors (20% of those at risk will not be identified) and a specificity of 68% (a 32% rate of false positives) [5]. On the 14-item scale, a score above 7 has sensitivity of 91% and a specificity of 69%. A copy of the SOAPP-24 questionnaire for clinical use can be obtained at http://www.emergingsolutionsinpain.com.

Tools to Identify Current Misuse

Many tools in development aim to detect misuse of opioids while opioids are prescribed for pain. Among these are the Prescription Drug Use Questionnaire (PDUQ) [2]; the Current Opioid Misuse Measure (COMM), a 17-item self-administered questionnaire [6]; the Pain Medication Questionnaire (PMQ), a 24-item self-administered questionnaire [16]; and the Addiction Behaviors Checklist (ABC), a 20-item, clinician-observed checklist [46]. The Drug Misuse Index, a combination of several measures, including SOAPP, COMM, urine toxicology, and other measures, has been used to predict and identify risk behaviors [42].

A recent evidence-based review of these evolving opioid risk prediction and aberrant use identification tools and others noted promise, but also significant limitations, in evidence supporting their validity and generalizability for clinical use in different settings [26].

Identification of Substance Use Disorders

A recent study of 904 chronic pain patients receiving opioid therapy in a primary care setting for an average of 6.4 years attempted to determine which aberrant drug use behaviors might best indicate an active SUD. The study found that a patient's reporting of four or more aberrant behaviors on a self-report survey of 12 questions was highly predictive of detection of an SUD with a structured clinical interview. Four specific behaviors were most strongly associated with SUD: oversedation on purpose, feeling intoxicated, obtaining early refills, and increasing the dose on one's own. Those who screened positive for cocaine use were 14 times more likely to have an SUD [14].

Improving Safety and Efficacy of Opioid Therapy by Addressing Risk

The concept of "universal precautions" for pain management, discussed in another chapter in this volume, includes screening and risk assessment as an important part of pain assessment [15]. The purpose is not to deny the use of opioids if they are deemed to be appropriate therapy for a patient's pain. Rather, it is to optimize outcome and reduce risk by assuring that all patients receive key components of care and that patients who may require more structured care are identified.

Persistent pain is a multidimensional experience that often includes biopsychosocial and functional dimensions. More complex chronic pain syndromes, especially in the higher-risk population, respond best to interdisciplinary care that encourages an active patient role with well-coordinated guidance from a team of diverse professionals. When opioid therapy is indicated for a higher-risk individual, an addiction professional, when available, may be an important participant in care. Interdisciplinary care has been demonstrated to reduce misuse of opioids in many patients over time [29]. In patients identified to be at higher risk or who demonstrate misuse of opioids, it is possible and prudent to adapt the structure of care to support safe and effective treatment [31]. Some broad elements of structure to consider include the following "5 S's":

• Setting of care (specialty vs. primary care, highly coordinated vs. routine)

• Selection of treatments (e.g., weighing the relative risk and benefit of opioids vs. other interventions; selecting quick-onset, intermittent opioids vs. steady-state, longer-acting opioids)

• Supply of opioid medications (prescribed vs. dispensed at intervals by trusted others, the frequency of medication provision, and the quantity released to the patient)

• Supportive care (recovery groups, psychotherapy, and counseling as indicated)

• Supervision (frequency of clinician visits, urine toxicology screens, and pill counts)

Some specific strategies that have been suggested for higher-risk patients include weekly or more frequent medication release, 24-hour-notice pill counts, substance abuse education worksheets, referral to pain and substance abuse websites, individual compliance counseling, completion of an opioid compliance checklist before receiving opioid prescriptions, and urine drug screens at each visit. Early identification of opioid misuse permits the introduction of strategies to reduce risk of addiction or harmful consequences.

Tightened structure of care appears effective in reducing risk behaviors in many patients and in identifying those for whom opioid therapy may not be appropriate. A Veterans Administration opioid renewal clinic that introduced structured care of patients with active aberrant drug-related behaviors found that at 1 year, 45.6% resolved such behaviors, 44.1% self-discharged or were discontinued from opioid therapy for nonadherence to the treatment plan, and 10.2% accepted referral for addiction treatment [44]. The structure of care may change over time in response to the patient's needs or behaviors.

Acknowledgments

Major portions of this paper were previously published by the author in Savage SR. Management of opioid medications in patients with chronic pain and risk of substance misuse. Curr Psychiatry Rep 2009;11:377–84. Dr. Savage has been on advisory boards for Registrat (chronic pain registry), Meda (Risk Evaluation and Mitigation Strategy (REMS) for Onsolis), and Ameritox (quantitative urine drug screens).

References

[1] Ballantyne J, LaForge K. Opioid dependence and addiction during opioid treatment of chronic pain. Pain 2007;129:235–55.

[2] Banta-Green CJ, Merrill JO, Doyle SR, Boudreau DM, Calsyn DA Measurement of opioid problems among chronic pain patients in a general medical population. Drug Alcohol Depend 2009;104:43–9.

[3] Berrocoso E, Sanchez-Blazquez P, Garzon J, Mico J. Opiates as antidepressants. Curr Pharm Des 2009;15:1612–22.

[4] Bieber CM, Fernandez K, Borsook D, Brennan MJ, Butler SF, Jamison RN, Osgood E, Sharpe-Potter J, Thomson HN, Weiss RD, Katz NP. Retrospective accounts of initial subjective effects of opioid in patients treated for pain who do or do not develop opioid addiction: a pilot case-control study. Exp Clin Psychopharmacol 2008;16:429–34.

[5] Butler S, Fernandez K, Benoit C, Budman SH, Jamison RN. Validation of the revised Screener and Opioid Assessment for Patients with Pain (SOAPP-R). J Pain 2008;9:360–72.

[6] Butler SF, Budman SH, Fernandez KC, Houle B, Benoit C, Katz N, Jamison RN. Development and validation of the Current Opioid Misuse Measure. Pain 2007;130:144–56.

[7] Chou R, Fanciullo GJ, Fine PG, Adler JA, Ballantyne JC, Davies P, Donovan MI, Fishbain DA, Foley KM, Fudin J, et al.; American Pain Society-American Academy of Pain Medicine Opioids Guidelines Panel. Clinical guidelines for the use of chronic opioid therapy in chronic noncancer pain. J Pain 2009;10:113–30.

[8] Chou R, Fanciullo G, Fine P, Miaskowski C, Passik SD, Portenoy RK. Opioids for chronic noncancer pain: prediction and identification of aberrant drug-related behaviors: a review of the evidence for an American Pain Society and American Academy of Pain Medicine clinical practice guideline. J Pain 2009;10:131–46.

[9] Chu LF, Angst MS, Clark D. Opioid-induced hyperalgesia in humans: molecular mechanisms and clinical considerations. Clin J Pain 2008;24:479–96.

[10] Dickenson AH, Suzuki R. Opioids in neuropathic pain: clues from animal studies. Eur J Pain 2005;9:113–6.

[11] Dowling K, Storr C, Chilcoat H. Potential influences on initiation and persistence of extramedical prescription pain reliever use in the US population. Clin J Pain 2006;22:776–83.

[12] Drug Abuse Warning Network. Emergency visits involving non medical use of selected pharmaceuticals. In: The New DAWN Report. Issue 23, 2006R. Drug Abuse Warning Network; 2006. Available at: http://dawninfo.samhsa.gov/files/TNDR/2006-07R/TNDR07EDVisitsNonMedicalUse.htm. Accessed 27 August 2009.

[13] Edlund MJ, Steffick D, Hudson T, Harris KM, Sullivan M. Risk factors for clinically recognized opioid abuse and dependence among veterans using opioid for chronic non-cancer pain. Pain 2007;129:355–62.

[14] Fleming M, Davis J, Passik S. Reported lifetime aberrant drug-taking behaviors are predictive of current substance use and mental health problems in primary care patients. Pain Med 2008;9:1098–106.

[15] Gourlay DL, Heit HA, Almahrezi A. Universal precautions in pain medicine: a rational approach to the treatment of chronic pain. Pain Med 2005;6:107–12.

[16] Holmes CP, Gatchel RJ, Adams LL, Stowell AW, Hatten A, Noe C, Lou L. An opioid screening instrument: long-term evaluation of the utility of the pain medication questionnaire. Pain Pract 2006;6:74–88.

[17] Ives TJ. Predictors of opioid misuse in patients with chronic pain: a prospective cohort study. BMC Health Serv Res 2006;6:46.

[18] Joranson DE, Gilson AM. Drug crime is a source of abused pain medications in the United States. J Pain Symptom Manage 2005;30:299–301.

[19] Kieffer B, Evans C. Opioid receptors: from binding sites to visible molecules in vivo. Neuropharmacology 2009;56:205–12.

[20] Koob G. Neurobiological substrates for the dark side of compulsivity in addiction. Neuropharmacology 2009;56(Suppl 1):S18–31.

[21] Layne R, Pellegrino R, Lerfald N. Prescription opioids and overdose deaths. JAMA 2009;301:1766–7.

[22] Manchikanti L, Singh A. Therapeutic opioids: a ten-year perspective on the complexities and complications of the escalating use, abuse, and nonmedical use of opioids. Pain Physician 2008;11:S63–88.

[23] Martins S, Keyes K, Storr C, Zhu H, Chilcoat HD. Pathways between nonmedical opioid use/dependence and psychiatric disorders: results from the National Epidemiologic Survey on Alcohol and Related Conditions. Drug Alcohol Depend 2009;103:16–24.

[24] McCabe SE, Boyd CJ, Teter CJ. Subtypes of nonmedical prescription drug misuse. Drug Alcohol Depend 2009;102:63–70.

[25] Meghani SH, Wiedemer NL, Becker WC, Gracely EJ, Gallagher RM. Predictors of resolution of aberrant drug behavior in chronic pain patients treated in a structured opioid risk management program. Pain Med 2009;10:858–65.

[26] Moore TM, Jones T, Browder JH, Daffron S, Passik SD. A comparison of common screening methods for predicting aberrant drug-related behavior among patients receiving opioids for chronic pain management. Pain Med 2009;10:1426–33.

[27] Morasco B, Dobscha S. Prescription medication misuse and substance use disorder in VA primary care patients with chronic pain. Gen Hosp Psychiatry 2008;30:93–9.

[28] Niikura K, Narita M, Narita M, Nakamura A, Okutsu D, Ozeki A, Kurahashi K, Kobayashi Y, Suzuki M, Suzuki T. Direct evidence for the involvement of endogenous beta-endorphin in the suppression of the morphine-induced rewarding effect under a neuropathic pain-like state. Neurosci Lett 2008;435:257–62.

[29] Passik SD. Issues in long-term opioid therapy: unmet needs, risks, and solutions. Mayo Clin Proc 2009;84:593–601.

[30] Rollason V, Samer C, Piguet V, Dayer P, Desmeules J. Pharmacogenetics of analgesics: towards individualization of prescription. Pharmacogenetics 2008;9:905–33.

[31] Savage SR, Kirsh KL, Passik SD. Challenges in using opioids to treat pain in persons with substance use disorders. Addict Sci Clin Pract 2008;4:4–25.

[32] Schwartz AC, Bradley R, Penza KM, Sexton M, Jay D, Haggard PJ, Garlow SJ, Ressler KJ. Pain medication use among patients with posttraumatic stress disorder. Psychosomatics 2006;47:136–42.

[33] Silverman SL. Opioid induced hyperalgesia: clinical implications for the pain practitioner. Pain Physician 2009;12:679–84.

[34] Somogyi A, Barratt D, Coller J. Pharmacogenetics of opioids. Clin Pharmacol Ther 2007;81:429–44.

[35] Substance Abuse and Mental Health Services Administration, Office of Applied Studies. Treatment Episode Data Set (TEDS). Available at: http://wwwdasis.samhsa.gov/webt/newmapv1.htm. Accessed August 27, 2009.

[36] Substance Abuse and Mental Health Services Administration. Results from the 2006 National Survey on Drug Use and Health: National Findings. Rockville, MD: Substance Abuse and Mental Health Services Administration, Office of Applied Studies; 2007.

[37] Turk D, Swanson K, Gatchel R. Predicting opioid misuse by chronic pain patients: a systematic review and literature synthesis. Clin J Pain 2008;24:497–508.

[38] Utah Department of Health. Utah clinical guidelines on prescribing opioids. Available at: http://www.health.utah.gov/prescription/pdf/Utah_guidelines_pdfs.pdf. Accessed August 12, 2009.

[39] Vadalouca A, Moka E, Argyra E, Sikioti P, Siafaka I. Opioid rotation in patients with cancer: a review of the current literature. J Opioid Manag 2008;4:213–50.

[40] Vorobeychik Y, Chen L, Bush M, Mao J. Improved opioid analgesic effect following opioid dose reduction. Pain Med 2008;9:724–7.

[41] Wasan AD, Butler SF, Budman SH, Fernandez K, Weiss RD, Greenfield SF, Jamison RN. Does report of craving opioid medication predict aberrant drug behavior among chronic pain patients? Clin J Pain 2009;25:193–8.

[42] Wasan AD, Butler SF, Budman SH, Benoit C, Fernandez K, Jamison RN. Psychiatric history and psychologic adjustment as risk factors for aberrant drug-related behavior among patients with chronic pain. Clin J Pain 2007;23:307–15.

[43] Webster L. Pharmacogenetics in pain management: the clinical need. Clin Lab Med 2008;28:569–79.

[44] Wiedemer NL, Harden PS, Arndt IO, Gallagher RM. The opioid renewal clinic: a primary care, managed approach to opioid therapy in chronic pain patients at risk for substance abuse. Pain Med 2007;8:573–84.

[45] Wilsey B, Fishman S, Tsodikov A, Ogden C, Symreng I, Ernst A. Psychological comorbidities predicting prescription opioid abuse among patients in chronic pain presenting to the emergency department. Pain Med 2008, 9:1107–1117.

[46] Wu SM, Compton P, Bolus R, Schieffer B, Pham Q, Baria A, Van Vort W, Davis F, Shekelle P, Naliboff BD. The addiction behaviors checklist: validation of a new clinician-based measure of inappropriate opioid use in chronic pain. J Pain Symptom Manage 2006;32:342–51.

[47] Zacny JP, Lichtor SA. Nonmedical use of prescription opioids: motive and ubiquity issues. J Pain 2008;9:473–86.

[48] Zacny JP, McKay MA, Toledano AY, Marks S, Young CJ, Klock PA, Apfelbaum JL. The effects of cold-water immersion stressor on the reinforcing and subjective effects of fentanyl in healthy volunteers. Drug Alcohol Depend 1996;42:133–42.

Correspondence to: Seddon R. Savage, MD, MS, Dartmouth Center on Addiction Recovery and Education, 7764 Parker House, Dartmouth College, Hanover, NH 03755, USA. Email: seddon.r.savage@dartmouth.edu.

Balancing Safety with Pain Relief When Prescribing Opioids

Jonathan Bannister, MB ChB, FFPMRCA

Tayside Pain Services, University of Dundee, Ninewells Hospital and Medical School, Dundee, Scotland, United Kingdom

Evidence indicates that opioids can be effective in managing long-term pain in some patients. We also know that opioid therapy can create challenging patient management problems for the clinician. Taking an approach of "prevention is better (or easier) than cure" when prescribing opioids may help us avoid problems or at least reduce their impact on the patient and on society.

Universal Precautions in Pain Management

Several authors have proposed using the concept of "Universal Precautions" in opioid prescribing for chronic noncancer pain [5]. The philosophy is based on the same precautions used to reduce the spread of infectious disease between patients and their caregivers. Since we cannot be sure if an individual patient carries a risk, we treat every patient as being a potential source of infection, and we take appropriate precautions—such as gloves, gowns, and masks—when there is any risk of exposure to bodily fluids. Likewise, because it is difficult to accurately predict which patients will become problematic opioid consumers, we can take some reasonable measures to reduce the risk in everyone.

Gourlay et al. [5] recommend the following 10 steps:

1) Make a diagnosis with an appropriate differential

2) Perform a psychological assessment including screening for risk of addictive disorders

3) Provide informed consent to use of opioids (verbal or written/signed)

4) Document a treatment agreement (verbal or written/signed)

5) Assess and document pain level and function before the start of treatment

6) Provide an appropriate trial of opioid therapy with or without adjunctive medication

7) Regularly reassess pain scores and level of function

8) Regularly assess the "four A's" of pain medicine:
Analgesia—using some type of pain scoring system
Activities—physical and psychosocial functioning
Adverse effects of treatment and suggested remedies
Ambiguous drug-related behaviors

9) Periodically review pain diagnosis and comorbid conditions, including risk for opioid misuse/addiction

10) Document, and in particular, carefully monitor opioid prescribing [5]

These recommendations, when seen in the format above, can be recognized simply as good clinical practice. All treatments in medicine should be undertaken with the informed consent of the patient, evaluated and adjusted as needed, and regularly reviewed. Unfortunately, this process does not seem to be common practice with the prescribing of long-term opioids, resulting in problems for patients, physicians, and society. There are many reasons for this deficiency, chief among them being the lack of adequate training in either pain or addiction medicine in health professional curricula.

Implicit within the above strategy is the informed cooperation of the patient. As with so much of pain medicine, we achieve better results when our patients understand their condition and its treatment. Patients should be informed of both the potential benefits and risks of opioids. They should understand that development of addictive behaviors will generate closer scrutiny by prescribers and may result in more restrictive prescribing or even withdrawal of opioids as a treatment option. The use of written opioid agreements, to help demonstrate informed consent, is more widespread in North American practice than in the U.K., which perhaps reflects medicolegal concerns on the part of the prescribers [3,4]. (Certainly, the incidence of doctors being prosecuted over inappropriate opioid prescribing is much less common in the U.K.) Although the use of treatment agreements is recommended in most guidelines for the prescribing of opioids for pain, not all clinicians are in agreement that they are ethical and that they accomplish the goal of reducing the misuse of opioids [1].

The issue of what constitutes an opioid of concern is interesting, and the answer may vary from country to country. In the U.K., many patients are already taking opioids, such as codeine, dihydrocodeine, and tramadol, when they are first assessed in the pain clinic. Little concern seems to be expressed by their primary care physicians about these drugs, yet they form part of almost every history heard by pain and addiction specialists. Should there be a written agreement in place before starting these "weak" opioids? What about the opioids available "over the counter"? The traditional descriptors of "strong" and "weak" opioids may describe analgesic effects, but not necessarily addiction potential. Should we view with more concern the patient taking 240 mg/day dihydrocodeine, or the one taking 40 mg/day of controlled-release morphine?

The role of urine drug testing remains controversial. It is one method of assessing what drugs—licit and illicit—the patient is taking, but it is of limited use in detecting patients who are diverting part of their prescription. Also, those who intentionally choose to misuse prescribed opioids develop various ingenious methods to attempt to fool urine drug screens, including dilution, adding a masking substance,

or substituting someone else's urine [6]. Therefore, if a patient is manifesting repeated "out-of-bounds" behaviors with normal urine drug screens, the clinician should suspect urine "doctoring" and focus instead on behaviors. The patient's reaction to a potential urine screen can be as informative as the result. Patients who are reluctant to have their urine tested are unlikely to comply with the boundaries of opioid treatment. On the other hand, for the high-risk patient who is genuinely trying to improve his/her life, who consistently demonstrates no ambiguous drug behaviors and clean urine samples, the clinician can use this information to advocate on the patient's behalf with law enforcement and social service agencies. (A urine drug testing monograph and information on opioid prescribing agreements can be downloaded from www.emergingsolutionsinpain.com or www.painedu.org.)

Implicit within the treatment agreement is that regular assessments will be made of pain relief and functional abilities. A structured pain and activity diary is probably the easiest way for patients to generate this information. Remember that all medications, including opioids, should be prescribed initially as a therapeutic trial. The clinician needs to see sustained improvement to continue prescribing. Recording the four A's (see above) is a pragmatic way to demonstrate effectiveness of treatment. There are also a number of short, validated assessment tools, such as the Brief Pain Inventory, the Pain Disability Index, and the Pain Assessment and Documentation Tool, that can facilitate documentation of patient improvement in a time-efficient manner [8].

Opioids are not usually considered the first line of treatment for most chronic pain conditions. Clinicians need to document adequate trials of nonopioid analgesics and adjuvant medications such as tricyclic antidepressants and anticonvulsants, either prior to or concurrent with opioid therapy. When available and possible, pharmacotherapy should always be combined with physical/rehabilitative and psychological methods of pain management. Opioids work best when titrated to effect. Due to genetic heterogeneity, the dose of opioid required to relieve pain in a given individual is unpredictable, and titration upward should continue unless the patient is exhibiting adverse effects or addictive behaviors. There is no pharmacological rationale for a dose ceiling for pure opioid agonists. Setting an arbitrary ceiling dose at which the prescriber will "bail out" does not constitute a proper trial. On the other hand, as the opioid dosage increases, more monitoring is required to demonstrate that the treatment is doing more good than harm.

The most common reason for the development of apparent iatrogenic opioid addiction is failure to screen for previous addiction history. The limited existing evidence suggests that the development of abuse or addiction with therapeutic opioids is unusual in patients without risk factors. Practical methods of risk assessment and stratification are addressed in another chapter in this volume.

Aberrant drug consumption is most commonly noticed from prescribing records—"lost" prescriptions and medications, repeated early requests for refills, seeking prescriptions from multiple physicians—which can be difficult when the pain clinician is not the primary prescriber. In these cases, close communication with the primary care physician is vital. In patients developing opioid addiction following prescription for chronic pain, one of the most common situations seen in our clinic is failure to adequately monitor, with subsequent loss of control of the prescription. From the patient's point of view, this dose escalation is seen as occurring with the doctor's approval. When the out-of-control behavior and excessive consumption suddenly become evident to the prescriber, it may lead to sudden reduction in prescription, withdrawal and failure of analgesia, and removal from the doctor's practice; effectively, the patient is abandoned when he or she most needs help. This approach is not just or humanitarian. An important part of prescribing opioids for pain is to understand how to taper opioids in a safe and humane fashion when required, and to maintain awareness of local addiction treatment resources where one can refer the patient for further assistance.

The importance of continued assessment of the patient's function, level of pain, and drug side effects cannot be overemphasized. As with all chronic conditions, pain can change over time, and new pathologies may develop.

Practical Strategies for Treating Pain in the High-Risk Patient

It is important to remember that patients who misuse substances experience pain just as acutely, and probably more so, than "normal" patients. Their lives tend to be chaotic and difficult, and they often suffer from concurrent mental health problems. Such problems increase these patients' stress and distress and may make their

experience of pain worse. Their coping mechanisms are heavily biased toward use of chemicals to deal with distress, and they may not respond easily to nonpharmaceutical measures for pain control. Addiction is a chronically relapsing illness, and we should expect our patients to respond accordingly. If a patient who has been stable and productive becomes unstable and chaotic again, it is not an indication of therapeutic failure and a signal to retreat; it means we have to change our management and try again. Addiction and chronic pain are rarely curable, just as diabetes is rarely curable. We are tasked with helping these patients to best manage their chronic diseases, and we should expect setbacks as much as we enjoy success.

In terms of therapeutic approaches, we can use any technique we would use in pain uncomplicated by addiction. Opioids do have analgesic effects in opioid misusers, even though popular myths have many patients believing otherwise. Methadone especially is commonly believed by the addict population not to have analgesic qualities, but it can be a good treatment option when dealing with mixed nociceptive and neuropathic pain. As in patients without addiction, tolerance to therapeutic opioids can develop, and doses need to be adjusted accordingly. Clinicians need to maintain awareness of the opioid hyperalgesia syndrome and be prepared to switch or taper opioids when indicated [2]. Controlled-release/long-acting opioids are generally preferred because they may have a lower potential than immediate-release/short-acting drugs for inducing tolerance and "fueling" dependence by rapid onset and offset. Various drug technologies are evolving to reduce patients' ability to disable the controlled-release mechanism of opioids by crushing, snorting, or injecting. Breakthrough opioid medication is usually inappropriate and more open to abuse, so other modalities (drug or nondrug) should be used to manage transient increases in pain. The high-risk patient on opioids requires more structured treatment, including more frequent follow-up, more monitoring, and dispensing of smaller amounts of medication on a more frequent basis, even daily if required.

When treating this challenging group of patients, we should follow some basic principles, whether we are seeing them in the chronic or the acute setting. Negative physician and nurse attitudes to addicted patients are unhelpful. We often find ourselves mistrusting such patients, failing to identify with them, and expecting to be duped. Addicted patients are used to this treatment, and in turn they may respond by dissembling, manipulating, and confronting. They often do not expect the doctors to care about or acknowledge their pain, and they expect to be treated poorly. We have an opportunity to begin to change this relationship, both by the way in which we interact with the patient and by educating our colleagues about the realities of addiction and acute or chronic pain. An open, respectful, professional relationship with honest communication is the key. We need to know what is happening to the patient, in terms of both pain and drug intake. Patients need to know that we want to make them as comfortable as possible and specifically minimize withdrawal symptoms. In the acute situation, such as a surgical admission, patients may need to be reassured that there is no plan to "treat" their addiction by acute detoxification. It is still surprising how often one comes across health professionals who think that an acute surgical admission is an opportunity to get a patient off drugs. It is also important to set ground rules about behavior (ward disruption or taking illicit substances) during an admission; equally, it is helpful to generate realistic expectations, aiming for good analgesia rather than a pain-free state. Clinicians need to be aware that opioid doses for acute pain in patients already dependent on opioids—licit or illicit—can be much higher than usual [7].

High-risk patients on appropriate opioid therapy can benefit from structured addiction treatment programs as long as the pain clinician can negotiate the continued use of opioids with a program that uses an abstinence-based model. The patient with both pain and addiction needs to commit to an ongoing program of recovery, so as to optimize the benefit and increase the safety of long-term opioid therapy. Good communication among health professionals is vital to optimal outcomes in patients with both pain and addiction. There should only be one prescriber for all mood-modifying medications, and each member of the team should know exactly what the prescription is. It is equally important to maintain continuity so that the patient does not run out of medication, a potent driver for seeking illicit drugs. With teamwork and structure, patients with both pain and addiction can make meaningful changes in their lives.

References

[1] Arnold RM, Han PK, Seltzer D. Opioid contracts in chronic nonmalignant pain management: objectives and uncertainties. Am J Med 2006;119:292–6.

[2] Chang G, Chen L, Mao J. Opioid tolerance and hyperalgesia. Med Clin North Am 2007;91:199–211.

[3] Fishman SM, Kreis PG. The opioid contract. Clin J Pain 2002;18(4 Suppl):S70–5.

[4] Fishman SM, Mahajan G, Jung SW, Wilsey BL. The trilateral opioid contract. Bridging the pain clinic and the primary care physician through the opioid contract. J Pain Symptom Manage 2002;24:335–44.

[5] Gourlay DL, Heit HA, Almahrezi A. Universal precautions in pain medicine: a rational approach to the treatment of chronic pain. Pain Med 2005;6:107–12.

[6] Jaffee WB, Trucco E, Levy S, Weiss RD. Is this urine really negative? A systematic review of tampering methods in urine drug screening and testing. J Subst Abuse Treat 2007;33:33–42.

[7] Jovey RD. Managing acute pain in the opioid-dependent patient. In: Flor H, Kalso E, Dostrovsky JO. Proceedings of the 11th World Congress on Pain. Seattle: IASP Press; 2006. p. 469–79.

[8] Passik SD, Kirsh KL, Whitcomb L, Schein JR, Kaplan MA, Dodd SL, Kleinman L, Katz NP, Portenoy RK. Monitoring outcomes during long-term opioid therapy for noncancer pain: results with the Pain Assessment and Documentation Tool. J Opioid Manag 2005;1:257–66.

Further Reading

[A] British Pain Society. Pain and substance misuse: improving the patient experience. A consensus statement prepared by The British Pain Society in collaboration with The Royal College of Psychiatrists, The Royal College of General Practitioners and The Advisory Council on the Misuse of Drugs. April 2007. Available at: www.britishpainsociety.org/book_drug_misuse_main.pdf. Accessed Mar 1, 2010.

[B] British Pain Society. British Pain Society's opioids for persistent pain: good practice. A consensus statement prepared on behalf of the British Pain Society, the Royal College of Anaesthetists, the Royal College of General Practitioners and the Royal College of Psychiatrists. January 2010. Available at: www.britishpainsociety.org/book_opioid_main.pdf. Accessed Mar 1, 2010.

[C] Smith HS, Passik SD, editors. Pain and chemical dependency. New York: Oxford University Press; 2008.

Correspondence to: Dr. Jonathan Bannister, Tayside Pain Services, Ninewells Hospital and Medical School, Dundee DD1 9SY, Scotland, United Kingdom. Email: j.bannister@dundee.ac.uk.

Part 15
Pathophysiology, Diagnosis, and Treatment of Persistent Abdominal/Pelvic Pain

Pathophysiology of Persistent Abdominal and Pelvic Pain

Emeran A. Mayer, MD

Center for Neurobiology of Stress, Departments of Medicine, Psychiatry and Physiology,
David Geffen School of Medicine at UCLA, Los Angeles, California, USA

Persistent abdominal and pelvic pain syndromes are part of a spectrum of complex syndromes that are characterized by persistent pain and discomfort referred to different visceral structures (the upper and lower gastrointestinal [GI] tract and urogenital system) and somatic structures (in particular muscles and joints) [23]. The most common constellation of symptoms has been clustered into subspecialty-specific syndromes, such as irritable bowel syndrome (IBS), functional abdominal pain syndrome (FAPS), painful bladder syndrome (PBS), and interstitial cystitis (IC). In the absence of reliable biological markers or a full understanding of their pathophysiology, these syndromes are currently defined by symptom criteria and sometimes by the exclusion of "organic" disease. In addition to overlapping with each other, these syndromes share several clinical and epidemiological features, including high comorbidity with symptoms of anxiety, depression, somatization, and enhanced stress sensitivity. These similarities have led to the concept that these syndromes share certain pathophysiological features, both central (e.g., central pain amplification) and peripheral (e.g., neuroimmune interactions), as well as common genetic and environmental vulnerability [23]. In addition, syndrome-specific environmental and genetic factors may be responsible for the manifestation of an individual syndrome.

Patients with persistent abdominal or pelvic pain are likely to belong to heterogeneous groups. This heterogeneity is reflected in clinical features and may reflect differences in underlying pathophysiological mechanisms. For example, some patients have long pain-free intervals, with recurrent bouts of pain and discomfort, are generally symptom-free during sleep, and often associate symptoms with end-organ function such as urination or defecation, or with specific triggers, for example, food or stress. Others report constant pain ("24/7") that is not related to any triggers. Mechanisms underlying these two general symptom patterns are likely to differ. There may be subsets of patients with different patterns of organ-specific peripheral abnormalities (involving epithelial permeability, mast cell abnormalities, and neurogenic inflammation), and with different mechanisms involved in central pain amplification (different impairment of endogenous pain modulation mechanisms).

The traditional view has focused on organ-specific changes in the GI or the urogenital tracts, and multiple plausible peripheral mechanisms leading to peripheral and central sensitization have been studied in rodent models of visceral hyperalgesia [38]. However, as discussed in this chapter, the peripheral mechanisms implicated show a remarkable similarity between syndromes, in particular between IBS and PBS/IC. It remains to be determined how many of the reported abnormalities found in humans (tissue, stool, urine) play a causative role in the pathophysiology of these syndromes, and how many are secondary manifestations of central alterations. This question is important because many novel treatment approaches aimed at the most plausible peripheral pain mechanisms (including inflammation or specific signaling systems in primary afferent neurons) have generally been disappointing. Because of the failure to develop effective novel therapies, more recent approaches have focused on understanding the mechanisms and vulnerability factors that are responsible for the transition from acute to persistent pain states.

There is solid evidence supporting the concept of enhanced perception of physiological and/or experimental stimuli in both IBS and PBS/IC, which is generally referred to as "visceral hypersensitivity." In human subjects, it is difficult to determine whether this phenomenon is related to sensitization of peripheral visceral afferent pathways, to central sensitization, or to some form of central (spinal or supraspinal) pain amplification. In this chapter I will first review evidence for peripheral mechanisms that have been implicated in such sensitization, then briefly discuss proposed mechanisms of central pain amplification, and finally propose an integrative model, which takes into account both peripheral and central mechanisms.

Peripheral, Organ-Specific Abnormalities

Sensitization of Primary Afferent Pathways

The role of sensitized primary sensory afferents in the symptoms of persistent or chronically recurrent abdominal and pelvic pain states in human patient populations is not known. Evidence from both IBS and PBS/IC biopsies suggests neuroplastic remodeling in the epithelium, which may affect primary afferents, altering their response properties [14]. Studies on primary afferents from an animal model of IC, feline IC, suggest electrophysiological alterations of DRG neurons innervating the bladder [36]. It is conceivable that in subsets of patients with epithelial abnormalities in neuroimmune interactions, as discussed in the following paragraphs, intermittent peripheral sensitization may occur and may play a role of acute bouts of abdominal/pelvic pain.

Infection and Microflora

The acute inflammatory epithelial changes associated with infections of the urinary or GI tract are associated with peripheral and central sensitization and with the resulting visceral hyperalgesia. An infectious etiology of persistent abdominal/pelvic pain syndrome has long been suspected; however, in the great majority of patients a causal relationship between acute or chronic infections cannot be established. In the case of PBS/IC, flares of symptoms are often indistinguishable from an acute urinary tract infection. However, it is highly unlikely that bacterial or viral infection is involved in the ongoing pathological process, or that antibiotic treatment is beneficial [14]. Nevertheless, it remains intriguing to speculate that host-microbial interactions in vulnerable individuals during the early phase of the disorder may result in permanently altered immune or host cell responses, or in changes in urothelial-neural interactions, which then continue to play a role in the persistence of symptoms, in the absence of the infectious organism [10,16]. In the case of IBS, several studies have reported the onset of IBS-like symptoms following established bacterial or viral infections of the GI tract [42]. This so-called "post-infectious IBS" (PI-IBS) occurs in about 10% of patients undergoing a documented infectious gastroenteritis, and risk factors for developing such symptom persistence are female sex, duration of the gastroenteritis, psychosocial stressors at the time of the infection, and psychological factors such as anxiety and depression. It is important to realize that the IBS-like symptoms do not typically arise in asymptomatic individuals, but rather in subjects with high somatization; that is, a history of other somatic symptoms. Thus, the "onset" of the IBS-like symptoms may in part represent an attentional shift from other somatic symptoms, or it may reflect the generalized central pain amplification state, which produces enhanced perception of signals coming from a slowly healing mucosa. In addition to PI-IBS, other microorganism-related mechanisms have been proposed to underlie symptoms in subsets of IBS patients [8,28]. Small-bowel overgrowth [42] and alterations in the colonic microflora (dysbiosis) have been implicated. However, a causal relationship between such alterations in microflora and IBS symptoms remains to be established.

Epithelial-Immune Activation

Immune/neuroimmune mechanisms have been implicated in the pathogenesis of both IBS and PBS/IC. It is important to point out that reported changes cannot be characterized as inflammation, since generally neither leukocyte infiltration or increased expression of inflammatory cytokines in the epithelium are observed. In both disorders, enhanced release of neuropeptides from primary sensory nerve endings (such as substance P and calcitonin gene-related peptide [CGRP]), as well as release of mast cell mediators (including serotonin, histamine, and proteases) have been implicated in the sensitization of primary afferent pathways, as well as in the release of nerve growth factor (NGF), which in turn can result in neuroplastic and morphological changes in the sensory and motor innervation of the bladder and colon [13,26]. Such neuroplastic changes may play a role in long-term symptoms long after the initial immune activation subsides.

Evidence for small increases in immune cells in the colon mucosa and in the bladder has been reported [14,25,42]. In IBS, such persistent immune activation has been demonstrated best in PI-IBS, and less consistently in other subtypes [25]. The results are conflicting if increased immune cell numbers are associated with an increase in proinflammatory cytokines, and if they play a role in symptoms. The strongest argument against such a pathophysiological role of the immune system was the negative outcome of a well-designed clinical trial in patients with PI-IBS comparing prednisolone with placebo. Even though the active treatment normalized the mucosal immune activation, this outcome was not accompanied by an improvement of IBS symptoms [12].

Mast Cells

Increased mast cell numbers or density, alterations in mast cell-nerve interactions, and increased release of mast cell products from epithelial biopsies have all been reported in both IBS and PBS/IC (for reviews, see [2,7,14,34]). However, mast cell abnormalities are not specific to either syndrome, since they have been implicated in a wide range of stress-sensitive disorders involving neuroimmune interactions, including multiple sclerosis, migraine, rheumatoid arthritis, and atopic dermatitis [43,44]. Mast cells can be activated by immunoglobulins, neuropeptides, and cytokines to secrete mediators without degranulation. They can release many signaling molecules, including histamine, serotonin, corticotropin-releasing factor (CRF), and proteases. Alterations in these signaling molecules have been implicated in the pathophysiology of both conditions, and respective receptor antagonists (targeted at histamine-, serotonin-, CRF-, and protease-activated receptors) have been evaluated as possible therapies. A particularly interesting aspect of mast cell regulation is the close interaction of mast cells with noradrenergic, cholinergic, and peptidergic nerve endings. Stress-induced degranulation of mast cells, along with increased release of mast cell products, has been reported both in preclinical and clinical studies [1,3,4].

However, despite the strong and converging experimental evidence in both IBS and PBS/IC for a prominent role of mast cells as a transducer between the central nervous system and the end organ, the clinical relationship between an increased number of mast cells and symptoms of IC or IBS has not been established, and no high-quality clinical trial data are available to unequivocally support a pathophysiological role. One of the reasons for the inconsistent correlation between end-organ mast cell numbers or density and symptoms may be the fact that activated mast cells lose their identifiable granules once degranulation occurs, and standard histological techniques may underestimate mast cell numbers [33].

Epithelial Permeability

In both IBS and PBS/IC there is solid evidence for increased epithelial permeability in some patients, even though a pathophysiological role of this abnormality by itself has not been demonstrated for either syndrome [11,14,18,27]. Based on both preclinical and clinical studies, different types of increased epithelial permeability with different molecular mechanisms can be distinguished, and different underlying mechanisms have been identified, including different types of stressors [40,41] and mucosal inflammation [24]. Mast cell products, such as CRF and proteases, have been implicated in mediating permeability changes in the GI tract [39]. Given that increased mucosal permeability has also been reported in asymptomatic individuals, it is likely that this epithelial abnormality, like several other reported peripheral findings, may play a pathophysiological role only in subsets of patients and may require the presence of other factors.

Central Pain Amplification

As shown in Fig. 1, there are multiple mechanisms by which the central nervous system can modulate afferent signals from the viscera, including increased activity of endogenous pain facilitation and reduced engagement of endogenous pain inhibitory systems. Endogenous pain modulation systems are likely to mediate the effects of affect, mood, and environmental context (such as stress) on pain perception. Three such mechanisms that may be relevant for visceral hypersensitivity are briefly reviewed below.

Enhanced Stress Responsiveness

Whereas acute, severe, inescapable stressors are typically associated with stress-induced analgesia, other types of uncertain, unpredictable, and milder stressors can be associated with stress-induced hyperalgesia [6,29,30]. There is considerable epidemiological evidence linking first symptom onset or symptom exacerbation in both disorders to certain types of psychosocial stressors, and acute laboratory stressors have shown to be associated with enhanced visceral perception in both IBS patients [22] and PBS/IC patients [17,31]. On the basis of these clinical findings, an upregulation of central stress and arousal circuits has been postulated [20]. An extensive amount of preclinical data support a role for the central (and to a certain degree the peripheral) CRF-CRF1-receptor-signaling system in mediating some forms of acute and chronic stress-induced visceral hyperalgesia of both bladder and colon [19,29,30]. The central CRF-CRF1-receptor-signaling system involves a brain network (a stress and arousal circuit) that has also been studied in human subjects using functional brain imaging techniques [21].

Neuroimmune Activation in the Spinal Cord

Evidence from preclinical models of visceral hyperalgesia have implicated activation of glia (microglia, astro-

cytes) as a possible mechanism underlying the chronicity of pain following a psychological stressor or peripheral inflammation (reviewed in [5]). Activation of glia can produce proinflammatory cytokines, such as tumor necrosis factor-alpha (TNF-α), and can result in the downregulation of the glutamate transporter on astrocytes, resulting in elevated synaptic glutamate concentrations. Both effects result in an upregulation of the glutamate/N-methyl-D-aspartate (NMDA) receptor-signaling system, thereby contributing to the development of central sensitization, even with non-noxious stimuli. It remains to be determined whether alterations in this spinal-neuroimmune interaction play a role in subsets of patients with persistent abdominal/pelvic pain, and whether this system comes into play during stress-induced flares, or following GI or bladder infections.

Central Pain Amplification

In IBS patients, evidence for both increased engagement of endogenous pain facilitatory mechanisms and compromised engagement of endogenous pain inhibitory mechanisms has been reported (reviewed in [21]). A recent meta-analysis of 17 functional magnetic resonance imaging (fMRI) studies reported differences in the brain's response to controlled rectal balloon distension in IBS patients. Across studies, there was consistent activation in regions associated with visceral afferent processing, emotional arousal, and attention among IBS patients and healthy controls. Patients show more consistent activations in regions associated with emotional arousal (the pregenual anterior cingulate cortex, parahippocampal gyrus/amygdala, and hypothalamus). Only patients show activation of a midbrain cluster, including regions involved in pain facilitation and inhibition. Female patients show greater engagement of the emotional arousal circuit during expectation of visceral pain compared to male patients. These findings are consistent with the hypothesis that changes in central pain modulation systems play a prominent role in the pathophysiology of persistent abdominal pain, and that the greater prevalence of these disorders in women may in part be related to sex-related differences in the engagement of an emotional arousal circuit. The stress and arousal circuit demonstrated in human subjects using fMRI shows significant homology with the stress circuit related to the CRF-CRF1-receptor-signaling system in rodents that was mentioned above.

There is also a growing body of evidence for gray matter abnormalities in patients with various persistent

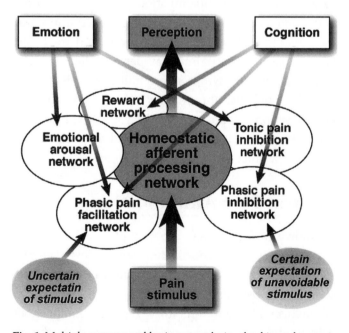

Fig. 1. Multiple systems and brain networks involved in endogenous pain modulation (adapted with permission from [23]).

pain disorders, including IBS [37]. IBS was associated with decreased gray matter density in widespread areas of the brain, including medial and lateral prefrontal regions. Compared with healthy controls, *increased* gray matter density in IBS patients was observed in the pregenual anterior cingulate cortex and the orbitofrontal cortex, both regions involved in the stress and arousal circuit. Analogous structural changes have been reported in other persistent pain disorders, including vulvodynia [35].

Summary and Conclusion

Despite significant progress during the past two decades in the characterization of peripheral and central candidate mechanisms that may play a role in the pathophysiology of persistent abdominal and pelvic pain states, it is becoming obvious that no single pathophysiological mechanism can explain symptoms in all patients. Nevertheless, the similarities in peripheral and central mechanisms implicated in IBS and PBS/IC are remarkable. Based on currently available information, it is likely that different patterns of dysregulation

in the interactions between the central nervous system and the respective abdominal and pelvic end organs are involved in different subsets of patients. Gene-environment interactions are likely to shape the vulnerability of individuals to develop chronic abdominal and pelvic pain states by altering the specific components of these neurovisceral interactions [9,32].

Some of plausible components of these interactions are illustrated in Fig. 2. The brain receives interoceptive input from abdominal and pelvic viscera and responds to these inputs in a reflexive way, taking into account contextual factors and other needs of the organism. In the healthy individual, most of this interoceptive input is not consciously perceived. However, alterations in the modulation of interoceptive input by stress and arousal circuits, and cortical input to these circuits, can alter both perception and feedback to these organs. The brain responds to the interoceptive input through the emotional motor system (EMS) [15], which refers to a set of parallel motor pathways governing somatic, autonomic, neuroendocrine, and pain modulatory motor responses associated with different emotions, including those associated with the stress response and emotional

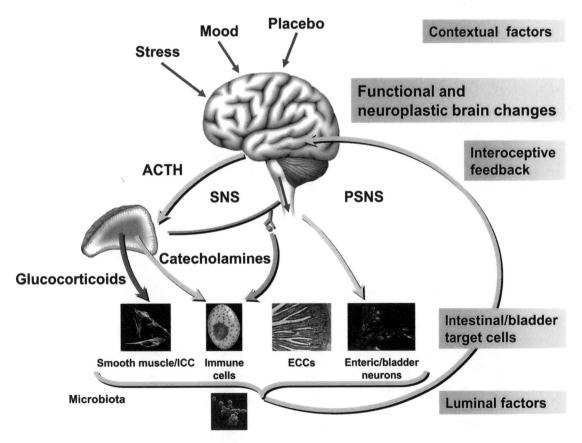

Fig. 2. Bidirectional brain-visceral interactions which may play a role in the pathophysiology of irritable bowel syndrome (IBS) and painful bladder syndrome/interstitial cystitis (PBS/IC). ACTH, adrenocorticotropic hormone; ECC, enterochromaffin cells; ICC, interstitial cells of Cajal; PSNS, parasympathetic nervous system; SNS, sympathetic nervous system.

states. Whereas acute, transient changes in EMS output can result in acute changes in organ function (motility, secretion, blood flow, and immune activity), persistent alterations can induce neuroplastic changes in specific cells within peripheral target organs. The peripheral changes reported in patients with IBS and PBS/IC, reviewed above, may represent such EMS-induced changes in immune cells (mast cell responsiveness) and neural cells (sensitization of primary afferents). These changes in turn will result in alterations in interoceptive feedback to the brain. In addition, "interoceptive memories" may develop over time, which may allow the brain to recall visceral experiences of discomfort and pain, even in the absence of acute interoceptive input.

Acknowledgments

Supported in part by grants from the National Institutes of Health DK 64531, DK 48351, and AT 00268.

References

[1]   Barbara G, Stanghellini V, De Giorgio R, Cremon C, Cottrell GS, Santini D, Pasquinelli G, Morselli-Labate AM, Grady EF, Bunnett NW, Collins SM, Corinaldesi R. Activated mast cells in proximity to colonic nerves correlate with abdominal pain in irritable bowel syndrome. Gastroenterology 2004;126:693–702.

[2]   Barbara G, Wang B, Stanghellini V, De Giorgio R, Cremon C, Di Nardo G, Trevisani M, Campi B, Geppetti P, Tonini M, Bunnett NW, Grundy D, Corinaldesi R. Mast cell-dependent excitation of visceral-nociceptive sensory neurons in irritable bowel syndrome. Gastroenterology 2007;132:26–37.

[3]   Bauer O, Razin E. Mast cell-nerve interactions. News Physiol Sci 2000;15:213–8.

[4]   Bienenstock J, MacQueen G, Sestini P, Marshall JS, Stead RH, Perdue MH. Mast cell/nerve interactions in vitro and in vivo. Am Rev Respir Dis 1991;143:S55–8.

[5]   Bradesi S. Role of spinal cord glia in the central processing of peripheral pain perception. Neurogastroenterol Motil;22:499–511.

[6]   Bradesi S, Schwetz I, Ennes HS, Lamy CM, Ohning G, Fanselow M, Pothoulakis C, McRoberts JA, Mayer EA. Repeated exposure to water avoidance stress in rats: a new model for sustained visceral hyperalgesia. Am J Physiol Gastrointest Liver Physiol 2005;289:G42–53.

[7]   Buhner S, Li Q, Vignali S, Barbara G, De Giorgio R, Stanghellini V, Cremon C, Zeller F, Langer R, Daniel H, Michel K, Schemann M. Activation of human enteric neurons by supernatants of colonic biopsy specimens from patients with irritable bowel syndrome. Gastroenterology 2009;137:1425–34.

[8]   Collins SM, Bercik P. The relationship between intestinal microbiota and the central nervous system in normal gastrointestinal function and disease. Gastroenterology 2009;136:2003–14.

[9]   Dimitrakov J, Guthrie D. Genetics and phenotyping of urological chronic pelvic pain syndrome. J Urol 2009;181:1550–7.

[10] Domingue GJ, Ghoniem GM, Bost KL, Fermin C, Human LG. Dormant microbes in interstitial cystitis. J Urol 1995;153:1321–6.

[11] Dunlop SP, Hebden J, Campbell E, Naesdal J, Olbe L, Perkins AC, Spiller RC. Abnormal intestinal permeability in subgroups of diarrhea-predominant irritable bowel syndromes. Am J Gastroenterol 2006;101:1288–94.

[12] Dunlop SP, Jenkins D, Neal KR, Naesdal J, Borgaonker M, Collins SM, Spiller RC. Randomized, double-blind, placebo-controlled trial of prednisolone in post-infectious irritable bowel syndrome. Aliment Pharmacol Ther 2003;18:77–84.

[13] Dupont MC, Spitsbergen JM, Kim KB, Tuttle JB, Steers WD. Histological and neurotrophic changes triggered by varying models of bladder inflammation. J Urol 2001;166:1111–8.

[14] Hanno PM, Wein AJ, Kavoussi LR, Novick AC, Partin AW, Peters CA. Painful bladder syndrome/interstitial cystitis and related disorders. In: Wein AJ, Kavoussi LR, Novick AC, Partin AW, Peters CA, editors. Campbell-Walsh urology. Philadelphia: W.B. Saunders; 2007.

[15] Holstege G, Bandler R, Saper CB, Holstege G, Bandler R, Saper CB. The emotional motor system. Amsterdam: Elsevier; 1996.

[16] Kau AL, Hunstad DA, Hultgren SJ. Interaction of uropathogenic *Escherichia coli* with host uroepithelium. Curr Opin Microbiol 2005;8:54–9.

[17] Lutgendorf SK, Kreder KJ, Rothrock NE, Ratliff TL, Zimmerman B. Stress and symptomatology in patients with interstitial cystitis: a laboratory stress model. J Urol 2000;164:1265–9.

[18] Marshall JK, Thabane M, Garg AX, Clark W, Meddings J, Collins SM. Intestinal permeability in patients with irritable bowel syndrome after a waterborne outbreak of acute gastroenteritis in Walkerton, Ontario. Aliment Pharmacol Ther 2004;20:1317–22.

[19] Martinez V, Taché Y. CRF1 receptors as a therapeutic target for irritable bowel syndrome. Curr Pharm Des 2006;12:4071–88.

[20] Mayer EA. The neurobiology of stress and gastrointestinal disease. Gut 2000;47:861–9.

[21] Mayer EA, Aziz Q, Coen S, Kern M, Labus JS, Lane R, Kuo B, Naliboff B, Tracey I. Brain imaging approaches to the study of functional GI disorders: a Rome working team report. Neurogastroenterol Motil 2009;21:579–96.

[22] Mayer EA, Bradesi S, Chang L, Spiegel BM, Bueller JA, Naliboff BD. Functional GI disorders: from animal models to drug development. Gut 2008;57:384–404.

[23] Mayer EA, Bushnell MC. Functional pain disorders: time for a paradigm shift? In: Mayer EA, Bushnell MC, editors. Functional pain syndromes: presentation and pathophysiology. Seattle: IASP Press; 2009. p. 531–65.

[24] Meddings JB. Intestinal permeability in Crohn's disease. Aliment Pharmacol Ther 1997;11(Suppl 3):47–53; discussion 53–46.

[25] Ohman L, Simren M. Pathogenesis of IBS: role of inflammation, immunity and neuroimmune interactions. Nat Rev Gastroenterol Hepatol;7:163–73.

[26] Ossovskaya VS, Bunnett NW. Protease-activated receptors: contribution to physiology and disease. Physiol Rev 2004;84:579–621.

[27] Piche T, Barbara G, Aubert P, Bruley des Varannes S, Dainese R, Nano JL, Cremon C, Stanghellini V, De Giorgio R, Galmiche JP, Neunlist M. Impaired intestinal barrier integrity in the colon of patients with irritable bowel syndrome: involvement of soluble mediators. Gut 2009;58:196–201.

[28] Rhee SH, Pothoulakis C, Mayer EA. Principles and clinical implications of the brain-gut-enteric microbiota axis. Nat Rev Gastroenterol Hepatol 2009;6:306–14.

[29] Robbins MT, DeBerry J, Ness TJ. Chronic psychological stress enhances nociceptive processing in the urinary bladder in high-anxiety rats. Physiol Behav 2007;91:544–50.

[30] Robbins MT, Ness TJ. Footshock-induced urinary bladder hypersensitivity: role of spinal corticotropin-releasing factor receptors. J Pain 2008;9:991–8.

[31] Rothrock NE, Lutgendorf SK, Kreder KJ, Ratliff T, Zimmerman B. Stress and symptoms in patients with interstitial cystitis: a life stress model. Urology 2001;57:422–7.

[32] Saito YA, Zimmerman JM, Harmsen WS, De Andrade M, Locke GR 3rd, Petersen GM, Talley NJ. Irritable bowel syndrome aggregates strongly in families: a family-based case-control study. Neurogastroenterol Motil 2008;20:790–7.

[33] Sant GR, Theoharides TC. The role of the mast cell in interstitial cystitis. Urol Clin North Am 1994;21:41–53.

[34] Santos J, Guilarte M, Alonso C, Malagelada JR. Pathogenesis of irritable bowel syndrome: the mast cell connection. Scand J Gastroenterol 2005;40:129–40.

[35] Schweinhardt P, Kuchinad A, Pukall CF, Bushnell MC. Increased gray matter density in young women with chronic vulvar pain. Pain 2008;140:411–9.

[36] Sculptoreanu A, de Groat WC, Buffington CA, Birder LA. Abnormal excitability in capsaicin-responsive drg neurons from cats with feline interstitial cystitis. Exp Neurol 2005;193:437–43.

[37] Seminowicz DA, Labus JS, Bueller JA, Tillisch K, Naliboff BD, Bushnell MC, Mayer EA. Regional gray matter density changes in brains of patients with irritable bowel syndrome. Gastroenterology 2010; Epub Mar 27.

[38] Sengupta JN. Visceral pain: the neurophysiological mechanism. Handb Exp Pharmacol 2009;31–74.

[39] Soderholm JD, Perdue MH. Stress and gastrointestinal tract. II. Stress and intestinal barrier function. Am J Physiol Gastrointest Liver Physiol 2001;280:G7–13.

[40] Soderholm JD, Yang PC, Ceponis P, Vohra A, Riddell R, Sherman PM, Perdue MH. Chronic stress induces mast cell-dependent bacterial adherence and initiates mucosal inflammation in rat intestine. Gastroenterology 2002;123:1099–108.

[41] Soderholm JD, Yates DA, Gareau MG, Yang PC, MacQueen G, Perdue MH. Neonatal maternal separation predisposes adult rats to colonic barrier dysfunction in response to mild stress. Am J Physiol Gastrointest Liver Physiol 2002;283:G1257–63.

[42] Spiller R, Garsed K. Postinfectious irritable bowel syndrome. Gastroenterology 2009;136:1979–88.

[43] Theoharides TC. Panic disorder, interstitial cystitis, and mast cells. J Clin Psychopharmacol 2004;24:361–4.

[44] Theoharides TC, Cochrane DE. Critical role of mast cells in inflammatory diseases and the effect of acute stress. J Neuroimmunol 2004;146:1–12.

Correspondence to: Emeran A. Mayer, MD, Center for Neurobiology of Stress, Division of Digestive Diseases, University of California, Los Angeles, 10945 Le Conte Avenue, Suite 2338, Room F, Los Angeles, CA 90095-6949, USA. Email: emayer@ucla.edu.

Diagnosis and Treatment of Persistent Pelvic Pain

35

Fred M. Howard, MS, MD

Department of Obstetrics and Gynecology, University of Rochester School of Medicine and Dentistry, Rochester, New York, USA

Chronic or persistent pelvic pain (CPP) in women is a common problem. It has a prevalence of about 4% in women, similar to the prevalence of migraine (2.1%), asthma (3.7%), and back pain (4.1%) [15,17,35]. CPP is the indication for 17% of all hysterectomies and over 40% of gynecological diagnostic laparoscopies [10,11]. It is estimated that direct and indirect costs of CPP in the United States are over $2 billion per year [17].

CPP may be defined as nonmenstrual pain of 6 or more months' duration that localizes to the anatomical pelvis, the anterior abdominal wall below the umbilicus, or the lumbosacral back and causes functional disability or requires medical or surgical treatment [1]. This definition excludes vulvar pain and the cyclical pain of dysmenorrhea. However, women with CPP often have vulvar pain or dysmenorrhea as part of their symptom complex.

More than 80% of women with CPP have had pain for more than a year when they seek medical care, and about one-third have had pain for more than 5 years [36]. About one-half of women with CPP have either urinary or gastrointestinal symptoms, or both, in addition to their pelvic pain. Reproductive tract symptoms are also very common.

Diagnosis

The number of potential diagnoses, the variety of anatomical sources of pain, the likelihood that the patient may have more than one diagnosis, and the potential that pain itself may be a diagnosis are only a few of the issues that make diagnostic evaluation challenging.

The history and physical examination are powerful diagnostic and therapeutic tools in CPP [12]. As diagnostic tools, a thorough history and examination may lead to accurate diagnosis, minimizing the need for expensive laboratory or imaging testing, or risky operative interventions. As therapeutic tools, a compassionately taken history, during which the patient talks and the physician listens, and a sensitively performed examination establish rapport and build trust that the physician is caring and competent, and allow the patient to leave the physician's office feeling better. Because the examination is often painful for the woman with CPP, it is important that the physician remember that even a "routine" pelvic examination is very emotionally stressful for many patients with CPP.

The diversity of potential etiological or associated diagnoses demands a multidisciplinary approach to diagnostic evaluation. Referrals to and consultations with other specialists may be needed. The history of the patient's pain must be thoroughly obtained, as must the review of systems, with particular attention to the gastrointestinal, reproductive, urological, neurological, and musculoskeletal systems. Psychological assessment is crucial, also. Because of the complexity of the history in most patients, intake questionnaires are extremely helpful in obtaining details of the history (www.pelvicpain.org). However, they should not replace allowing patients to tell their story.

Establishing the location of the patient's pain can be crucial to accurate diagnosis. An ideal way to do this is to have the patient mark the location(s) of the pain on a pain map. A pain map may show both ventral and dorsal pain, suggesting intrapelvic pathology, whereas dorsal lower back pain only suggests an orthopedic or musculoskeletal origin. A pain map may show a dermatomal distribution of pain, suggesting a central neurological source, or it may show a unilateral cutaneous distribution along the anterior lower abdominal wall into the labia or upper inner aspect of the thigh, suggesting neuropathic pain of the iliohypogastric or ilioinguinal nerves. A pain map may show a very diffuse distribution, consistent with visceral pain.

Exploring the nature of the onset of pain may aid in diagnosis. For example, an immediately antecedent trauma, such as a fall, surgery, or motor vehicle accident, suggests that a musculoskeletal cause is likely. Pain that started with a pregnancy or immediately postpartum may suggest peripartum pelvic pain syndrome. Pain that started at or soon after menarche as dysmenorrhea, progressed to premenstrual pain, and then became constant, suggests endometriosis. If pain started soon after a physical or sexual assault, it may have significant musculoskeletal or psychological components.

Finding out if there is any temporal pattern to the pain may be helpful. Cyclicity related to menses suggests gynecological pain but is not pathognomonic of gynecological disease. The same pattern may occur with pain of intestinal, urological, or musculoskeletal origin. A history of pain or increased pain with coitus is frequently present and may be due to a variety of disorders, including psychological disease, marital problems, endometriosis, vulvodynia, interstitial cystitis, and irritable bowel syndrome (IBS). If intercourse is painful, it is important to find out if pain is with entry at the outermost part of the vagina, with deeper penetration high in the vagina or pelvis, or both.

Finding out about any prior treatments for CPP and the response to those treatments is crucial part of the history. It may be important to know about any prior surgery, not just surgical treatment for pain, as pain may be a risk factor for or a cause of CPP.

Ideally, a thorough psychosocial history should be obtained on every patient with CPP. An extensive evaluation by a psychologist, or similarly educated professional, is not always possible. However, a basic psychosocial history is always important, especially asking about depression and anxiety. Depression is one of several predictors of pain severity in women with CPP, and it is also a significant indicator of responsiveness to treatment [9]. Asking about abuse is another important part of the psychosocial history. There is a significant association of physical and sexual abuse with the development of chronic pain [6].

The physical examination should seek to find the exact anatomical locations of any areas of tenderness and, as much as possible, correlate these with areas of pain. This type of "pain mapping" examination requires a systematic and methodical attempt to elicit the patient's pain by palpation, positioning, or bodily movement. At any tender areas or painful positions, the patient should be asked whether the pain produced is the same as the chronic pain. The examination should evaluate the musculoskeletal, gastrointestinal, urinary, and neurological systems, not just the reproductive tract. It facilitates the examination to divide it into standing, sitting, supine, and lithotomy components.

One of the aspects of the "pain mapping" examination that differs from the traditional examination is the use of single-digit palpation of the back, abdomen, and pelvis. The single-digit examination is particularly useful looking for myofascial or trigger point pain. The abdominal wall tenderness test (Carnett test) is also a useful technique in pain mapping and may be used to distinguish abdominal wall tenderness from visceral tenderness [5,29]. In this test, while the area of abdominal tenderness is palpated, the patient voluntarily tenses the abdominal muscles, which is readily accomplished by having her raise her head or legs. If the pain is increased, it suggests that the pain is of abdominal wall origin. If the pain is decreased or unchanged, it suggests that the pain is most likely of visceral origin.

A single-digit examination, using only one hand, is also how the pelvic examination should be initiated. The introital bulbocavernosus and transverse perineal muscles, then the levator ani muscles, should be palpated for tone, spasm, and tenderness. In patients with pelvic floor pain, palpation may cause pain consistent with at least part of the patient's clinical pain symptoms. Pelvic floor pain may also result from trigger points of one or more of the muscles of the pelvis. The piriformis, coccygeus, and obturator internus muscles should be thoroughly evaluated using a single-digit examination.

The anterior vaginal, urethral, and trigonal areas should be palpated to elicit any areas of tenderness, induration, discharge, or thickening suggestive of chronic urethritis, chronic urethral syndrome, urethral diverticulum, vaginal wall cyst, trigonitis, or interstitial cystitis. With deeper palpation the cervix, paracervical areas, and vaginal fornices should be palpated with the single digit for tenderness or trigger points suggestive of problems such as repeated cervical trauma (usually from intercourse), pelvic infection, endometriosis, ureteral pain, or trigger points.

The uterus usually can be adequately evaluated for tenderness by direct palpation with a single digit. Significant uterine tenderness may be consistent with diseases such as adenomyosis, pelvic congestion syndrome, pelvic infection sequelae, endometriosis, or premenstrual syndrome. A uterus that is immobile and fixed in position, especially a retroflexed one, may suggest endometriosis or adhesions. The coccyx should also be palpated with a single digit, and an attempt should be made to move it 30° or less. This movement may be easier to evaluate during the rectovaginal examination. Normally the coccyx moves 30° without eliciting pain, but in patients with coccydynia this movement elicits pain. The ureteral and the adnexal areas should be palpated next, still using a single digit without the use of the abdominal hand. All of the above are "monomanual, monodigital" evaluations—that is, only one finger of one hand is used. No abdominal palpation with the other hand is involved.

Examination with a moistened cotton-tipped swab may be more useful than the single-digit examination to evaluate the vulva and the vulvar vestibule for tenderness. This technique is particularly useful in patients with localized vulvodynia (previously known as vulvar vestibulitis), who have exquisite tenderness in localized areas at the minor vestibular glands just external to the hymen, with normal sensation in adjacent vulvar areas. Sometimes palpation with a cotton-tipped swab also can elicit allodynia in a neural distribution in women with pudendal neuralgia. In post-hysterectomy patients, the full vaginal cuff should be similarly palpated for tenderness with a cotton-tipped swab.

The traditional visual, speculum, and bimanual examinations are still needed for a thorough evaluation, but usually they should follow the single-digit examination. The pain or tenderness elicited with the bimanual examination is less specific, as it involves stimulation of all layers of the abdominal wall, the parietal peritoneum, and the palpated organ(s). Including the rectovaginal examination is important in most women with CPP, looking particularly for nodularity and tenderness, which would suggest endometriosis.

Irritable Bowel Syndrome

IBS appears to be the most common diagnosis in women with CPP [36], with symptoms suggestive of the syndrome in 50–80%. The diagnosis is based on the history; usually extensive laboratory and radiological tests are not necessary.

Some of the findings that mandate more extensive diagnostic testing to rule out more serious pathology are blood in the stool, weight loss, ascites, watery bowel movements more than three times per day, an abdominal mass, or fever.

Interstitial Cystitis/Painful Bladder Syndrome

Interstitial cystitis/painful bladder syndrome (IC/PBS) is pelvic pain, pressure, or discomfort related to the bladder, associated with the persistent urge to void, in the absence of urinary infection or other pathology, such as bladder carcinoma or cystitis induced by radiation or medication.

Traditionally, IC/PBS was diagnosed only in severe cases, characterized by severely reduced bladder capacity and cystoscopic findings of Hunner's ulcer or glomerulations [14,18]. It is now clear that the bladder can be a source of pelvic pain without these clinical findings. IC/PBS appears to occur more commonly among women than men, and it is a frequent diagnosis in women with CPP. For example, in our gynecology-based pain clinic, about 30% of all women are diagnosed with IC/PBS (unpublished data).

Voiding frequency with IC/PBS is usually every 2 hours or less during the day and two or more times at night. Incontinence is not a common symptom. Evaluation should show the absence of objective evidence of another urinary tract disease that could cause the symptoms. Bladder tumors, especially carcinoma in situ, may cause symptoms similar to those of interstitial cystitis.

Cystoscopy with hydrodistension causes mucosal hemorrhages, called glomerulations, in patients with IC/PBS, although there are false-positive cystoscopies. In addition to glomerulations, linear cracking and Hunner's ulcer may also be noted. Because significant bladder distension is needed, which is very painful in women with IC/PBS, general or spinal anesthesia is usually necessary.

The potassium sensitivity test has been proposed as an office screening test for IC/PBS. This test evaluates pain and urgency after intravesical instillation of 40 mL of potassium chloride (0.4 mEq/mL) compared to symptoms with 40 mL of water. It is reportedly positive in 70–90% of patients with IC/PBS. As many as 85% of women evaluated by gynecologists for CPP may have positive intravesical potassium sensitivity tests [21].

It has been suggested that decreased pain with intravesical instillation of local anesthetic agents, such as lidocaine or bupivacaine, can be used to confirm the diagnosis. Finally, in cases that are clearly IC/PBS clinically, the diagnosis may be made without any interventional testing.

Endometriosis

Endometriosis is the presence of ectopic endometrial glands and stroma, that is, endometrium located outside of the endometrial cavity. Classically, the woman with endometriosis presents with one or more of the following triad: an adnexal mass (endometrioma), infertility, or pelvic pain. Estimates are that 5% to 40% of women with endometriosis have CPP. Endometriosis-associated pain almost always starts as menstrual pain, then progresses to include the luteal phase, and in many women progresses to constant pain with premenstrual and menstrual exacerbation. Most women with endometriosis-associated pelvic pain have severe dysmenorrhea as a component of their pain symptoms. Dyspareunia is present in at least 40%. The clinical diagnosis of endometriosis based on the history and physical examination is accurate in about 85% of women with CPP, but for absolute confirmation of the diagnosis there must be histological confirmation of ectopic endometrium. A solely visual diagnosis at the time of laparoscopy has a significant false-positive rate.

Pelvic Inflammatory Disease

Fifteen to 30% of all women with acute pelvic inflammatory disease subsequently develop CPP [19]. Pelvic inflammatory disease is most frequent among teenagers and women less than 25 years of age, which is about a decade younger than the mean age of women with CPP. CPP secondary to prior pelvic inflammatory disease is usually related to coitus and physical activity, and is acyclic, although sometimes there may be premenstrual or menstrual exacerbation. The diagnosis is based on past history of pelvic inflammatory disease and on operative findings consistent with prior pelvic inflammatory disease, such as adnexal adhesions, tubo-ovarian complexes, tubal agglutination and phimosis, and hydrosalpinges. Little is known about the actual mechanisms by which CPP results from pelvic inflammatory disease. Some evidence suggests that it is related to the severity of adnexal adhesions and damage [34]. Antibiotic treatment is often empirically tried in women with suspected "chronic pelvic inflammatory disease" or subclinical, chronic pelvic infection. There is scant evidence that any pathogenic microorganisms persist in the uterus or tubes after pelvic inflammatory disease, and there is no published evidence of efficacy of empiric antibiotic treatment of CPP when there is no suggestion of active, acute infection.

Although it is not a common diagnosis in the United States, tuberculous pelvic inflammatory disease must be remembered as a potential diagnosis in patients with CPP, especially as the incidence of tuberculosis has increased in association with human immunodeficiency virus-autoimmune deficiency disease (HIV-AIDS).

Pelvic Congestion Syndrome

Pelvic congestion syndrome is characterized by CPP, pelvic varicosities, and venographically documented evidence of venous congestion [3]. It is a controversial diagnosis among pelvic pain experts.

Pain associated with pelvic congestion is typically worst premenstrually. Pain is usually dull and aching, similar in quality to the leg pain produced by leg varicosities. It is usually not constant and may be brought on by simple acts such as walking or changing posture. Occasional acute, severe exacerbations of sharp pain may occur. Backache is common; it is characteristically sacral in position and is made worse by standing. Deep dyspareunia is present in three-quarters of women with pelvic congestion syndrome. Postcoital aching pain, lasting in some cases up to 24 hours, is present in 65% of cases.

Abdominal palpation at the ovarian point, which lies at the junction of the upper and middle thirds of a line drawn from the anterior superior iliac spine to the pubic symphysis, reproduces pelvic pain in 80% of women with pelvic congestion syndrome. Diffuse pelvic tenderness, particularly at the adnexa, is characteristic at bimanual pelvic examination.

The diagnosis is confirmed by pelvic venography showing venous stasis, dilation, and plexus formation of the ovarian or uterine vessels. Venography can be performed by transuterine injection of the myometrium or by retrograde injection of the ovarian veins.

Adhesions

Adhesions are aberrant fibrous tissues that abnormally attach anatomical structures to one another. In women, the major causes of adhesions are surgery, pelvic inflammatory disease, appendicitis, endometriosis, inflammatory bowel disease, and neoplasia.

It is generally accepted that adhesions can cause intestinal obstruction and infertility, but their role as a cause of CPP is not clear. There is an association of adhesions and CPP, as intra-abdominal and pelvic adhesions are found more often in women with CPP than in women without pain, but this association does not prove causation. Laparoscopic conscious pain mapping has demonstrated that at least one-third of patients with adhesions have focal, dramatic tenderness of some of their adhesions [13]. This finding suggests that adhesions cause pain in some, but not all, women with pelvic adhesions.

Pelvic pain due to adhesions is usually consistent in its location and may be exacerbated by sudden movements, intercourse, or certain physical activities. A history of pelvic inflammatory disease, endometriosis, perforated appendix, prior abdominopelvic surgery, or inflammatory bowel disease makes adhesive disease a more likely diagnosis. A history of at least one of these conditions is present in only 50% of women with adhesions, however.

The only definitive way to diagnose adhesions is by surgical visualization. Laparoscopy, not laparotomy, is the gold standard for diagnosing pelvic adhesive disease.

Chronic Abdominal Wall Pain

Chronic pain emanating from the abdominal wall is frequently unrecognized or confused with visceral pain, often leading to extensive diagnostic testing before an accurate diagnosis is achieved. Such pain is most often due to myofascial pain syndrome with trigger points. Other causes may be muscular injury or strain, hernias, or nerve injury. Chronic abdominal wall pain occurs in 7–9% of women after a Pfannenstiel incision [16].

Pelvic Floor Tension Myalgia

Pelvic floor tension myalgia is caused by involuntary spasm of the pelvic floor muscles (e.g., piriformis, levator ani, iliopsoas, and obturator internus). In particular, the levator ani muscle group can undergo pain-causing processes observed in other muscle groups, such as hypertonus, myalgia, overuse, and fatigue. The etiology includes any inflammatory painful disorder, childbirth, pelvic surgery, and trauma. In addition to dyspareunia, there may be aching pelvic pain, which is aggravated by sitting for prolonged periods and is relieved by heat and

lying down with the hips flexed. There is evidence that women with CPP have decreased thresholds to pain in the pelvic floor muscles, suggesting that pelvic floor tension myalgia may sometimes be a direct sequela of CPP due to other disorders, such as endometriosis or IC/PBS [30].

Depression

The etiological relationship of depression and chronic pain is complex and confusing. Regardless, depression is one of the major findings that leads to a diagnosis of chronic pain syndrome, and it is a major predictor of pain severity and response to treatment [9]. It is important to seek evidence of depression in women with CPP.

Treatment

There are two primary approaches to the treatment of CPP: (1) treatment of pain (pain-specific treatment) and (2) treatment of specific diseases responsible for CPP (disease-specific treatment). There are randomized clinical trials of treatment of several of the common diagnoses associated with CPP, such as endometriosis, IBS, and IC/PBS. Pain-specific treatment of CPP is not as well studied.

Disease-Specific Treatment

Endometriosis

Endometriosis may be treated surgically, medically, or with combined surgical and medical therapy. Medical treatment usually is hormonal with oral contraceptives, danazol, progestins, or gonadotropin-releasing hormone agonists. Randomized clinical trials confirm effective pain relief with danazol, gonadotropin-releasing hormone (GnRH) agonists (nafarelin, goserelin, and leuprolide), continuous oral contraceptives, subcutaneous and oral medroxyprogesterone acetate, and norethindrone acetate. Side effects observed with medical therapy include breakthrough bleeding, mood changes, depression, hot flushes, weight gain, and irritability. Danazol may also cause androgenic side effects. Loss of bone density is a concern with GnRH agonists. To minimize loss of bone density, add-back treatment with estrogen and/or progestagen may be used.

Laparoscopic surgical treatment by destruction of endometriotic lesions and lysis of adhesions relieves pain in 60–85% of patients [2,26]. Although hysterectomy and bilateral salpingo-oophorectomy are thought to be curative for endometriosis, no clinical trials of hysterectomy or salpingo-oophorectomy for endometriosis-associated pelvic pain have been reported. It is important that all endometriosis be resected or destroyed at the time of hysterectomy and bilateral salpingo-oophorectomy to minimize the potential of recurrence.

Pain-specific neurolytic procedures, particularly uterosacral ligament transections and presacral neurectomy, are sometimes performed to treat endometriosis-associated pelvic pain. Controlled clinical trials suggest that presacral neurectomy (excision of the superior hypogastric plexus) gives a small improvement in pain relief compared with excision of endometriosis alone, with a number needed to treat (NNT) for presacral neurectomy of 4.8 [37]. However, transection of the uterosacral ligaments showed no efficacy in the treatment of endometriosis-associated pelvic pain over that obtained with only surgical excision of lesions in randomized clinical trials [25,32].

Interstitial Cystitis/Painful Bladder Syndrome

Dimethylsulfoxide (DMSO) was the first U.S. Food and Drug Administration (FDA)-approved drug indicated for IC/PBS. Intravesical treatments with DMSO are usually repeated at 1- to 2-week intervals. The NNT for DMSO therapy of IC/PBS-associated pelvic pain is estimated at 3.6 [22]. DMSO treatments result only in remission of disease, not cure. Other intravesical therapies for IC/PBS have been less extensively studied, and none other than DMSO has FDA approval for treatment of interstitial cystitis.

The other FDA-approved treatment of IC/PBS is oral pentosan polysulfate sodium, a polyanionic analogue of heparin. One randomized clinical trial showed an NNT of 3.7 for decreased pelvic pain [20]. Amitriptyline also has shown efficacy in a clinical trial, but is not FDA-approved [31].

The primary surgical treatment of IC/PBS is hydrodistension of the bladder. This procedure can be performed at the time of diagnostic cystoscopy if general or spinal anesthesia is used. Observational studies suggest that about 50% of patients have a successful response to hydrodistension. Remission generally lasts for 6 to 10 months, with a gradual recurrence of symptoms in almost all patients. Retreatment with hydrodistension has a greatly diminished success rate.

Approximately 5% of patients have unresponsive, intractable, incapacitating symptoms. Such patients usually have small-capacity bladders (<400 mL), void 18–20 times per day, and have severe, uncontrolled pain. Augmentation cystoplasty or cystectomy-urethrectomy-continent diversion have been the most successful and acceptable radical surgical treatments.

Irritable Bowel Syndrome

Dietary interventions constitute the initial approach to IBS. Lactose, fructose, and sorbitol can contribute to symptoms and should be eliminated from the diet, at least on a trial basis. Caffeinated products, carbonated beverages, and gas-producing foods (such as broccoli, cabbage, brussels sprouts, asparagus, cauliflower, and beans) may contribute to bloating and should be avoided if possible. Smoking and chewing gum lead to more swallowed air and may increase gas and bloating as well. Excessive alcohol consumption may lead to increased rectal urgency. Fiber supplementation is often useful, for both diarrhea and constipation symptoms.

Pharmacological treatment is not specific to the disease, but rather is directed to relief of symptoms. Patients may be divided into one of three major symptom categories, depending on which symptoms are dominant. The three symptom categories are: (1) abdominal pain, gas, and bloating; (2) constipation predominant; and (3) diarrhea predominant. Unfortunately, many patients do not fall clearly into one of these three groups, but have overlapping symptoms. The severity of the symptoms also influences the choice of pharmacological treatment. Details of treatment are discussed in the presentation on abdominal pain.

Adhesions

The traditional treatment of abdominopelvic adhesions is surgical adhesiolysis. The only randomized trial of adhesiolysis for CPP failed to show any significant improvement after lysis of adhesions by laparotomy, compared to a control group that did not undergo adhesiolysis [23]. Only when a subgroup analysis of 15 women with severe, stage IV adhesions was performed was there any detectable improvement in pain that could be attributed to adhesiolysis. A randomized trial of laparoscopic adhesiolysis for abdominal pain (in men and women) suggested a difference between surgically treated versus untreated patients, but the difference was not statistically significant [28].

A problem with studies of surgical adhesiolysis is that there are no effective methods for preventing recurrence of adhesions. Adhesions will most likely remain a cause for some cases of CPP until a method to prevent them is found.

Musculoskeletal Pain Syndromes

Abdominal myofascial pain syndrome and pelvic floor tension myalgia are the most commonly encountered musculoskeletal diagnoses in women with CPP. Both are probably best treated by physical therapy, although trigger point infections and nerve blocks are sometimes useful. Empirical evidence suggests that muscle relaxants are sometimes helpful.

Pain-Specific Treatment

Pain-specific treatment is directed not to the noxious stimulus that triggers the nociceptive pathway, but rather to the fundamental processes involved in the nociceptive pathway—transduction, transmission, modulation, or perception. Pain-specific treatment can be a crucial component of therapy because disease-specific treatment often gives inadequate pain relief. Pain-specific treatment may be pharmacological, psychological, physical, or neuroablative.

Pharmacological Treatment

The mosaic of neural elements and chemical mediators involved in pain perception make it possible to decrease pain with medications with different pharmacological profiles and mechanisms. Oral analgesics are particularly important in the treatment of pain, yet optimization of analgesic medications is sometimes overlooked in the initial treatment of CPP. Optimization of analgesia is usually best accomplished with a scheduled regimen, not with a pro re nata (p.r.n.) or "as needed" regimen. However, a scheduled regimen also presents some hazards. For example, with nonsteroidal anti-inflammatory drugs (NSAIDs) it may lead to gastric irritation or renal damage, and with opioids it may lead to constipation, sedation, habituation, addiction, or diminished analgesic potency.

Analgesics include acetaminophen, NSAIDs, and opioids. Opioid maintenance treatment for CPP is controversial and generally should only be used after all traditional attempts at pain control have failed. Before opioid treatment is initiated there should be a written or documented verbal agreement with the patient that includes at least the following particulars: (1) the treating doctor is the sole provider of opioids; (2) the patient has seen this physician before having the opioid prescription refilled; (3) lost medications or prescriptions will not be refilled; and (4) the patient agrees to actively participate in strategies to develop alternative pain therapies.

Some physicians have advocated inclusion of random urine drug testing as a condition of opioid maintenance therapy. Antidepressants, particularly tricyclic antidepressants (TCAs), have been used to treat a number of chronic pain syndromes including arthritis, diabetic neuropathy, headache, back pain, and cancer pain. TCAs may result in improved pain levels at doses much lower than those typically used for the treatment of depression. Pain levels generally are decreased by 20–50% in chronic pain syndromes, although it is not clear that TCAs are effective in all pain syndromes. There are no randomized clinical trials of TCAs for treatment of CPP. One open-label study suggested that nortriptyline at 100 mg per day was effective, but the dropout rate due to side effects was 50% [33]. Depression is common in women with CPP, and when it is diagnosed it should be treated with an appropriate antidepressant in most cases.

Combination drug therapy uses medications with different sites or mechanisms of action to improve the treatment of pain. For example, combining a centrally acting opioid analgesic and a peripherally acting NSAID often gives better pain relief than either analgesic alone. Similarly, combining two medications that act centrally but have different mechanisms, such as a TCA and an opioid analgesic, might result in better pain relief than monotherapy. Combination drug therapy may improve pain relief, but it also increases adverse effects and potential drug interactions.

Psychological Treatment

Ideally, psychological evaluation and treatment would be part of the care of every patient with CPP. Patients with chronic pain develop psychological changes that maintain or increase the distress of their pain regardless of the degree of physical trauma or disease. Combining psychotherapy (usually cognitive-behavioral therapy) with traditional surgical or medical treatment results in better outcomes than those obtained with surgical or medical treatment alone [4,7,8,24,27]. Unfortunately, many patients are unable to afford or reluctant to accept referral to a psychologist or psychiatrist for evaluation and treatment.

Complementary Treatments

Other treatments, especially complementary treatments, are often used by women with CPP. Most complementary treatments are not well-studied for CPP. Relaxation therapy, music therapy, transcutaneous electrical nerve stimulation (TENS), acupuncture, massage therapy, chiropractic manipulation, reflexology, magnetic field therapy, hypnosis, spiritual or religious treatments, and general comfort measures (heat packs, hot baths or whirlpools, ice packs, back rubs, etc.) are examples of complementary therapies.

Key Points

• CPP is a common disorder in women, with an estimated prevalence of 4%.

• Disorders of the gastrointestinal, urological, and musculoskeletal systems are at least as common as reproductive system disorders in women with CPP.

• Chronic pain differs from acute pain in that it serves no known biological function and frequently is a diagnosis, not a symptom.

• CPP may be treated in a disease-specific manner or in a pain-specific manner; in many women it is more effective to treat both specific diseases (e.g., endometriosis) and pain.

• A thorough history and physical examination are crucial in the evaluation and treatment of women with CPP.

References

[1] ACOG Practice Bulletin No. 51. Chronic pelvic pain. Obstet Gynecol 2004;103:589–605.

[2] Abbott J, Hawe J, Hunter D, Holmes M, Finn P, Garry R. Laparoscopic excision of endometriosis: a randomized, placebo-controlled trial. Fertil Steril 2004;82:878–84.

[3] Beard RW, Highman JH, Pearce S, Reginald PW. Diagnosis of pelvic varicosities in women with chronic pelvic pain. Lancet 1984;2:946–9.

[4] Farquhar CM, Rogers V, Franks S, Pearce S, Wadsworth J, Beard RW. A randomized controlled trial of medroxyprogesterone acetate and psychotherapy for the treatment of pelvic congestion. Br J Obstet Gynaecol 1989;96:1153–62.

[5] Gray DW, Dixon JM, Seabrook G, Collin J. Is abdominal wall tenderness a useful sign in the diagnosis of non-specific abdominal pain? Ann R Coll Surg Engl 1988;70:233–4.

[6] Green CR, Flowe-Valencia H, Rosenblum L, Tait AR. The role of childhood and adulthood abuse among women presenting for chronic pain management. Clin J Pain 2001;17:359–64.

[7] Guthrie E, Creed F, Dawson D, Tomenson B. A controlled trial of psychological treatment for the irritable bowel syndrome. Gastroenterology 1991;100:450–7.

[8] Guthrie E, Creed F, Dawson D, Tomenson B. A randomised controlled trial of psychotherapy in patients with refractory irritable bowel syndrome. Br J Psychiatry 1993;163:315–21.

[9] Hartmann KE, Ma C, Lamvu GM, Langenberg PW, Steege JF, Kjerulff KH. Quality of life and sexual function after hysterectomy in women with preoperative pain and depression. Obstet Gynecol 2004;104:701–9.

[10] Hillis SD, Marchbanks PA, Peterson HB. The effectiveness of hysterectomy for chronic pelvic pain. Obstet Gynecol 1995;86:941–5.

[11] Howard FM. The role of laparoscopy in chronic pelvic pain: promise and pitfalls. Obstet Gynecol Surv 1993;48:357–87.

[12] Howard FM. Chronic pelvic pain. Obstet Gynecol 2003;101:594–611.

[13] Howard FM, El-Minawi AM, Sanchez RA. Conscious pain mapping by laparoscopy in women with chronic pelvic pain. Obstet Gynecol 2000;96:934–9.

[14] Hunner GL. A rare type of bladder ulcer in women: report of cases. Boston Med Surg 1915;172.

[15] Lippman SA, Warner M, Samuels S, Olive D, Vercellini P, Eskenazi B. Uterine fibroids and gynecologic pain symptoms in a population-based study. Fertil Steril 2003;80:1488–94.

[16] Loos MJ, Scheltinga MR, Mulders LG, Roumen RM. The Pfannenstiel incision as a source of chronic pain. Obstet Gynecol 2008;111:839–46.

[17] Mathias SD, Kuppermann M, Liberman RF, Lipschutz RC, Steege JF. Chronic pelvic pain: prevalence, health-related quality of life, and economic correlates. Obstet Gynecol 1996;87:321–7.

[18] Messing EM, Stamey TA. Interstitial cystitis: early diagnosis, pathology, and treatment. Urology 1978;12:381–92.

[19] Ness RB, Soper DE, Holley RL, Peipert J, Randall H, Sweet RL, Sondheimer SJ, Hendrix SL, Amortegui A, Trucco G, et al. Effectiveness of inpatient and outpatient treatment strategies for women with pelvic inflammatory disease: results from the Pelvic Inflammatory Disease Evaluation and Clinical Health (PEACH) Randomized Trial. Am J Obstet Gynecol 2002;186:929–37.

[20] Parsons CL, Benson G, Childs SJ, Hanno P, Sant GR, Webster G. A quantitatively controlled method to study prospectively interstitial cystitis and demonstrate the efficacy of pentosanpolysulfate. J Urol 1993;150:845–8.

[21] Parsons CL, Bullen M, Kahn BS, Stanford EJ, Willems JJ. Gynecologic presentation of interstitial cystitis as detected by intravesical potassium sensitivity. Obstet Gynecol 2001;98:127–32.

[22] Perez-Marrero R, Emerson LE, Feltis JT. A controlled study of dimethyl sulfoxide in interstitial cystitis. J Urol 1988;140:36–9.

[23] Peters AA, Trimbos-Kemper GC, Admiraal C, Trimbos JB, Hermans J. A randomized clinical trial on the benefit of adhesiolysis in patients with intraperitoneal adhesions and chronic pelvic pain. Br J Obstet Gynaecol 1992;99:59–62.

[24] Peters AA, van Dorst E, Jellis B, van Zuuren E, Hermans J, Trimbos JB. A randomized clinical trial to compare two different approaches in women with chronic pelvic pain. Obstet Gynecol 1991;77:740–4.

[25] Sutton C, Pooley AS, Jones KD, Dover RW, Haines P. A prospective, randomized, double-blind controlled trial of laparoscopic uterine nerve ablation in the treatment of pelvic pain associated with endometriosis. Gynaecol Endoscopy 2001;10:6.

[26] Sutton CJ, Ewen SP, Whitelaw N, Haines P. Prospective, randomized, double-blind, controlled trial of laser laparoscopy in the treatment of pelvic pain associated with minimal, mild, and moderate endometriosis. Fertil Steril 1994;62:696–700.

[27] Svedlund J. Psychotherapy in irritable bowel syndrome: a controlled outcome study. Acta Psychiatr Scand Suppl 1983;306:1–86.

[28] Swank DJ, Swank-Bordewijk SC, Hop WC, van Erp WF, Janssen IM, Bonjer HJ, Jeekel J. Laparoscopic adhesiolysis in patients with chronic abdominal pain: a blinded randomised controlled multi-centre trial. Lancet 2003;361:1247–51.

[29] Thomson WH, Dawes RF, Carter SS. Abdominal wall tenderness: a useful sign in chronic abdominal pain. Br J Surg 1991;78:223–5.

[30] Tu FF, Fitzgerald CM, Kuiken T, Farrell T, Harden RN. Comparative measurement of pelvic floor pain sensitivity in chronic pelvic pain. Obstet Gynecol 2007;110:1244–8.

[31] van Ophoven A, Pokupic S, Heinecke A, Hertle L. A prospective, randomized, placebo controlled, double-blind study of amitriptyline for the treatment of interstitial cystitis. J Urol 2004;172:533–6.

[32] Vercellini P, Aimi G, Busacca M, Apolone G, Uglietti A, Crosignani PG. Laparoscopic uterosacral ligament resection for dysmenorrhea associated with endometriosis: results of a randomized, controlled trial. Fertil Steril 2003;80:310–9.

[33] Walker EA, Roy-Byrne PP, Katon WJ, Jemelka R. An open trial of nortriptyline in women with chronic pelvic pain. Int J Psychiatry Med 1991;21:245–52.

[34] Westrom L. Chronic pain after acute PID. In: Belfort P, Pinotti J, Eskes T, editors. Advances in gynecology and obstetrics. Proceedings of the XIIth FIGO World Congress of Gynaecology and Obstetrics, Oct. 1988, Rio de Janeiro. New York: Parthenon; 1989.

[35] Zondervan KT, Yudkin PL, Vessey MP, Dawes MG, Barlow DH, Kennedy SH. Prevalence and incidence of chronic pelvic pain in primary care: evidence from a national general practice database. Br J Obstet Gynaecol 1999;106:1149–55.

[36] Zondervan KT, Yudkin PL, Vessey MP, Jenkinson CP, Dawes MG, Barlow DH, Kennedy SH. Chronic pelvic pain in the community: symptoms, investigations, and diagnoses. Am J Obstet Gynecol 2001;184:1149–55.

[37] Zullo F, Palomba S, Zupi E, Russo T, Morelli M, Cappiello F, Mastrantonio P. Effectiveness of presacral neurectomy in women with severe dysmenorrhea caused by endometriosis who were treated with laparoscopic conservative surgery: a 1-year prospective randomized double-blind controlled trial. Am J Obstet Gynecol 2003;189:5–10.

Correspondence to: Fred M. Howard, MS, MD, Department of Obstetrics and Gynecology, University of Rochester School of Medicine and Dentistry, 601 Elmwood Avenue, Box 668, Rochester, NY 14642, USA. Email: fred_howard @ urmc.rochester.edu.

Diagnosis and Treatment of Persistent Abdominal Pain

Kirsten Tillisch, MD

Center for Neurobiology of Stress, Division of Digestive Diseases, David Geffen School of Medicine, UCLA, Los Angeles, California, USA

Persistent abdominal pain is a common presenting symptom that can be caused by a multitude of factors, both functional and organic (see Table I). A key differentiation to be made by the clinician is whether an intervention can be made to eliminate the underlying cause of the pain, or whether symptomatic management will be the primary goal. A complete history and physical examination are essential for determining the correct diagnosis, guiding further testing, and choosing a therapeutic approach. Many patients with persistent abdominal pain will have already undergone investigation at the time that the pain was acute. Review of this investigation is essential because some patients may require no further diagnostic testing. However, persistent pain that changes in character over time may require further evaluation.

History

Chronology of Pain

A careful history can be the most useful diagnostic tool. Thorough discussion of the first episode of pain may give insight into its pathophysiology. This discussion includes a review of temporally related illness, surgical procedures, sick contacts, and life events (e.g., travel, geographic relocation, diet changes, or stressful experiences). Determining whether prior episodes or similar symptoms predate the current problem is important. While an episode may feel "acute" to a patient, a history of prior self-limited episodes may be recalled with prompting. Eliciting a history of repeated bouts of visceral or somatic pain over the lifespan, especially with negative diagnostic evaluations, is highly suggestive of a functional rather than organic disorder. Pain that has been present for many years is similarly reassuring. However, slowly progressive pain over a few months may be more concerning for organic disorders, particularly malignancy.

Pain Location and Extent

Persistent abdominal pain can either be localized in a distinct, reproducible area, which suggests somatic or abdominal wall pain, or it may be diffuse, which is more consistent with visceral pain. Compared to the somatic innervation of the abdominal wall, a smaller number of mechanically sensitive spinal afferents innervates the viscera, converging onto spinal neurons at several spinal segments. Thus, the perceived site of visceral pain tends to be referred to general areas such as the epigastrium (stomach, duodenum, pancreas, and biliary tree), periumbilical or mid-abdominal area (jejunum and ileum, and ascending colon) and suprapubic or lower abdomen (descending colon, sigmoid colon, and rectum). Pain from functional disorders may have an inconsistent location, may move from place to place, or may even cross anatomical boundaries, such as upper abdominal pain radiating to an entire side of the body.

Table I
Causes of persistent abdominal pain

Inflammatory
Peptic ulcer disease
Ulcerative colitis
Crohn's disease
Celiac disease
Vasculitis
Chronic cholecystitis
Chronic pancreatitis
Malignant
Colorectal carcinoma
Small-bowel carcinoma
Hepatoma/hepatocellular carcinoma
Pancreatic carcinoma
Carcinoid tumor
Structural
NSAID strictures
Postsurgical strictures
Adhesions
Functional
Functional abdominal pain
Functional dyspepsia
Irritable bowel syndrome
Chronic intestinal pseudo-obstruction
Other
Porphyria
Lead poisoning
Familial Mediterranean fever
Intestinal ischemia

A greater referral area to pain has been described experimentally in patients with irritable bowel syndrome (IBS), in whom referral areas on the abdomen from a rectal stimulation are larger in extent compared to controls receiving the same stimulus [13].

Characteristics of Pain

It can be useful to determine if pain is constant or colicky. Obstructive pain from the intestines tends to be colicky, due to modulation of the intensity by peristaltic waves. Similarly, pain from the biliary tree and ureters can be colicky. Pain from inflammation or from the distension of a solid organ capsule, as in hepatitis or hepatic tumor, tends to be more constant in nature.

Modulating Factors

Pain that is modulated by food intake suggests involvement of the luminal gastrointestinal tract. However, this modulation can be seen in both organic disorders (such as peptic ulcer disease or symptomatic gallstones) and functional disorders (such as dyspepsia or IBS). Because of this variability, the traditional beliefs that ulcer

pain improves with food, and biliary pain worsens with fatty food, are likely to offer little diagnostic specificity. Psychosocial stressors and depressed mood can aggravate pain of any kind, but this feature tends to be most prominent in functional disorders, which may have a component of central pain amplification.

Associated Symptoms

Fever, weight loss, signs of gastrointestinal bleeding, and abnormal laboratory studies are unlikely in functional pain disorders and are considered alarm symptoms [3]. These symptoms should prompt a more thorough evaluation for an organic cause of pain. Concomitant fever suggests an inflammatory component such as chronic infection, familial Mediterranean fever, or Crohn's disease. Weight loss may occur in functional disorders, but it is more characteristic of malignancy. Jaundice can be associated with persistent abdominal pain from chronic liver or biliary disease. Altered bowel habits in conjunction with abdominal pain are most suggestive of IBS, but they also occur in inflammatory bowel disease or malabsorptive syndromes.

Additional Medical History

A history of multiple pain syndromes (such as interstitial cystitis, fibromyalgia and chronic fatigue syndrome) is suggestive of a functional cause, given the high frequency of comorbidity of the functional disorders [16]. A history of vascular disease, hypercoagulable state, and tobacco use should prompt a careful evaluation for mesenteric ischemia. Multiple surgeries, intermittent symptoms, abdominal distension, or vomiting may indicate adhesive disease or intestinal stricture. Psychosocial stressors, depression, and anxiety have been associated with chronic functional pain syndromes, but they may also exacerbate pain from organic sources and drive health care utilization.

Drug History

Many medications can cause nonspecific abdominal discomfort and pain. A careful evaluation of the temporal correlation between pain onset and initiation of medications is necessary. Chronic use of nonsteroidal anti-inflammatory drugs (NSAIDs) is associated with pain from ulcer disease, most commonly in the upper gastrointestinal tract. Intestinal webs or strictures can also develop with chronic NSAID use, leading to chronic obstructive symptoms. Chronic opiate use can lead to both subtle and overt withdrawal symptoms, often with abdominal pain as a prominent feature. Heavy alcohol use or intravenous drug use should prompt an evaluation for hepatic disease.

Physical Examination

The physical examination is complementary to the history and should be guided by the knowledge gained during the interview. Vital signs may be abnormal in during acute exacerbations of pain. The presence of muscle wasting or cachexia is suggestive of organic disease such as malignancy or chronic ischemia. Visual inspection of the abdomen should be performed to assess for distension, hernias, or scars. Bowel sounds should be evaluated prior to palpation. Percussion should be performed to assess for ascites or distension of the abdomen with air. During palpation, involuntary guarding may suggest inflammatory disease with peritoneal irritation. Rebound tenderness is unusual in the setting of chronic abdominal pain. Assessment for point tenderness versus diffuse or nonreproducible tenderness may also be useful. Carnett's test should be performed (palpation of the abdomen with tensed abdominal muscles) to determine whether there is predominant abdominal wall pain. Palpation of a mass or localized fullness should prompt a radiological evaluation. A tender palpable sigmoid colon is frequently described in IBS, potentially due to sigmoid colon spasm. Rectal examination is useful to assess for a mass, abscess, fissure, fistula, or other findings suggesting an organic disorder, particularly in the setting of pelvic or perineal pain. The stool should be assessed for occult blood. A pelvic examination can help in differentiating gastrointestinal from gynecological disease.

Diagnostic Testing

Diagnostic tests should be tailored to the individual history and physical examination. When a functional disorder in the absence of alarm symptoms is the likely diagnosis, very little testing needs to be done. Current guidelines for IBS suggest that routine endoscopic and laboratory testing, other than screening for anemia and celiac sprue, may be unnecessary, and this advice may extend to the other functional disorders as well [3,18]. If an organic disorder is suggested by the history and physical examination, then endoscopic, radiological, and laboratory testing should be performed to target the suspected disease process.

Differential Diagnosis and Treatment of Persistent Abdominal Pain

Most organic causes of pain, such as malignancy, inflammatory bowel disease, pancreaticobiliary disease, structural abnormalities, and infection will be identified with the evaluation outlined above. A small percentage of patients will have more obscure causes of pain such as heavy metal poisoning, carcinoid tumors, familial Mediterranean fever, or porphyria. These may be more difficult to identify, and specialized testing is necessary if the suspicion is high. Once the specific diagnosis is reached, the treatment approach should be targeted based on ameliorating the underlying disease process when possible, as well as relieving symptoms. The remaining patients with persistent abdominal pain are likely to fall into the categories of abdominal wall pain or functional syndromes (most commonly dyspepsia, IBS, and functional abdominal pain syndrome [FAPS]), which will be discussed in more detail below.

Abdominal Wall Pain

Abdominal wall pain may account for 10% to 30% of chronic abdominal pain presentations to pain clinics [14,19]. Cutaneous abdominal nerve entrapment may occur after surgery or an injury, but it can occur in the absence of these factors. Unlike functional visceral pain, a common misdiagnosis, cutaneous nerve entrapment generally has a single localized maximal point of tenderness. The pain is generally sharp or burning in nature, and it may be exacerbated by positional changes. As noted above, a positive Carnett's sign, along with localized pain, is diagnostic of cutaneous abdominal nerve entrapment. Injection of a local anesthetic at the site with temporary resolution of pain is confirmatory. Multiple tender points can be seen in myofascial pain syndromes and should be treated as such. Treatments are not well established but may include intermittent local injection with an anesthetic, physical therapy, analgesic medication, or surgical intervention to free the entrapped nerves [9,15].

Functional Abdominal Pain Syndromes: Diagnosis and Treatment

Despite distinct diagnostic criteria, IBS, FAPS, and functional dyspepsia (FD) probably all share common pathophysiological mechanisms (see the chapter on pathophysiology by Mayer). The diagnostic criteria for the individual disorders are shown in Tables II–V, and

Table II
Rome III diagnostic criteria for irritable bowel syndrome (IBS)

Recurrent abdominal pain or discomfort at least 3 days per month in the last 3 months (but with symptom onset for at least 6 months) associated with 2 or more of the following:

1) Improvement with defecation
2) Onset associated with a change in frequency of stool
3) Onset associated with a change in form (appearance) of stool

Symptoms that cumulatively support the diagnosis of IBS:

    Abnormal stool frequency:
        fewer than 3 bowel movements per week
        or more than 3 bowel movements per day
    Abnormal stool form: lumpy/hard stool or loose/watery stool
    Straining during defecation
    Urgency
    Feeling of incomplete bowel movement
    Passing mucus
    Bloating or feeling of abdominal distension

Source: See [6].

collectively they will be referred to as functional gastrointestinal disorders (FGIDs) [6]. The specific diagnosis must be made within the context of the history and physical examination, and should include screening for alarm symptoms. Patients 50 years or older should have a colonoscopy as part of routine screening. If there is a family history of gastrointestinal cancer or inflammatory bowel disease, or if the patient develops symptoms for the first time at the age of 50 years or above, additional testing should be considered. Upper endoscopy should be considered for patients with suspected FD, particularly those over the age of 50. However, while the Rome III diagnostic criteria dictate that structural lesions must be ruled out, in clinical practice not all younger patients under go an invasive workup because it is expensive and of low yield [20].

Treatment of all three FGIDs is based on symptom reduction and improving quality of life, although current modalities are often suboptimal. A positive physician-patient relationship involving education and

Table III
Rome III diagnostic criteria for functional dyspepsia

1) One or more of:
    Bothersome postprandial fullness
    Early satiation
    Epigastric pain
    Epigastric burning
    AND
2) No evidence of structural disease (including at upper endoscopy) that is likely to explain the symptoms

The criteria must be fulfilled for the last 3 months, with symptom onset at least 6 months before diagnosis.

Source: See [6].

Table IV
Rome III diagnostic criteria for functional dyspepsia subgroups

Postprandial Distress Syndrome

One or both of the following:

1) Bothersome postprandial fullness, occurring after ordinary-sized meals, at least several times per week
2) Early satiation that prevents finishing a regular meal, at least several times per week

The criteria must be fulfilled for the last 3 months, with symptom onset at least 6 months before diagnosis.

Supportive criteria:

1) Upper abdominal bloating or postprandial nausea or excessive belching can be present
2) Epigastric pain syndrome may coexist

Epigastric Pain Syndrome

Must include all of the following:

1) Pain or burning localized to the epigastrium of at least moderate severity at least once per week
2) The pain is intermittent
3) Not generalized or localized to other abdominal or chest regions
4) Not relieved by defecation or passage of flatus
5) Not fulfilling criteria for gallbladder and sphincter of Oddi disorders

The criteria must be fulfilled for the last 3 months, with symptom onset at least 6 months before diagnosis.

Source: See [6].

reassurance about the benign prognosis of the disorder is helpful. All pharmacological treatments for FD and FAPS are used "off label," as are most of those for IBS symptoms, the current exceptions being alosetron and lubiprostone. FGIDs comprise heterogeneous combinations of symptoms, and as such the treatment plan needs to be tailored for the specific patient's needs. While not well studied, a combination of pharmacological treatment and psychological therapy may be the optimal approach for many FGID patients.

Table V
Rome III diagnostic criteria for functional abdominal pain

Must include all of the following:

1) Continuous or nearly continuous abdominal pain
2) No or only occasional relationship of pain with physiological events (e.g., eating, defecation, or menses)
3) Some loss of daily functioning
4) The pain is not feigned
5) Insufficient symptoms to meet criteria for another functional gastrointestinal disorder that would explain the pain

The criteria must be fulfilled for the last 3 months with symptom onset at least 6 months before diagnosis.

Source: See [6].

Pharmacological Therapy

Traditional analgesics tend to be poor choices for FGIDs. Acetaminophen and NSAIDS are not generally effective. Opiates, while helpful for some patients, are problematic for a number of reasons. Rigorous clinical studies are lacking, though most experts agree that opiates have limited efficacy for FGID-related pain. Additionally, opiates may worsen the underlying gastrointestinal symptoms, and given the chronicity of the disorders, the use of opiates could be associated with a risk of dependence and abuse.

Centrally targeted treatments may be effective in modulating visceral afferent input signals as well as acting on emotional arousal circuitry in the brain. The most commonly used are low-dose tricyclic antidepressants (TCAs) and selective serotonin reuptake inhibitors (SSRIs). TCAs have been shown to benefit IBS in several clinical trials, with a number-needed-to-treat (NNT) of 4 [3]. They are best started at lower doses and increased gradually, due to the occurrence of side effects at higher doses. Patients treated for pain symptoms may do well at doses considered subtherapeutic for depression. Interestingly, in addition to their presumed central mechanisms of action, TCAs have also been found to have an analgesic effect on visceral afferent neurons as well as an effect on neuropathic pain. SSRIs have also shown efficacy over placebo, with an NNT of 3.5 [3]. Since SSRIs are generally used at full doses for FGIDs, they also can be effective in treatment of concomitant anxiety and depression. While some studies of SSRIs have carefully tried to evaluate psychological symptoms, reporting this outcome has not been universal; thus, it is not clear whether global symptom improvements seen with these agents are due to improvement in mood and affect or represent a direct effect on the brain-gut axis. Combined serotonin/norepinephrine reuptake inhibitors (SNRIs) have not been well studied in FGIDs. While it expected that they would have similar or even better efficacy compared to SSRIs, one well-designed trial in FD showed no benefit over placebo [21].

Gabapentin and pregabalin, used for neuropathic pain, have been shown in small studies of IBS patients to improve rectal hypersensitivity [10,11]. However, studies of these agents on pain or other symptoms in FGIDs are lacking. While there is little support for their use in the literature, benzodiazepines have been used for FGIDs, with the goal of decreasing pain-associated anxiety and possibly having direct effects on gastrointestinal smooth muscle activity or the brain-gut axis. With this rationale, a combination of clidinium (an anticholinergic, antispasmodic agent) with chlordiazepoxide has been used for IBS and other FGIDs. While selected patients may benefit from benzodiazepines, the risk of abuse is higher than that of other, more rigorously

studied agents, and they are not generally recommended. Dextofisopam, which binds benzodiazepine receptors, has been studied in IBS with potential benefit, though further study is warranted [12].

Other central agents that have been in development for use in FGIDs include neurokinin antagonists and corticotropin-releasing factor type 1 receptor antagonists. While the preclinical evidence for these disorders has been strong, early efficacy studies have been disappointing.

Peripherally acting drugs are targeted at specific symptoms, and thus recommendations vary across the specific FGIDs. FD-related pain may respond to acid suppression with histamine type 2 receptor antagonists or proton pump inhibitors [20]. Prokinetic agents have been used for symptoms of nausea or bloating in FD and IBS, but with questionable efficacy. In IBS, abdominal pain is linked to bowel dysfunction, and thus treatment of associated constipation or diarrhea is a reasonable first step [3]. While this approach is useful, the management of bowel symptoms alone is generally not adequate to relieve the pain or discomfort associated with IBS. An exception to this generalization has been alosetron, a 5-HT_3-receptor antagonist with both central and peripheral effects, which is indicated for women with severe diarrhea-predominant IBS. This agent has both antidiarrheal and potent analgesic effects, but its use is limited by potential side effects of severe constipation and ischemic colitis [1].

Psychological Treatment

Several trials have shown the benefit of different forms of psychological therapy for FGID [2,4,5,7,8,17], with most using hypnotherapy and cognitive-behavioral therapy. These treatments have the advantage of no reported "side effects," and persistent benefit has been documented over time. One of the difficulties of psychological therapy, however, is that it depends largely on the skills of the therapist. Potential out-of-pocket cost to patients and lack of availability of specifically trained therapists has limited the widespread use of these treatments for FGIDs.

Conclusions

In summary, persistent functional abdominal pain and associated disorders remain a significant clinical problem without adequate pharmacological therapies. Current optimal treatment consists of a personalized approach to designing a treatment plan. While not well studied, the combination of psychological and pharmacological treatments in the setting of a supportive patient-physician interaction maybe the optimal approach for many patients.

References

[1] Andresen V, Montori VM, Keller J, West CP, Layer P, Camilleri M. Effects of 5-hydroxytryptamine (serotonin) type 3 antagonists on symptom relief and constipation in nonconstipated irritable bowel syndrome: a systematic review and meta-analysis of randomized controlled trials. Clin Gastroenterol Hepatol 2008;6:545–55.

[2] Brandt LJ, Bjorkman D, Fennerty MB, Locke GR, Olden K, Peterson W, Quigley E, Schoenfeld P, Schuster M, Talley N. Systematic review on the management of irritable bowel syndrome in North America. Am J Gastroenterol 2002;97(11 Suppl):S7–26.

[3] Brandt LJ, Chey WD, Foxx-Orenstein AE, Schiller LR, Schoenfeld PS, Spiegel BM, Talley NJ, Quigley EM. An evidence-based position statement on the management of irritable bowel syndrome. Am J Gastroenterol 2009;104(Suppl 1):S1–35.

[4] Calvert EL, Houghton LA, Cooper P, Morris J, Whorwell PJ. Long-term improvement in functional dyspepsia using hypnotherapy. Gastroenterology 2002;123:1778–85.

[5] Creed F, Fernandes L, Guthrie E, Palmer S, Ratcliffe J, Read N, Rigby C, Thompson D, Tomenson B, North of England IBSRG. The cost-effectiveness of psychotherapy and paroxetine for severe irritable bowel syndrome. Gastroenterology 2003;124:303–17.

[6] Drossman DA. The functional gastrointestinal disorders and the Rome III process. Gastroenterology 2006;130:1377–90.

[7] Drossman DA, Camilleri M, Mayer EA, Whitehead WE. AGA technical review on irritable bowel syndrome. Gastroenterology 2002;123:2108–31.

[8] Drossman DA, Toner BB, Whitehead WE, Diamant NE, Dalton CB, Duncan S, Emmott S, Proffitt V, Akman D, Frusciante K, et al. Cognitive-behavioral therapy versus education and desipramine versus placebo for moderate to severe functional bowel disorders. Gastroenterology 2003;125:19–31.

[9] Greenbaum DS, Greenbaum RB, Joseph JG, Natale JE. Chronic abdominal wall pain. Diagnostic validity and costs. Dig Dis Sci 1994;39:1935–41.

[10] Houghton LA, Fell C, Whorwell PJ, Jones I, Sudworth DP, Gale JD. Effect of a second-generation alpha2delta ligand (pregabalin) on visceral sensation in hypersensitive patients with irritable bowel syndrome. Gut 2007;56:1218–25.

[11] Lee KJ, Kim JH, Cho SW. Gabapentin reduces rectal mechanosensitivity and increases rectal compliance in patients with diarrhoea-predominant irritable bowel syndrome. Aliment Pharmacol Ther 2005;22:981–8.

[12] Leventer SM, Raudibaugh K, Frissora CL, Kassem N, Keogh JC, Phillips J, Mangel AW. Clinical trial: dextofisopam in the treatment of patients with diarrhoea-predominant or alternating irritable bowel syndrome. Aliment Pharmacol Ther 2008;27:197–206.

[13] Mayer EA, Gebhart GF. Basic and clinical aspects of visceral hyperalgesia. Gastroenterology 1994;107:271–93.

[14] McGarrity TJ, Peters DJ, Thompson C, McGarrity SJ. Outcome of patients with chronic abdominal pain referred to chronic pain clinic. Am J Gastroenterol 2000;95:1812–6.

[15] Paajanen H. Does laparoscopy used in open exploration alleviate pain associated with chronic intractable abdominal wall neuralgia? Surg Endosc 2006;20:1835–8.

[16] Riedl A, Schmidtmann M, Stengel A, Goebel M, Wisser AS, Klapp BF, Monnikes H. Somatic comorbidities of irritable bowel syndrome: a systematic analysis. J Psychosom Res 2008;64:573–82.

[17] Soo S, Moayyedi P, Deeks J, Delaney B, Lewis M, Forman D. Psychological interventions for non-ulcer dyspepsia. Cochrane Database Syst Rev 2001;4:CD002301.

[18] Spiller R, Aziz Q, Creed F, Emmanuel A, Houghton L, Hungin P, Jones R, Kumar D, Rubin G, Trudgill N, Whorwell P. Guidelines on the irritable bowel syndrome: mechanisms and practical management. Gut 2007;56:1770–98.

[19] Srinivasan R, Greenbaum DS. Chronic abdominal wall pain: a frequently overlooked problem. Practical approach to diagnosis and management. Am J Gastroenterol 2002;97:824–30.

[20] Talley NJ, Vakil N. Guidelines for the management of dyspepsia. Am J Gastroenterol 2005;100:2324–37.

[21] van Kerkhoven LA, Laheij RJ, Aparicio N, De Boer WA, Van den Hazel S, Tan AC, Witteman BJ, Jansen JB. Effect of the antidepressant venlafaxine in functional dyspepsia: a randomized, double-blind, placebo-controlled trial. Clin Gastroenterol Hepatol 2008;6:746–52.

Correspondence to: Kirsten Tillisch, MD, Center for Neurobiology of Stress, Division of Digestive Diseases, David Geffen School of Medicine, 100 UCLA Medical Plaza, Suite 700, UCLA, Los Angeles, CA 90095, USA. Email: ktillisch@mednet.ucla.edu.

Part 16
Basics, Management, and Treatment of Low Back Pain

Basics, Management, and Treatment of Low Back Pain

37

Paul J. Watson, FCSP, PhD,[a] **Chris J. Main, PhD,**[b] **and Rob J.E.M. Smeets, MD, PhD**[c,d]

[a]*Department of Health Sciences, University of Leicester, Leicester, United Kingdom;* [b]*Arthritis Research Campaign National Primary Care Centre, Keele University, Keele, United Kingdom;* [c]*Department of Rehabilitation Medicine, Maastricht University Medical Centre, Maastricht, The Netherlands;* [d]*Adelante Care Group, Hoensbroek, The Netherlands*

The majority of people in the industrialized world will experience an episode of low back pain during their life. Of all these persons with acute low back pain, 10–50% will experience pain lasting more than 3 months, which is defined as chronic pain [46]. There is also an increase in the economic and societal burden caused by chronic low back pain, such as high medical and nonmedical costs, the latter mainly due to absence from work.

It is estimated that 85% of these patients have nonspecific back pain with no known specific underlying disease or pathology [30]. Diagnosing back pain is problematic in primary care, and the lack of a clear biomedical model to legitimize the pain and direct initial treatment decisions can be frustrating for patients and practitioners alike. Back pain for many is characterized as a persistent or recurrent condition with periods relatively free from pain and disability and with occasional acute episodes. A relatively small number of people will go on to have chronic disabling back pain where their day-to-day function is severely compromised [27].

Low back pain is common in the working population. In a recent survey of over 1,100 working people, 18.5% reported back pain at the time of the study, but most (approximately 57%) of them reported that the pain had little or no effect on their activities (including their work); around 18% of those with back pain reported that it affected their activities significantly [13].

Most absences from work due to low back pain are brief, and the majority of workers will return to work within 3 or 4 weeks. It has often been concluded that this provides the evidence for the mantra "80% of back pain recovers within weeks" and represents low back pain recovery; it does not. Symptomatic workers with acute back pain return to work, and many will remain symptomatic a year later [46]; if the pain persists longer than 3 months, the chance of returning to work is substantially less and the incidence of pain at 1 year is much higher [73]. A significant number of people (between 18% and 44%) will be absent from work due to low back pain again within the year [124], and subsequent absences are likely to be longer and more costly [123,127].

Interestingly, little is known about why patients with low back pain seek care and what they expect from the health care provider. In a recent review, 10 population-based studies could be identified showing that women and patients with a previous history of back pain were more likely to seek care for their back pain [34]. Back pain intensity was only slightly associated with consultation, whereas patients with high levels of disability were nearly eight times more likely to seek care. Due to the small number of studies and their heterogeneity, the role of psychological and social factors could not be assessed. These results seem to indicate that the disability experienced rather than the pain intensity itself is a major reason to seek care. Nevertheless, the major and primary goal of the health care system and its providers is to reduce pain levels. Relative little attention is paid to the reduction or prevention of development of disability. This emphasis is also reflected in the literature, in which treatments mostly based on the biomedical model (and often monodisciplinary) are used to try and fix a somatic problem. This situation continues, despite many years of exhortations to consider low back pain within a biopsychosocial model incorporating not only biomedical features but also the psychological reaction to the condition and the social environment in which the patients live.

Evidence-based guidelines for nonspecific back pain in primary care highlight the need to consider prognostic clinical indicators [111]. Although there is evidence that clinicians' global prognostic assessment compares favorably with that of formal epidemiological prediction rules [53], identifying specific indicators as appropriate targets of primary care treatment has proved problematic [68]. It is still far from common practice for clinicians to perform a systematic assessment of modifiable obstacles to recovery, which are mainly psychosocial.

Screening as a Basis for Treatment Decision Making in Low Back Pain

Concepts of Risk

Risk identification as a precursor to screening is a cornerstone of clinical medicine, but it has a different objective in different contexts. *Epidemiological* studies, whether of the general public or of clinical populations, defined by a particular illness or symptom, are primarily descriptive rather than explanatory in nature, and they may include appraisal of a wide range of demographic, clinical, psychological, and socioeconomic factors. *Clinical* studies tend to focus on health care outcomes, and although they have a narrower focus, they potentially provide a clear focus for clinical management of the individual patient, or patients with a common condition. *Occupational* risk factor studies traditionally have focused on the identification of factors in the workplace associated with industrial diseases such as asbestosis, but in recent years they have broadened their focus to include consideration of factors associated with work absence and performance.

In the treatment/management of low back pain, however, during the last two decades, there have been four important developments. First, in terms of concepts of illness, there has been a shift from the narrow biomedical (and biomechanical) "disease" model to more integrative biopsychosocial models. Second, there has been an increasing focus not just on primary prevention and treatment/rehabilitation, but on *secondary prevention*, a refocusing driven not only by the harsh realities of rising costs of back pain to both the individual and society, but also by compelling research evidence for the powerful influence of psychosocial factors on health care consulting, treatment adherence, and outcome. Third, the distinguishing of modifiable from unmodifiable risk factors has broadened the focus for intervention beyond disease and pathology to include obstacles to recovery, such as in the original "Yellow Flags" initiative [56]. Finally, the somewhat disappointing results of randomized controlled trials (RCTs) into early psychosocial interventions, in terms of specific effects, has led to reappraisal of the generally adopted "one-size-fits all approach" and recommendation of specific clinical targeting as a precursor to intervention. Interventions specifically targeting risk factors have been developed [101,103], along with specific risk-factors-based screening tools [48,60], as included in the Startback study, the first low back pain RCT incorporating an intervention specifically linked with risk-factor identification.

While screening can have a number of purposes, the primary purpose of yellow flag screening is to identify potentially modifiable risk factors. The identification of risk factors may enable us to select subgroups of patients, whether in terms of possible benefit from treatment ("screening in") or unlikely to benefit from treatment ("screening out"). Furthermore, identification of risk factors may lead to the identification of new and different approaches to treatment for groups of patients with differing presenting characteristics or at different stages of pain chronicity [113]. However, whether or not such interventions are effective at the individual level can depend upon broader contextual factors as well as individual motivational considerations [72].

Methods of Screening

The value of screening depends not only on the content of the items, but on the manner in which the information is collected and the way the information is integrated. Thus, more individualized and clinically relevant information may be collected using questionnaires or telephone or face-to-face interviews than can be obtained using actuarial approaches.

Timing

In addition to the concerns raised by von Korff et al. [115], different challenges may be associated with screening at different times. Waddell et al. [118] illustrated the importance of timing in consideration of the prediction of incapacity, whereby at the initial presentation, the task for a screening tool may be to identify the 1–2% of individuals who will go on to develop long-term incapacity from among the 98–99% with relatively simple problems, most of whom are likely to return to work quite rapidly, more or less irrespective of any intervention. However, at 26 weeks after onset, the task may be to identify the 40% likely to continue on long-term benefits from those who might (or could) return to work.

Accuracy versus Cost

In some circumstances it may be preferable to be overinclusive to minimize the chances of missing a positive case, but as Waddell et al. [117] pointed out, this may come at a cost. Thus, if it is extremely important to identify all possible cases of a particular condition, it may be considered justifiable to also include a large number of those who do not have the condition. Conversely, if the costs of screening are prohibitively expensive, a lower "hit rate" in terms of identifying those with the condition may be considered acceptable because a lot of unnecessary costs (false positives) will have been saved. Judgments of acceptability in screening may thus involve political and ethical considerations as well as statistical computations.

Content of Screening

There are many measurement instruments and assessment schedules containing psychosocial elements [106] that might be used for classification purposes. Many, however, are too long and cumbersome, and many were designed primarily as research instruments and are unsuitable for use in routine clinical contexts or require specialist assessment skills. Others were really developed for people with chronic pain conditions and go well beyond the usual time frame of primary care. There are, however, a plethora of potentially useful assessment tools.

In the field of pain and disability assessment, a wide range of measurement instruments are available [66,118], with content ranging from highly specific pain scales to multidimensional inventories. There is also wide variation in the extent of psychosocial content. Many instruments have a specific psychological focus. A pain compendium recently produced by the Accident and Compensation Corporation in New Zealand [1] offers a comprehensive contemporaneous description and evaluation of available instruments currently in use for assessment of persistent pain.

A number of instruments were recommended specifically for assessment of pain characteristics or specific psychological concomitants of pain, such as fear, catastrophizing, and depression. There is, however, widespread evidence that outcome of treatment is multifactorial, and thus attempts to derive a somewhat broader approach to classification would seem to have appeal.

Linking Screening with Targeting

Over time there has been a gradual awareness of the need to broaden assessment and identify risk factors for poor outcome. However, even when clinicians identify negative prognostic indicators, they appear not to tailor patient management accordingly [9]. Investigators increasingly advocate effective early secondary prevention of back pain in primary care through better identification of prognostic indicators that require treatment [12,52].

Several back pain classification tools have been developed to aid clinical decision making [20,78], and such tools may improve clinical outcomes when subgrouping guides treatment [29,37]. However, the conceptual purposes of these tools vary substantially, with most designed for the occupational setting or to identify patients for specific treatment modalities. There is a need for a brief, easy-to-score, adequately validated screening tool that allocates and prioritizes treatment for the entire spectrum of patients with nonspecific low back pain presenting to primary care, on the basis of treatment-modifiable indicators.

The key objectives of the screening tool are: (1) to identify patients with potentially treatment modifiable prognostic indicators using a brief, user-friendly tool; and (2) to validate cut-off scores for subgrouping patients into one of three initial treatment options in primary care: a low-risk subgroup (patients with few negative prognostic indicators, suitable for primary care management according to best-practice guidelines, such as analgesia, advice, and education); a medium-risk subgroup (patients with an unfavorable prognosis, with high levels of physical prognostic indicators, appropriate for physiotherapy); and a high-risk subgroup (patients with a very unfavorable prognosis, with consistently high levels across psychosocial prognostic indicators, appropriate for management by a combination of physical and cognitive-behavioral approaches).

Key Messages Regarding Screening

The key messages from review of the utility of screening are:

1) A variety of instruments and screening tools are available.

2) It is important to be clear about the purpose and content of screening.

3) In selecting a screening strategy it is important to be guided by the overall conceptual framework connecting the information captured by the instrument and its intended use.

4) The utility of screening instruments is context dependent.

5) Traditionally, screening has been used to prevent the development of disease, but the identification of potentially modifiable factors associated with the persistence of pain and development of disability offers new possibilities for secondary prevention.

6) Linking screening with the targeting of interventions addressing modifiable prognostic factors appears to be a promising strategy meriting further evaluation.

Early Interventions for Secondary Prevention of Disability Related to Chronic Back Pain

The shift from the disease model of illness to the biopsychosocial model of pain and disability is evidenced in practice by the development of multifaceted interdisciplinary pain management [66], by the shift in focus from cures of pain to pain management (in a broad sense), and by recognition of the powerful psychological and social influences on the outcome of clinical treatment. This shift has led to the identification and targeting of potentially *modifiable* risk factors, among which psychological factors appear to exert a particularly powerful influence. The broadening in focus has led to new types of intervention perhaps better described as psychologically informed reactivation,

adopting a cognitive-behavioral approach rather than pain treatment as previously understood.

During the last 20 years, since the beginning of systematic interventions of the effectiveness of physiotherapy, there has been increasing interest in the nature of such interventions. Common themes have been the need to remobilize patients, based on a biomechanical appraisal of their pain-associated limitations, and provision of recommendations for reactivation, incorporating a range of therapeutic modalities, accompanied by some sort of attention to the psychosocial component.

Wave 1, 2, and 3 Studies

In an attempt to synthesize the results of recent research studies, Main et al. [66] distinguished Wave 1, Wave 2 or Wave 3 studies, the criteria for which are outlined here:

Wave 1
- Educational approaches (e.g., back schools)
- Assumption of a knowledge deficit
- Generic approach
- No assessment of competency in cognitive-behavioral approach

Wave 2
- Specific cognitive and behavioral content
- Generic approach
- No specific training in yellow flag elicitation

Wave 3
- Specific yellow flag training
- Competencies assumed
- Individualized approach

Conclusions from Studies on Early Psychosocial Intervention

It appears that even with relevant training and a defined intervention protocol, it cannot be assumed that the intervention has been carried out in the population identified or in the manner intended. It seems clear that in intervention trials of the type recently undertaken, a clear picture in terms of treatment outcome cannot be obtained without careful attention to factors such as treatment adherence and protocol violation as major potential confounders. The recent research studies have not been powered to elucidate, or control for, such confounders. Unfortunately, in "real-life" clinical trials there is a perpetual difficulty in deciding how much cost in terms of clinical service delivery and generalizability of findings is acceptable to ensure tighter experimental control.

The principal lessons learned from the recent research studies into psychosocial interventions are:

1) A biopsychosocial approach to management appears to be acceptable to such patients and to be beneficial (although to a different extent in different studies).

2) To date, biopsychosocial approaches have not been shown to be superior either to usual care (whether delivered by general practitioners or by physiotherapists) or to other specific physiotherapeutic approaches.

3) There are number of possible reasons for this lack of a better outcome, but the strongest contenders appear to be: (i) Insufficient training to guarantee competent assessment and intervention protocol violation in terms of delivery of intervention, resulting in similarities outweighing the differences in the content of interventions. (ii) Lack of information about the treatment processes. (iii) Insensitive or inappropriate outcome measures. (iv) Lack of comparability in treatment cohorts across trials.

Suggestions for a Way Forward: Wave 4

Moving from a "one-size-fits-all" approach to more individualized pain management clearly requires not only a way of grouping patients in terms of potentially modifiable factors, but also a way to address these factors in the intervention. Sullivan et al. [103], for example, found that a structured psychological intervention by psychologists for injured workers, who had been selected on the basis of their having one or more elevated psychological risk factors, was significantly more effective in achieving return to work than a usual-care comparison sample treated earlier. In addition, Sullivan et al. [101] reported that a similar intervention conducted mainly by physiotherapists and occupational therapists, the Progressive Goal Attainment Program (PGAP), appeared quite effective. This program was aimed at reducing risk factors for prolonged work disability (e.g., pain catastrophizing, fear of movement and re-injury, and perceived disability), with individuals selected on the basis of elevated scores on measures of these psychological risk factors. In that (nonrandomized) clinical trial with a sample of individuals who had been work-disabled due to whiplash symptoms, 75% of individuals in the PGAP group returned to work, compared to 50% who followed usual treatment [101].

More recently, Hay et al. have investigated the possibility of early intervention targeted treatment based on a screening tool developed specifically to categorize patients in terms of risk factors for chronicity [48]. Further research is underway to determine the validity of tailoring treatments based upon the relative perceived risk in primary care.

Key messages are as follows:

1) We still do not know whether, how, or for whom psychosocial interventions are effective. There are a number of possible reasons for this lack of definitive findings, but the appropriateness of the "one-size-fits-all" approach, as evidenced to date in the design of RCTs evaluated primarily by a comparison of group means, while appropriate for certain types of intervention, appears ill-suited to psychosocial interventions, which by their very nature are complex, and interactions between patient characteristics and response to treatment might be anticipated.

2) We need to clearly define the competencies we require for the outcomes we desire.

3) We need to develop and validate the training required to establish the necessary competencies, in association with the "dose-response curves" required for various levels of risk reduction.

4) In order to develop more effective interventions, we have still a lot to learn about the influence of psychosocial factors on change across time and on the development of chronicity, but at least the nature of the task is becoming clearer.

5) If linking screening, targeting, and customizing interventions accordingly leads to improved clinical outcome, it offers the promise of developing a much more "patient-centered approach" to clinical management.

Health Care and Workplace Barriers to Successful Work Reintegration

Roles and Responsibilities of Health Care Professionals, Patients/Workers, and Employers

The discussion thus far has focused primarily on clinical parameters, and the "social" part of the framework has not been given specific attention. The social context of pain can be investigated in terms of influences on pain perception, adjustment, and adaptation, or in terms of the impact of pain on family and society. Arguably, the most important impact of pain and pain-associated limitations is on participation in activities, of which the most important is work. Although the importance of work was recognized within the original flags framework [56], the primary focus of attention was on clinical obstacles to recovery.

The Occupational Agenda

Characteristics of work and the work environment have emerged as predictors of back pain and disability, even after investigators control for a host of other psychosocial, demographic, and health variables [28,91]. Although consensus treatment guidelines for back pain have underscored the importance of occupational factors [99], the development and dissemination of specific methods for clinicians to assess and intervene in these factors have been limited. Even among specialists in occupational medicine and rehabilitation, many obstacles exist for intervening in the workplace, including barriers to employer communication, limited information about job tasks and prospects for modifying work, and employers who are unwilling or unable to provide modified or transitional work [61,83]. Thus, more research is needed to support optimal methods for interpreting and intervening in occupational factors. In particular, authors have emphasized the need to reduce the growing list of workplace variables to a manageable set of core factors, improve the accuracy and utility of patient screening, and develop effective and plausible intervention strategies to address workplace concerns [90].

In recent years, this system has been refined in scope and concept [67], and workplace factors that were previously included as yellow flags now occupy two separate categories: "black flags," or contextual factors (which include actual workplace conditions that can affect disability), and "blue flags," or individual perceptions about work, whether accurate or inaccurate, that can affect disability.

Shaw et al. [90] reviewed the scientific literature on the role of occupational variables as prognostic factors, representative of seven types of screening methods that had been developed. The types of workplace factors identified yielded a total of 27 occupational variables that were included in at least one of these screening methods. The authors further categorized these 27 variables into four groups that connote different intervention strategies. Four variables described physical demands of work, five described psychological demands, 12 represented social/managerial factors, and six included general workplace perceptions [90]. They observed that psychological factors may require cognitive-behavioral strategies to cope with job strain, and they found that personal perceptions that work is dissatisfying, dangerous, or likely to cause re-injury might be important mediators of back disability. They concluded by recommending a focus on seven key workplace factors, each linked with a sample interview question and a number of possible courses of action. Whereas a number of factors are most appropriately tackled in the actual workplace with workplace personnel, consideration of blue flags as potential obstacles to return to optimal occupational function should be the responsibility of health care practitioners as well. Given that one of the important "drivers" of consultation about musculoskeletal symptoms is concern about work, it is important that clinical management addresses such concerns directly if possible. Clinicians can by addressing mistaken beliefs both about the possible impact of musculoskeletal symptoms on work capability and concerns about the perceived possible adverse effects on the physical demands of work on musculoskeletal symptoms, but also by encouraging patients to establish appropriate communication with their employer regarding development of a return-to-work strategy.

Challenges in Implementation

With regard to blue flags, the Decade of the Flags conference made four key recommendations to facilitate more widespread implementation: (1) expand the responsibilities of clinicians (or their agents) to include workplace concerns; (2) design easily administered tools that require minimal time and interpretation; (3) improve access to early intervention for high-risk cases; and (4) avoid stigma to workers identified as "high risk" [57].

However, also identified were a number of challenges. In current clinical practice, clinicians rarely communicate with the workplace, few assess workplace concerns, and there are only infrequent attempts to facilitate early intervention targeting the workplace. Reasons that have been suggested for reluctance to explore workplace issues include personal style, clinical training background, perceived conflicts of interest, and the policies and procedures of insurance or government benefit systems. The use of allied health professionals (e.g., case managers) to coordinate or facilitate return to work is one method that may provide a very important and necessary link between clinicians and employers when back-injured workers are at high risk for long-term disability [89].

In addressing this challenge, we need an approach linking individually focused, worker-centered interventions with interventions at an organizational level. In this process, early identification of modifiable risk factors is a key first step. Designing interventions targeted on such factors, and thereby turning potential obstacles into opportunities for change, requires a systems approach such as that advocated by the Flags framework. Detailed recommendations for appropriate roles for health care professional, employees, and employers, based on the early identification of risk factors (primarily yellow and blue flags), but with consideration of the contextual factors or "black flags," within an overall systems approach, are offered in the Flags Monograph [57].

Key points regarding the health care/occupational interface are as follows:

1) Occupational concerns are a major driver of health care consultation among a significant proportion of patients with musculoskeletal symptoms.

2) We now know the principal "blue flags" associated with suboptimal response to treatment.

3) These flags need to be identified and addressed as early as possible after the development of symptoms.

4) Many clinicians feel ill-equipped to address occupational factors within the clinical consultation, but failure to do so will have an adverse effect on outcome.

5) There is a twin role for the clinician: first in addressing mistaken beliefs about the impact of pain on work capability and on the impact of physical demands on symptoms, and second in persuading their patients to develop appropriate lines of communication with their workplace (possibly even offering to facilitate the process).

6) Finally, since many employees have recurrent or chronic pain, there is a role for the health care professional in work retention (i.e., in secondary prevention) as well as in rehabilitation back into work by assisting patients in minimizing the impact of their symptoms. If, as seems probable, the number of older people in the workforce increases over the next decades, identification and management of yellow and blue flags will increase in importance.

Treatment Options for Low Back Pain

The last two decades have seen the publication of many systematic reviews and meta-analyses of studies evaluating the effectiveness of different types of exercise, cognitive-behavioral therapy, and combinations of these treatments for patients with chronic low back pain

(CLBP), and the number is growing. For the health care provider who tries to select the most effective treatment for patients with CLBP seeking care for their back pain and evolving consequences, the results of these reviews and meta-analyses are difficult to interpret and apply in clinical practice. This part of the chapter aims to (1) provide an overview of the current evidence of the above-mentioned treatments and (2) present a best-evidence synthesis for the intervention for each particular patient with CLBP.

Once pain persists for several months and is associated with marked interference in daily activities, depressed mood, catastrophizing, and/or fear-avoidance beliefs, the risk is very high for continuing deterioration of pre-injury lifestyles, including absence from work. The first part of the chapter has clearly described the importance of identifying and treating patients considered to be at risk of this secondary disability as soon as possible. In this phase a psychosocial or biopsychosocial perspective is preferably used to identify the factors that are associated with reduced activities and participation problems. Very often, cognitive and behavioral approaches are used, sometimes with one or more types of exercise. While pain relief is often unlikely to be achieved, other goals may be more feasible. These are quality-of-life goals, including work, home, and social activities as well as daily life activities. However, the question is whether these treatments are effective, or at least more effective than no treatment, regular care, or other types of treatment. To answer this question, the results of systematic reviews and meta-analyses are needed, because these methods provide the strongest proof of evidence.

However, while interpreting the results of reviews and meta-analyses, the health care provider should always take into account the characteristics of the population in which a particular treatment was studied in order to decide whether the results could apply to the individual patient visiting the clinic. Furthermore, and even more importantly, the care provider must clarify the patient's treatment goals, expectations, attributions, and motivation. And last but not least, the care provider has to consider whether he or she is sufficiently skilled to select and provide this particular treatment.

Exercise

Exercise is defined as any form of treatment that includes the performance of any physical activity in order to influence the body (or part of it) with the goal of improving health. Eligible treatments are therapeutic exercises designed to improve muscle function (strength, power, endurance, control, etc.), range of motion/flexibility, cardiorespiratory fitness, and tolerance to activity. Up until recently only one meta-analysis had been conducted to provide a quantitative estimate of the size of the effect of exercise interventions for patients with CLBP [43]. The authors found that exercise improved pain and disability outcomes by a small amount when compared to no treatment or other conservative treatments. The same group conducted a meta-regression analysis [44] and found that an individually designed program, high exercise doses (preferably stretching or strengthening for ≥20 hours), supervision of home exercise, and inclusion of additional conservative treatment with the exercise treatment were all associated with improvements in pain and disability. Because only studies up until 2004 were included and a considerable number of trials have been published since, and because Hayden et al. also included studies with mixed symptom duration, neck complaints, and treatment combinations where exercise was not the main component, we performed an update including only patients with CLBP, and with exercise being the main component [34A]. A total of 41 studies up until August 2008 were included, and the following study variables were assessed: (1) population features (baseline severity of symptoms), (2) dosage (number of exercise hours and sessions), (3) program features (supervision, individual tailoring, and cognitive-behavioral components), (4) methodological features (intention to treat, concealment of allocation). Thirty studies reported the effects on pain, and 34 on disability. In general, pooled estimates show that exercise is only slightly better than no treatment and minimal care in reducing pain and disability immediately after treatment (e.g., on a scale of 0–100, mean difference = 9.3, 95% CI = 1.6 to 17 for pain; mean difference = 3.3, 95% CI = 1.9 to 4.8 for disability) and up to 12 months' follow-up, but these differences are too small to be clinically relevant. Exercise is equally effective as other conservative treatments. Although individual study variables partially explain between-trial heterogeneity, only the number of sessions was associated with exercise effect sizes of pain immediately after the end of treatment in a statistically significant (although not clinically relevant) manner.

Although passive types of treatment such as massage, application of heat/cold, laser therapy, transcutaneous electrical nerve stimulation, traction, and manual therapy are normally not regarded as exercise treatments, they are provided by physiotherapists. Specific Cochrane reviews on these treatments report no proof that these treatments are effective, with the exception of massage (especially when combined with exercises and education) and manual therapy, which are reported as being equally effective compared to other conservative treatments such as exercise. The latest review on manual therapy was published in 2004 [3], and an update is currently being undertaken [84].

Reviews that only include specific types of exercise show similar results to the reviews discussed above, although the weighted mean differences when comparing exercise to no treatment/minimal intervention are a bit higher, reaching moderate levels at best. For example, Macedo et al. [64] reviewed the effectiveness of motor control exercise for CLPB of at least 6 weeks' duration. It appeared that motor control is superior to minimal interventions and confers benefit when added to another therapy at short- and long-term follow-up for pain (e.g., mean difference 14.4 points, 95% CI = 5.7 to 23.1) and in reducing disability at long-term follow-up (10.8 points, 95% CI = 2.8 to 18.7). Motor control exercises are not any more effective than manual therapy or other forms of exercise. A recently published placebo-controlled trial showed similar results, except for pain levels showing no difference between the active and placebo treatment [25]. Therapeutic aquatic exercises are equally effective as other types of exercise, although the methodological quality of the 37 trials included was rather low [121].

Cognitive-Behavioral Interventions

The problem with evaluating the efficacy of cognitive-behavioral interventions is that many definitions appear in the published studies. Often the term "psychological treatment" is used, even though this term might be rather confusing as many of these treatments are not provided by psychologists. Cognitive-behavioral therapy (CBT) is based on a multidimensional model of pain that includes physical, affective, cognitive, and behavioral components. According to the Cochrane collaboration, CBT may include education about a multidimensional view of pain; identification of pain-eliciting and pain-aggravating thoughts, feelings, and behavior; identification and modification of maladaptive cognitions; and the use of coping strategies, relaxation, and electromyographic biofeedback [79].

A Cochrane review published in 2005 concluded that combined respondent-cognitive therapy and progressive relaxation therapy are more effective than waiting-list controls for short-term pain relief [79]. However, it is unknown whether these results are sustained in the long term. No significant differences could be detected between CBT and exercise therapy. An update [47] shows similar results, with CBT being equally effective as exercise therapy regarding pain and functional status. Operant therapy also appears to be effective for short-term pain reduction, but not any more effective than other types of CBT. These results are similar to the Cochrane review of psychological therapies for the management of chronic musculoskeletal pain, including CLBP in adults, showing that CBT and operant treatment have weak effects in improving pain and minimal effect on functional status (disability). These treatments are effective in altering mood, with some evidence that this improvement is maintained at 6 months [32]. A Cochrane review on individual patient education shows that its effectiveness is still unclear [33], although it should be noted that this treatment is often provided alongside other types of treatment.

Cognitive-behavioral models propose that pain-related fear, kinesiophobia, and unhelpful beliefs about back pain are primary factors leading to increased pain and decreased level of activity and functioning [112]. Graded activity and graded exposure are interventions commonly used and even propagated in clinical guidelines for the management of CLBP, although their effectiveness is not well established. Therefore, we recently performed a systematic review [65]. Both treatments incorporate behavioral and cognitive approaches to improve activity tolerance. The primary difference between the two interventions is that with graded exposure, patients are asked to create a hierarchy of feared activities. The exposure starts with the least feared activity, and the therapist helps the patient to appraise the exposure and its consequences, and then address irrational and counterproductive beliefs, leading to reductions in the anxiety associated with the activity. Once the negative associations are extinguished, activities associated with higher levels of anxiety are addressed in the same way. In the graded activity program, operant conditioning principles are used to reinforce healthy behaviors. The program focuses on functional activities and progresses in a time-contingent manner regardless of pain, to achieve functional goals and increased activity. Principles of quotas, pacing, and self-reinforcement

are key features of this program. The overall conclusion is that graded activity is slightly more effective in reducing pain and disability than a minimal intervention, but not any more effective than other forms of exercise. The limited evidence suggests that graded exposure is as effective as minimal treatment or graded activity. Because of the poor reporting within many of the studies, it is often unclear precisely how interventions were implemented.

Multidisciplinary Treatment

Multidisciplinary treatment of at least 100 hours, combining exercise, functional restoration, and CBT, appeared promising compared to other nonmultidisciplinary treatments, whereas multidisciplinary programs of less than 30 hours failed to show improvements in pain and function [40]. However, there is a lack of a clear consensus about the content, intensity, and frequency of the different treatment components of a multidisciplinary treatment [54], and the results of this Cochrane review were based on a relatively low number of studies. This review was later withdrawn from the Cochrane library, and so far no update has been done.

In another Cochrane review, multidisciplinary treatment was defined as consisting of a physician's consultation plus a psychological, social, or vocational intervention, or a combination of these interventions [54]. The authors found moderate evidence for the effectiveness of multidisciplinary treatment for subacute low back pain, although there were some methodological shortcomings. They noted that several expensive programs are commonly used for uncomplicated low back pain problems. The moderate effectiveness of multidisciplinary treatment was confirmed by Haldorsen et al., who divided patients into three subgroups according to an algorithm for prognosis [41].

One systematic review (including 10 studies) on the long-term effect of multidisciplinary back training based on the biopsychosocial model of pain and including several disciplines showed effectiveness for work participation and quality of life, but not for pain and functional status. The intensity of the intervention (less than or more than 30 hours) had no substantial influence on its effectiveness [108].

In a recent cluster-randomized controlled trial, we examined whether a combination of a physical training and an operant-behavioral graded activity with problem solving training is more effective than either alone. During the 1-year follow-up, there were no significant differences between each single treatment and the combination treatment on pain and disability [94]. A cost-effectiveness analysis showed that the operant-behavioral graded activity with problem-solving training was cost-effective compared to the combination treatment and physical training only [92]. Another randomized trial comparing a function-centered with a pain-centered multidisciplinary in-patient treatment showed that the total costs were similar over the whole 3-year follow-up [4].

Conclusion

There is fair-to-good evidence that exercise, CBT, and multidisciplinary treatment are moderately effective for CLBP, which is congruent with the recent national guidelines in both the United States and the United Kingdom [21,85]. However, the magnitude of the effect reported in more recent reviews is lower than reported in the aforementioned guidelines, and none seems better than the other. Furthermore, looking at individual patients with at least moderate levels of disability, about half or even more of the patients do not experience a clinically relevant improvement in their health status, whether expressed as pain or functional status (disability).

Synthesis

Many treatments, especially exercise treatments, try to resolve the problems in function, such as pain or loss of strength, coordination, and aerobic capacity, despite the fact that there is no strong evidence that there is a "deconditioning syndrome" causing the physiological deficits [96]. Nevertheless, these treatments are effective, as they reduce pain and improve level of functioning, although they do so only moderately and sometimes not even to a clinically relevant degree. There is some evidence that the positive effect of exercise is mediated by the reduction of catastrophizing thoughts [95]. Nevertheless, there is sufficient scientific basis to use this type of treatment.

Despite the clear and plausible rationale of the biopsychosocial model, the results of CBT either alone or in combination with more biomedically oriented exercise treatment are at least somewhat disappointing, especially regarding improvement in functioning. Compared to exercise alone, they are not any more effective. Furthermore, for a rather large number of patients with CLBP, the treatment provided—whether it is exercise, CBT or a combination—is not successful.

Some have argued that we need more "component-type" analyses of comprehensive multidisciplinary programs to dissect the relative contributions of the various components [38]. However, due to relatively minor differences in effectiveness between different treatment modalities, and hence low power, such studies require high numbers of patients, seriously diminishing their feasibility. It is also remarkable that no trials have addressed the optimal selection and sequencing of therapies, and methods for tailoring treatment to individual patients are still in early stages of development [22].

Otherwise, one should realize that the results of reviews and meta-analyses apply to groups of patients and not to individuals, meaning that although the effectiveness of a specific treatment is only moderate, it may still be very effective for a particular patient. A better approach, therefore, may be to study prognostic factors for a particular treatment. A meta-analysis found consistent evidence for the predictive value of pain intensity (more pain results in worse outcome), work-satisfaction (high satisfaction results in better outcome), and active coping style (less active coping results in better outcome) for the outcome of biopsychosocial multidisciplinary programs [107]. Two more recent studies showed that treatment expectancy might be an important prognostic factor for all kinds of treatment provided to patients with CLBP [39,93]. It is still impossible to define a generic set of predictors of outcome of multidisciplinary or other types of treatment, and large confirmatory studies are needed to test the value of these supposed predictors.

Despite the lack of moderating variables, a growing number of researchers and health care providers, especially those working in multidisciplinary teams, have been arguing that the treatment offered should specifically focus on the factors important for the persistence of the CLBP-associated problems for each individual patient. Hence, a thorough assessment of all potentially relevant biopsychosocial factors should be made in order to select the appropriate treatment modules. Thus, we need to consider not only the nature of the pain but also the person in pain and his or her perspectives, abilities, and goals (or desires), as well as the context in which he or she lives—the workplace, the home, and even the broader social environment including available social support systems. The World Health Organization's International Classification of Functioning, Disability, and Health (ICF) model (see Fig. 1) provides a holistic model to access all relevant biopsychosocial factors, as it identifies three concepts described from the perspective of body systems (body functions and structures), the individual (activity), and society (participation).

After the (preferably multidisciplinary) assessment, the problems identified and the interrelationship of factors must be discussed with the patient, who should be invited to indicate want he or she wants to change or achieve, given the explanation that there is probably no treatable cause or relief for the pain complaint itself. This type of process is essential in establishing a working alliance with the patient in order to enhance the probability for a successful rehabilitation [122]. A client-centered approach, in which the client is invited to participate in decision making and takes more responsibility for solving the problem, has been shown to be more effective than the traditional clinician-centered care in other patient groups [7,77]. Motivational interviewing might be another successful way to increase treatment adherence and effectiveness [55].

Despite the inherent difficulties in providing combined treatment modalities, evidence is emerging that a strategy of combining treatments aimed at different targets in CLBP can lead to better results. In an uncontrolled trial, Molloy et al. [74] reported significant reduction of disability for patients diagnosed with failed back surgery syndrome after being treated with an implanted spinal cord stimulator plus a multidisciplinary CBT program compared to either modality used alone. This finding suggests that such combined approaches are possible, but no RCTs have been reported.

When environmental factors (e.g., the patient's spouse or employer) seem to be important in perpetuating the chronic pain-related disability, treatment probably should not commence unless these persons are willing and able to attend specific treatment modalities. A recent review questioned the degree to which the social component is included in intervention studies [11].

Each health care provider should consider whether he or she is sufficiently capable to provide a particular type of treatment as it is known that clinician attitudes and beliefs do influence treatment content and outcome. For example, clinicians with more biomedical orientations may give advice that results in a less active lifestyle [10,49].

As pain rehabilitation aims to change the patient's management of the chronic condition, and extensive evidence is available that the pain complaint hardly ever disappears or even diminishes, it is remarkable how little research has been done on the effectiveness and timing of relapse prevention or refresher courses [75]. Sorensen [97] performed a study of the effect of addition of home visits by specially trained nurses after discharge from a multidisciplinary pain care program. Although the investigators did not find differences in health status, the intervention group tended to use fewer health care resources, and the costs of the intervention were more than balanced out by savings in other health care resources after the 2-year intervention period.

Back Pain and Work

It is well established that low back pain is costly to countries with well-established health and social welfare systems. The cost of treating low back pain is substantial, but social benefit costs including wage replacement and lost production are many times greater [69,109]. There is a political and fiscal imperative in many countries that interventions should be not only clinically effective but also cost effective; therefore, work loss and social costs associated with back pain should be considered in treatment outcomes. However, health care interventions, although very necessary in the management and rehabilitation of low back pain, are not sufficient to assure that the person with back pain returns to work in a timely manner. An integrated response involving the worker, health care practitioners, the employer, and the funder is required to ensure

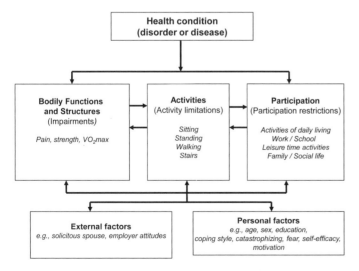

Fig. 1. The World Health Organization (WHO) International Classification of Functioning, Disability, and Health model. Reprinted with permission of WHO.

success. Earlier in this chapter the obstacles to recovery were elucidated. We will now present the evidence for effective management of the person with back pain to enable early and sustained return to work.

The management of work and low back pain falls generally into the following main areas:

1) The prevention of injury and the reduction of biomechanical stress and management of the work environment to prevent the development of low back pain.

2) The management of those who are symptomatic but continue to work with pain.

3) Rehabilitative efforts to return to work those who have been absent due to their symptoms.

4) Rehabilitation for the person with chronic pain who might have withdrawn from the employment market and is unemployed or on disability/incapacity benefits or pensions.

The services available and how they are delivered are usually determined by the health and social benefits system of each country, and this in itself complicates analysis of the data and identification of the "best" solution for successfully managing low back pain and work loss. Workers' compensation systems usually require the demonstration of a workplace injury to access treatment and benefits. Social health care systems, such as those in many European countries, offer a more universal access to health care irrespective of the cause of injury. There is insufficient space in this chapter to address the advantages and disadvantages of these approaches. This section will not address primary prevention of low back pain other than to say the prevention of injuries to workers should be one of the duties of a good employer. Work may not be the cause of much low back pain, but it undoubtedly affects the symptoms. In the case of work-related low back pain, there continues to be difficulty in identifying the primary causative mechanism, and although certain physical risk factors for the development of low back pain have been identified, the direct relationship between risk factor modification and prevention of low back pain remains problematic [71].

Occupational Health Care

It might be understood that a caring employer should provide support and perhaps even health care for employees who become injured in the course of their work or who find it difficult to perform their duties due to pain, and some employers do so. More and more people are employed in small-to-medium-sized businesses (see www.census.gov/epcd/www/smallbus. html). In the United Kingdom there is only one occupational health specialist employed for every 35 medium-sized businesses (defined as having between 50 and 250 employees) and only 1 for every 1,506 small businesses (with fewer than 50 employees) [35]. The coverage in other European Union countries is considerably higher, and comprehensive access to occupational health services reaches 90%. In some countries, health care associated with workplace injuries is covered by a workers' compensation insurance system. However, tensions exist in all health care systems between the perceived role of the care provider, the family physician, the therapist, the occupational health service, the employer, and the third-party payer determined to manage costs tightly. All can mitigate to some degree against the provision of the best care [2].

Rehabilitation: A Philosophy

Waddell and Watson [120] suggested that there was a difference in emphasis between health care and (work) rehabilitation approaches to the treatment of back pain. They suggested that in health care, back pain was a symptom; the aim of the clinician was to make people better (pain free) through identifying the cause of the symptom and the resultant disability. Treatment was focused on the symptom, with the intention that resolution of the symptom would result in a return to normal activities. A rehabilitation approach, on the other hand, regards low back disability as restricted function. The aim of rehabilitation is to restore function directly through a combination of clinical, psychosocial, and work-related interventions; success is measured in sustained return to regular work [120]. In short, the success of vocational rehabilitation (occupational or work rehabilitation) is measured by success in employment outcomes. It is important to note that rehabilitation requires the participation of more than health care practitioners. There is now strong evidence for the effectiveness of vocationally orientated rehabilitation [117] in reducing work loss due to low back pain.

Although the focus of vocational rehabilitation is on improving function, the very important role of treating pain and the provision of adequate analgesia cannot be denied. The main reason people with low back pain consult a health care practitioner is to seek some sort of relief from their pain, and pain treatment is integral to vocational rehabilitation. However, there is very little evidence that health care focusing on symptoms alone is effective in helping people return to work, especially in those who have had a chronic condition with long work absences [117].

Health Care Practitioners' Beliefs about Back Pain and Work

In recent years there has been a burgeoning interest in the role health care practitioners play in advising people with low back pain about their ability to work with their symptoms. Differences have been noted between different professions in encouraging patients to maintain normal activities.

A number of researchers have suggested that concerns regarding recommending physical activity will result in different advice regarding work. This suggestion is predicated on the findings that some practitioners show concern about being physically active with low back pain. Houben et al. [50,51] demonstrated two distinct groups in studies of physical therapists, who were described as having either a biomedical or psychosocial orientation to the management of low back pain. Those with a biomedical orientation were more likely to believe that back pain had a specific cause, and they were more likely to suggest activity restriction, including recommending work restrictions. Clinicians with a biopsychosocial orientation were less likely to recommend activity and work restriction. A similar conclusion has been drawn from studies in physicians [26,82]: restrictions on activity were commonly reported, and these restrictions appear to relate to the fear-avoidance beliefs about activity and work on the part of the clinicians [51].

The research on fear-avoidance beliefs in physicians and the influence that it has on recommendations about activity and work is not without its problems. Most of the research has been conducted using health care practitioner beliefs questionnaires that have not been fully validated. The most frequently used questionnaire, the Practitioner Attitudes and Beliefs Scale (PABS), has been through a number of iterations and has been found to have poor psychometric properties, although a newer version has been demonstrated to be robust [126]. Furthermore, the research has used case studies, vignettes, or videos to test recommendations about activity; actual clinician behavior has not been assessed [10,126]. Watson et al. found no direct relationship between family practitioner beliefs and sickness certification for back pain; instead, the practitioners'

propensity for sickness certification for back pain was best explained by their propensity to issue sickness certificates for other common health conditions [126]. However, the likely influence of both practitioner beliefs and patient beliefs, within the context of the consultation and the eventual outcome with regard to advice to be absent from work, is currently under investigation.

In a very recent study, patient and practitioner variables were used to predict the issuing of a sick note following a primary care consultation in a group of patients attending for low back pain. All patients were working at the time of the consultation and had not been absent from work in this episode at that point. The patient variables of previous work loss due to low back pain and high scores on the fear avoidance beliefs questionnaire about work were predictive of being given a sickness certificate by their practitioner. Practitioner beliefs alone were weak predictors of sickness certification. However, practitioner and patient beliefs combined were highly predictive, yielding an 85% correct prediction of receiving a sickness certificate as an outcome of the consultation [76].

It might seem obvious that, if beliefs and attitudes about back pain are predictive of work absence, then an intervention to change the beliefs about the relationship between physical activity and work to engender more positive cognitions about the benefits of activity and remaining at work might be a fruitful way of reducing sickness absence. Indeed, there is a literature that appears to demonstrate that approaches to promote more positive messages about low back pain in a local workforce [104] or in a general population, including family physicians [15,16,119], do appear to produce positive changes in people's beliefs about back pain. The evidence that this approach results in a sustained reduction in people being absent from work is contradictory, however, with very similar interventions demonstrating a reduction in work loss [16] and no effect [119]. The general consensus is that information only has only a weak effect [17] and probably has no effect on work absence in isolation [45].

Early Interventions in Those at Risk of Developing Chronicity

Most vocational rehabilitation is triggered once the worker is absent from work. In workers' compensation systems, the intervention is only triggered if the back pain is related to a workplace incident. A preemptive approach was developed by Linton and

Anderson [59], in which workers who had previously been absent from work for short periods of time due to low back pain were screened using a musculoskeletal screening questionnaire, to identify those who were likely to be at greatest risk of developing long-term work absence based upon many of the risk factors identified in this chapter. Subjects received either a systematic low back pain cognitive-behavioral program of approximately 12 hours' duration over six sessions, a back pain education intervention, or a simple leaflet on low back pain. The results demonstrated a 9-fold reduction in the development of long-term work loss and reduced physician and physical therapy visits over the next year in those who underwent the CBT intervention [59]. Most health care and health insurance systems, and indeed most employers, do not have the organizational systems in place to implement an early screening and intervention program, and interventions are most likely to be triggered once absence from work occurs.

Early Intervention and Secondary Prevention

As was discussed earlier, the majority of people who miss work for low back pain return within a matter of a few weeks, and most of these workers will not be absent again within a year of their return. The natural rate of return to work is high, with most workers returning within a month or so. Furthermore, the number who are absent briefly is large, and to implement a comprehensive program of rehabilitation for all would prove costly. Not all people with low back pain require comprehensive treatment programs, particularly in the first few weeks after onset or work absence [41]; many will fare equally well with simple workplace-based interventions. There is good evidence that some of these simple measures to encourage early return to work are beneficial for most people with low back pain [8,14].

Secondary prevention involves alleviating symptoms, minimizing disability, and identifying and addressing the factors that might lead to a recurrence of back pain symptoms. The focus is on maximizing recovery. Secondary prevention aims at preventing the person from becoming stuck in the sick role, as well as reducing inactivity, psychological sequelae, and long-term disability and work loss.

Reviews have provided suggested care pathways for early intervention, which include early contact with the worker to discuss the problem, assessing the possibility of returning to work, and involving a health care professional as required with simple analgesic pain re-

lief. If there is no recovery after 2 weeks, this plan reviewed with the employer and employee, with advice to the employee to commence increasing activity. Increasing activity refers to restoring normal activity levels and activities of daily living, and does not necessarily mean performing specific back exercises [8,14]. A Cochrane review concluded that exercise programs alone probably have no effect in the acute phase of low back pain with respect to shortening work absence [88].

A trial of a very similar approach, in which workers were contacted by occupational health nurses within 1 week of work loss and managed with a psychosocial intervention package linked with communication with the line manager regarding modified work, reduced the mean work loss from 10 to 6 days [72]. Similar success has been reported in a workers' compensation system targeting those perceived to be at risk of poor outcome in the early stages of work loss, and further demonstrated the redundancy of expensive integrated programs for low-risk workers [87].

Shortened work loss in the early stages is also related to the actions of the family physician; being given a date for a return to work, having a discussion of the prevention of recurrences, and the physician contacting the workplace have been associated with a shorter work absence [58]. Franche et al. [36] also conclude that there is strong evidence that contact between the health care provider and the workplace shortens work absence. The same author also found moderate evidence that contact from the workplace with the worker had the potential to reduce work loss and improve outcome.

Workplace Modifications

A review of workplace interventions alone for the prevention of work disability found moderate but reasonably consistent evidence that interventions such as workplace modification and involvement of the employer were more effective than treatment as usual in reducing time to return to work and total work days lost [110]. Workplace interventions in this review were defined as "either changes to the workplace or equipment, changes in work design and organization, changes in working conditions or work environment, and occupational (case) management with active stakeholder involvement of (at least) the worker and the employer." This disability management program aims to facilitate early return to work by addressing some of the obstacles, in particular "blue flags," to working with pain. The review by van Oostrom et al. [110] did not demonstrate any clear improvements in health outcomes, which has led to concerns that workers might be returning to work at a cost to themselves. Reviews of modified work and transitional arrangements have repeatedly demonstrated that they shorten work absence without an increase in recurrence rates; in fact, recurrence rates may be reduced in industries with such arrangements in place. This latter point helps to reduce the concern that people are encourage to return to work too early or that "presenteeism" (working when unfit and/or working with reduced productivity) may be encouraged with this type of intervention [128]. Presenteeism is more likely if functional problems are not recognized and addressed.

Some of these interventions obviously require the employer to provide modifications and implement appropriate advice in the workplace. Many people rely on their family physician or a therapist for advice about workplace modifications; these practitioners might feel unable or unwilling to offer advice [23,81]. In many systems the family physician is also the gatekeeper to sickness certification. Patients report vague or poor advice regarding returning to work, with practitioners relying on workers to be the best judge of their own ability to work. The vague advice to "take it easy" and "go back when you feel ready" is too often the default position for health care practitioners [23,24]. Such advice is not helpful and might present an obstacle to return to work, particularly if modified work is readily available [19]. An additional problem is the availability of modified work in small businesses with few job positions or in heavy industries such as construction [6].

Most of the early interventions are low cost or even cost-neutral to the employer provided there is appropriate cooperation between the employer, the employee, and the health care practitioner [18]. Successful implementation might require a change in the organizational culture of the employer as much as a change in how the employee is managed.

Exercise Interventions

There are some indications that early referral to physiotherapy or manual therapy interventions can reduce the duration of work loss over treatment as usual. However, the effect of such interventions is small because of the natural improvement with time of low back pain, and most people return to work relatively quickly even if they are symptomatic. Providing more than simple advice as outlined above to all workers may not be cost-effective; indeed Staal et al. [98] found that treatment provided too early (in this case, exercise therapy) was no more effective than usual care until the patient had been absent for over 50 days. Zigenfus et al. [129] found that early referral to physiotherapy (in less than 7 days) was more effective than treatment as usual. The treatment delivered consisted of a mixed package emphasizing physical conditioning, encouraging an expectation of returning to work, reducing the risk of recurrence, and engaging in activity. This mixed approach, incorporating many of positive messages recommended in early management, may have been the important influence. A self-referral physiotherapy vocational program with similar content was recently completed, concluding that such an approach was cost-effective in terms of health care and societal costs [80]. It would appear that routine referral may have only limited effect over and above structured advice and encouragement to remain in work. Whether this advice is delivered more effectively in the setting of a physical therapy consultation is an interesting research question.

There has been much debate on when is the appropriate time to intervene with a more structured intervention beyond those described above. There is a general and clear consensus that, should an employee fail to return to work within 4 to 12 weeks, the risk of not returning in the next year increases considerably. It is at this point that most guidelines and reviews recommend the adoption of the next step in a stepwise management plan [99]. Von Korff and Moore [114] recommend that those who do not respond to simple measures such as simple analgesics, advice, education, and encouragement to remain active and at work should receive a brief structured intervention.

A biopsychosocial approach is recommended where the potential obstacles to return to work are identified and addressed. The most successful programs incorporate a combination of graded activity or exercise, the use of cognitive-behavioral principles to address psychosocial barriers, and a workplace context or focus [120]. Reviews of graded exercise programs have demonstrated an effect on occupational outcomes [42] in subacute low back pain patients, and Waddell and Watson [120] argue that the addition of cognitive-behavioral therapy with an occupational focus improves return to work.

Although some guidelines recommend a multidisciplinary approach to those who fail to return to work after a few weeks, increasing evidence shows that effective rehabilitation can be provided by a suitably trained professional (a psychologist or physiotherapist) linked to the workplace or a case management system. Intensive multidisciplinary rehabilitation programs are expensive, and it is not clear if the provision of such intense interventions is cost-effective at this stage without effective screening to target only those with high risk of poor outcome. Relatively low-cost reactivation programs may be more cost-effective at this stage [31,41].

Sullivan and coworkers have developed two interventions predicated on a program of activity scheduling, increasing physical activity, and specifically targeting risk factors such as fear of movement/re-injury and perceived disability. The programs are run in the community by trained psychologists (Pain Disability Program [PDP]) [102] or physiotherapists (Progressive Goal Attainment Program [PGAP]) [101]. Workers are screened for their risk of developing chronic disability, and those considered at high risk are referred for individual treatment in addition to usual care. These approaches have been demonstrated to be more successful in returning people to work than usual care, although the PGAP has yet to be evaluated in the management of low back pain.

The Worker with Prolonged Work Loss

Despite early management, a relatively small number of workers will develop prolonged work loss. Often this group has not received the evidence-based approaches described above, and routine management has failed to help them return to work. Occupational guidelines recommend comprehensive multidisciplinary interventions for this group of workers, such as vocationally orientated pain management programs or functional restoration programs, and there is good evidence that these intensive programs are effective in returning people to work even with prolonged work absence [8,31]. One might be tempted to look at relatively brief programs such as the one used by Linton and Andersson [59], but although such programs are effective in those with short-term work loss (2–6 months) they were not found to be effective in people with prolonged work loss (>12 months) [70]. Indeed, outcomes from other programs of relatively moderate intensity have reported similar findings [100].

Intensive rehabilitation programs for the rehabilitation of employees with prolonged work loss due to back pain are supported by a considerable amount of literature, and there is some evidence that prolonged programs are more effective than those of short duration. These programs are generally expensive, and they are typically multidisciplinary, intensive, and of long duration (3 or 4 weeks). Haldorsen et al. [41] demonstrated that an intensive rehabilitation program was most effective for those who were at high risk of poor outcome. Those judged as low risk did well from routine management and did not do better if treated in more multidisciplinary programs. Those of medium risk did equally well with a brief or an intense multidisciplinary rehabilitation program. From this and similar studies, it would appear that expensive and intense programs should be reserved for those who are deemed to be at high risk of poor outcome.

An Integrated Approach

One example of an integrated approach tested empirically is the Sherbrooke model for the community practice approach to the management of low back pain [63], which represents a good example of a community stepped-care approach. The original program was developed in 31 workplaces and involved an occupational intervention at 6 to 10 weeks of absence from work, involving a consultation with an occupational physician, examination, advice, and treatment as suggested by the physician. It also included a participatory ergonomics intervention and modified duties as indicated. Contact was developed and maintained between the worker, ergonomist, and work supervisor to implement the program. If the worker did not return to work within 6 to 8 weeks of absence, the second step focused on further investigation, reassurance (or intervention), and attendance at a "back school." Should this step not result in a return to work within 12 weeks, a functional restoration or therapeutic return-to-work program was instigated.

This model has been adapted to a two-step, community-based model of work disability diagnosis by a physician and occupational therapist. Step 1 identifies red flags and possible barriers to return to work, followed if necessary by Step 2, which is a therapeutic return-to-work program, based on the needs of the individual [62].

The Chronically Disabled Person with Back Pain

A small minority of people will eventually be classed as incapable of doing their job, and they may subsequently go on to long-term wage replacement benefits, early retirement, or disability pension. This group increased considerably, particularly in European countries, at the end of the 20th century [116], and there have been considerable efforts to change social security systems to address this problem. The main problems faced by this group are dislocation from the workforce and the need to adopt new skills, find opportunities to re-engage in the workplace, and be given encouragement to withdraw from social benefits. Integrated programs aimed at identifying transferable skills, skills training, work experience, and financial support to encourage the transition from benefit dependency to work have been demonstrated to have some effect [5,125]. However, these programs require major investment and commitment by social security payers and governments at a national and regional level, and there is only limited evidence on how they should be implemented [105].

Communication among All Players

A coordinated approach to return to work requires communication among all those involved: the health care practitioner, occupational health services, the employer, and the payer. Tensions occur between those involved in the care of the patient with back pain, and poor communication is a common feature particularly between primary care physicians, occupational health services, and employers. A more recent assessment of family physicians' perceptions of their role in helping people return to work demonstrated that they feel they lack the skills to perform this role, even though it is one that, by default, is often expected of them [23]. Primary care physicians in particular have a conflicting role between patient advocacy, supporting sickness absence, and being part of the rehabilitation process.

Employers are often immediately affected by reduced production and the expense of providing replacement workers. They often find it difficult to see how modified work and graded return to work or the provision of changes to the workplace can be cost-effective. This problem is brought into sharp relief when the role of line managers or supervisors is considered, where there is often perceived conflict between maintaining production and accommodating return-to-work programs.

A recent review of collaborative approaches between health care and the workplace demonstrates that these approaches are not only effective but are also cost-effective for employers and more cost-effective than health care alone when the wider, societal costs

are considered [18]. Unfortunately, to date most of the cost-effectiveness studies have been performed among large employers, often with access to a range of facilities, and there remains a lack of information from small and medium-sized employers, which form the majority of employers in most countries.

Even if all involved understand and appreciate innovative approaches to vocational rehabilitation, having all players "on side," while necessary, may not be sufficient to ensure success [86]. Barriers to implementation may exist at the systems level—the so-called black flags referred to earlier. Case management systems have been adopted in many countries to attempt improve communication among all parties. The results in workers' compensation systems are mixed, and at worst workers refer to disempowerment, delay, and frustration at the decisions made [6]. To date, there does not seem to be even one system that has squared the circle of effective engagement of all stakeholders.

Conclusion

Despite many years of research, low back pain has remained stubbornly problematic to manage, and the associated health care and societal costs have remained high and continue to rise. Research has started to demonstrate some approaches to rehabilitation that have merit. The key challenges for the future are how we integrate these approaches, and in particular, how we can effectively target treatments to patient subgroups through the identification of specific presenting features including obstacles to recovery.

Although there is a continuous exhortation to apply a biopsychosocial approach in the management of disability associated with the condition, we remain unclear as to specifically what the elements are and how they should be assessed and structured in individualized treatment. This lack of clarity is particularly pertinent in the management of the "social" component of the model.

Vocational rehabilitation approaches have been investigated and models of care developed. Nevertheless, back pain continues to be one of the main reasons why people are absent from work in different health and social care systems. Research to date has identified specific types of programs or interventions that are effective. There has been conspicuously little research into how these effective treatments can be integrated. Knowing what to do is of little value if we do not know how to implement it. A systems approach to the application of evidence into practice and the science of implementation requires much greater attention in future studies.

References

[1] Accident and Compensation Corporation. Persistent pain assessment instruments: a compendium. Wellington: Accident and Compensation Corporation of New Zealand; 2008.

[2] Anema JR, Van Der Giezen AM, Buijs PC, Van Mechelen W. Ineffective disability management by doctors is an obstacle for return-to-work: a cohort study on low back pain patients sicklisted for 3–4 months. Occup Environ Med 2002;59:729–33.

[3] Assendelft WJ, Morton SC, Yu EI, Underwood M. Review: spinal manipulative therapy is not better than standard treatments for low back pain. Evid Based Med 2004;9:171.

[4] Bachmann S, Wieser S, Oesch P, Schmidhauser S, Knusel O, Kool J. Three-year cost analysis of function-centred versus pain-centred inpatient rehabilitation in patients with chronic non-specific low back pain. J Rehabil Med 2009;41:919–23.

[5] Bambra C, Whitehead M, Hamilton V. Does "welfare to work" work? A systematic review of the effectiveness of the UK's welfare to work programmes for people with disability or chronic illness. Soc Sci Med 2005;60:1905–18.

[6] Baril R, Clarke J, Friesen M, Stock S, Cole D, Work-Ready G. Management of return-to-work programs for workers with musculoskeletal disorders: a qualitative study in three Canadian provinces. Soc Sci Med 2003;57:2101–14.

[7] Bauman A, Fardy H, Harris P, Anderson R, Mullen P. Getting it right: why bother with patient-centred care? In diabetes care, moving from compliance to adherence is not enough. Something entirely different is needed. Compliance becomes concordance. Med J Aust 2003;179:253–6.

[8] Bevan S, Quadrello T, McGee R, Mahdon M, Vavrovsky A, Barham L. Fit for work? Musculoskeletal Disorders in the European Workforce. The Work Foundation; 2009.

[9] Bishop A, Foster NE. Do physical therapists in the United Kingdom recognize psychosocial factors in patients with acute low back pain? Spine 2005;30:1316–22.

[10] Bishop A, Foster NE, Thomas E, Hay EM. How does the self-reported clinical management of patients with low back pain relate to the attitudes and beliefs of health care practitioners? A survey of UK general practitioners and physiotherapists. Pain 2008;135:187–95.

[11] Blyth FM, Macfarlane G, Nicholas MK. The contribution of psychosocial factors to the development of chronic pain: the key to better outcomes for patients? Pain 2007;129:8–11.

[12] Boersma K, Linton SJ. Screening to identify patients at risk: profiles of psychological risk factors for early intervention. Clin J Pain 2005;21:38–43; discussion 69–72.

[13] Bowey-Morris J, Davies S, Purcell-Jones G, Watson PJ. Beliefs about back pain: results of a population survey of working age adults. Clin J Pain 2010; in press.

[14] Breen A, Langworthy J, Baghurst J. Improved early pain management for musculoskeletal disorders. London: HSE Books; 2007.

[15] Buchbinder R, Jolley D. Effects of a media campaign on back beliefs is sustained 3 years after its cessation. Spine 2005;30:1323–30.

[16] Buchbinder R, Jolley D, Wyatt M. Population based intervention to change back pain beliefs and disability: three part evaluation. BMJ 2001;322:1516–20.

[17] Burton AK, Waddell G. Educational and informational approaches. Amsterdam: Elsevier; 2002.

[18] Caroll C, Rick J, Pilgrim H, Cameron J, Hillage J. Workplace involvement improves return to work rates among employees with back pain on long-term. Disabil Rehabil 2010; in press.

[19] Carter J, Birrell L. Occupational health guidelines for the management of low back pain at work: evidence review and recommendations. London: Faculty of Occupational Medicine; 2000.

[20] Childs J, Fritz J, Flynn T, Irrgang J, Johnson K, Majkowski G, Delitto A. A clinical prediction rule to identify patients with low back pain most likely to benefit from spinal manipulation: a validation study. Ann Intern Med 2004;141:920–8.

[21] Chou R, Atlas SJ, Stanos SP, Rosenquist RW. Nonsurgical interventional therapies for low back pain: a review of the evidence for an American Pain Society clinical practice guideline. Spine 2009;34:1078–93.

[22] Chou R, Huffman LH, American Pain S, American College of P. Nonpharmacologic therapies for acute and chronic low back pain: a review of the evidence for an American Pain Society/American College of Physicians clinical practice guideline. Ann Intern Med 2007;147:492–504.

[23] Coole C, Watson PJ, Drummond A. Work problems due to low back pain: what do GPs do? A questionnaire survey. Fam Pract 2010;27:31–7.

[24] Corbett M, Foster NE, Ong B. GP attitudes and self reported behaviour in primary care consultations for low back pain. Fam Pract 2009;26:359–64.

[25] Costa LO, Maher C, Latimer J, Hodges PW, Herbert RD, Refshauge KM, McAuley JH, Jennings MD. Motor control exercise for chronic low back pain: a randomized placebo-controlled trial. Phys Ther 2009;89:1275–86.

[26] Coudeyre E, Rannou F, Tubach F, Baron G, Coriat F, Brin S, Revel M, Poiraudeau S. General practitioners' fear-avoidance beliefs influence their management of patients with low back pain. Pain 2006;124:330–7.

[27] Croft PR, Macfarlane GJ, Papageorgiou AC, Thomas E, Silman AJ. Outcome of low back pain in general practice: a prospective study. BMJ 1998;316:1356–9.

[28] Crook J, Milner R, Stringer B. Determinants of occupational disability following a low back injury: a critical review of the literature. J Occup Rehabil 2002;12:277–95.

[29] Denison E, Asenlof P, Sandborgh M, Lindberg P. Musculoskeletal pain in primary health care: subgroups based on pain intensity, disability, self-efficacy, and fear-avoidance variables. J Pain 2007;8:67–74.

[30] Deyo RA, Weinstein JM. Low back pain. N Engl J Med 2001;344:363–70.

[31] EASHAW. Work-related musculoskeletal disorders: back to work report. Office for Official Publications of the European Communities; 2007.

[32] Eccleston C, Williams ACDC, Morley S. Psychological therapies for the management of chronic pain (excluding headache) in adults. Cochrane Database Syst Rev 2009;2:CD007407.

[33] Engers A, Jellema P, Wensing M, van der Windt DAWM, Grol R, van Tulder MW. Individual patient education for low back pain. Cochrane Database Syst Rev 2008;1:CD004057.

[34] Ferreira ML, Machado G, Latimer J, Maher C, Ferreira PH, Smeets RJ. Factors defining care-seeking in low back pain: a meta-analysis of population based surveys. Eur J Pain 2009; Epub Dec 23.

[34A] Ferreira M, Smeets RJEM, Kamper S, Ferreira P, Machado L. Can we explain heterogeneity among exercise randomised clinical trials in chronic back pain? A meta-regression of randomized controlled trials. Phys Ther 2010;in press.

[35] Faculty of Occupational Medicine. Position statement: provision of occupational health services to small and medium-sized enterprises (SMEs). London: Faculty of Occupational Medicine; 2006.

[36] Franche RL, Baril R, Shaw W, Nicholas M, Loisel P. Workplace-based return-to-work interventions: optimizing the role of stakeholders in implementation and research. J Occup Rehabil 2005;15:525–42.

[37] Fritz JM, Brennan GP, Clifford S, Hunter S, Thackeray A. An examination of the reliability of a classification algorithm for subgrouping patients with low back pain. Spine 2006;31:77–82.

[38] Gatchel RJ, Rollings KH. Evidence-informed management of chronic low back pain with cognitive behavioral therapy. Spine J 2008;8:40–4.

[39] Goossens ME, Vlaeyen JW, Hidding A, Kole-Snijders A, Evers SM. Treatment expectancy affects the outcome of cognitive-behavioral interventions in chronic pain. C J Pain 2005;21:18–26; discussion 69–72.

[40] Guzman J, Esmail R, Karjalainen K, Malmivaara A, Irvin E, Bombardier C. Multidisciplinary biopsychosocial rehabilitation for chronic low back pain. Cochrane Database Syst Rev 2002;1:CD000963.

[41] Haldorsen E, Grasdal A, Skouen J, Risa A, Kronholm K, Ursin H. Is there a right treatment for a particular patient group? Comparison of ordinary treatment, light multidisciplinary treatment, and extensive multidisciplinary treatment for long term sick-listed employees with musculoskeletal pain. Pain 2002;95:49–63.

[42] Hayden JA, van Tulder MW, Malmivaara A, Koes BW. Exercise therapy for treatment of non-specific low back pain. Cochrane Database Syst Rev 2005;3:CD000335.

[43] Hayden JA, van Tulder MW, Malmivaara AV, Koes BW. Meta-analysis: exercise therapy for nonspecific low back pain. Ann Intern Med 2005;142:765–75.

[44] Hayden JA, van Tulder MW, Tomlinson G. Systematic review: strategies for using exercise therapy to improve outcomes in chronic low back pain. Ann Intern Med 2005;142:776–85.

[45] Henrotin YE, Cedraschi C, Duplan B, Bazin T, Duquesnoy B. Information and low back pain management: a systematic review. Spine 2006;15:E326–34.

[46] Henschke N, Maher CG, Refshauge KM, Herbert RD, Cumming RG, Bleasel J, York J, Das A, McAuley JH. Prognosis in patients with recent onset low back pain in Australian primary care: inception cohort study. BMJ 2008;337.

[47] Henschke N, Ostelo RW. Behavioural treatment for chronic low back-pain. Cochrane Review Update. June 2010.

[48] Hill JC, Dunn KM, Lewis M, Mullis R, Main CJ, Foster NE, Hay EM. A primary care back pain screening tool: identifying patient subgroups for initial treatment. Arthritis Care Res 2008;59:632–41.

[49] Houben RM, Gijsen A, Peterson J, de Jong PJ, Vlaeyen JW. Do health care providers' attitudes towards back pain predict their treatment recommendations? Differential predictive validity of implicit and explicit attitude measures. Pain 2005;114:491–8.

[50] Houben RM, Ostelo RW, Vlaeyen JW, Wolters PM, Peters M, Stomp-van den Berg SG. Health care providers' orientations towards common low back pain predict perceived harmfulness of physical activities and recommendations regarding return to normal activity. Eur J Pain 2005;9:173–83.

[51] Houben RMA, Ostelo R, Vlaeyen JWS, Wolters P, Peters M, Stomp-van Den Berg SGM. Health care providers' orientations towards common low back pain predict perceived harmfulness of physical activities and recommendations regarding return to normal activity. Eur J Pain 2005;9:173–83.

[52] Jellema P, van der Horst HE, Vlaeyen JWS, Stalman WAB, Bouter LM, van der Windt DAWM. Predictors of outcome in patients with (sub)acute low back pain differ across treatment groups. Spine 2006;31:1699–1705.

[53] Jellema P, van der Windt DA, van der Horst HE, Stalman WA, Bouter LM. Prediction of an unfavourable course of low back pain in general practice: comparison of four instruments. Br J Gen Pract 2007;57:15–22.

[54] Karjalainen K, Malmivaara A, van Tulder M, Roine R, Jauhiainen M, Hurri H, Koes B. Multidisciplinary biopsychosocial rehabilitation for subacute low back pain among working age adults. Cochrane Database Syst Rev 2003;2:CD002193.

[55] Keefe FJ, Abernethy AP, C Campbell L. Psychological approaches to understanding and treating disease-related pain. Annu Rev Psychol 2005;56:601–30.

[56] Kendall N, Linton SJ, Main CJ. Guide to assessing psychosocial yellow flags in acute low back pain: risk factors for long-term disability and workloss. Wellington: Accident Rehabilitation and Compensation Insurance Corporation of New Zealand and the National Health Committee, Ministry of Health; 1997.

[57] Kendall NAS, Burton AK, Watson P, Main CJ. Tackling musculoskeletal problems: the psychosocial flags framework—a guide for the clinic and workplace. London: The Stationary Office; 2009.

[58] Kosny A, Franche RL, Pole J, Krause N, Cote P, Mustard C. Early healthcare provider communication with patients and their workplace following a lost-time claim for an occupational musculoskeletal injury. J Occup Rehabil 2006;16:27–39.

[59] Linton SJ, Andersson T. Can chronic disability be prevented? A randomized trial of a cognitive-behavior intervention and two forms of information for patients with spinal pain. Spine 2000;25:2825–31.

[60] Linton SJ, Hallden K. Can we screen for problematic back pain? A screening questionnaire for predicting outcome in acute and subacute back pain. Clin J Pain 1998;14:209–15.

[61] Loisel P, Durand MJ, Baril R, Gervais J, Falardeau M. Interorganizational collaboration in occupational rehabilitation: perceptions of an interdisciplinary rehabilitation team. J Occup Rehabil 2005;15:581–90.

[62] Loisel P, Durand MJ, Diallo B, Vachon B, Charpentier N, Labelle J. From evidence to community practice in work rehabilitation: the Quebec experience. Clin J Pain 2003;19:105–13.

[63] Loisel P, Gosselin L, Durand P, Lemaire J, Poitras S, Abenhaim L. Implementation of a participatory ergonomics program in the rehabilitation of workers suffering from subacute back pain. Appl Ergon 2001;32:53–60.

[64] Macedo L, Maher CG, Latimer J, McAuley JH. Motor control exercise for persistent, nonspecific low back pain: a systematic review. Phys Ther 2009;89:9–25.

[65] Macedo L, Smeets RJEM, Maher CG, Latimer J, McAuley JH. Graded activity and graded exposure for persistent non-specific low back pain: a systematic review. Phys Ther 2010; in press.

[66] Main C, Sullivan MJL, Watson PJ. Pain management: practical applications of the biopsychosocial perspective in clinical and occupational settings. Edinburgh: Churchill Livingstone; 2008.

[67] Main CJ. Concepts of treatment and prevention in musculoskeletal disorders. In: Linton S, editor. New avenues for the prevention of chronic musculoskeletal pain and disability. Vol. 12. Amsterdam: Elsevier; 2002. p. 47–63.

[68] Main CJ, Williams AC de C. Musculoskeletal pain. BMJ 2002;325:534–7.

[69] Maniadakis N, Gray A. The economic burden of back pain in the UK. Pain 2000;84:95–103.

[70] Marhold C, Linton SJ, Melin L. A cognitive-behavioral return-to-work program: effects on pain patients with a history of long-term versus short-term sick leave. Pain 2001;91:155–63.

[71] Martimo K, Verbeek J, Karppinen J, Furlan AD, Kuijer P, Viikari-Juntura E, Takala EP, Juahiainen M. Manual material handling advice and assistive devices for preventing and treating back pain in workers. Cochrane Database Syst Rev 2007;3:CD005958.

[72] McCluskey S, Burton AK, Main CJ. The implementation of occupational health guidelines principles for reducing sickness absence due to musculoskeletal disorders. Occup Med (Lond) 2006;56:237–42.

[73] Menezes-Costa L, Maher CG, McAuley JH, Hancock MJ, Herbert RD, Refshauge KM, Henschke N. Prognosis for patients with chronic low back pain: inception cohort study. BMJ 2009;339:3829.

[74] Molloy A, Nicholas MK, Asghari A, Beeston L, Dehghani M, Cousins M, Brooker C, Tonkin L. Does a combination of intensive cognitive-behavioral pain management and a spinal implantable device confer any advantage? A preliminary examination. Pain Pract 2006;6:96–103.

[75] Morley S. Relapse prevention: still neglected after all these years. Pain 2008;134:239–40.

[76] Morris J, Watson PJ. Investigating decisions to absent from work with low back pain: a study combining patient and general practitioner factors. Eur J Pain 2010; in press.

[77] Mullen P. Mullen PD. Compliance becomes concordance. BMJ 1997;314:691–2.

[78] Neubauer E, Junge A, Pirron P, Seeman H, Schiltenwolf M. HKF-R 10: screening for predicting chronicity in acute low back pain (LBP). A prospective clinical trial. Eur J Pain 2006;10:559–66.

[79] Ostelo RWJG, van Tulder MW, Vlaeyen JWS, Linton SJ, Morley SJ, Assendelft WJJ. Behavioural treatment for chronic low-back pain. Cochrane Database Syst Rev 2005;1:CD002014.

[80] Phillips C, Buck R, Aylward M, Main CJ, Watson PJ. An evaluation of the Welsh Assembly government Occupational Health Physiotherapy Project. Swansea University; 2009.

[81] Pincus T, Woodcock A, Vogel S. Returning back pain patients to work: how private musculoskeletal practitioners outside the National Health Service perceive their role (an interview study). J Occup Rehabil 2010; in press.

[82] Poiraudeau S, Rannou F, Le Henanff A, Coudeyre E, Rozenberg S, Huas D, Martineau C, Jolivet-Landreau I, Revel M, Ravaud P. Outcome of subacute low back pain: influence of patients' and rheumatologists' characteristics. Rheumatology 2006;45:718–23.

[83] Pransky G, Shaw W, Franche RL, Clarke A. Disability prevention and communication among workers, physicians, employers, and insurers: current models and opportunities for improvement. Disabil Rehabil 2004;26:625–34.

[84] Rubinstein SM, van Middelkoop M, Assendelft WJJ, de Boer M, van Tulder MW. Spinal manipulative therapy for chronic low-back pain (protocol). Cochrane Database Syst Rev 2009;CD008112.

[85] Savigny P, Kuntze S, Watson P, Underwood M, Ritchie G, Cotterell M, Hill D, Browne N, Buchanan E, Coffey P, et al. Low back pain: early management of persistent non-specific low back pain. London: Royal College of General Practitioners; 2009.

[86] Scheel IB, Hagen KB, Oxman AD. Active sick leave for patients with back pain: all the players onside, but still no action. Spine 2002;27:654–9.

[87] Schultz IZ, Crook J, Berkowitz J, Milner R, Meloche GR, Lewis ML. A prospective study of the effectiveness of early intervention with high-risk back-injured workers: a pilot study. J Occup Rehabil 2008;18:140–51.

[88] Shaafsma F, Schonstein E, Whelan K, Ulvestad E, Kenny D, Verbeek JH. Physical conditioning programs for improving work outcomes in workers with back pain. Cochrane Database Syst Rev 2010;1:CD001822.

[89] Shaw W, Hong Q-N, Pransky G, Loisel P. A literature review describing the role of return-to-work coordinators in trial programs and interventions designed to prevent workplace disability. J Occup Rehabil 2008;18:2–15.

[90] Shaw W, van der Windt DA, Main CJ, Loisel P, Linton SJ. Early patient screening and intervention to address individual-level occupational factors (Blue Flags) in back disability. J Occup Rehabil 2009;19:64–80.

[91] Shaw WS, Pransky G, Fitzgerald TE. Early prognosis for low back disability: intervention strategies for health care providers. Disabil Rehabil 2001;23:815–28.

[92] Smeets RJ, Severens JL, Beelen S, Vlaeyen JW, Knottnerus JA. More is not always better: cost-effectiveness analysis of combined, single behavioral and single physical rehabilitation programs for chronic low back pain. Eur J Pain 2009;13:71–81.

[93] Smeets RJEM, Beelen S, Goossens MEJB, Schouten EGW, Knottnerus JA, Vlaeyen JWS. Treatment expectancy and credibility are associated with the outcome of both physical and cognitive-behavioral treatment in chronic low back pain. Clin J Pain 2008;24:305–15.

[94] Smeets RJEM, Vlaeyen JWS, Hidding A, Kester ADM, van der Heijden GJMG, Knottnerus JA. Chronic low back pain: physical training, graded activity with problem solving training, or both? The one-year post-treatment results of a randomized controlled trial. Pain 2008;134:263–76.

[95] Smeets RJEM, Vlaeyen JWS, Kester ADM, Knottnerus JA. Reduction of pain catastrophizing mediates the outcome of both physical and cognitive-behavioral treatment in chronic low back pain. J Pain 2006;7:261–71.

[96] Smeets RJEM, Wade D, Hidding A, Van Leeuwen PJCM, Vlaeyen JWS, Knottnerus JA. The association of physical deconditioning and chronic low back pain: a hypothesis-oriented systematic review. Disabil Rehabil 2006;28:673–93.

[97] Sorensen J, Frich L. Home visits by specially trained nurses after discharge from multi-disciplinary pain care: a cost consequence analysis based on a randomised controlled trial. Eur J Pain 2008;12:164–71.

[98] Staal JB, Hlobil H, Twisk JW, Smid T, Koke AJ, van Mechelen W. Graded activity for low back pain in occupational health care: a randomized, controlled trial. Ann Intern Med 2004;140:77–84.

[99] Staal JB, Hlobil H, van Tulder MW, Waddell G, Burton AK, Koes BW, van Mechelen W. Occupational health guidelines for the management of low back pain: an international comparison. Occup Environ Med 2003;60:618–26.

[100] Sullivan MJ, Adams H, Tripp D, Stanish WD. Stages of chronicity and treatment response in patients with musculoskeletal injuries and concurrent symptoms of depression. Pain 2008;135:151–9.

[101] Sullivan MJL, Adams H, Rhodenizer T, Stanish WD. A psychosocial risk factor-targeted intervention for the prevention of chronic pain and disability following whiplash injury. Phys Ther 2006;86:8–18.

[102] Sullivan MJL, Stanish WD. Psychologically based occupational rehabilitation: the Pain-Disability Prevention Program. Clin J Pain 2003;19:97–104.

[103] Sullivan MJL, Ward LC, Tripp D, French DJ, Adams H, Stanish WD. Secondary prevention of work disability: community-based psychosocial intervention for musculoskeletal disorders. J Occup Rehabil 2005;15:377–92.

[104] Symonds TL, Burton AK, Tillotson KM, Main CJ. Absence resulting from low back trouble can be reduced by psychosocial intervention at the work place. Spine 1995;20:2738–45.

[105] Thornton P, Zeitzer I, Bruyere S, Golden T, Houtenville A. What works and looking ahead: a comparative study of UK and US policies and practices facilitating return to work for people with disabilities. New York: Cornell University; 2003.

[106] Turk DC, Melzack R. Handbook of pain assessment. New York: Guilford; 2001.

[107] van der Hulst M, Vollenbroek-Hutten MM, Ijzerman MJ. A systematic review of sociodemographic, physical, and psychological predictors of multidisciplinary rehabilitation or back school treatment outcome in patients with chronic low back pain. Spine 2005;30:813–25.

[108] van Geen J-W, Edelaar MJA, Janssen M, van Eijk JTM. The long-term effect of multidisciplinary back training: a systematic review. Spine 2007;32:249–55.

[109] van Leewen M, Blyth F, March L, Nicholas MK, Cousins M. Chronic pain and reduced work effectiveness: the hidden cost to Australian employers. Eur J Pain 2006;10:161–6.

[110] van Oostrom SH, Driessen MT, de Vet HCW, Franche R-L, Schonstein E, Loisel P, van Mechelen W, Anema JR. Workplace interventions for preventing work disability. Cochrane Database Syst Rev 2009;2:CD006955.

[111] Van Tulder M, Becker A, Bekkering T, Breen A, del Real M T, Hutchinson A, Koes B, Laerum E, Malmivaara A. European Guidelines for the management of acute non-specific low back pain in primary care. Eur Spine J 2006;15:S169–91.

[112] Vlaeyen JW, Kole-Snijders AM, Boeren RG, van Eek H. Fear of movement/(re)injury in chronic low back pain and its relation to behavioral performance. Pain 1995;62:363–72.

[113] Vlaeyen JW, Morley S. Cognitive-behavioral treatments for chronic pain: what works for whom? Clin J Pain 2005;21:1–8.

[114] Von Korff M, Moore JC. Stepped care for back pain: activating approaches for primary care. Ann Intern Med 2001;134(9 Pt 2):911–7.

[115] Von Korff M, Russell E, Sharpe M. Organising care for chronic illness. BMJ 2002;325:92–4.

[116] Waddell G, Aylward M, Sawney P. Back pain, incapacity for work and social security benefits: an international literature review and analysis. London: Royal Society of Medicine Press; 2002.

[117] Waddell G, Burton AK, Kendall N. Vocational rehabilitation. What works for whom, and when? London: The Stationary Office; 2008.

[118] Waddell G, Burton KA, Main JC. Screening people at risk of long-term incapacity: a conceptual and scientific review. London: Royal Society of Medicine; 2003.

[119] Waddell G, O'Connor M, Boorman S, Tornsey B. Working Back Scotland: a public and professional health education campaign for back pain. Spine 2007;32:2139–43.

[120] Waddell G, Watson P. Rehabilitation. The back pain revolution. Edinburgh: Churchill Livingstone; 2004. p. 371–99.

[121] Waller B, Lambeck J, Daly D. Therapeutic aquatic exercise in the treatment of low back pain: a systematic review. Clin Rehabil 2009;23:3–14.

[122] Wampold B, Brown G. Estimating variability in outcomes attributable to therapists: a naturalistic study of outcomes in managed care. J Consult Clin Psychol 2005;73:914–23.

[123] Wasiak R, Kim J, Pransky G. Work disability and costs caused by recurrence of low back pain: longer and more costly than in first episodes. Spine 2006;31:219–25.

[124] Wasiak R, Pransky G, Verma S, Webster B. Recurrence of low back pain: definition-sensitivity analysis using administrative data. Spine 2003;28:2283–91.

[125] Watson PJ, Booker CK, Moores L, Main CJ. Returning the chronically unemployed with low back pain to employment. Eur J Pain 2004;8:359–69.

[126] Watson PJ, Bowey J, Purcell-Jones G, Gales T. General practitioner sickness absence certification for low back pain is not directly associated with beliefs about back pain. Eur J Pain 2008;12:314–20.

[127] Watson PJ, Main CJ, Waddell G, Gales TF, Purcell-Jones G. Medically certified work loss, recurrence and costs of wage compensation for back pain: a follow-up study of the working population of Jersey. Br J Rheumatol 1998;37:82–6.

[128] Williams RM, Westmoreland M, Lin C, Schmuck G, Creen M. Effectiveness of workplace rehabilitation interventions in the treatment of work related low back pain: a systematic review. Disabil Rehabil 2007;29:607–24.

[129] Zigenfus GC, Yin J, Giang GM, Fogarty WT. Effectiveness of early physical therapy in the treatment of acute low back musculoskeletal disorders. J Occup Environ Med 2000;42:35.

Correspondence to: Paul J. Watson, FCSP, PhD, Department of Health Sciences, University of Leicester, Gwendolen Road, Leicester, LE5 4PW, United Kingdom. Email: pjw25@le.ac.uk.

Part 17
Basics, Management, and Treatment of Pain in Children

The Development of Pain Mechanisms, Pain Effects, and Pain Experiences in Infants and Children

38

Maria Fitzgerald, PhD

Department of Neuroscience, Physiology and Pharmacology, University College London, London, United Kingdom

We are born with the ability to detect noxious stimulation, and even very young infants are capable of displaying a robust physiological response to tissue injury. Recent research has highlighted the fact that this nociceptive response is not simply a rudimentary form of the more complex pain adult experience, but rather has its own characteristic features that are appropriate to the age of the child. Thus, important changes in pain processing take place throughout development from infancy through to adolescence. These developmental events occur at every level of the pain pathway, from nociceptor transduction and transmission through to cortical pain mapping and integration. Understanding these processes is essential for the appropriate measurement and treatment of children's pain and for understanding how it may shape future pain experience in adulthood.

Historically, infant and childhood pain has been undertreated [28,66], and even now, when pain management in children is benefiting from increased evidence-based data, many treatments for the youngest patients continue to be empirically rather than scientifically based [21]. Change will come from a better understanding of the developmental neurobiology of pain processing, new quantitative methods of pain assessment, and improved measures of analgesic efficacy in young children.

Pain is processed at several different levels of the nervous system (Fig. 1), beginning with the *transduction* of intense physical stimuli into neural activity at nociceptor terminals and the *transmission* of neural activity along peripheral sensory nerves. This information undergoes *integration* and *modulation* by nociceptive circuits in the dorsal horn and trigeminal nuclei, under powerful *supraspinal control* from descending pathways arising in the brainstem. Finally *cortical processing* of centrally transmitted nociceptive activity, together with emotional and environmental inputs, produces the final *pain experience* [6].

Furthermore, at every level, nociceptive processing is subject to modulation by factors and mechanisms activated by tissue and nerve injury and inflammation, such as may follow multiple skin-breaking procedures or surgery, leading to hyperalgesia, allodynia, and prolonged pain states (Fig. 1). It is this modulation that forms the major emphasis of current pain research in laboratories and clinics all over the world.

Differences are found in immature and mature nociceptive processing at every level of the nociceptive pathway that are likely to have an impact upon infant and childhood pain experience and treatment. Evidence is also emerging that modulation by tissue damage and inflammation is also age-dependent, suggesting that the pattern and degree of hyperalgesia and allodynia and characteristics of pain states will differ in young and adult subjects.

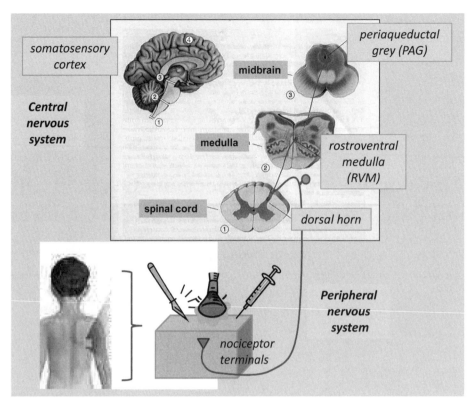

Fig. 1. Key sites of pain transmission and modulation in children.

Peripheral Nociceptive Mechanisms

Nociceptor Transduction and Transmission

Pain generally begins with the activation of nociceptors in peripheral organs, which detect noxious mechanical, thermal, or chemical stimuli through a set of specific transduction molecules. An important family of transduction molecules is the transient receptor potential (TRP) family of ion channels, which transduce physical and chemical stimuli into action potentials in nociceptor sensory nerves in the tissue. TRPV1, TRPM8, and TRPA1 are directly activated by heat, cold, chemical stimuli, and mechanical force, and can also act as local integrators of several noxious stimuli [56]. It has recently been discovered that the full complement of TRP channels are not present in young mammals. TRPV1 channels are not expressed in one group of nociceptors (the so-called nonpeptidergic, IB4-positive group) until well into postnatal life in a rat. Even more striking is the fact that TRPA1 channels are not expressed in nociceptors at all in the first weeks of life [27], which explains the absence of nociceptive reflex responses to the TRPA1 agonist mustard oil (allyl isothiocyanate) in young animals [18]. The importance of this finding for pain in children is not

yet clear, but it is likely that nociceptor transduction is less robust in younger patients.

Conduction velocities in immature afferent sensory nerves are lower than in mature nerves as the axons are smaller and incompletely myelinated. As a result nociceptive transmission through Aδ- and C-fiber axons and innocuous sensory transmission through Aβ axons will inevitably be slower in young children [31]. Frequency of action potential firing is also lower due to immature ion channel properties [36], leading to less reliable stimulus frequency coding. Whereas clear and distinguishable patterns of spike activity can be evoked by noxious and innocuous skin stimulation in the fetus and neonate [16], there are some activity patterns that are not normally observed in adults [15,36]. Somatosensory activity in young mammals is of special importance because it is required for the normal synaptic development of mature nociceptive pathways [24,55,65]. Local anesthetic block of A-fiber touch receptor activity in young rats delays the maturation of nociceptive reflexes [65].

Nociceptor Sensitization

Mechanical hyperalgesia at the site of surgical injury or inflammation is evident from birth in both rat pups and human infants [3,47,48,60]. The nociceptor sensitization to repeated noxious stimulation or inflammatory mediators [30,71] that is a feature of even the most immature nociceptors [35] undoubtedly contributes to this hyperalgesia. TRPA1 is also implicated in mechanical hyperalgesia [56], and the lack of TRPA in infant rats may explain the observation that acute mechanical (but not thermal) hypersensitivity following surgical incision recovers more quickly in young compared to adult rats [48]. Neurotrophins, a family of molecules that are crucial for the normal development of nociceptors [34], are upregulated in tissue inflammation and play a key role in altered transduction in inflammatory and postsurgical pain. The neurotrophins have therefore become a target for the development of new pain therapies [11]. Nerve growth factor (NGF), one of the most important pain neurotrophins, induces hyperalgesia in both young and adult animals, but this sensitization is brought about by different mechanisms in neonatal and adult rats. NGF treatment at postnatal days 0–14 results in a profound and long-lasting sensitization of Aδ nociceptive afferents to mechanical (but not thermal) stimuli, but this outcome does not occur older animals, which develop mechanical and thermal hyperalgesia apparently through a combination of C-fiber sensitization and central changes [38]. This difference is important because the upregulation of NGF is significantly higher following skin injury in young compared to adult animals [12].

A major difference in peripheral nociceptor response to tissue injury in young animals is the fact that the effects long outlast the injury itself, beyond the healing process and into adulthood. Prolonged hyperinnervation of skin wounds that outlasts wound healing occurs in young animals. Hyperinnervation also occurs following adult wounding, but it resolves when the wound has healed [46]. The longer-lasting neonatal hyperinnervation may result from a downregulation of inhibitory molecules that normally act to control nerve terminal growth in early life [42].

Nerve terminal sprouting may contribute to another very important consequence of early tissue injury, namely "priming" of the pain response. Skin incision made during a critical stage in neonatal pups leads to a greater response to subsequent injury in later life [69]. Thus, when an initial incision is performed in the first week of life, the degree of hyperalgesia following repeat incision 2 weeks later is greater than in animals having a single incision at the same age. Skin incisions in older animals do not have this lasting effect. The "priming" in young animals is blocked by perioperative local anesthetic block [69], highlighting the important role of sensory activity at the time of the first injury in triggering this phenomenon. Interestingly, continuous recording from single dorsal horn cells both before and after skin incision shows that the initial afferent-evoked spike activity is greater in young compared to adult animals [47].

Summary and Translational Implications

Nociceptors are capable of transducing and transmitting noxious information in children, but the incomplete complement of transduction proteins and immature channel kinetics may limit the nociceptors' efficiency, particularly in the preterm neonate. The modulation of nociceptors by tissue damage matures over childhood. Key neurotrophins, such as NGF, are released in very high levels after neonatal tissue damage, resulting in long-lasting hyperinnervation. Importantly, wounds and inflammation in early life may lead to a heightened sensitivity to further wounding in later life, which may have important implications for childhood surgery, but this possibility remains to be established.

Spinal Nociceptive Circuits

Central Nociceptive Processing

Nociceptors and low-threshold touch receptors form their first synaptic connections with neurons in the dorsal horn of the spinal cord. In the young rat's spinal cord, the central terminals of low-threshold tactile inputs are more diffuse and initially overlap with those of nociceptive C fibers in lamina II of the neonatal dorsal horn, slowly becoming pruned over the postnatal period [7,24]. The separation of the two types of sensory terminals is not complete until the rats are 3–4 weeks old; before that time, discrimination between noxious and non-noxious stimuli is less efficient.

Nociceptors excite a heterogenous population of dorsal horn neurons, consisting of excitatory and inhibitory interneurons and some projection neurons, which together form what is commonly called a nociceptive circuit. This circuit undergoes considerable changes over postnatal life [17]. Excitatory receptive fields (the area of skin that, when stimulated, evokes activity) of dorsal horn neurons remain plastic and changeable throughout life, but they are notably tuned over development. These excitatory fields are relatively larger at birth and only gradually diminish in size with age [17,47,61]. Furthermore, sensory neurons in the dorsal horn respond at longer and more variable latencies in young animals, due to immature myelination, slower synaptic transmission, and immature channel kinetics, which results in less synchronized responses to peripheral stimulation [19,59].

Nociceptive inputs also recruit inhibitory interneurons in the circuit. These inhibitory neurons powerfully control evoked spike activity and regulate dorsal horn cell receptive field size [73], and their synaptic connections are developmentally regulated [5]. The major inhibitory neurotransmitter, γ-aminobutyric acid (GABA), can produce a similar functional inhibition of spinal nociceptive circuits to that seen in adults [9], but the inhibitory receptive fields are spatially defined such that they are not precisely matched with excitatory fields [10]. This differing circuitry explains the poor spatial organization of spinal nociceptive reflexes and the high incidence of poorly directed nociceptive reflex movements in young mammals [65].

Central Sensitization

An important feature of the dorsal horn is that it is the site of central sensitization, a key mechanism underlying the pain and hyperalgesia following tissue damage. Relatively brief trains of activity in peripheral nociceptors have the ability to trigger long-term changes in dorsal horn nociceptive circuitry and cause prolonged states of hypersensitivity. This "central sensitization" contributes to an amplification of the noxious input (hyperalgesia), a spread of pain into areas outside the original damaged region, and the onset of pain from normally innocuous stimuli (allodynia) [70]. Central sensitization arises from prolonged increases in membrane excitability, strengthened excitatory synaptic inputs, and reduction of inhibitory interneuronal activity [32,50,72], which in turn are regulated by shifts in gene expression, by the production and trafficking of key receptors and channels, and by downstream neuronal signaling pathways [49].

The central pathways responsible for sensitization and hyperalgesia are functional in the newborn but appear to differ in magnitude and time course from those in adults. Observational studies have shown that newborn infants who undergo repeated painful procedures react more during a painful procedure than normal infants [58]. Nevertheless, secondary hyperalgesia (spread of pain to the area surrounding the injury) and referred hyperalgesia (pain in distant body areas) are weak in very young infants and increase with postnatal age [4,68]. Nevertheless, at the cellular level, tissue damage and inflammation in young animals are especially effective at modulating excitatory synapses in spinal nociceptive circuits. Surgical skin incision in the first weeks of life selectively increases excitatory synaptic activity in the dorsal horn 2–3 days after injury, without altering inhibitory activity, an effect that is not observed in older animals [39].

Central sensitization is mediated by the excitatory neurotransmitter glutamate via N-methyl-D-aspartate (NMDA) receptors, which, despite undergoing developmental changes in subunit content [41], are fully functional in pain circuits from birth [33]. Brain-derived neurotrophic factor (BDNF) is upregulated and released in the dorsal horn following peripheral inflammation and has been implicated in spinal mechanisms of sensitization. BDNF functions at the spinal level to enhance synaptic efficacy in young dorsal horn neurons and is therefore likely to contribute to central sensitization and exaggerated pain states in children as well as adults [22]. There are likely to be developmental differences in the cascade of enzymes and signaling proteins that mediate central sensitization, including protein kinase C (PKC). The isozyme PKCε, for example, mediates inflammatory pain at all ages, but the isozyme PKCγ does not contribute in young animals [57].

Central sensitization spreads beyond neuronal circuits to involves glial cells and neuroimmune pathways in the dorsal horn [1]. Nerve injury or C-fiber stimulation causes release of chemokines and other factors into the dorsal horn, triggering the recruitment and activation of microglia and T cells [13]. This process, in turn, can amplify and prolong neuronal activity, which itself releases more inflammatory factors and activates more glial cells. This positive feedback control loop plays a major role in chronic pain states, especially those involving nerve damage [14]. Interestingly, neither rat nor human infants develop mechanical allodynia following nerve injury [2,29]. Since both are capable of acute and chronic inflammatory pain behavior from an early neonatal age, it appears that the mechanisms underlying neuropathic pain are differentially regulated over a prolonged postnatal period. We have shown that the immune response to nerve injury and C-fiber stimulation differs in young and adult animals and that microglial activation does not occur in young rats [26,43,64]. Our recent transcriptome analysis of the dorsal horn at different ages revealed that a greater number of immune-related genes are regulated in the adult compared to young rats after nerve injury and that the pattern of cytokine activation is different in young animals, suggesting a protective anti-inflammatory response that is down-regulated with maturity [13].

Summary and Translational Implications

Central pain processing in children is robust but is likely to be less predictable and organized than in adults. Central sensitization can occur, leading to hyperalgesia and allodynia, but underlying mechanisms are likely to differ from those in adults. Notably, peripheral nerve damage is unlikely to trigger a strong neuroimmune response in children. Identifying the molecular mechanisms responsible for age-specific patterns of hyperalgesia will inform the rational development of novel therapeutic strategies for treating pediatric pain.

Supraspinal Descending Control Pathways

The Changing Role of the Rostroventral Medulla

An important aspect of central nervous system (CNS) pain processing is the system of endogenous control that modulates nociceptive activity through descending modulatory systems and endogenous opioids [8,23,45]. In this way, a noxious stimulus or injury not only excites neuronal networks but also activates local inhibitory circuits and alters the balance of brainstem descending inhibitory and excitatory activity, thus contributing to a homeostatic feedback mechanism of control [62]. These descending and endogenous pain modulatory pathways are the mechanisms by which factors such as attention and distraction, suggestion and expectation, stress and anxiety, context and past experience influence pain responses [40]. It is well established that rat pups have less descending inhibitory tone from higher CNS centers in the first weeks of life [20] and that as a result, no analgesia is produced from periaqueductal gray stimulation until 3 weeks of age [63]. However, recent research has shown that the situation in young animals is more strikingly different that was previously appreciated. The rostroventral medulla (RVM), which is the main output nucleus for brainstem descending control, undergoes a remarkable maturational switch after day P21 [25]. Both lesioning and electrical stimulation of RVM at different postnatal ages reveal that RVM control over spinal nociceptive

circuits switches from being entirely facilitatory before day P21 to inhibitory at older ages. Between days P25 and P35, descending inhibition begins to dominate, but it is not as powerful as in the adult until day P40. This gradual change is observed in the changing influence of the RVM over spinal nociceptive reflexes and dorsal horn neuronal activity over this critical periadolescent developmental period.

Neurotransmitters and Neuromodulators

Descending inhibition is mediated, in part, through the neurotransmitters 5-hydroxytryptamine (serotonin) and norepinephrine, but it is unlikely that major changes in the actions of these neurotransmitters are responsible for altering the balance of descending controls. Investigation of age-related effects of epidural dexmedetomidine has been used to evaluate postnatal function of noradrenergic pathways in rat pups using a quantitative model of nociception and C-fiber-induced hyperalgesia. Dose requirements were lower in the youngest pups, suggesting that noradrenergic activity is, if anything, more efficient [67]. Neonatal inflammation increases β-endorphin and met/leu-enkephalin protein levels and decreases opioid receptor expression in the periaqueductal gray of the adult rat, suggesting that early noxious insult can produce long-lasting alterations in endogenous opioid tone [37].

Summary and Translational Implications

Childhood may represent a time when the normal balance, rather than the absolute onset, of descending brainstem controls is established. A lack of balance or stability between inhibitory and excitatory supraspinal controls in early life may mean that young children are less able to mount effective endogenous control over noxious inputs compared to adults.

Cortical Pain Processing

Although we frequently use the term "pain" when discussing the mechanisms and responses at every level of this process, it is important to remember, especially when considering very young infants, that evidence of nociceptive activity at the level of the spinal cord or brainstem cannot be equated with pain experience. While input to the spinal cord and brain is necessary for perception of pain, it is not sufficient. Activity in the spinal cord, brainstem, and subcortical midbrain structures is sufficient to generate reflex behaviors and hormonal responses but is not sufficient to support pain awareness.

Activation of central nociceptive circuits in the spinal cord and brainstem is transmitted to the thalamus and brain, including the somatosensory cortex, cingulate cortex, and amygdala, which together contribute to the "pain matrix," the basis of pain experience [44,62]. Nothing is known about the maturation of the pain matrix over infancy and childhood in humans or laboratory animals, but we know from recent studies that nociceptive activity is processed at the level of the cortex from a very young age. Specific cortical hemodynamic and electrical (EEG) responses can be recorded from preterm and term infants in response to noxious heel lance [52,54], and while these responses are often correlated with behavioral and physiological responses, this is not always the case [51], showing that observational measures alone are insufficient to measure pain. Understanding cortical pain processing requires quantitative electrophysiological and functional neuroimaging in infants and children.

The infant cortical pain response appears highly plastic: there is evidence that intensive care influences cerebral pain processing even before a preterm infant leaves intensive care. Infants who are born prematurely and who have experienced at least 40 days of intensive or special care have increased brain neuronal evoked potential responses to noxious stimuli compared to healthy newborns at the same postmenstrual age [53].

Summary and Translational Implications

Understanding the changing nature of infant and children's pain experience requires a multidisciplinary approach. Little laboratory work has been done in this area. Nevertheless, our ability to quantify experience-dependent changes in infant and childhood cortical pain processing using neurophysiological methods will allow us to carry out controlled studies of analgesic efficacy with clear, objective outcome measures.

References

[1]   Abbadie C, Bhangoo S, De Koninck Y, Malcangio M, Melik-Parsadaniantz S, White FA. Chemokines and pain mechanisms. Brain Res Rev 2009;60:125–34.

[2]   Anand P, Birch R. Restoration of sensory function and lack of long-term chronic pain syndromes after brachial plexus injury in human neonates. Brain 2002;125:113–22.

[3]   Andrews K, Fitzgerald M. Wound sensitivity as a measure of analgesic effects following surgery in human neonates and infants. Pain 2002;99:185–95.

[4]   Andrews KA, Desai D, Dhillon HK, Wilcox DT, Fitzgerald M. Abdominal sensitivity in the first year of life: comparison of infants with and without prenatally diagnosed unilateral hydronephrosis. Pain 2002;100:35–46.

[5]   Baccei ML, Fitzgerald M. Development of GABAergic and glycinergic transmission in the neonatal rat dorsal horn. J Neurosci 2004;24:4749–57.

[6]   Basbaum AI, Bautista DM, Scherrer G, Julius D. Cellular and molecular mechanisms of pain. Cell 2009;139:267–84.

[7]   Beggs S, Torsney C, Drew LJ, Fitzgerald M. The postnatal reorganization of primary afferent input and dorsal horn cell receptive fields in the rat spinal cord is an activity-dependent process. Eur J Neurosci 2002;16:1249–58.

[8]   Bodnar RJ. Endogenous opiates and behavior: 2006. Peptides 2007;28:2435–513.

[9]   Bremner L, Fitzgerald M, Baccei M. Functional GABA$_A$-receptor-mediated inhibition in the neonatal dorsal horn. J Neurophysiol 2006;95:3893–7.

[10] Bremner LR, Fitzgerald M. Postnatal tuning of cutaneous inhibitory receptive fields in the rat. J Physiol 2008;586:1529–37.

[11] Cattaneo A. Tanezumab, a recombinant humanized mAb against nerve growth factor for the treatment of acute and chronic pain. Curr Opin Mol Ther 2010;12:94–106.

[12] Constantinou J, Reynolds ML, Woolf CJ, Safieh-Garabedian B, Fitzgerald M. Nerve growth factor levels in developing rat skin: upregulation following skin wounding. Neuroreport 1994;5:2281–4.

[13] Costigan M, Moss A, Latremoliere A, Johnston C, Verma-Gandhu M, Herbert TA, Barrett L, Brenner GJ, Vardeh D, Woolf CJ, Fitzgerald M. T-cell infiltration and signaling in the adult dorsal spinal cord is a major contributor to neuropathic pain-like hypersensitivity. J Neurosci 2009;29:14415–22.

[14] Costigan M, Scholz J, Woolf CJ. Neuropathic pain: a maladaptive response of the nervous system to damage. Annu Rev Neurosci 2009;321–32.

[15] Fitzgerald M. Cutaneous primary afferent properties in the hindlimb of the neonatal rat. J Physiol 1987;383:79–92.

[16] Fitzgerald M. Spontaneous and evoked activity of fetal primary afferents in vivo. Nature 1987;326:603–5.

[17] Fitzgerald M. The development of nociceptive circuits. Nat Rev Neurosci 2005;6:507–20.

[18] Fitzgerald M, Gibson S. The postnatal physiological and neurochemical development of peripheral sensory C-fibres. Neuroscience 1984;13:933–44.

[19] Fitzgerald M, Jennings E. The postnatal development of spinal sensory processing. Proc Natl Acad Sci USA 1999;96:7719–22.

[20] Fitzgerald M, Koltzenburg M. The functional development of descending inhibitory pathways in the dorsolateral funiculus of the newborn rat spinal cord. Brain Res 1986;389:261–70.

[21] Fitzgerald M, Walker S. Infant pain management: a developmental neurobiological approach. Nat Clin Pract Neurol 2009;5:35–50.

[22] Garraway SM, Petruska JC, Mendell LM. BDNF sensitizes the response of lamina II neurons to high threshold primary afferent inputs. Eur J Neurosci 2003;18:2467–76.

[23] Gebhart GF. Descending modulation of pain. Neurosci Biobehav Rev 2004;27:729–37.

[24] Granmo M, Petersson P, Schouenborg J. Action-based body maps in the spinal cord emerge from a transitory floating organization. J Neurosci 2008;28:5494–503.

[25] Hathway G, Koch S, Low L, Fitzgerald M. The changing balance of brainstem-spinal cord modulation of pain processing over the first weeks of rat postnatal life. J Physiol 2009;587:2927–35.

[26] Hathway GJ, Vega-Avelaira D, Moss A, Ingram R, Fitzgerald M. Brief, low frequency stimulation of rat peripheral C-fibres evokes prolonged microglial-induced central sensitization in adults but not in neonates. Pain 2009;144:110–8.

[27] Hjerling-Leffler J, Alqatari M, Ernfors P, Koltzenburg M. Emergence of functional sensory subtypes as defined by transient receptor potential channel expression. J Neurosci 2007;27:2435–43.

[28] Howard RF. Current status of pain management in children. JAMA 2003;290:2464–9.

[29] Howard RF, Walker SM, Mota PM, Fitzgerald M. The ontogeny of neuropathic pain: postnatal onset of mechanical allodynia in rat spared nerve injury (SNI) and chronic constriction injury (CCI) models. Pain 2005;115:382–9.

[30] Hucho T, Levine JD. Signaling pathways in sensitization: toward a nociceptor cell biology. Neuron 2007;55:365–76.

[31] Issler H, Stephens JA. The maturation of cutaneous reflexes studied in the upper limb in man. J Physiol 1983;335:643–54.

[32] Ji RR, Kohno T, Moore KA, Woolf CJ. Central sensitization and LTP: do pain and memory share similar mechanisms? Trends Neurosci 2003;26:696–705.

[33] King TE, Barr GA. Spinal cord ionotropic glutamate receptors function in formalin-induced nociception in preweaning rats. Psychopharmacology (Berl) 2007;192:489–98.

[34] Koltzenburg M. The changing sensitivity in the life of the nociceptor. Pain 1999;Suppl 6:S93–102.

[35] Koltzenburg M, Lewin GR. Receptive properties of embryonic chick sensory neurons innervating skin. J Neurophysiol 1997;78:2560–8.

[36] Koltzenburg M, Stucky CL, Lewin GR. Receptive properties of mouse sensory neurons innervating hairy skin. J Neurophysiol 1997;78:1841–50.

[37] Laprairie JL, Murphy AZ. Neonatal injury alters adult pain sensitivity by increasing opioid tone in the periaqueductal gray. Front Behav Neurosci 2009;3:31.

[38] Lewin GR, Ritter AM, Mendell LM. Nerve growth factor-induced hyperalgesia in the neonatal and adult rat. J Neurosci 1993;13:2136–48.

[39] Li J, Walker SM, Fitzgerald M, Baccei ML. Activity-dependent modulation of glutamatergic signaling in the developing rat dorsal horn by early tissue injury. J Neurophysiol 2009;102:2208–19.

[40] Melzack R, Wall PD. The challenge of pain. London: Penguin Books; 1966.

[41] Molnar E, Isaac JTR. Developmental and activity dependent regulation of ionotropic glutamate receptors at synapses. ScientificWorldJournal 2002;2:27–47.

[42] Moss A, Alvares D, Meredith-Middleton J, Robinson M, Slater R, Hunt SP, Fitzgerald M. Ephrin-A4 inhibits sensory neurite outgrowth and is regulated by neonatal skin wounding. Eur J Neurosci 2005;22:2413–21.

[43] Moss A, Beggs S, Vega-Avelaira D, Costigan M, Hathway GJ, Salter MW, Fitzgerald M. Spinal microglia and neuropathic pain in young rats. Pain 2007;128:215–24.

[44] Price DD. Central neural mechanisms that interrelate sensory and affective dimensions of pain. Mol Interv 2002;2:392–403, 339.

[45] Ren K, Dubner R. Descending modulation in persistent pain: an update. Pain 2002;100:1–6.

[46] Reynolds M, Fitzgerald M. Long-term sensory hyperinnervation following neonatal skin wounds. J Comp Neurol 1995;358:487–98.

[47] Ririe D, Bremner L, Fitzgerald M. Comparison of the immediate effects of surgical incision on dorsal horn neuronal receptive field size and responses during postnatal development. Anesthesiology 2008;109:698–706.

[48] Ririe DG, Vernon TL, Tobin JR, Eisenach JC. Age-dependent responses to thermal hyperalgesia and mechanical allodynia in a rat model of acute postoperative pain. Anesthesiology 2003;99:443–8.

[49] Salter MW. Cellular signalling pathways of spinal pain neuroplasticity as targets for analgesic development. Curr Top Med Chem 2005;5:557–67.

[50] Sandkuhler J. Understanding LTP in pain pathways. Mol Pain 2007;3:9.

[51] Slater R, Cantarella A, Franck L, Meek J, Fitzgerald M. How well do clinical pain assessment tools reflect pain in infants? PLoS Med 2008;5:e129.

[52] Slater R, Cantarella A, Gallella S, Worley A, Boyd S, Meek J, Fitzgerald M. Cortical pain responses in human infants. J Neurosci 2006;26:3662–6.

[53] Slater R, Fabrizi L, Worley A, Meek J, Boyd S, Fitzgerald M. Premature infants display increased noxious-evoked neuronal activity in the brain compared to healthy age-matched term-born infants. Neuroimage 2010;52:583–9.

[54] Slater R, Worley A, Fabrizi L, Roberts S, Meek J, Boyd S, Fitzgerald M. Evoked potentials generated by noxious stimulation in the human infant brain. Eur J Pain 2010;14:321–6.

[55] Spitzer NC. Electrical activity in early neuronal development. Nature 2006;444:707–12.

[56] Stucky CL, Dubin AE, Jeske NA, Malin SA, McKemy DD, Story GM. Roles of transient receptor potential channels in pain. Brain Res Rev 2009;60:2–23.

[57] Sweitzer SM, Wong SM, Peters MC, Mochly-Rosen D, Yeomans DC, Kendig JJ. Protein kinase C epsilon and gamma: involvement in formalin-induced nociception in neonatal rats. J Pharmacol Exp Ther 2004;309:616–25.

[58] Taddio A, Shah V, Gilbert-MacLeod C, Katz J. Conditioning and hyperalgesia in newborns exposed to repeated heel lances. JAMA 2002;288:857–61.

[59] Takahashi T. Postsynaptic receptor mechanisms underlying developmental speeding of synaptic transmission. Neurosci Res 2005;53:229–40.

[60] Torsney C, Fitzgerald M. Age-dependent effects of peripheral inflammation on the electrophysiological properties of neonatal rat dorsal horn neurons. J Neurophysiol 2002;87:1311–7.

[61] Torsney C, Fitzgerald M. Spinal dorsal horn cell receptive field size is increased in adult rats following neonatal hindpaw skin injury. J Physiol 2003;550:255–61.

[62] Tracey I, Mantyh PW. The cerebral signature for pain perception and its modulation. Neuron 2007;55:377–91.

[63] van Praag H, Frenk H. The development of stimulation-produced analgesia (SPA) in the rat. Brain Res Dev Brain Res 1991;64:71–6.

[64] Vega-Avelaira D, Moss A, Fitzgerald M. Age-related changes in the spinal cord microglial and astrocytic response profile to nerve injury. Brain Behav Immun 2007;21:617–23.

[65] Waldenstrom A, Thelin J, Thimansson E, Levinsson A, Schouenborg J. Developmental learning in a pain-related system: evidence for a cross-modality mechanism. J Neurosci 2003;23:7719–25.

[66] Walker SM. Pain in children: recent advances and ongoing challenges. Br J Anaesth 2008;101:101–10.

[67] Walker SM, Fitzgerald M. Characterization of spinal alpha-adrenergic modulation of nociceptive transmission and hyperalgesia throughout postnatal development in rats. Br J Pharmacol 2007;151:1334–42.

[68] Walker SM, Meredith-Middleton J, Lickiss T, Moss A, Fitzgerald M. Primary and secondary hyperalgesia can be differentiated by postnatal age and ERK activation in the spinal dorsal horn of the rat pup. Pain 2007;128:157–68.

[69] Walker SM, Tochiki KK, Fitzgerald M. Hindpaw incision in early life increases the hyperalgesic response to repeat surgical injury: critical period and dependence on initial afferent activity. Pain 2009;147:99–106.

[70] Woolf CJ. Central sensitization: uncovering the relation between pain and plasticity. Anesthesiology 2007;106:864–7.

[71] Woolf CJ, Ma Q. Nociceptors: noxious stimulus detectors. Neuron 2007;55:353–64.

[72] Zeilhofer HU. Loss of glycinergic and GABAergic inhibition in chronic pain: contributions of inflammation and microglia. Int Immunopharmacol 2008;8:182–7.

[73] Zhou HY, Zhang HM, Chen SR, Pan HL. Increased C-fiber nociceptive input potentiates inhibitory glycinergic transmission in the spinal dorsal horn. J Pharmacol Exp Ther 2008;324:1000–10.

Correspondence to: Maria Fitzgerald, PhD, Department of Neuroscience, Physiology and Pharmacology, University College London, Gower Street, London WC1E 6BT, United Kingdom. Email: m.fitzgerald@ucl.ac.uk.

Management and Treatment of Pain in Infants

Denise Harrison, RN, RM, PhD

Centre for Nursing and the Child Health Evaluative Sciences, Hospital for Sick Children, Toronto, Canada;
Lawrence S. Bloomberg Faculty of Nursing, University of Toronto, Canada;
Department of Neonatology, Royal Children's Hospital, Melbourne, Australia

"If a new skin in old people be tender, what is it you think in a newborn Babe? Doth a small thing pain you so much on a finger, how painful is it then to a Child, which is tormented all the body over, which hath but a tender new grown flesh? If such a perfect Child is tormented so soon, what shall we think of a Child, which stayed not in the wombe its full time? Surely it is twice worse with him."

Felix Wurtz, 1612, *The Children's Book*

Burden of Pain

All infants and young children are exposed to painful procedures from the time of birth. For healthy infants and children, painful procedures comprise capillary or venous blood sampling within a few days after birth, and a series of intramuscular (i.m.) injections during scheduled childhood immunizations. These procedures are known to be painful, and they have the potential to cause anxiety and distress for infants and children as well as their parents. Longer-term fears of needle pain, parental non-adherence to vaccination administration, and avoidance of medical care have been described [72]. For sick hospitalized infants and children, repeated episodes of minor painful procedures, major surgical procedures, and other painful stimuli throughout the period of hospitalization contribute to a significant burden of pain [10,19,54,77,88]. Hospitalized children have reported that procedures involving needles caused extreme pain and were scary [54], and sick infants and children continue to undergo large numbers of painful procedures, mainly with no or minimal use of pain reduction strategies [19,35,38,49,70,77,88]. Immediate consequences of untreated pain in sick infants include behavioral distress and physiological changes, often with prolonged recovery [32]. Potential longer-term risks include altered responses to subsequent pain; increased risk of adverse neurodevelopmental, behavioral, and cognitive outcomes [8,32]; and altered temperament [53]. Health care professionals have a responsibility to ensure that effective and safe pain management strategies during painful procedures are consistently applied in diverse pediatric settings where painful procedures take place. It is by reducing exposure to painful events, and ensuring provision of best pain management strategies, that the burden of pain can be lessened, and advances can be made in reducing risks of long-term adverse consequences of pain.

Effective Pain Reduction Strategies

There is abundant evidence to support the effectiveness of various pain reduction strategies in infants [41,95] and children [82] during painful procedures. Although there are still vital research gaps, the key challenge today is to translate current best evidence into practice in diverse clinical settings. Without a doubt, the most effective strategy to reduce pain is to prevent pain. A key recommendation of the American Academy of Pediatrics and the Canadian Paediatric Society is to reduce painful procedure occurrence [4]. Based on the ongoing reports of large numbers of painful procedures in infants [19], this recommendation does not seem to have been successfully implemented. Ongoing exposure of hospitalized infants to large numbers of painful procedures continues, despite the move toward less invasive methods of assisted ventilation and the availability of less invasive methods of monitoring. Paradoxically, although early weaning of invasive mechanical ventilation in a neonatal intensive care unit (NICU) was associated with reduced respiratory-related painful procedures, including airway suctioning, an increase in the number of invasive heel lance procedures performed for capillary blood sampling was noted [9]. This increase in invasive monitoring, in the face of less invasive care, highlights that although health care professionals need to ensure vigilant assessment, they also need to remain cognizant of the need to reduce pain exposure. A coordinated plan throughout an organization, which includes reducing the need for multiple episodes of blood sampling, evaluating the need for intravenous (i.v.) line insertions, and carefully assessing the need for distressing procedures such as airway suctioning, is required for a sustained reduction in painful procedures to occur.

Evidence supporting each of the strategies in the acronym "Be SWEET to Babies" will be presented in the remainder of this chapter:

Breast feeding (or kangaroo care)

Sucrose

With

Entertainment

EMLA (and other topical anesthetics), and

Technique (for blood sampling and i.m. injections)

In addition, due to current debate and conflicting or limiting evidence, a brief discussion on epidural anesthetics for postoperative pain and opioid analgesics for acute procedural pain in infants will be included.

Breastfeeding

Breastfeeding profoundly reduces pain in infants during venipuncture, heel lance [17,21,48,73,93], and immunization [24,26,68]. Analgesic mechanisms involved are probably multifactorial, including a combination of skin-to-skin contact, suckling, pleasant taste [31], and intake of naturally occurring endorphins present in breast milk [15,69,96]. Promoting the practice of breastfeeding during painful procedures when feasible requires families, clinicians, and organizational leaders to strongly advocate for this method of pain management. In order for breastfeeding to be integrated into accepted pain management practices, breastfeeding mothers need to be allowed, and encouraged, to feed their infants during all non-emergency blood tests, i.v. catheter placements, and injections. In addition, a policy that reinforces the conduct of these procedures only when mothers are available and able to feed, and is fully endorsed and supported by all involved parties, is required for successful implementation of this practice. Recommendations for future research include rates of adoption of this pain reduction strategy into clinical practice in diverse acute care and community settings, as well as its feasibility and effectiveness in sick infants during painful procedures. As current evidence for analgesic effects of breastfeeding is limited to infants up to 12 months [68], studies of analgesic benefits, acceptance to mothers, and feasibility of breastfeeding toddlers beyond 12 months of age during painful procedures are warranted.

Kangaroo Care

A growing body of evidence supports skin-to-skin contact, or kangaroo care, as an effective pain reduction strategy for preterm and term newborn infants during heel lance and i.m. injection [2,23,50-52,55,60]. Mechanisms involved are thought to be the combination of maternal heartbeat, maternal voice, rocking, containment [58] and release of oxytocin, a hormone closely associated with the endogenous opioid system [59,78]. The key practical challenge is the integration of kangaroo care into routine practice during non-emergency painful procedures. A policy outlining that non-emergency minor painful procedures are performed only when mothers, fathers, or designated family or friends are available for kangaroo care is necessary to facilitate the adoption of such care into accepted pain-management practices. Infant pain, plus the loss of the parental role, are considered the most stressful aspects for mothers of infants in intensive care [27]. Implementing breastfeeding and kangaroo care for pain management of sick infants in hospitals would help parents and their families to play an active role in supporting their infants. Recommendations for future research include evaluating the effectiveness and feasibility of kangaroo care during procedures, as well as during the postoperative period in sick hospitalized infants. Audits of the use of kangaroo care during painful procedures will inform the degree of adoption into normalized pain management practices and address issues of feasibility.

Sweet-Tasting Solutions

Although the first randomized controlled trial of sweet-tasting solutions during painful procedures was not published until 1991, there are numerous historical references describing calming and analgesic effects of sweet substances. Around 632 C.E., Prophet Mohammed recommended giving infants a well-chewed date [47], and in 1545, Thomas Phaire recommended "and if ye can gette any syrup of popye, geue it the chylde to licke" [67]. Three centuries later, sugar solutions, most often mixed with a combination of alcohol and cocaine or opium, were used to calm infants [42,66]. In the early 1900s, sugar mixed with alcohol was used during circumcision [13]; "Perry Davis pain killer," a mix of sugar, alcohol and opium, was used to cure colic and minor injuries [42]; and "a sucker consisting of a sponge dipped in some sugar water" was used for infants during surgery [89]. There are now over 125 studies evaluating the analgesic effects of sweet taste in infants [34,80,90], with the large majority of studies including healthy preterm or term neonates, during a single episode of heel lance, venipuncture, or i.m. injection. Overwhelming evidence from these large numbers of trials shows that sucrose or glucose effectively reduces crying duration, facial expressions of pain, and composite pain scores.

As there is no longer a state of equipoise relating to sweet-taste analgesia during heel lance, venipuncture, and i.m. injections, it is unethical to conduct further trials with placebo or nontreatment arms during single episodes of these painful procedures in medically stable preterm infants, healthy term newborns, and infants up to 12 months of age [29,34]. Priorities for clinicians and researchers need to shift to translating this research into clinical practice in settings where infants experience painful procedures. To successfully translate research into practice, recommendations with clear clinical practice guidelines are required. In this case, guidelines advising to administer the solutions in small increments over the entire duration of prolonged and stressful procedures, such as ophthalmology examinations and urethral catheterizations, would ensure that the short-acting analgesic effects of sweet solutions are optimized.

There do however, remain important knowledge gaps concerning the effectiveness and safety of sweet solutions for pain management. These include (1) prolonged use in preterm and sick infants, (2) effectiveness in the context of concomitant opioid analgesics, and (3) effectiveness in older babies and children.

1) Prolonged use. Only three studies have evaluated sucrose over prolonged periods. Stevens et al. [79] reported that sucrose remained effective and safe when given for all painful procedures in preterm infants in the first month of life. Mucignat et al. [64] reported that sucrose, in conjunction with the topical anesthetic EMLA®, effectively reduced pain scores in healthy preterm infants over a 6-week period during subcutaneous injections. Harrison et al. [36] reported ongoing effectiveness of sucrose during heel lancing in sick preterm and term infants over an entire hospitalization ranging from 4 weeks to 5 months. Further studies evaluating the ongoing effectiveness and safety of sweet solutions in sick infants, including extremely low birth weight infants, are warranted. To build on the understudied area of sucrose analgesia, longer-term outcomes should include evaluation of necrotizing enterocolitis, neurodevelopmental outcomes, pain responses during subsequent painful procedures, and infant and early childhood temperament.

2) Effectiveness with opioids. There is limited knowledge about effectiveness of sweet solutions given concomitantly with opioid or other strong analgesics. For health care professionals caring for sick hospitalized infants, this knowledge gap is important and clinically relevant. Safety concerns of opioid use, especially in preterm infants [6,11], and questionable analgesic effects of background morphine during acute painful procedures [18] warrant investigation of safe and effective pain management strategies to use in the context of background opioid delivery. Given that sweet-taste analgesic effects are considered to be due to endogenous opioid release [14], it is not understood if this mechanism can occur in the presence of exogenous opioids. Further observational and experimental research focusing on this knowledge gap is required.

3) Effectiveness in older babies and children. A frequently asked question is: Do sweet solutions effectively reduce pain in older babies and children? Sucrose and glucose, in sufficiently sweet concentrations, are effective in infants up to 12 months of age [40,75]. In toddlers, the evidence is less clear. There are only two studies, both of which used a 12% sucrose solution, generally considered to be insufficiently sweet to exert the sweet-taste-mediated analgesic effect [3]. The oldest of the two studies, published 14 years ago, demonstrated minimal analgesic effects beyond the neonatal period [3], yet more recently, 12% sucrose was shown to effectively reduce pain during immunizations in toddlers and preschool children aged 13 months to 4 years [24]. Such opposing findings from only two studies using the same sucrose concentration, volume, and placebo prevent sound recommendations from being made.

What about sweet-taste analgesia in school-aged children? Four published studies have included school-aged children: two during the cold pressor test [62,63], one during i.m. injection for immunization [57], and one during venipuncture [57]. Miller et al. [63] reported that 24% sucrose (held in the mouth) effectively delayed cold threshold (i.e., time at which the children indicated discomfort), but had no effect on cold tolerance (i.e., the time at which the arm was removed from the cold water) or self-report of pain [63]. Mennella et al. [62] reported, however, that sucrose did not increase pain threshold; however it did increase pain tolerance, but only in a subgroup of children categorized as non-depressed [62]. Both studies were limited by missing cold tolerance data (as the majority of children kept their arm in the water for the full 4-minute study period), by incomplete pain scoring [63], or by a failure to understand or complete the tasks [62]. To evaluate analgesic effects of sweet taste during needle-related procedures in school-aged children, Lewkowski et al. used sweet or non-sweet chewing gum [57]. Results showed that sweet-tasting gum either prior to, or during, the two procedures had no effect on self-reported pain ratings compared to non-sweet gum [57].

In summary, there is abundant evidence of sweet-taste analgesia in the newborn period, sufficient evidence up to 12 months of age, but beyond the first year of life, the evidence is limited and conflicting. Although further studies are warranted in toddlers and young children, there are more appropriate and effective strategies to use with school-aged children. As sweet-tasting solutions have been extensively studied, priorities must now be to consistently implement these solutions in clinical practice. Future research should focus on addressing knowledge gaps, while avoiding replication of studies where there is already high-quality evidence.

Entertainment

A number of studies, plus two systematic reviews [20,91] and a review of systematic reviews [82], have reported on psychological interventions to reduce procedural pain in infants and children. A systematic review of interventions to reduce needle-related pain in children from 2 to 19 years old showed that distraction was the most frequently studied and most effective intervention [91]. More recently, a systematic review focused on interventions to reduce pain during immunization only, and included studies with infants from one month of age [20]. Distraction with age-appropriate toys and breathing exercises, including using breathing as a distraction in children as young as 3 years of age, by having them blow bubbles or party blowers, was shown to be effective [20]. Recommendations arising from other studies have included encouraging parents and staff to use developmentally appropriate distraction techniques, non-procedural talk [16], and cartoon videos [22]. Interestingly, parent-led distraction was less effective in reducing pain responses in toddlers and children, in contrast to the demonstrated effectiveness of nurse-led distraction [20]. This finding seems to be related to parent behavior: specifically, the use of reassurance. Although it seems counterintuitive, toddlers as young as 18 months and older children may be more distressed when parents offer reassurance, apology, or comfort [16,61,84]. Potential mechanisms for this effect are well summarized by McCurtry et al. [61] and include the possibilities that (1) parental anxiety and reassurance warn the child that something bad is going to happen, (2) reassurance and comfort reinforce distress behaviors, and (3) reassurance by parents gives children "permission" to overtly convey their distress. Recommendations include parental encouragement and training to use effective distraction methods and minimize less effective reassuring behaviors. As the most effective methods to teach parents these skills remain uncertain, further research in this area is warranted. In the meantime, supporting parents to effectively reduce their child's pain needs to be considered part of the health care professional's role while performing, or assisting with, painful procedures.

Topical Anesthetics

Topical anesthetic agents are known to reduce pain in newborn infants during circumcision [56,87,95], and in infants and young children during immunization [75]. There are no analgesic effects during heel lancing, and inconclusive effects during venipuncture, arterial puncture, lumbar puncture and percutaneous peripheral line placement [56]. In studies that compared sweet solutions with topical anesthetics in newborn infants during venipuncture, sucrose and glucose were more effective in reducing pain than EMLA® [1,30], and concomitant use of EMLA® with oral sucrose was no more effective than oral sucrose alone. Topical anesthetic agents seem to have the most analgesic effect in children aged 4–6 years compared to both younger and older children, although this finding could be attributed to the methods of pain assessment in the different age groups [94]. Despite early childhood immunizations being a significant cause of pain and fear [72,86], and despite good evidence to support analgesic benefits of topical anesthetics during i.m. injection [75], topical anesthetics have not been integrated into clinical practice during immunization [86]. Physicians identified the long application time needed for effectiveness, the cost, and concerns that parents would not correctly apply the topical local anesthetics as barriers to the use of topical anesthetics during scheduled childhood immunizations, although these concerns were not substantiated by parents [86]. Although cost and feasibility barriers may preclude making recommendations to use topical anesthetics routinely for all immunizations, their use should be considered for infants and children who may require multiple invasive procedures in the future, are particularly anxious and distressed about the pending injection, and for children with a fear of needles [72]. In contrast, wherever feasible, topical anesthetics should be integrated into normal pain management practices for needle-related procedures in hospitalized children.

Technique

Techniques used for blood sampling, especially in infants, and for administering i.m. injections may substantially affect the severity of pain. Heel lancing has been shown to be more painful than venipuncture in neonates [74]; nevertheless, heel lances continue to be more frequently performed for routine blood sampling than the less painful venipuncture method [19] [37]. In sick infants, concerns about venous access for purposes of medication, fluids, and nutrition deter health care professionals from using venipuncture for blood sampling [37]. For healthy infants, the need for additional training to perform venipuncture, or having the procedures performed by a skilled phlebotomist, may also deter organizations from implementing venipuncture as the first-line method of blood collection in routine practice.

The i.m. injection technique, the choice of vaccine, and the order of vaccines injected during multiple vaccination episodes also have the potential to significantly affect severity of pain and self-reports of pain ratings in children. Injecting the most painful injection last reduced overall pain responses in infants [45], and injecting one brand of measles-mumps-rubella vaccine over another brand reduced pain in infants [43] and children aged 4–6 years [44]. A rapid i.m. injection technique without aspiration also resulted in less pain, during and following the procedure in infants, than the "standard" slower injection technique [46]. Recommendations for practice include a reexamination of i.m. injection techniques and a revision of vaccination guidelines to incorporate the least painful methods of injection.

Regional Anesthetics

Epidural anesthesia in infants and children was first reported on in 1936, followed in 1954 by publication of a series of 77 cases of epidural anesthesia in infants and children, the large majority of which were considered successful [71]. The key advantage of epidural anesthesia over general anesthesia and postoperative systemic opioid analgesics is the avoidance of respiratory depression and delayed tracheal extubation [76]. Since the case series of successful epidural anesthetics in infants was published over half a century ago, there have been few studies of epidural anesthesia for intra- and postoperative pain management in infants. A small number of case series highlights the benefits of epidurals, especially in preterm and former preterm infants in terms of successful intra- and postoperative analgesia, systemic opioid sparing, avoidance of extubation delay, avoidance of need for postoperative ventilation, and minimal adverse effects [65,76]. In a case series of 44 low birth weight infants, postoperative pain, as assessed first by physiological parameters, and later in the study with the Neonatal Pain and Sedation scale (N-PASS), was described as successfully managed with no use of systemic opioid analgesics. A pain-free postoperative course was reported for 33 (75%) cases and mild pain was reported for 11 (25%) cases, which was resolved following epidural boluses. The epidural infusate included an opioid (fentanyl) and a local anesthetic (bupivacaine). Further published case series as well as experimental studies are warranted to fully inform health care professionals about the best analgesic choices for infants undergoing surgery.

Opioid Analgesics

The use of opioid analgesics in sick infants is a conundrum. Evidence supports selective use of i.v. morphine in critically ill infants, as indicated by clinical judgment and pain assessment [11], but there is insufficient knowledge concerning the safety and effectiveness for long-term management of procedural and disease-related pain in infants with complex medical conditions [6,12,39,85]. The evidence is also conflicting concerning the analgesic effectiveness of background infusions of opioid analgesics during episodes of minor painful procedures [5,18]. Such findings pose difficulties for clinicians working to ensure safe and effective pain management for preterm and sick infants within a limited evidential base. As morphine and fentanyl have been targeted as high research priorities by the Neonatal Pain Control Group [7], we should see some of the complex questions relating to safety and effectiveness of prolonged opioid use in sick infants being addressed in the future.

Pain Assessment

The use of pain reduction strategies requires ongoing systematic evaluation to ensure their effectiveness (or demonstrate their ineffectiveness) in the management of pain in diverse populations of infants and children in diverse clinical settings. Although further discussion is beyond the scope of this chapter, there are four detailed reviews of pain assessment tools for use in the neonatal and pediatric populations to which readers are referred [25,81,83,92], as well as critical commentaries regarding integration of suitable pain assessment methods into normalized pain management practices [28,33].

Conclusion

A key priority for families, clinicians, researchers, health care organizations, and health care leaders is to reduce the impact of painful procedures on infants and young children. Consistent utilization of strategies with known effectiveness, along with further research focusing on current evidence gaps, will ensure advancements toward addressing this priority.

Acknowledgments

The CIHR Systematic Review of Sweet Solutions for Acute Pain Relief in Infants Knowledge Synthesis Team (KRS91774), the Pain in Child Health Strategic Training Initiative (STP53885), and the CIHR Team Grant in Children's Pain (CTP-79854 and MOP-86605) are thanked for their support in this review.

References

[1] Abad F, Diaz-Gomez NM, Domenech E, Gonzalez D, Robayna M, Feria M. Oral sucrose compares favourably with lidocaine-prilocaine cream for pain relief during venepuncture in neonates. Acta Paediatr 2001;90:160–5.

[2] Akcan E, Yigit R, Atici A. The effect of kangaroo care on pain in premature infants during invasive procedures. Turk J Pediatr 2009;51:14–8.

[3] Allen KD, White DD, Walburn JN. Sucrose as an analgesic agent for infants during immunization injections. Arch Pediatr Adolesc Med 1996;150:270–4.

[4] American Academy of Pediatrics Committee on Fetus and Newborn, American Academy of Pediatrics Section on Surgery, Canadian Paediatric Society Fetus and Newborn Committee; Batton DG, Barrington KJ, Wallman C. Prevention and management of pain in the neonate: an update. Pediatrics 2006;118:2231–41.

[5] Anand KJ, Barton BA, McIntosh N, Lagercrantz H, Pelausa E, Young TE, Vasa R. Analgesia and sedation in preterm neonates who require ventilatory support: results from the NOPAIN trial. Neonatal Outcome and Prolonged Analgesia in Neonates. Arch Pediatr Adolesc Med 1999;153:331–8.

[6] Anand KJ, Hall RW, Desai N, Shephard B, Bergqvist LL, Young TE, Boyle EM, Carbajal R, Bhutani VK, Moore MB, Kronsberg SS, Barton BA; NEOPAIN Trial Investigators Group. Effects of morphine analgesia in ventilated preterm neonates: primary outcomes from the NEOPAIN randomised trial. Lancet 2004;363:1673–82.

[7] Anand KJ, Johnston CC, Oberlander TF, Taddio A, Lehr VT, Walco GA. Analgesia and local anesthesia during invasive procedures in the neonate. Clin Ther 2005;27:844–76.

[8] Anand KJS, Soriano SG. Anesthetic agents and the immature brain: are these toxic or therapeutic? Anesthesiology 2004;101:527–30.

[9] Axelin A, Ojajärvi U, Viitanen J, Lehtonen L. Promoting shorter duration of ventilator treatment decreases the number of painful procedures in preterm infants. Acta Paediatr 2009;98:1751–5.

[10] Barker DP, Rutter N. Exposure to invasive procedures in neonatal intensive care unit admissions. Arch Dis Child 1995;72:F47–8.

[11] Bellu R, de Waal KA, Zanini R. Opioids for neonates receiving mechanical ventilation. Cochrane Database Syst Rev 2008;1:CD004212.

[12] Bhandari V, Bergqvist LL, Kronsberg SS, Barton BA, Anand KJ; NEOPAIN Trial Investigators Group. Morphine administration and short-term pulmonary outcomes among ventilated preterm infants. Pediatrics 2005;116:352–9.

[13] Blanton M, G. The behavior of the human infant during the first thirty days of life. Psychol Rev 1917;24:456–83.

[14] Blass E, Ciaramitaro V. A new look at some old mechanisms in human newborns. Monogr Soc Res Child Dev 1994;59:1–81.

[15] Blass EM, Blom J. Beta-casomorphin causes hypoalgesia in 10-day-old rats: evidence for central mediation. Pediatr Res 1996;39:199–203.

[16] Blount RL, Corbin SM, Sturges JW, Wolfe VV, Prater JM, James LD. The relationship between adults' behavior and child coping and distress during BMA/LP procedures: a sequential analysis. Behav Ther 1989;20:585–601.

[17] Brovedani P, Montico M, Shardlow A, Strajn T, Demarini S. Suckling and sugar for pain reduction in babies. Lancet 2007;369:1429–30.

[18] Carbajal R, Lenclen R, Jugie M, Paupe A, Barton BA, Anand KJS. Morphine does not provide adequate analgesia for acute procedural pain among preterm neonates. Pediatrics 2005;115:1494–500.

[19] Carbajal R, Rousset A, Danan C, Coquery S, Nolent P, Ducrocq S, Saizou C, Lapillonne A, Granier M, Durand P, et al. Epidemiology and treatment of painful procedures in neonates in intensive care units. JAMA 2008;300:60–70.

[20] Chambers CT, Taddio A, Uman LS, McMurtry CM, Team. H. Psychological interventions for reducing pain and distress during routine childhood immunizations: a systematic review. Clin Ther 2009;31(Suppl 2):S77–103.

[21] Codipietro L, Ceccarelli M, Ponzone A. Breastfeeding or oral sucrose solution in term neonates receiving heel lance: a randomized, controlled trial. Pediatrics 2008;122:e716–21.

[22] Cohen LL, Blount RL, Panopoulos G. Nurse coaching and cartoon distraction: an effective and practical intervention to reduce child, parent, and nurse distress during immunizations. J Pediatr Psychol 1997;22:355–70.

[23] de Sousa Freire NB, Santos Garcia JB, Carvalho Lamy Z. Evaluation of analgesic effect of skin-to-skin contact compared to oral glucose in preterm neonates. Pain 2008;139:28–33.

[24] Dilli D, Küçük I, Dallar Y. Interventions to reduce pain during vaccination in infancy. J Pediatr 2009;154:385–90.

[25] Duhn LJ, Medves JM. A systematic integrative review of infant pain assessment tools. Adv Neonatal Care 2004;4:126–40.

[26] Efe E, Ozer ZC. The use of breast-feeding for pain relief during neonatal immunization injections. Appl Nurs Res 2007;20:10–6.

[27] Franck LS, Allen A, Cox S, Winter I, Franck LS, Allen A, Cox S, Winter I. Parents' views about infant pain in neonatal intensive care. Clin J Pain 2005;21:133–9.

[28] Franck LS, Bruce E. Putting pain assessment into practice: why is it so painful? Pain Res Manag 2009;14:13–20.

[29] Freedman B. Equipoise and the ethics of clinical research. N Engl J Med 1987;317:141–5.

[30] Gradin M, Eriksson M, Holmqvist G, Holstein A, Schollin J. Pain reduction at venipuncture in newborns: oral glucose compared with local anesthetic cream. Pediatrics 2002;110:1053–7.

[31] Gray L, Miller LW, Philipp BL, Blass EM. Breastfeeding is analgesic in healthy newborns. Pediatrics 2002;109:590–3.

[32] Grunau RE, Holsti L, Haley DW, Oberlander T, Weinberg J, Solimano A, Whitfield MF, Fitzgerald C, Yu W. Neonatal procedural pain exposure predicts lower cortisol and behavioral reactivity in preterm infants in the NICU. Pain 2005;113:293–300.

[33] Harrison D. Implementation matters: pain assessment: not yet normalized practice. IASP Special Interest Group on Pain in Childhood Newsletter 2009;August:4–5.

[34] Harrison D, Bueno M, Adams-Webber T, Yamada J, Stevens B. Analgesic effects of sweet tasting solutions in infants: do we have equipoise yet? Proceedings of the 8th International Symposium on Pediatric Pain, Acapulco; 2010.

[35] Harrison D, Loughnan P, Johnston L. Pain assessment and procedural pain management practices in neonatal units in Australia. J Paediatr Child Health 2006;42:6–9.

[36] Harrison D, Loughnan P, Manias E, Gordon I, Johnston L. Repeated doses of sucrose in infants continue to reduce procedural pain during prolonged hospitalizations. Nurs Res 2009;58:427–34.

[37] Harrison D, Loughnan P, Manias E, Johnston L. Pain management practices during minor painful procedures in a cohort of infants with a prolonged length of stay. Pain Res Manag 2006;11(Suppl B):40–9.

[38] Harrison D, Loughnan P, Manias E, Johnston L. Analgesics administered during minor painful procedures in a cohort of hospitalized infants: a prospective clinical audit. J Pain 2009;10:715–22.

[39] Harrison D, Loughnan P, Manias E, Johnston L. Utilization of analgesics, sedatives, and pain scores in infants with a prolonged hospitalization: a prospective descriptive cohort study. Int J Nurs Stud 2009;46:624–32.

[40] Harrison D, Stevens B, Bueno M, Yamada J, Adams-Webber T, Beyene J, Ohlsson A. Efficacy of sweet solutions for analgesia in infants between one and 12 months of age: a systematic review. Arch Dis Child 2010;95:406–13.

[41] Harrison D, Yamada J, Stevens B. Strategies for the prevention and management of neonatal and infant pain. Curr Pain Headache Rep 2010;14:113–23.

[42] Holbrook S. The golden age of quackery. New York: Macmillan; 1959.

[43] Ipp M, Cohen E, Goldbach M, Macarthur C. Effect of choice of measles-mumps-rubella vaccine on immediate vaccination pain in infants. Arch Pediatr Adolesc Med 2004;158:323–6.

[44] Ipp M, Cohen E, Goldbach M, Macarthur C. Pain response to M-M-R vaccination in 4–6 year old children. Can J Clin Pharmacol 2006;13:e296–9.

[45] Ipp M, Parkin PC, Lear N, Goldbach M, Taddio A. Order of vaccine injection and infant pain response. Arch Pediatr Adolesc Med 2009;163:469–72.

[46] Ipp M, Taddio A, Sam J, Gladbach M, Parkin PC. Vaccine-related pain: randomised controlled trial of two injection techniques. Arch Dis Child 2007;92:1105–8.

[47] Islamic Voice. Relief of pain: a medical discovery. Accessed March 1, 2010. Available at: http://www.islamicvoice.com/april.2001/quran.htm.

[48] Iturriaga GS, Unceta-Barrenechea AA, Zarate KS, Olaechea IZ, Nunez AR, Rivero MM. [Analgesic effect of breastfeeding when taking blood by heel-prick in newborns.] An Pediatr (Barc) 2009;71:310–3.

[49] Johnston CC, Collinge JM, Henderson SJ, Anand KJ. A cross-sectional survey of pain and pharmacological analgesia in Canadian neonatal intensive care units. Clin J Pain 1997;13:308–12.

[50] Johnston CC, Filion F, Campbell-Yeo M, Goulet C, Bell L, McNaughton K, Byron J. Enhanced kangaroo mother care for heel lance in preterm neonates: a crossover trial. J Perinatol 2009;29:51–6.

[51] Johnston CC, Filion F, Campbell-Yeo M, Goulet C, Bell L, McNaughton K, Byron J, Aita M, Finley GA, Walker CD. Kangaroo mother care diminishes pain from heel lance in very preterm neonates: a crossover trial. BMC Pediatr 2008;8:13.

[52] Kashaninia Z, Sajedi F, Rahgozar M, Noghabi FA. The effect of Kangaroo Care on behavioral responses to pain of an intramuscular injection in neonates. J Spec Pediatr Nurs 2008;13:275–80.

[53] Klein VC, Gaspardo CM, Martinez FE, Grunau RE, Linhares MB. Pain and distress reactivity and recovery as early predictors of temperament in toddlers born preterm. Early Hum Dev 2009;85:569–76.

[54] Kortesluoma RL, Nikkonen M. 'I had this horrible pain': the sources and causes of pain experiences in 4- to 11-year-old hospitalized children. J Child Health Care 2004;8:210–31.

[55] Kostandy RR, Ludington-Hoe SM, Cong X, Abouelfettoh A, Bronson C, Stankus A, Jarrell JR. Kangaroo Care (skin contact) reduces crying response to pain in preterm neonates: pilot results. Pain Manag Nurs 2008;9:55–65.

[56] Lehr VT, Taddio A. Topical anesthesia in neonates: clinical practices and practical considerations. Semin Perinatol 2007;31:323–9.

[57] Lewkowski MD, Barr RG, Sherrard A, Lessard J, Harris AR, Young SN. Effects of chewing gum on responses to routine painful procedures in children. Physiol Behav 2003;79:257–65.

[58] Ludington-Hoe SM, Swinth JY. Developmental aspects of Kangaroo care. J Obstet Gynecol Neonatal Nurs 1996;25:691–703.

[59] Lund I, Yu LC, Uvnas-Moberg K, Wang J, Yu C, Kurosawa M, Agren G, Rosen A, Lekman M, Lundeberg T. Repeated massage-like stimulation induces long-term effects on nociception: contribution of oxytocinergic mechanisms. Eur J Neurosci 2002;16:330–8.

[60] Marin Gabriel MA, Lopez Escobar A, Galan Redondo M, Fernandez Bule I, del Cerro Garcia R, Llana Martin I, de la Cruz Bertolo J, Lora Pablos D. Evaluation of pain in a neonatal intensive care unit during endocrine-metabolic tests. An Pediatr (Barc) 2008;69:316–21.

[61] McMurtry CM, McGrath PJ, Chambers CT. Reassurance can hurt: parental behavior and painful medical procedures. J Pediatr 2006;148:560–61.

[62] Mennella JA, Pepino MY, Lehmann-Castor SM, Yourshaw LM. Sweet preferences and analgesia during childhood: effects of family history of alcoholism and depression. Addiction 2010;105:666–75.

[63] Miller A, Barr RG, Young SN. The cold pressor test in children: methodological aspects and the analgesic effect of intraoral sucrose. Pain 1994;56:175–83.

[64] Mucignat V, Ducrocq S, Lebas F, Mochel F, Baudon JJ, Gold F. [Analgesic effects of EMLA cream and saccharose solution for subcutaneous injections in preterm newborns: a prospective study of 265 injections.] Arch Pediatr 2004;11:921–5.

[65] Murrell D, Gibson PR, Cohen RC. Continuous epidural analgesia in newborn infants undergoing major surgery. J Pediatr Surg 1993;28:548–52; discussion 552–43.

[66] Norberry J. Illicit drugs, their use and the law in Australia. Canberra: Parliament of Australia, Department of the Parliamentary Library; 1996.

[67] Phaire T. The boke of chyldren. Edinburgh: E. & S. Livingstone; 1955. (Reprinted from: The boke of chyldren, 1553).

[68] Razek AA, El-Dein AN. Effect of breast-feeding on pain relief during infant immunization injections. Int J Nurs Pract 2009;15:99–104.

[69] Ren K, Blass EM, Zhou Q, Dubner R. Suckling and sucrose ingestion suppress persistent hyperalgesia and spinal Fos expression after forepaw inflammation in infant rats. Proc Natl Acad Sci USA 1997;94:1471–5.

[70] Rennix C, Manjunatha CM, Ibhanesebhor SE. Pain relief during common neonatal procedures: a survey. Arc Dis Child Fetal Neonatal Ed 2004;89:F563.

[71] Ruston FG. Epidural anaesthesia in infants and children. Can Anaesth Soc J 1954;1:37–44.

[72] Schechter NL, Zempsky WT, Cohen LL, McGrath PJ, McMurtry CM, Bright NS. Pain reduction during pediatric immunizations: evidence-based review and recommendations. Pediatrics 2007;119:e1184–98.

[73] Shah PS, Aliwalas LI, Shah V. Breastfeeding or breast milk for procedural pain in neonates. Cochrane Database Syst Rev 2006;3:CD004950.

[74] Shah V, Ohlsson A. Venepuncture versus heel lance for blood sampling in term neonates. Cochrane Database Syst Rev 2007;4:CD001452.

[75] Shah V, Taddio A, Rieder MJ. Effectiveness and tolerability of pharmacologic and combined interventions for reducing injection pain during routine childhood immunizations: systematic review and meta-analyses. Clin Ther 2009;31(Suppl 2):S104–51.

[76] Shenkman Z, Hoppenstein D, Erez I, Dolfin T, Freud E. Continuous lumbar/thoracic epidural analgesia in low-weight paediatric surgical patients: practical aspects and pitfalls. Pediatr Surg Int 2009;25:623–34.

[77] Simons SHP, Van Dijk M, Anand KS, Roofthooft D, van Lingen RA, Tibboel D. Do we still hurt newborn babies? A prospective study of procedural pain and analgesia in neonates. Arch Pediatr Adolesc Med 2003;157:1058–64.

[78] Sofroniew MV. Morphology of vasopressin and oxytocin neurones and their central and vascular projections. Prog Brain Res 1983;60:101–14.

[79] Stevens B, Yamada J, Beyene J, Gibbins S, Petryshen P, Stinson J, Narciso J. Consistent management of repeated procedural pain with sucrose in preterm neonates: Is it effective and safe for repeated use over time? Clin J Pain 2005;21:543–8.

[80] Stevens B, Yamada J, Ohlsson A. Sucrose for analgesia in newborn infants undergoing painful procedures. Cochrane Database Syst Rev 2010;1:CD001069.

[81] Stevens BJ, Pillai-Ridell RR, Oberlander T, Gibbins S. Assessment of pain in neonates and infants. In: Anand KJS, Stevens BJ, McGrath P, editors. Pain in neonates and infants. Toronto: Elsevier; 2007. p. 67–90.

[82] Stinson J, Yamada J, Dickson A, Lamba J, Stevens B. Review of systematic reviews on acute procedural pain in children in the hospital setting. Pain Res Manag 2008;13:51–7.

[83] Stinson JN, Kavanagh T, Yamada J, Gill N, Stevens B, Stinson JN, Kavanagh T, Yamada J, Gill N, Stevens B. Systematic review of the psychometric properties, interpretability and feasibility of self-report pain intensity measures for use in clinical trials in children and adolescents. Pain 2006;125:143–57.

[84] Sweet SD, McGrath PJ. Relative importance of mothers' versus medical staffs' behavior in the prediction of infant immunization pain behavior. J Pediatr Psychol 1998;23:249–56.

[85] Taddio A. Opioid analgesia for infants in the neonatal intensive care unit. Clin Perinatol 2002;29:493–509.

[86] Taddio A, Manley J, Potash L, Ipp M, Sgro M, Shah V. Routine immunization practices: use of topical anesthetics and oral analgesics. Pediatrics 2007;120:e637–43.

[87] Taddio A, Ohlsson K, Ohlsson A. Lidocaine-prilocaine cream for analgesia during circumcision in newborn boys. Cochrane Database Syst Rev 1999;3:CD000496.

[88] Taylor EM, Boyer K, Campbell FA. Pain in hospitalized children: a prospective cross-sectional survey of pain prevalence, intensity, assessment and management in a Canadian pediatric teaching hospital. Pain Res Manag 2008;13:25–32.

[89] Thorek M. Modern surgical technique, Vol. 111. Montreal: Lippincott; 1938.

[90] Tsao JCI, Evans S, Meldrum M, Altman T, Zeltzer LK. A review of CAM for procedural pain in infancy. Part I. Sucrose and non-nutritive sucking. Evid Based Complement Alternat Med 2008;5:371–81

[91] Uman LS, Chambers CT, McGrath PJ, Kisely S. Psychological interventions for needle-related procedural pain and distress in children and adolescents. Cochrane Database Syst Rev 2006;4:CD005179.

[92] von Baeyer CL, Spagrud LJ. Systematic review of observational (behavioral) measures of pain for children and adolescents aged 3 to 18 years. Pain 2007;127:140–50.

[93] Weissman A, Aranovitch M, Blazer S, Zimmer EZ. Heel-lancing in newborns: behavioral and spectral analysis assessment of pain control methods. Pediatrics 2009;124:e921–6.

[94] Wrzosek T, Hogan ME, Taddio A. Age and efficacy of topical anesthetics. Pediatr Pain Letter 2009;11:8–11.

[95] Yamada J, Stinson J, Lamba J, Dickson A, McGrath PJ, Stevens B. A review of systematic reviews on pain interventions in hospitalized infants. Pain Res Manag 2008;13:413–20.

[96] Zanardo V, Nicolussi S, Carlo G, Marzari F, Faggian D, Favaro F, Plebani M. Beta endorphin concentrations in human milk. J Pediatr Gastroenterol Nutr 2001;33:160–4.

Correspondence to: Denise Harrison, RN, RM, PhD, Centre for Nursing, Hospital for Sick Children, 555 University Avenue, Toronto, ON M5G 1X8, Canada. Email: denise. harrison@utoronto.ca.

Psychological Interventions for Chronic Pediatric Pain

Christiane Hermann, PhD

Department of Clinical Psychology and Psychotherapy, Justus-Liebig University, Giessen, Germany

Chronic Pain in Children: What Is the Scope of the Problem?

Children and adolescents experience pain from a number of different sources. Pediatric pain problems that have been the target of medical or psychological interventions include procedure-related pains (e.g., venipuncture or bone marrow aspiration), disease- or trauma-related chronic pain (e.g., rheumatoid arthritis, cancer, sickle cell anemia, or burns), and recurrent pain of benign origin (e.g., primary headaches or abdominal pain).

Aside from acute pain, recurrent pain without an underlying disease is the most common type of pain during childhood and adolescence. The prevalence of headache, and especially migraine, has been most extensively studied. According to a recent population-based study in 7–14-year-old children and adolescents in Germany, headaches have a 6-month prevalence of 53.2%, with a strong age-related increase [27]. Weekly headache was reported by 6.5% of the participants, with girls older than 11 years being affected significantly more often than boys. According to the International Classification of Headache Disorders-II criteria [13], migraine was diagnosed in 7.5% and tension-type headache in 18.5% of the participants. The observed prevalence for migraine matches well with previously reported rates of 3–10%,

depending on age and sex [34]. In the past decade, a number of well-controlled school- and population-based studies have been conducted in several countries worldwide, suggesting that chronic pain is common and may affect between 25% and 35% of children and adolescents, with a pronounced increase during adolescence [24,44]. The most common chronic pain problems, aside from migraine and tension-type headaches, are recurrent abdominal pain (RAP) and musculoskeletal pain. Chronic pain is associated with reduced quality of life, greater school absenteeism, higher use of medication, and more frequent physician visits [45]. Adolescents with frequent pain are likely to experience greater frustration with school and self-acceptance goals [36]. Such frustration with important individual goals is particularly detrimental to the adolescent's emotional well-being when blaming oneself or others or rumination are the primary coping strategies. Clearly, not all affected children necessarily seek treatment. Among individuals reporting chronic pain, only about 5% have moderate-to-severe pain [24].

Far less is known about the prognosis of chronic pain in children. The few existing prospective studies have mostly focused on childhood headache, abdominal pain, and unspecified musculoskeletal pain. Childhood headache has been found to persist in approximately 40–80% of children and adolescents, with follow-up periods ranging from 1 to 20

Pain 2010—An Updated Review: Refresher Course Syllabus
edited by Jeffrey S. Mogil
IASP Press, Seattle, © 2010

years [e.g., 3,8,31,32]. An impressive 40-year follow-up of Swedish pediatric migraineurs revealed that about 30% of the children continued to experience migraine throughout the 40-year period, about 20% had at least some migraine-free years, and about 45% were migraine-free during the complete follow-up period [2]. Notably, headache diagnosis is not necessarily stable. In one study, when assessed 10 years after their initial assessment between 10 and 14 years of age, about 42% of children and adolescents with migraine had continued to experience migraine, 20% had developed tension-type headache, and 38% were headache-free [41]. At a 5-year follow-up, children with RAP were more likely to have abdominal pain and other somatic symptoms and reported higher levels of functional disability than control children [53,54]. Moreover, pediatric RAP may be a precursor of chronic pain (e.g., irritable bowel syndrome) or other health and emotional problems in adulthood [e.g., refs. 4,22,23,50,53]. In children between the age of 9 and 12 years, nonspecific musculoskeletal pains are reported to persist in about 50% of cases at least for 1 year [39,40].

Taken together, these studies suggest that recurrent pain may persist in a substantial number of children and adolescents well into early adulthood. Consistent with the higher prevalence of chronic pain in women, several studies have confirmed that female sex heightens the risk for persisting pain. Also, similar to adults, there is increasing evidence for the importance of psychosocial variables as risk factors. At least in pediatric headache and RAP sufferers, anxiety and depression predict further ongoing pain [49]. Thus, recurrent pain during childhood may increase the risk of a lifetime of chronic pain, at least in a subgroup of children. From this perspective, the treatment of recurrent pain in children and adolescents is not only important as a primary intervention (at least for some of the children), but may also constitute an important measure of secondary prevention.

Psychological Interventions for Chronic Pediatric Pain and Their Empirical Support

Virtually all psychological interventions for chronic pediatric pain that have been developed over the years were adapted from interventions for pain management in adults. As a consequence, both treatment strategies and treatment components for children with chronic pain are almost identical to those in adults, the main difference being that the materials and the therapist-patient interaction are adjusted for children and adolescents. Given the strong focus on adult pain management, it is perhaps less of a puzzle that rather little is known about parental involvement in treatment.

Most of what we know about the efficacy comes from treatment studies in childhood headache, which probably reflects its high prevalence in youth. Psychological intervention programs typically address children and adolescents between the ages of 8 and 16 years, with very few attempts to treat children below the age of 6–7 years. Consistent with treatment approaches in adults, all available psychological treatments for chronic pediatric pain require the child to engage in active and self-initiated coping attempts. This effort requires an understanding of how one's own thinking and doing influences experienced pain and well-being. Below the age of about 7–8 years, due to their cognitive development, most children are not capable of doing this. During this stage, children focus on specific and concrete situations and have only a rudimentary understanding of body functions. They cannot flexibly shift between perspectives or change the focus of their attention, and they find it difficult to distinguish between one's own and others' perspective and feelings. Most importantly, they have a limited understanding of causality, and they experience pain primarily as a phenomenon caused by some external event. Hence, below the age of about 7–8 years, children have a limited ability to be self-reliant and to engage, on their own, in cognitive or behavioral strategies to cope with ongoing pain or prevent pain episodes. Interestingly, while a number of interventions for procedural pain are available for these younger children [16], interventions specifically targeting recurrent pain in this age group have not been systematically evaluated. In general, little is known about the occurrence of recurrent pain without an underlying organic disease in these young children.

Psychological treatments for chronic pediatric pain were first developed in the late 1980s. Consistent with psychosocial pain treatments for adult pain patients, psychological treatments for children and adolescents with chronic pain entail behavioral, cognitive, and cognitive-behavioral therapy (CBT) interventions. Specifically, relaxation training, biofeedback, and cognitive techniques have most often been empirically evaluated. In addition, parent training based on the operant model of chronic pain is available.

Relaxation

Progressive muscle relaxation (PMR) is one of the most frequently used relaxation techniques for pediatric pain, either as single intervention or as part of a comprehensive CBT treatment program. Typically, relaxation training comprises 8 to 10 sessions led by a trained therapist on an individual basis or in groups of 3 to 5 children. Based on Öst's concept of applied relaxation [42], children learn to use PMR when experiencing stress or pain. Children are first taught to progressively relax, and then practice cue-controlled and differential relaxation so they can readily use these relaxation techniques in their everyday life. At least for recurrent migraine and tension-type headache, there is robust evidence for the efficacy of PMR, even when used as single intervention (e.g., refs. [18,43]). Relaxation can also be taught in a self-help format. Children and adolescents receive relaxation tapes and information materials with no or minimal contact with a therapist. When offered in a school setting, self-help relaxation has been shown to be effective [30]. However, when headaches are frequent, therapist-guided relaxation training is superior to self-help relaxation.

Biofeedback

Biofeedback (BFB) has been studied almost exclusively as a treatment for recurrent headache. For both migraine and tension-type headache, electromyographic (EMG)-BFB from the frontalis muscle has been shown to be effective (e.g., refs. [20,43]). EMG-BFB is usually taught as BFB-assisted relaxation. During 8 to 10 sessions, children learn to reduce muscle activity as a means to induce a state of relaxation. During a session, children typically receive visual or auditory feedback of the EMG activity for 15–20 minutes and are encouraged to try out different mental strategies to reduce muscular activity. EMG-BFB is often combined with PMR in order to facilitate the transfer of the relaxation response acquired in the session into the child's daily life.

For migraine, various BFB modalities are available, all of which were designed to modify the presumed underlying pathophysiological processes. Thermal BFB ("hand warming") is supposed to reduce autonomic hyperarousal by voluntarily inducing peripheral vasodilatation and is used to prevent migraine attacks from occurring. By contrast, vasoconstriction training (i.e., learned voluntary constriction of extracranial blood vessels) was developed as a

BFB technique that may abort a migraine when the first signs of an attack are noticed. Based on the notion that migraine is associated with cortical hyperexcitability, a specific form of electroencephalography (EEG)-BFB has been developed. Specifically, children learn to reduce the contingent negative variation (CNV), a slow cortical potential that, interictally, is enhanced in migraine. The effectiveness of thermal BFB alone in the treatment of pediatric migraine has been demonstrated in several randomized controlled trials (RCTs) [20,43], and there is initial evidence from an RCT for its efficacy when combined with a high-fiber diet in the treatment of RAP [26]. Because vasoconstriction training for migraine has only been offered in combination with CBT, its specific efficacy has yet to be demonstrated. CNV-BFB seems to be more effective compared to a waiting-list control [48], but thus far no RCT is available. Also, different BFB modalities have not been evaluated against each other.

While BFB is undoubtedly effective in the treatment of chronic pediatric pain (at least for headaches), the mediating mechanisms have yet to be identified. Consistent with the original rationale, the effectiveness of BFB has been attributed to learned control of dysregulated physiological processes (e.g., elevated muscle tension). However, there is little empirical support for this contention. For example, several studies failed to observe a close correlation between treatment success and learned physiological control. In adults, BFB has been associated with increased self-efficacy or reduced pain catastrophizing, suggesting cognitive mediation of BFB (e.g., ref. [7]). In children and adolescents, this hypothesis has not yet been tested. In the past few years, surprisingly few studies have been published on BFB, despite its well-documented efficacy, at least in the treatment of recurrent childhood headache.

Cognitive-Behavioral Treatment

In the past 15 years, CBT has increasingly been the treatment of choice for chronic pediatric pain. This development is illustrated by the increasing number of RCTs that have evaluated CBT not only for the treatment of recurrent headache, but also for abdominal pain or fibromyalgia (for reviews see refs. [6,43]). CBT treatment packages for chronic pediatric pain are highly similar to adult programs. They typically comprise four major components: (1) education about the pain (e.g., migraine); (2) learning of cognitive and behavioral pain coping skills such as imagery, thought stopping, distraction, focused attention, and relaxation; (3) stress management, i.e., identifying and coping with stressful situations using strategies such as thought stopping, cognitive restructuring ("helpful thoughts"), assertiveness, and problem solving; and (4) relapse prevention. CBT for pediatric pain has been provided individually or in groups, and it typically entails 8 to 10 sessions. Recently, a CBT program specifically tailored for adolescents with pain and depressive symptoms was presented with the specific aim of improving functioning at school [35]. As substantiated by various systematic reviews and a recent meta-analysis [43], CBT is efficacious for reducing pain activity in different chronic pediatric pain conditions.

In adults, CBT approaches to the treatment of chronic pain in adults increasingly take into account recent CBT developments, in particular acceptance and commitment therapy (ACT; ref. [12]). According to the theory behind ACT, experiential avoidance is a core problem in emotional disorders (and chronic pain), leading to disability and reduced quality of life. This experiential avoidance is a result of maladaptive cognitions and feelings being treated as reality and acted upon (denoted as "cognitive fusion"). Exposure to avoided situations and activities is a core intervention, with the focus on the acceptance of negative responses (thoughts, emotions, and body sensations such as pain) rather than on changing or controlling them. In addition, engagement in personally meaningful activities is promoted; that is, it is a goal to increase patients' flexibility so that they pursue personally meaningful values despite interfering cognitions, feelings, and body symptoms. A recent RCT by Wicksell and colleagues [55] in children and adolescents between the ages of 10 to 18 years who had various chronic pain conditions (headache, back or neck pain, widespread musculoskeletal pain, complex regional pain syndrome [CRPS], or visceral pain) demonstrated that a series of approximately 10 ACT sessions (range: 7 to 20 sessions; $N = 16$ patients) was superior to a multidisciplinary pain management program combined with antidepressant medication ($N = 16$ patients) with regard to improvements in functional disability, pain intensity, pain-related distress, fear of injury or re-injury, pain-related interference, and quality of life at post-treatment and at follow-ups at 3.5 and 6 months. Unlike in previous RCT studies, the patients in the Wicksell et al. [55] study had different chronic pain syndromes, varied greatly with regard to age, and were severely impaired. Moreover,

the multidisciplinary pain management program did not entail a specified treatment package; rather, individuals received treatment based on perceived individual needs. Whether ACT may indeed have additional benefits above and beyond CBT (alone or as part of a multidisciplinary program) or other single psychological interventions in children and adolescents, especially if they are less severely affected, remains to be demonstrated. Clearly, ACT seems promising in the treatment of youth severely affected by pain.

Role of Parents and Parent Training

The operant model of chronic pain postulates that chronic pain is maintained by operant reinforcement of pain behaviors such as verbal and nonverbal expressions of pain, guarding, limping, resting and reduced activity. In children, interventions to modify (pain) behavior based on the operant model have mostly been used as an additive to CBT or biofeedback protocols. Sanders et al. [46] was one of the first to demonstrate that six sessions of family CBT significantly improved pain activity in children with recurrent RAP. Operant treatment is typically provided as brief parent training (1–3 sessions) as part of a more comprehensive CBT program. Parents are taught principles of contingency management with the aim of minimizing positively reinforcing responses (e.g., paying attention) or negatively reinforcing responses (e.g., excuse from daily chores) to the child's pain behaviors. Moreover, parents learn to support and encourage their children in practicing and using pain coping skills and maintaining normal daily activities during pain episodes. Overall, surprisingly little is known about the differential contribution of parent training when provided in combination with CBT or BFB. For example, parent training as an adjunct to BFB has been found to enhance treatment success in some studies [1], but not in others [28]. While there is consensus that a child's experience of pain is modulated by social context, it is less clear which pain-related parental behaviors are adaptive and which are not. One obstacle for determining the differential impact of parental behavior has been a lack of assessment tools. Only recently have questionnaires been developed to assess pain-related parent behavior, including Adult Responses to Children's Symptoms (ARCS) (parent version) [52]; The Inventory of Parent/Caregiver Responses to the Children's Pain Experience (IRPEDNA) (parent version only) [25]; and the Pain-Related Parent Behavior Inventory (PPBI) (child and parent version) [19]. Thus far, the findings of studies evaluating the impact of parent training are difficult to interpret because, due to the lack of available instruments, the investigators did not systematically assess exactly which parental behaviors were related to the child's pain activity prior to treatment, which behaviors were changed by treatment, and how altered parent behavior may have mediated the child's clinical improvement. Nonetheless, on an individual basis, a fine-grained behavioral analysis based on the operant model is helpful for understanding how parental behavior may reinforce the child's pain and contribute to pain maintenance and pain-related disability.

Even in cases when operant processes may not be considered as primarily relevant, it is important to involve parents in their child's treatment. First, parents should be educated about their child's pain, which will help them not to engage in excessive catastrophizing. As Vervoort, Goubert, and colleagues have shown in several studies (e.g., ref. [10]), parental pain catastrophizing influences how much pain parents perceive their child is having, which eventually will determine the parents' response to the pain [9]. Second, especially in younger children, parents should learn about what the child is taught in order to be able to encourage and prompt the child to use the coping strategies, given that in younger children self-regulatory skills are still developing.

Are Psychological Interventions for Chronic Pediatric Pain Effective?

As outlined above, relaxation, BFB, and CBT are efficacious, at least for the treatment of recurrent headache [43]. However, several questions remain. First, the differential efficacy of the various psychological interventions when compared to each other or to pharmacological interventions remains to be determined. Thus far, direct comparisons between treatments are scarce. Second, the long-term outcome (>6 months) of such psychological pain management has been evaluated in very few studies. If psychological interventions for pediatric pain do have long-term effectiveness, they may indeed hold promise as a measure of secondary prevention. Third, traditionally, pain management programs have aimed at reducing pain activity (i.e., frequency and/or intensity and/or duration). Accordingly, it is mostly the change in pain activity that has been used as the primary and only outcome measure, with little attention to disability, other somatic complaints, coping efforts,

and emotional and social adjustment. A recent meta-analysis of RCTs revealed that psychological interventions have led to substantial improvement in pain activity, whereas disability and emotional functioning have shown little change (when they were assessed in the respective studies). To some extent, this finding may reflect that these outcome measures were only assessed in a few studies. It may also reflect that children and adolescents participating in RCTs evaluating outpatient pain management trainings may experience low-to-moderate levels of disability and emotional distress. For example, Eccleston et al. [5] reported that, after participating in an interdisciplinary pain management program for adolescents with longstanding chronic pain that included physical, occupational, and cognitive therapy as well as pain education, adolescents with chronic pain reported significantly less disability, lower levels of anxiety and somatic awareness, and better physical functioning. Taken together, psychological interventions should be considered a core intervention for management of chronic pediatric pain of benign origin.

Current Developments

Having established a number of more or less simple psychological interventions that are effective for reducing recurrent pediatric pain, research has increasingly focused on systematically evaluating more complex treatment packages and different and potentially more efficient formats of treatment delivery.

Multimodal Treatments

Multimodal and multidisciplinary inpatient and outpatient treatment programs are increasingly available for children and adolescents. In most programs, participants receive medical treatment, psychological interventions, and physical therapy. Some programs entail additional services such as occupational therapy, consultations by social workers, and schooling by teachers in the clinic. For example, programs for children with CRPS in Philadelphia [47] and Boston [33], with a heavy focus on physiotherapy, have reported excellent outcomes. Inpatient interdisciplinary pain management programs for children and adolescents are also established in Germany (Vodafone Stiftungsinstitut für Kinderschmerztherapie und Palliativmedizin, Datteln) and the United Kingdom (Bath Pain Management Program). Both of these programs offer treatment for children with chronic headaches, musculoskeletal pain, fibromyalgia, CRPS, and rheumatic diseases. Both programs are effective in reducing pain activity, functional disability, affective distress, and parental distress and yield impressive return-to-school rates, both in children [14] and adolescents [5,15].

Self-Help and Internet-Based Treatments

There have been efforts to develop treatment formats with minimal therapist contact ("home-based treatment") or self-help programs. For example, McGrath and colleagues published a self-help booklet for pediatric migraine in 1990, which proved to be just as successful as therapist-administered treatment [37,38]. Consistent with this observation, home-based thermal BFB led to improvements in headache activity in children with migraine that did not significantly differ from those of clinic-based thermal BFB [11,17], although the intervention had lower success rates than some of the earlier studies reporting success rates of up to 90–100% [29]. Home-based thermal BFB entailed four clinic sessions with a therapist, a manual for four sessions at home, and a portable temperature device for practicing the acquired hand-warming skills at home.

Today, self-help programs are increasingly offered as Internet-based CBT programs. Hicks et al. [21] were the first to report that about 70% of children (aged 9–16 years) who had recurrent pain (mostly headache and abdominal pain) showed at least a 50% reduction of pain after completing the program. This self-help program comprises a total of seven weekly modules, which are equivalent to McGrath and colleagues' self-help booklet. The contents include education about headache and stomachaches, self-monitoring, various relaxation techniques (deep breathing, PMR, and imagery), physical pain management methods, the tension-pain vicious cycle, changing dysfunctional thoughts, social and physical activities, self-management of pain episodes, managing pain at school, and maintaining treatment gains. Similarly, an Internet-delivered family CBT (i.e., CBT including parent training) significantly reduced pain activity and pain-related disability in adolescents with various recurrent pains (e.g., headache, abdominal pain, and leg pain) [43]. Children and their parents accessed two separate websites and were required to complete one module and one assignment per week (duration: 30 minutes) for 8 weeks. Assignments were handed in and were commented on by a therapist. The children's

modules were: (1) education, (2) recognizing stress, (3) deep breathing and relaxation, (4) distraction, (5) cognitions, (6) sleep, (7) activities, and (8) relapse prevention. The parents' modules were: (1) education, (2) recognizing stress and negative emotions, (3 and 4) operant strategies, (5) modeling, (6) sleep hygiene, (7) communication, and (8) relapse prevention. Interestingly, parental solicitousness diminished from pre- to post-treatment in both groups; that is, no treatment-specific change was observed. Since little is known about the stability of parent behavior, this finding is difficult to interpret. Both the Hicks et al. [21] and the Palermo et al. [43] studies compared Internet-based CBT to a wait list control, and hence these findings essentially replicate the efficacy of self-help CBT. As stated earlier, there is a dearth of studies comparing efficacious psychological interventions. Gassmann et al. [51] conducted an RCT comparing Internet-based CBT (with weekly email support by a therapist), self-help applied relaxation, and an attention placebo (pain education and regular e-mail contacts with a therapist) in children and adolescents with recurrent headache. CBT was superior to applied relaxation and an attention placebo post-treatment. However, at 6-month follow-up, responder rates were not significantly different (CBT: 63%, relaxation: 56%, placebo: 55%). These findings highlight that it is far from clear whether there is indeed differential efficacy of psychological interventions. The study also underlines the need for long-term follow-ups. The observed success rate in the attention placebo group may be due to an actual placebo effect; it may also reflect the natural course of recurrent headaches in youth. Unlike in adult chronic pain patients, recurrent pain in children does not necessarily persist over a longer period of time, even when untreated.

Perspective

A sizable number of children and adolescents are affected by recurrent pains, mostly headache, abdominal pain, and musculoskeletal pain. Fortunately, in most of these children, pain and pain-related interference is not severe. Nonetheless, recurrent pain in childhood bears a substantial risk for persistence into adulthood. Several efficacious psychological interventions for chronic pediatric pain are available. Aside from determining what works best for which type of pediatric pain problem, at what age, and for whom, the greatest challenge is to make such treatments available for those who need it. Given that the greatest barrier for psychological interventions for pediatric pain is their availability in a given health care system, Internet-based programs are particularly promising.

References

[1] Allen KD, Shriver MD. Role of parent-mediated pain behavior management strategies in biofeedback treatment of childhood migraines. Behav Ther 1998;29:477–90.

[2] Bille B. A 40-year follow-up of school children with migraine. Cephalalgia 1997;17:488–91.

[3] Brna P, Dooley J, Gordon K, Dewan T. The prognosis of childhood headache: a 20-year follow-up. Arch Pediatr Adolesc Med 2005;159:1157–60.

[4] Campo JV, Di LC, Chiappetta L, Bridge J, Colborn DK, Gartner JC, Jr., Gaffney P, Kocoshis S, Brent D. Adult outcomes of pediatric recurrent abdominal pain: do they just grow out of it? Pediatrics 2001;108:E1.

[5] Eccleston C, Malleson PN, Clinch J, Connell H, Sourbut C. Chronic pain in adolescents: evaluation of a programme of interdisciplinary cognitive behaviour therapy. Arch Dis Child 2003;88:881–5.

[6] Eccleston C, Yorke L, Morley S, Williams AC, Mastroyannopoulou K. Psychological therapies for the management of chronic and recurrent pain in children and adolescents. Cochrane Database Syst Rev 2003;CD003968.

[7] Flor H, Birbaumer N. Comparison of the efficacy of electromyographic biofeedback, cognitive-behavioral therapy, and conservative medical interventions in the treatment of chronic musculoskeletal pain. J Consult Clin Psychol 1993;61:653–8.

[8] Gassmann J, Morris L, Heinrich M, Kröner-Herwig B. One-year course of paediatric headache in children and adolescents aged 8-15 years. Cephalalgia 2008;28:1154–62.

[9] Goubert L, Craig KD, Vervoort T, Morley S, Sullivan MJ, de CWA, Cano A, Crombez G. Facing others in pain: the effects of empathy. Pain 2005;118:285–8.

[10] Goubert L, Vervoort T, Sullivan MJ, Verhoeven K, Crombez G. Parental emotional responses to their child's pain: the role of dispositional empathy and catastrophizing about their child's pain. J Pain 2008;9:272–9.

[11] Guarnieri P, Blanchard EB. Evaluation of home-based thermal biofeedback treatment of pediatric migraine headache. Biofeedback Self Regul 1990;15:179–84.

[12] Hayes SC, Luoma JB, Bond FW, Masuda A, Lillis J. Acceptance and commitment therapy: model, processes and outcomes. Behav Res Ther 2006;44:1–25.

[13] Headache Classification Subcommittee of the International Headache Society. The International Classification of Headache Disorders, 2nd edition. Cephalalgia 2004;24:9–160.

[14] Hechler T, Blankenburg M, Dobe M, Kosfelder J, Hübner B, Zernikow B. Effectiveness of a multimodal inpatient treatment for pediatric chronic pain: a comparison between children and adolescents. Eur J Pain 2010;14:97.e1–9.

[15] Hechler T, Dobe M, Kosfelder J, Damschen U, Hubner B, Blankenburg M, Sauer C, Zernikow B. Effectiveness of a 3-week multimodal inpatient pain treatment for adolescents suffering from chronic pain: statistical and clinical significance. Clin J Pain 2009;25:156–66.

[16] Hermann C. Psychological treatment of pain in children. In: Schmidt RF, Willis W, editors. Encyclopedic reference of pain. Berlin: Springer; 2007. p. 2037–9.

[17] Hermann C, Blanchard EB, Flor H. Biofeedback treatment for pediatric migraine: prediction of treatment outcome. J Consult Clin Psychol 1997;85:611–6.

[18] Hermann C, Kim M, Blanchard EB. Behavioral and prophylactic pharmacological intervention studies of pediatric migraine: an exploratory meta-analysis. Pain 1995;60:239–56.

[19] Hermann C, Zohsel K, Hohmeister J, Flor H. Dimensions of pain-related parent behavior: Development and psychometric evaluation of a new measure for children and their parents. Pain 2008;137:689–99.

[20] Hermann C, Blanchard EB. Biofeedback in the treatment of headache and other childhood pain. Appl Psychophysiol Biofeedback 2002;27:143–62.

[21] Hicks CL, Von Baeyer CL, McGrath PJ. Online psychological treatment for pediatric recurrent pain: a randomized evaluation. J Pediatr Psychol 2006;31:724–36.

[22] Hotopf M, Carr S, Mayou R, Wadsworth M, Wessely S. Why do children have chronic abdominal pain, and what happens to them when they grow up? Population-based cohort study. BMJ 1998;316:1196–200.

[23] Howell S, Poulton R, Talley NJ. The natural history of childhood abdominal pain and its association with adult irritable bowel syndrome: birth-cohort study. Am J Gastroenterol 2005;100:2071–8.

[24] Huguet A, Miro J. The severity of chronic pediatric pain: an epidemiological study. J Pain 2008;9:226–36.

[25] Huguet A, Miro J, Nieto R. The Inventory of Parent/Caregiver Responses to the Children's Pain Experience (IRPEDNA): development and preliminary validation. Pain 2008;134:128–39.

[26] Humphreys PA, Gevirtz RN. Treatment of recurrent abdominal pain: components analysis of four treatment protocols. J Pediatr Gastr Nutr 2000;31:47–51.

[27] Kröner-Herwig B, Heinrich M, Morris L. Headache in German children and adolescents: a population-based epidemiological study. Cephalalgia 2007;27:519–27.

[28] Kröner-Herwig B, Mohn U, Pothmann R. Comparison of biofeedback and relaxation in the treatment of pediatric headache and the influence of parent involvement on outcome. Appl Psychophysiol Biofeedback 1998;23:143–57.

[29] Labbé EE, Williamson DA. Treatment of childhood migraine using autogenic feedback training. J Consult Clin Psychol 1984;52:968–76.

[30] Larsson B, Carlsson J, Fichtel A, Melin L. Relaxation treatment of adolescent headache sufferers: results from a school-based replication series. Headache 2005;45:692–704.

[31] Larsson B, Sund AM. One-year incidence, course, and outcome predictors of frequent headaches among early adolescents. Headache 2005;45:684–91.

[32] Laurell K, Larsson B, Mattsson P, Eeg-Olofsson O. A 3-year follow-up of headache diagnoses and symptoms in Swedish schoolchildren. Cephalalgia 2006;26:809–15.

[33] Lee BH, Scharff L, Sethna NF, McCarthy CF, Scott-Sutherland J, Shea AM, Sullivan P, Meier P, Zurakowski D, Masek BJ, Berde CB. Physical therapy and cognitive-behavioral treatment for complex regional pain syndromes. J Pediatr 2002;141:135–40.

[34] Linet MS, Stewart WF, Celentano DD, Ziegler D, Sprecher M. An epidemiologic study of headache among adolescents and young adults. JAMA 1989;261:2211–6.

[35] Logan DE, Simons LE. Development of a group intervention to improve school functioning in adolescents with chronic pain and depressive symptoms: a study of feasibility and preliminary efficacy. J Pediatr Psychol 2010; Epub Feb 18.

[36] Massey EK, Garnefski N, Gebhardt WA. Goal frustration, coping and well-being in the context of adolescent headache: a self-regulation approach. Eur J Pain 2009;13:977–84.

[37] McGrath PJ, Cunningham SJ, Lascelles MA, Humphreys P. Help yourself: a treatment for migraine headaches. Ottawa: University of Ottawa Press; 1990.

[38] McGrath PJ, Humphreys P, Keene D, Goodman JT, Lascelles MA, Cunningham SJ, Firestone P. The efficacy and efficiency of a self-administered treatment for adolescent migraine. Pain 1992;49:321–4.

[39] Mikkelsson M, Salminen JJ, Kautiainen H. Non-specific musculoskeletal pain in preadolescents. Prevalence and 1-year persistence. Pain 1997;73:29–35.

[40] Mikkelsson M, Salminen JJ, Sourander A, Kautiainen H. Contributing factors to the persistence of musculoskeletal pain in preadolescents: a prospective 1-year follow-up study. Pain 1998;77:67–72.

[41] Monastero R, Camarda C, Pipia C, Camarda R. Prognosis of migraine headaches in adolescents: a 10-year follow-up study. Neurology 2006;67:1353–6.

[42] Öst LG. Applied relaxation: description of a coping technique and review of controlled studies. Behav Res Ther 1987;25:397–409.

[43] Palermo TM, Eccleston C, Lewandowski AS, Williams ACDC, Morley S. Randomized controlled trials of psychological therapies for management of chronic pain in children and adolescents: an updated meta-analytic review. Pain 2010;148:387–97.

[44] Perquin CW, Hazebroek-Kampschreur AA, Hunfeld JA, Bohnen AM, Suijlekom-Smit LW, Passchier J, van der Wouden JC. Pain in children and adolescents: a common experience. Pain 2000;87:51–8.

[45] Perquin CW, Hazebroek-Kampschreur AA, Hunfeld JA, van Suijlekom-Smit LW, Passchier J, van der Wouden JC. Chronic pain among children and adolescents: physician consultation and medication use. Clin J Pain 2000;16:229–35.

[46] Sanders MR, Shepherd RW, Cleghorn G, Woolford H. The treatment of recurrent abdominal pain in children: a controlled comparison of cognitive-behavioral family intervention and standard pediatric care. J Consult Clin Psychol 1994;62:306–14.

[47] Sherry DD, Wallace CA, Kelley C, Kidder M, Sapp L. Short- and long-term outcomes of children with complex regional pain syndrome type I treated with exercise therapy. Clin J Pain 1999;15:218–23.

[48] Siniatchkin M, Hierundar A, Kropp P, Kuhnert R, Gerber W-D, Stephani U. Self-regulation of slow cortical potentials in children with migraine: An exploratory study. Appl Psychophysiol Biofeedback 2000;25:13–32.

[49] Stanford EA, Chambers CT, Biesanz JC, Chen E. The frequency, trajectories and predictors of adolescent recurrent pain: a population-based approach. Pain 2008;138:11–21.

[50] Stordal K, Nygaard EA, Bentsen BS. Recurrent abdominal pain: a five-year follow-up study. Acta Paediatr 2005;94:234–6.

[51] Trautmann E, Kröner-Herwig B. A randomized controlled trial of Internet-based self-help training for recurrent headache in childhood and adolescence. Behav Res Ther 2010;48:28–37.

[52] Van Slyke DA, Walker LS. Mothers' responses to children's pain. Clin J Pain 2006;22:387–91.

[53] Walker LS, Garber J, Van Slyke DA, Greene JW. Long-term health outcomes in patients with recurrent abdominal pain. J Pediatr Psychol 1995;20:233–45.

[54] Walker LS, Guite JW, Duke M, Barnard JA, Greene JW. Recurrent abdominal pain: a potential precursor of irritable bowel syndrome in adolescents and young adults. J Pediatr 1998;132:1010–5.

[55] Wicksell RK, Melin L, Lekander M, Olsson GL. Evaluating the effectiveness of exposure and acceptance strategies to improve functioning and quality of life in longstanding pediatric pain: a randomized controlled trial. Pain 2009;141:248–57.

Correspondence to: Christiane Hermann, PhD, Department of Clinical Psychology and Psychotherapy, Justus-Liebig-University Giessen, Otto-Behaghel-Str. 10F, D-35394 Giessen, Germany. Email: christiane.hermann@psychol.uni-giessen.de.

Part 18
Preclinical and Clinical Challenges in Drug Development

Overview of the Drug Development Process and Regulatory Approval for New Drugs

Steve Quessy, PhD

qd consulting, LLC, Durham, North Carolina, USA

Background

The process of drug discovery through approval and delivery of safe, effective, and useful medicines to society relies on a partnership between the pharmaceutical industry, public health authorities, regulatory agencies and national health services, the medical profession and caregiver groups, pharmacists, patients, and society as a whole. There are natural tensions amongst the stakeholders in these groups, not the least of which concern intellectual property, the approval process itself, risk/benefit assessment for both intended and unintended populations, cost effectiveness, promotional claims, and access.

The development of new drugs and the process leading to approval for marketing are complex, expensive, time-consuming, and subject to intense regulatory controls. An approved product is the culmination of a long and risky road that begins with drug discovery (see Fig. 1). Failure and attrition at all stages along the road are the norm rather than the exception [3] (see Figs. 2, 3). It is estimated that for every 5,000 to 10,000 potential new medicines identified by drug discovery groups, only about 250 (2.5–5%) reach extensive testing in animals, about 5 (1%) reach clinical testing in humans, and only 1 becomes an approved medicine [4]. This process can span 15 years and require substantial investment. The average research and development cost per approved medicine is estimated at US$800 million (€1,300 million), and the major proportion of this investment is incurred at later stages of development [1–4].

The purpose of this chapter is to provide a brief overview of the typical process and decision points of drug development from drug discovery to approval and introduction of a new medicine, including the major regulatory controls and types of documentation and the agencies involved in this process. The development of a new analgesic closely follows the scheme shown in Fig. 1. The illustrations presented here highlight those that relate to U.S. and European processes (through the International Conference on Harmonization; ICH). Japan is also a signatory to the agreements of ICH, and many other countries have adopted the same principles of controls and standards embodied in ICH. A primer of the various acronyms used, along with definitions of the functions of institutions and documents referred to in this overview, is provided in Table I.

Drug Discovery and Development

Drug Discovery

Drug discovery involves the application of scientific and medical basic research to identify targets for specific diseases and to identify molecules that interact with these targets in an appropriate way. Once a lead compound is identified, there is a considerable optimization effort to refine structures to balance the best chance for "on-target" selectivity and activity and improvement over other therapies. This stage is systematic, high-tech, and often highly automated, but low-yield.

Candidate Selection

One or more lead compounds are explored in more extensive in vitro and in vivo preclinical testing against a comprehensive set of developability criteria (e.g., cost/ease of synthesis in pure form, pharmacokinetic profile, options for a dose form, primary and secondary pharmacology, and toxicology profile). This stage is highly experience- and information-based, with considerable modeling against reference compounds to predict performance in humans and select out compounds that are unlikely to have the desired characteristics. It may take several cycles through drug discovery to arrive at a suitable drug candidate.

Clinical Development

The designation of clinical development into phases is somewhat arbitrary but is used ubiquitously. The terminology can be confusing without qualification, because a given drug can be in more than one phase simultaneously, and the number and timing of actual trials conducted within each phase can vary. For example: a drug in Phase 3 for one indication may enter Phase 2 for a different indication; a drug completing Phase 2 may undergo Phase 1 trials for a new formulation that is hoped to be the one brought to market or for a definitive QTc (the heart rate-corrected QT interval evaluation on the electrocardiogram); an oral drug in Phase 2 or III may be being investigated in Phase 1 for a different route of administration. However, it is generally accepted that a new medicine will progress through these three phases before gaining approval.

Phase 1

Phase 1 can usually be described as safety testing in healthy human subjects (some drugs or routes of administrations are tested in the target patient population if the risk to healthy volunteers is considered too great). This applies to a new chemical entity, a new salt or form of an existing drug, a new dose formulation, or a new route of administration. The objectives in Phase 1 are to establish a safe dose range for testing in patients, to study the pharmacokinetics of the drug and its metabolites in humans, to evaluate relevant biomarker or pharmacodynamic endpoints where possible, and to perform special safety evaluations (such as drug interactions, QTc safety, and elderly and pediatric safety). It is usual to begin with single-dose evaluations in a small number of subjects and progress to repeat dosing for 1–2 weeks. Phase 1 studies are conducted in a very controlled environment,

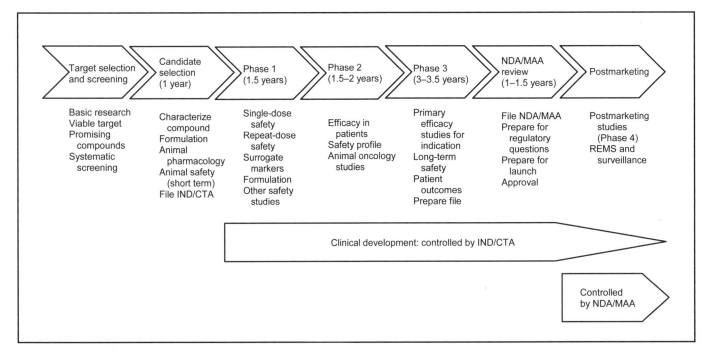

Fig. 1. Schematic describing the various stages for typical drug development. See Table I for abbreviations.

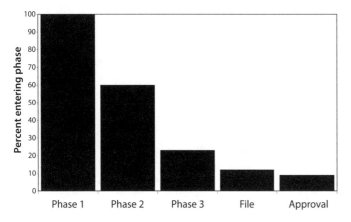

Fig. 2. Attrition rates by development phase for drugs entering Phase 1 during the period 1991–2000. Adapted from Kola and Landis [3].

with intense monitoring for safety, and usually on an inpatient basis. Individual studies rarely expose more than 12–30 subjects, and crossover designs are common. In addition to assessing safety, many of the objectives in Phase 1 have added value in improving the ability to design scientifically valid experiments to test efficacy in Phase 2.

Phase 2

Phase 2 can be described as investigating whether a desired level of efficacy for a new drug (or formulation or route of administration) can be achieved with an acceptable level of tolerability in patients with a disease relevant to the target indication. The objectives in Phase 2 are to decide whether the drug profile warrants further investigation, based on medical need and competitive standing against alternative treatments, and to establish a suitable dose range for Phase 3 study. The size of Phase 2 trials can vary considerably depending on the objectives and design of the trial. In some cases the first Phase 2 trial (often labeled Phase 2a) might be a small, short-term "proof-of-concept" trial to determine if it is worth pursuing further clinical study, followed in series by a larger Phase 2 trial (Phase 2b). Phase 2 may involve exposure of several hundred patients for a given indication for periods of usually less than 6 weeks. Recent design tendencies toward greater statistical power and multiple doses means that it is not uncommon for many analgesic Phase 2 trials to involve 200–300 patients in studies of 4 weeks' duration or longer. The subjects in Phase 2 trials are carefully selected for safety reasons, and although most Phase 2 trials are conducted on an outpatient basis, there are frequent clinic visits for monitoring progress.

Phase 3

Phase 3 can be described as confirming safety and efficacy projections from Phase 2, and evaluating long-term effects of the drug. In general it is trials from Phase 3 that form the clinical basis for regulatory approval in an indication (so-called "pivotal trials"), and thus the primary objective of Phase 3 is to generate the necessary efficacy and safety data to support the dossier that is submitted for review by regulatory agencies to gain marketing authorization. Phase 3 studies can be numerous, very large, and of long duration. Phase 3 trials may expose several thousand patients, depending on the number of doses planned and the scope of the indication sought (examples of the safety exposure data in initial dossiers: celecoxib >6,000 patients, rofecoxib >5,000 patients, pregabalin >9,000 patients). For an analgesic aimed at indications in chronic pain, study durations of 12 weeks to 6 months may be required for demonstration of efficacy. In line with ICH guidance on the requirements for demonstration of safety, it is usually necessary to run long-term safety trials with cumulative exposure in patients for a year or more, such that the dossier can report on safety in at least 300 patients for 6 months or more, and 100 patients for 12 months or more, at the highest dose to be recommended for marketing. The patient population studied in Phase 3 should match the target population for intended use as closely as possible. The data generated in Phase 3 very much shape the clinical sections of approved labels (U.S. package insert and European summary of product characteristics). There is an increasing tendency to

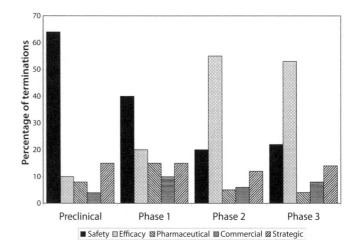

Fig. 3. Reasons for development termination by development phase. Adapted from an European Federation of Pharmaceutical Industries and Associations workshop, Nov. 27, 2009.

Table I
A primer of common terms and definitions

Acronym	Definition	Brief Description
AARP	Anesthesia, Analgesia and Rheumatology Products	FDA division of the Center for Drug Evaluation and Research that reviews most analgesic NDAs.
API	Active Pharmaceutical Ingredient	ICH term for drug substance.
CHMP	Committee for Medicinal Products for Human Use	Group within the EMEA that reviews applications for medicinal products.
CFR	U.S. Code of Federal Regulations	In particular, Title 21 includes regulations governing food and drugs.
CTA	Clinical Trials Application	A request made to a "Competent National Authority" for authorization to conduct a clinical trial of a medicinal product for human use in a specific European member state. A CTA is required for each trial and each country in which a trial is planned (no centralized process for multi-country protocols). Similar submissions and dossiers are required in other countries that support investigational clinical trials.
EC	European Commission	The body with authority for the licensing of products in Europe. Issues EPAR.
EFPIA	European Federation of Pharmaceutical Industries and Associations	European industry association. Website: www.efpia.org.
EMEA	European Medicines Agency	European agency responsible for assessing marketing applications. Website: www.ema.europa.eu.
EPAR	European Public Assessment Report	Public report on the basis of approvals, issued by the European Commission.
FDA	U.S. Food and Drug Administration	The agency of the U.S. Government authorized to approve and license medicines. Website: www.fda.gov.
GCP	Good clinical practice	A standard for the design, conduct, performance, monitoring, auditing, recording, analysis, and reporting of clinical trials, providing assurance that reported data are credible and accurate, and that the rights and confidentiality of trial subjects are protected. Website: www.fda.gov.
IB	Investigators brochure	A compilation of the clinical and nonclinical data on the investigational product that is relevant to the study of the product in human subjects.
ICH	International Committee on Harmonization of Technical Requirements for Registration of Pharmaceuticals for Human Use	Organization that includes regulatory and industry authorities from Europe, Japan, and the United States to harmonize the interpretation and application of technical guidelines for the development of drugs. Website: www.ich.org.
IND	Investigational New Drug application	A submission required by the FDA for the investigational use of a drug product not previously authorized for marketing in the United States. A living dossier that summarizes essential properties, animal and human safety, and efficacy information for investigational use.
IEC/IRB	Independent Ethics Committee or Institutional Review Board	An independent body with the responsibility to ensure the protection of the rights, safety, and wellbeing of human subjects involved in a trial and to provide public assurance of that protection.
MAA	Marketing Authorization Application	The application through which drug sponsors formally seek approval of a new pharmaceutical for licensing in European Union member states. Dossier that compiles all data in support of licensing in Europe.
NDA	New Drug Application	The application through which drug sponsors formally seek FDA approval of a new pharmaceutical for sale and marketing in the United States. Dossier that compiles all data in support of licensing in the United States.
NICE	National Institute for Clinical Excellence	A U.K.-based independent organization that produces guidance on promoting good health and preventing ill health; on the use of new and existing medicines, treatments and procedures; and on appropriate care and treatment of patients with specific diseases and conditions. Website: www.nice.org.uk.
PDUFA	Prescription Drug User Fee Act	The law that authorizes the FDA to collect fees from companies that produce certain human drugs and biological products. The 2010 fee for an original NDA is $1.4 million.
PhRMA	Pharmaceutical Research Manufacturers Association	U.S. industry association. Website: www.phrma.org.
REMS	Risk evaluation and mitigation strategy	An FDA-approved postmarketing drug safety program that serves to assure the safe use of a drug product and ensure that benefits outweigh risks. A REMS may include more than the approved medication guide, e.g., communication and education plans, additional clinical trials, patient registries, and distribution controls. REMS outcomes must be measurable and are reassessed at 18 months, 3 years, and 7 years after implementation.
SmPC	Summary of product characteristics	European-approved product label.

include patient-reported functional or quality-of-life outcomes and health economic measures in Phase 3 trials, to meet the expectations of other institutional groups that set pricing, tiered access to treatment, or treatment guidelines (e.g., national health systems, health maintenance organizations, and the United Kingdom National Institute for Clinical Excellence).

Regulatory Agency Review

An application for approval to market a new medicine requires filing a dossier with the appropriate regulatory reviewing agency. In the United States, a new drug application (NDA) is filed with the FDA (most analgesic drug dossiers are reviewed by the AARP division), and in European Union member states an MAA is filed with the EMEA (the dossier is assessed by the CHMP, which issues a recommendation for the European Commission, an authority that controls licensing of medicines for the member states) (see Table I for acronym definitions). The content and format of all the information required in a NDA is governed by U.S. law and regulations (21CFR314) and by ICH guidelines. The NDA/MAA dossier covers drug substance (synthesis, manufacture, properties, purity, and stability), the dose form (composition, manufacture, properties, purity, and stability), pharmacology (intended and unintended effects in animals), animal toxicology (acute and chronic toxicities, oncogenicity, and reproductive effects), animal pharmacokinetics, human pharmacokinetics, all human safety data, and human efficacy in the intended population. NDA/MAA dossiers contain massive amounts of data and summary documents and may be equivalent to 100,000 pages (fortunately, electronic submission is now common). At the end of this process, the essential information is distilled down into a few printed pages of the approved prescribing information. The PDUFA performance goal for FDA is to review and act on 90% of all applications within 10 months (6 months if priority review is granted). The median time to approval for standard NDAs in 2006 was just over 10 months, but the timeframe can be much longer for individual products. Over the period of 2002–2007, the rate of approval during the first review cycle was 36% for non-priority NDAs and 67% for priority applications. In Europe, the timeline to regulatory action is 210 days, but there are several specified "clock stop" points along the way. One common reason for delay is a request for additional data or analyses by the regulatory agency at the action date.

Postmarketing

Drug development does not stop with approval. In the immediate post-marketing period, the drug sponsor may be required to conduct a number of specific clinical trials or surveillance protocols to assess the safety of the product in the real-world environment. Trials may be initiated to compare the effectiveness of the new treatment against alternative treatments. Postmarketing experience may provide new insights into best use of a new therapy or leads about new indications or patient populations that warrant clinical trial (e.g., the use of gabapentin as an analgesic developed from astute clinical observation in its use in epilepsy). Risk of failure also does not stop at approval. There have been many notable product withdrawals for safety findings as experience accumulated in the population at large. Postmarketing attrition among analgesic products includes the product withdrawals of bromfenac, rofecoxib, valdecoxib, and lumiracoxib from the markets around the world in which each drug was approved.

Control of the Clinical Trial Process

Clinical development is not possible without patient populations willing to volunteer to participate in trials. The clinical trial process is a contract between the trial sponsor, the investigator, the patient, the ethics committee (IRB or IEC), regulatory agencies, and society. This contract is embodied by the trial protocol, good clinical practice, and the informed consent process. An investigational clinical trial of a new medicine or non-approved use of an existing medicine is controlled by investigational new drug (IND) or CTA regulations, which concern a formal notification, approval and reporting process to initiate a clinical protocol and review safety as development progresses. All investigational trials are filed to this dossier, and the essential information to aid safe use by investigators is embodied in the investigator brochure (IB), which is a living document that is updated regularly. In the United States, the conduct of postmarketing clinical trials consistent with the approved use is controlled by the NDA and the approved package insert. In this case, trials and safety findings are filed to the NDA, and the accumulated experience can result in modifications to the approved package insert (or product label in Europe) and conditions of licensing for the product.

The framework of the discovery and development process works well, but success is influenced by the high degree of attrition and investment required to bring drugs to market. However, regulatory hurdles tend to evolve at a rate faster than the clinical development cycle time, such that the final goal can be a moving target. There remains a fine balance between maintaining high standards of safety and effectiveness and the need for rapid development and approval of new drugs.

References

[1]   Adams CP, Brantner VV. Estimating the cost of drug development. Is it really $802 million? Health Affairs 2006;25:420–8.

[2]   Congressional Budget Office. Research and development in the pharmaceutical industry. Publication number 2589 (October 2006). Available at: www.cbo.gov/publications. Accessed 3 March 2010.

[3]   Kola I, Landis J. Can the pharmaceutical industry reduce attrition rates? Nat Rev Drug Discover 2004;3:711–15.

[4]   Pharmaceutical Research Manufacturer's Association. Discovering new medicines. Available at: www.phrma.org/education. Accessed 3 March 2010.

Correspondence to: Steve Quessy, PhD, 20 Wythebrook Lane, Durham, NC 27713, USA. Email: quessy@qd-consulting.com.

Predicting Analgesic Efficacy from Animal Models of Peripheral Neuropathy and Nerve Injury: A Critical View from the Clinic

Andrew S.C. Rice, MB BS, MD, FRCA, FFPMRCA

Department of Anaesthetics, Pain Medicine and Intensive Care, Imperial College London,
and Chelsea and Westminster Hospital, London, United Kingdom

In this chapter, I will critically discuss the role of animal models in predicting analgesic efficacy in humans, as measured by the use of randomized controlled trials (RCTs). By way of illustration, I will focus on neuropathic pain, but many of the issues I will discuss are equally pertinent to the development of analgesic drugs for other types of pain. A theme that will be developed in the chapter is an attempt to construct arguments based on comparing and contrasting the ethics, methods, and standards employed when assessing novel analgesics in animal models and human RCTs. The emphasis will be on discussing the behavioral outcome measures employed in animal models, but the points made can perhaps be equally be applied to other outcome measures such as electrophysiology and image analysis of histologically derived images. Furthermore, these comments may also have relevance outside of the immediate topic of drug development, into areas such as the use of animal models to identify pain mechanisms and thus novel drug targets.

I will start by outlining the perspective from which this is written. I have been active in academic laboratory research using animal models of pain for over 20 years, and these models continue to form the core tool in my laboratory research. I am also active in clinical practice and see patients with neuropathic pain, predominantly in the context of peripheral nerve injuries, HIV-related polyneuropathies, and postherpetic neuralgia. Finally, I have been involved in the design, conduct, and meta-analysis of RCTs of novel analgesic agents for many years.

What is the Utility of Current Animal Models for Prediction of Efficacy in RCTs?

Kola and Landis undertook a review of attrition rates in drug development using data from 10 large pharmaceutical companies during the period 1991–2000 [55]. They concluded that there was a major attrition of candidate molecules between Phase 1 and registration, across a number of therapeutic areas. They estimated that only about 11% of drugs that enter Phase 1 clinical trials eventually proceeded to successfully acquire regulatory approval; specifically for pain and arthritis this figure was about 16%. Traditionally, the justification to undertake Phase 1/2 clinical trials in humans is heavily reliant on the efficacy data from "clinical trials" of efficacy conducted in animal models. It is worth reflecting on this strategy in the light of the fact that a lack of efficacy accounts for approximately 30% of the attrition between Phase 1 and regulatory approval. Therefore, it would appear that, in general, animal models, or how they are used, are not very efficient in predicting efficacy in RCTs. A similar figure of ~30% attrition is due to failures to adequately predict critical issues relating to toxicology and safety [55]. Higher attrition rates were evident in areas such as oncology and central nervous system diseases, where animal models are notoriously unpredictive for efficacy. Conversely, during the period 1991–2000, some disciplines had dramatically improved their contribution to the success rate of development compounds in achieving registration; in 1991 problems with pharmacokinetics and bioavailability accounted for about 40% of all attrition, but by 2000 improvements in this area had resulted in these factors contributing to attrition in only about 10% of failures [55]. This figure demonstrates that attention to certain factors can indeed result in beneficial changes in the drug development process.

Similarly, in 2004 the U.S. Food and Drug Administration commissioner Lester M. Crawford estimated that success rates of drugs entering Phase 1 trials in achieving registration had fallen from 14% to 8% (cited in [59]). He also estimated that "a mere 10% improvement in predicting products' failures in clinical trials could save $100 million in development costs per drug." There is little evidence that this situation has improved in 2010.

Another, perhaps somewhat philosophical and self-evident, but nevertheless important introductory point to make is the necessity to adequately differentiate between the *model* (i.e., what is done to an animal in order to create a reflection of the clinical condition of which pain is a feature) and the *outcome measures* (i.e., the procedures that are performed in order to determine, for example, the nature and severity of a sensory perturbation and the effect of a therapeutic intervention thereon). I suggest that, for the avoidance of confusion, the term "model" should be reserved solely for the purpose of describing the clinical lesion or disease being mirrored—e.g., peripheral nerve injury, antiretroviral-induced polyneuropathy, or diabetic polyneuropathy. In much of the literature, these models tend to be described as models of "neuropathic pain," which is dangerous because it can lead to a tacit assumption that pain is indeed a feature of these models—an assumption that is very difficult to test because of the difficulty of reliably measuring pain, especially spontaneous pain, in rodents. Usually, of course, the "clinical" feature of the model that leads to the indirect inference that it reflects aspects of clinical pain is usually the appearance of certain evoked phenomena, such as mechanical hypersensitivity, which are also observed in some patients with neuropathic pain as mechanical allodynia

or hyperalgesia. With regard to outcome measures, the clinical symptom or sign that is being replicated should be properly described as such (e.g., spontaneous pain, mechanical hypersensitivity, or pain-associated anxiety) and not simply as "pain." Again, sometimes the literature does not adequately make this distinction.

Some years ago, Willner proposed a method for assessing the validity of animal models of depression [111]. Such critical analyzes are rarely systematically undertaken when models of painful disease and pain-related outcome measures are characterized. I suggest that this approach should be systematically undertaken for existing and new animal models of neuropathic pain. Willner assessed the validity of animal models using three sets of relatively independent criteria: (1) *Face validity* refers to the degree of symptomatic resemblance between the model (or outcome measure) and the clinical condition. (2) *Construct validity* describes the theoretical rationale of the model or outcome measure. (3) *Predictive* (or *pharmacological*) *validity* concerns the extent to which the model/outcome measure responds appropriately to drugs that are clinically effective and to those that are not. It is important to remember that when selecting agents to test pharmacological validity, investigators should use only the highest-quality clinical evidence from high-quality RCTs or meta-analyses, or else they may draw erroneous conclusions about the clinical efficacy of drugs. Jadad (with a later modification [48,84]) has described a simple tool to evaluate the quality of RCTs, which is now in widespread use in the clinical systematic review field. If adequate measurements of pharmacological validity are performed, then it is possible to calculate the *sensitivity* (ability to correctly detect a true positive) and *specificity* (ability to correctly detect a true negative) of a model or outcome measure. These factors are essential in the validation and comparison of models and outcome measures. (For a useful online calculator of sensitivity and specificity, see: http://faculty.vassar.edu/lowry/clin1.html).

In addition, the *reliability* (*reproducibility*) of a model or outcome measures, which might include: "test-retest," "interobserver," and "intercenter" (laboratory) reliability, should be systematically assessed. It is salutary to reflect whether the robust and systematic approach adopted by the German Neuropathic Pain Network to control these factors in quantitative sensory testing of humans [89] would be of benefit to the animal model field. (See www.neuro.med.tu-muenchen.de/dfns/e_index.html.)

Efficiency of Current Models and Outcome Measures in Predicting Efficacy in RCTs

Do animal models and outcome measures of neuropathic pain efficiently predict efficacy in RCTs? The increasingly widespread adoption of such animal models for this purpose since the first peripheral nerve injury models were described two decades ago [12,52,53,95] would suggest that perhaps there is a degree of utility in these models. Or does this practice rather reflect something of a "herd" mentality inherent in the drug development process or the lack of credible and well-validated alternative approaches? The analysis by Kola and Landis [55] would suggest that there is plenty of room for improved efficiency.

A useful method of assessing evidence across a wide number of studies is to conduct a systematic review and meta-analysis. (See the Bandolier website for much useful information on this topic: www.medicine.ox.ac.uk/bandolier.) This method has become the standard approach for clinical evidence synthesis. Such an exercise was attempted by Kontinen and Meert, who analyzed results from 119 reports of estimates of analgesic efficacy studies in models of neuropathic pain. They then compared these data to evidence from corresponding RCTs [56]. Their analysis suggested that, for the prediction of efficacy in RCTs, the chronic constriction model (CCI) has 88% sensitivity, compared to 68% for spinal nerve ligation (SNL), 61% for partial sciatic nerve ligation (PSNL), and 70% for the streptozotocin model of diabetic polyneuropathy (STZ). CCI was reported as having 0% specificity (possibly reflecting a bias from the low number of "negative" reports that were identified), with 60% for SNL and 66% for STZ. The authors were unable to estimate specificity for the PSNL model. However, this analysis had a number of fundamental limitations.

First, a lack of availability of evidence from "negative" studies generates an inevitable source of publication bias. While this phenomenon is widely recognized as a problem compromising the assessment of clinical evidence [36], it is probably even more of an issue with evidence synthesis for animal model efficacy studies. There have been calls for a more open approach to this issue in the clinical pain field [91], and encouragement to register RCTs is beginning to mitigate against this problem. "Negative" animal efficacy studies from either academic or industry sources are rarely published in the peer-reviewed literature, and there is an understandable, but detrimental to the "greater good," reluctance of the pharmaceutical industry to publish data on development compounds. Publication bias would have comprised specificity estimates in particular.

Second, not only publication bias, but also study selection bias probably overestimated specificity: this review did not use robust methodological quality criteria [48,84] for selecting which RCTs were included in the comparator; this is a fundamental tenet of the systematic review process. Similarly, it is widely recognized that inconsistent and unclear reporting standards for studies in animal models make it very difficult to assess the methodological quality of these studies, and therefore to exclude from the analysis studies of low methodological quality with inherent bias [42,72,82]. This is one of the reasons why we have called for more uniformity and transparency in the reporting of animal studies of pain [86].

We still have much to learn from the stroke field in this area [64,96], and it is salutary to reflect on the impact of the widespread adoption of the CONSORT reporting standards for clinical RCTs and the consequential ability to conduct high-quality systematic reviews of the clinical literature [93]. CONSORT [93] (and the related PRISMA for systematic reviews and meta-analyzes [61]) provide a framework (including a useful checklist and suggestion for a flow chart) for the minimal methodological information to be included with a publication of a clinical trial. This process allows reviewers and readers to rapidly determine the methodological quality of a clinical trial or systematic review from the published data. Most major journals have now adopted this policy. (For more information, see www.consort-statement.org and www.prisma-statement.org.)

Although a general problem of animal models not adequately predicting efficacy in RCTs across a number of disease areas has been highlighted [22,42,65,72,82,96,97], it is difficult to find thorough, critical, and systematic assessments discussing the direct relevance of this issue to the pain field. However, one example in the field is the failure of neurokinin-1 receptor antagonists to achieve efficacy in pain RCTs, despite a sound scientific rationale and strong evidence from studies in animal models, including the use of transgenic mice [17,46].

Nevertheless, it is worthwhile critically reflecting on the clinical evidence base for the effectiveness of compounds in neuropathic pain [31,38,45]. This evidence reveals that tricyclic and dual reuptake inhibitors of both serotonin and norepinephrine, calcium channel $\alpha_2\delta_1$ ligands (i.e., gabapentin and pregabalin), opioids, and topical sodium channel blockers and capsaicin have effectiveness across a number of neuropathic pain conditions. However, very few of these drugs were *primarily* developed for pain using the conventional approach of identifying a drug "target" from animal model studies of pain mechanisms, and proceeding to demonstrate the efficacy of molecules directed at that target in animal models in order to justify the conduct of Phase 2–3 clinical effectiveness studies. Perhaps the one exception to this statement is topical capsaicin, in various concentrations; all the others were either long-established drugs (e.g., opioids or tricyclic antidepressants) or drugs that were initially developed for other disease areas (e.g., $\alpha_2\delta_1$ ligands for epilepsy) that were subsequently tested in pain RCTs. Conversely, the preceding statement needs to be balanced by the recognition that nearly all of the above compounds have been demonstrated, retrospectively at least, to have efficacy in animal models (e.g., refs. [41,43,105,107,108]). This situation could suggest that these models have sensitivity for the detection of clinical effectiveness, but that their specificity is largely unknown, as discussed above, although a robust systematic analysis would have to be conducted to prove the point.

How Can the Efficiency of Current Models and Outcome Measures Be Improved?

The foregoing discussion suggests that there is room for further development and refinement of animal models of neuropathic pain in order to improve their validity and reliability for the purposes of predicting efficacy in RCTs. Aspects of this issue have been reviewed elsewhere [75,86,101,110], and because of space limitations this chapter will cover only some of the more important aspects.

Choice of Animals/Species

In the majority of cases, rats and mice are the experimental species of choice for modeling neuropathic pain. At a generic level, it is reasonable to question whether rodents are indeed a reasonable species in which to conduct studies of complex human diseases. A rebuttal to this criticism is that no valid and reliable

alternative experimental approach for replacing animals has been yet offered for such studies. Most essential studies that are conducted in rodents would not be ethically justifiable or scientifically feasible in human volunteers or patients, particularly when novel agents of unknown toxicity are being evaluated. Furthermore, public opinion and economic considerations discourage the widespread experimental use of higher species such as primates, which may be scientifically more appropriate for modeling human disease. There has also been some interest in using animals with naturally occurring painful diseases for prehuman investigation of novel analgesics [86].

By and large, the rodents used for neuropathic pain models are usually previously healthy, young, and genetically similar males [74]. Conversely, human neuropathic pain often presents in the context of chronic disease (e.g., diabetes, HIV, or cancer) or in the elderly (e.g., postherpetic neuralgia). Rodent age has an important impact on the development of pain-related signs after peripheral nerve injury [83]. The strain of rodent can also have a major impact on the ability to model pain, and although we are only just beginning to understand this complex area [20,73,112], the investigator does need to carefully consider the strain and supplier of rodents when designing a study.

Chronicity

There is a general temporal disconnection between the duration of disease in rodent models and that of humans with neuropathic pain. For example, the median duration of disease of patients entering a major postherpetic neuralgia RCT was about 4 years [85], similar to that in a cross-sectional survey (4.8 years) [24]. This contrasts with reports of a rodent model of herpes zoster-associated pain where the maximum period over which measurements was made was 10 weeks [41] and where pharmacological interventions were studied at only 2–4 weeks after viral infection [41,43]. One potential consequence of this disconnection is that most animal model studies are conducted in the initiation/acute injury phase of the disease, whereas the mechanisms of pain and comorbidities and functional expression of drug targets maybe entirely different in the patients usually selected for inclusion in RCTs—patients who have suffered from the disease in question and have had chronic pain for many years. However, it should also be considered that the relative lifespans of laboratory rodents and humans differ by a factor of about 35, which may mitigate against the above criticisms [86].

Incidence of Pain

Most patients who experience a condition that puts them at risk of developing neuropathic pain (e.g., peripheral nerve trauma, diabetes, or HIV disease) do *not* in fact go on to develop chronic pain. For example, only ~9% of patients with acute herpes zoster have pain a year later (i.e., postherpetic neuralgia) [94]. Conversely, existing animal models of neuropathic pain have been selected to give a very high incidence of "pain responses," which does not accurately reflect the clinical situation. However, it is difficult to see an easy solution that would circumvent the important ethical and economic issues posed by accurately modeling a pain condition in which a large number of animals would have to be excluded from further study because they did not develop signs of pain.

Disease/Lesion

There is an increasing appreciation that there is a greater degree of heterogeneity among patients suffering from neuropathic pain than was previously thought. Both within and between different diseases or injuries associated with a risk of developing neuropathic pain, there are clusters of different patterns of symptoms and signs [3,4,10,89,92]. Therefore, it would seem logical, if using the currently conventional approach of disease-specific RCTs, to match the animal model as closely as possible with the condition to be studied in the RCT. Historically, this has not been the case. Over the past two decades, partial sciatic nerve injury models have become the industry standard for the preclinical assessment of novel analgesics targeted at neuropathic pain. In order to make a comparison with the diseases studied in RCTs, we extracted data [86] from the 123 interventions assessed in the 105 neuropathic pain RCTs included in a meta-analysis [38]. Sixty-five RCTs (53%) were conducted in patients with peripheral polyneuropathies, and 17 (21%) were in postherpetic neuralgia patients. In contrast, only 11 RCTs (9%) studied patients with peripheral nerve injury. Fortunately, there has been considerable activity in recent years in developing a range of animal models that reflect many of the diseases studied in RCTs, including cancer or antiretroviral therapy [5–7,13,19,29,39,50,51,62,63,67,107], HIV-associated peripheral neuropathy [14,108], diabetic peripheral neuropathy [21,66], varicella zoster infection

[40,41,43,70], multiple sclerosis [1], and lumbar radiculopathy [79]. Although the predictive validity of these models remains to be fully proven, it is reasonable to argue that for drug development the animal model should be matched, as far as possible, to the disease that is proposed for the RCT. However, because the literature regarding the more conventional peripheral nerve injury models is now so vast, it is probably also important to retain representation of the models in any drug development program, if only for compatibility purposes. Therefore, the best approach would probably be to examine development drugs in a range of different animal models rather than rely only on peripheral nerve injury.

Outcome Measures

Before attempting to compare and contrast the outcome measures used in RCTs of neuropathic pain with those employed in animal models, it is important to first remind ourselves of the distinction between symptoms and clinical signs. *Symptoms* are subjective features of an illness experienced by a patient. A physician elicits symptoms from a patent when taking a clinical history. Pain is a symptom. The term *clinical sign* is reserved for objective aspects of the disease, including behaviors, that are detected by a physician during the process of a clinical examination. Signs may or may not be evident to the patient. Measurement of sensory function, including sensory gain phenomena such as allodynia and hyperalgesia, is an example of the elicitation of clinical signs. Self-evidently, symptoms are subjective and their elicitation requires a level of communication between patient and physician that is impossible between a rodent and experimental scientist. Therefore, outcome measures in most animal models are, of necessity, reliant upon the measurement of features that reflect human clinical signs rather than symptoms. For many disease areas this does not pose a significant difficulty—for example, studies of hypertension generally rely upon measuring the same clinical sign (blood pressure) in human and animal studies. However, there is a difficulty when dealing with a highly subjective symptom such as pain. As a broad generalization, the primary efficacy variable in neuropathic pain RCTs is nearly always some aspect of pain symptomatology (e.g., self-report of pain intensity), whereas hypersensitivity of withdrawal reflexes to a range of sensory stimuli is the usual measure employed in animals. This measure probably reflects an aspect of sensory gain (e.g., allodynia or hyperalgesia), which is a sign observed only in subsets of patients suffering from neuropathic pain [8]. It is easy to see why the widespread use of these reflex measures has persisted over many years, given their simplicity and reproducibility.

Neuropathic RCTs only rarely select patients (or even phenotype them at baseline for subsequent post hoc responder analysis) on the basis of their sensory profile; rather, the level of pain intensity is the important factor. Therefore, inevitably in many RCTs there will be only a subset of patients to whom the animal outcome measure of sensory gain is relevant. This lack of direct comparability of measurements is further compounded by the infrequency of reports of clinical signs (e.g., allodynia and hyperalgesia), and the impact of some therapeutic intervention thereon, being robustly assessed in RCTs, although the ability to undertake such assessments is developing [90].

A second comparability factor to consider is the *range* of measures used to determine the effect of a therapeutic intervention in human and animal studies. As pointed out above, the conventional single outcome measure in animal studies is assessment of reflex hypersensitivity, although methodological aspects of such techniques, particularly when obtained with von Frey filaments, have been criticized [16]. It is rare for any other measures to be reported. In contrast to animal studies, the predominant clinical feature in neuropathic pain, and therefore the primary efficacy measure in many neuropathic pain RCTs, is not evoked pain, but spontaneous pain (continuous and/or paroxysmal) [34], a feature that is not generally explored in animal studies (see ref. [76]). Furthermore, in high-quality RCTs the primary efficacy measure is supported by a portfolio of secondary outcome measures, which when considered together give a holistic impression of the effect of an intervention on the patients' health. Neuropathic pain has a wide impact on many aspects of quality of life, psychological state, and ability to function [24,30,49,71]. For secondary outcome measures in RCTs, a broad range of symptoms and signs are usually measured, reflecting other measures of pain intensity, pain descriptors and characteristics (spontaneous, paroxysmal, and evoked), psychological and other comorbidities (e.g., sleep disturbance, anxiety, or depression), physical function, quality of life, and adverse effect; the domains that should be assessed in chronic pain RCTs have been enunciated in recommendations from the IMMPACT group [33]. The continuous evolution of clinical study

design should also be borne in mind when considering these factors [35,78]. Table I compares the generic outcome domains generally measured in animal studies of neuropathic pain and RCTs. Furthermore, patients with neuropathic pain display a range of sensory signs, of which sensory gain is just one example. As mentioned above, evidence of heterogeneity of symptoms and signs in neuropathic pain is increasing [3,4,10,89,92], and consequently the choice of outcome measures in both RCTs and animal model studies must reflect this heterogeneity.

The need for refinement of the range of outcome measures used in animal pain studies has been discussed in detail elsewhere [15,75,76,101,110], and space precludes a detailed discussion of that important topic here. However, there have now been reports of attempts to measure a range of complex pain-related behaviors in animal models of neuropathic pain, including those based on operant function, which all reflect differing and important aspects of human pain comorbidity. These include various approaches to place preference (possibly reflecting spontaneous pain or global impression) [54,57,58,80,81,100–103], anxiety-like behavior (possibly also reflecting spontaneous pain) [43,68,87,88,105–108], circadian rhythm disturbance [2,77], and depression [47]. Such behaviors are perhaps easier to assess in rats than in mice [23,44]. It is also important to note that there has been less success in measuring other behaviors, such as ultrasound vocalization, which on face value would be likely to be associated with pain [109]; it is important to publish such "negative" studies to avoid publication bias. An important recent paper has described a method for assessing

Table I
Comparison of the generic outcome domains generally measured in animal studies of neuropathic pain and corresponding clinical trials

Outcome Domain	Animal Efficacy Studies	Human RCTs
Evoked hypersensitivity	+	+/–
Spontaneous continuous pain	–	+*
Spontaneous paroxysmal pain	–	+/–
Comorbidity	–	+
Physical function	–	+
Emotional function	–	+
Circadian rhythm disturbance	–	+
Adverse events	–	+
Global impression	–	+

* The usual primary efficacy measure.

pain in mice using analysis of facial expression, a common technique used in nonverbal humans [60]. This technique was useful for detecting analgesic-sensitive abnormalities in a range of acute and inflammatory pain models, but it did not detect any similar behaviors in peripheral nerve injury models. This finding may reflect some ability to adapt behavior away from using facial grimaces in chronic as opposed to acute pain, in humans and rodents. Alternatively, perhaps the models of traumatic nerve injury used may only have an evoked hypersensitivity component (and possibly spontaneous paroxysmal pain) without a sufficient element of spontaneous continuous pain to evoke facial grimacing. Finally, the utility of electrophysiological parallel human and animal measures of sensory neuronal excitability is worthy of further exploration [69,98,99].

The implication of the above discussion for the choice of outcome measures in animal studies is that it would be logical to attempt to match the range of outcome measures in the animal study to the range of primary and secondary efficacy measures and patient sensory phenotypes that one intends to measure in the eventual RCT. However, the feasibility, validity, reproducibility, and economics of such routine use of such complex measures for routine drug development studies remains to be fully evaluated. It is also important to consider the meaning of such measurements in the context of the world of the laboratory rat and resist the temptation to "over-anthropomorphize" in the interpretation of these behaviors [23,111]. The documentary film made by Berdoy of the behavioral consequences of laboratory rats being released into a "wild" environment is worthy viewing for anyone designing, conducting, or analyzing animal experiments (see www.ratlife.org), as are the major reference tomes discussing rat behavior [9]. Housing, handling, and other aspects of animal husbandry, species and strain, and the test environment also need to be considered as important variables in the design of behavioral experiments [20,23,27,104]. Additionally, when designing outcome measures for use in animal models, it might be pertinent to reflect on what the survival advantage might be to a prey species, such as rat, in displaying overt "pain behavior," when to do so could reveal it as potential prey.

Experimental Bias

Experimental bias has variously been defined as "any process which systematically overestimates or underestimates a parameter" [25] or in the excellent Bandolier guide to bias as "a systematic disposition of certain trial designs to produce results consistently better or worse than other trial designs" (www.medicine.ox.ac.uk/bandolier/extraforbando/bias.pdf).

High-quality RCTs [26,93], and indeed other methods of clinical evidence synthesis, such as meta-analyses [61], have reached a high level of sophistication in terms of methodological quality and reporting transparency in an attempt to minimize the influence of bias. McQuay, Moore, and colleagues [32] have estimated the magnitude of "overestimation of treatment effect" attributable to common sources of bias in clinical pain studies, which are summarized in Fig. 1. The effect size attributable to these sources of bias is of similar magnitude to the ≥30% decrease in pain intensity, which has been estimated to be of "moderate clinical importance" [32].

Does bias confound animal studies in the same way as it does clinical studies? There is certainly evidence to suggest that it does so in other disease areas [72,82]. Probably the best-evaluated area in this regard is the field of stroke, thanks largely to the laudable efforts of the Camarades collaboration (see www.camarades.info). Having assessed the general failure of animal models of stroke to predict efficacy in clinical trials, these investigators have concluded that a systemic failure to minimize the impact of various forms of experimental bias in animal studies is a major contributing factor [11,22,28,65,82,96,97].

We undertook a simple exploratory exercise to investigate where tools to minimize experimental bias were reported in animal pain studies [86]. We searched some recent volumes of *Pain* for papers in which a pharmacological intervention was assessed in an animal pain model, and identified 14 such reports. We subjected these reports to a modified form of the "Jadad" quality scoring tool [84]. Of the 14, only 5 were described as blinded, 4 as randomized, and only 1 reported withdrawals and dropouts. None described a power calculation. Although 5 out of a possible 7 points or more would normally be required for a study to be included in a clinical systematic review, none of the animal studies scored more than one point. In the same review [86], we also reanalyzed unpublished data from a previous systematic review [56] and revealed that only 29% of the 125 studies were described as randomized and only 28% were described as blinded. Furthermore, only a few papers described how randomization and blinding were performed. Does this mean that widespread experimental bias confounds

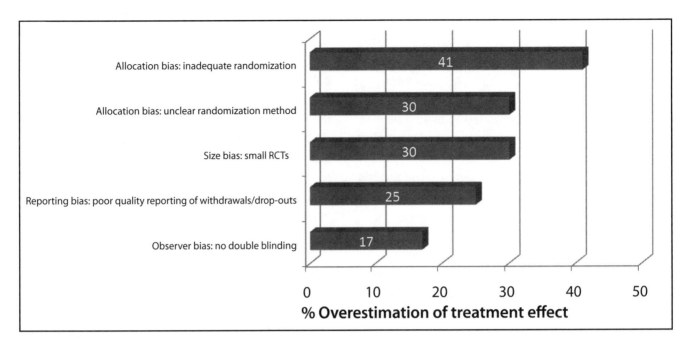

Fig. 1. The overestimation of treatment effect compiled from analyses of pain studies. Adapted from Carroll et al. [18] and Ernst and White [37] and from the *Bandolier Bias Guide* (www.medicine.ox.ac.uk/bandolier/extraforbando/bias.pdf).

animal pain model studies? Not necessarily, because there are several possible interpretations: (1) Experimental bias does not confound animal model efficacy studies in the same way that it does in clinical trials, and thus the use of bias reduction methods is not necessary. (2) Experimental bias does confound animal model efficacy studies, and adequate experimental bias reduction techniques are already used, but they are not transparently reported in the methods. (3) Experimental bias does confound animal model efficacy studies the same way as it does in clinical trials, and bias reduction methodologies should be employed and transparently reported.

However, it will be impossible to ascertain which of the above factors is closest to the truth until widespread adequate methodology information is included in reports of animal studies and systematic reviews are possible. CONSORT-type reporting standards for animal studies would certainly assist the transparency of descriptions of methods and permit systematic reviews to be conducted. We have called for more uniformity and transparency in the reporting of animal studies of pain, and we have suggested a checklist (Extended Methods Form) that authors could include when submitting with their manuscripts (see Fig. 2) [86]. The Camarades collaboration has published a code of "Good Laboratory Practice" for animal model studies in the stroke field [64]. I suggest

that pain studies would benefit greatly from a similar approach (see Table II).

Table II
Key domains of good laboratory practice for animal studies

Information about animals (species, strain, gender, age, source, etc.) should be given. Details of the environmental conditions in which the animals were housed and experiments conducted should also be stated.

Details of the sample size (power) calculation must be given.

Explicit inclusion and exclusion criteria, determined in the protocol before commencement of the study, should be stated.

Randomization: Clear details of the methods used to allocate animals to experimental groups must be given.

Allocation concealment: Details of how the allocation of animals to experimental groups was concealed from the investigator who was responsible for the induction of the pain state (e.g., peripheral nerve surgeon).

Reporting of animals excluded from analysis: The stage at which any animals were excluded and the reasons for that exclusion (e.g., the animal died) should be clearly stated. CONSORT-type flow charts are useful for this purpose.

Blinded measurement, assessment, and analysis of outcome measures should be conducted and reported. The methods used to blind investigators who perform and analyze the outcome measures should be explicitly stated. The point at which the blinding codes were broken should also be stated.

Potential conflicts of interest and study funding should be stated.

Source: Adapted from Macleod et al. [64].

Extended **M**ethods **F**orm

Rice ASC, Cimino-Brown D, Eisenach JC, Kontinen VK, LaCroix-Fralish ML, Machin I, Mogil JS, Stöhr T. Animal models and the prediction of efficacy in clinical trials of analgesic drugs: a critical appraisal and call for uniform reporting standards. *Pain 2008;139(2):241-5*

1. Experimental design

Experiments blinded

  - what

  - how

Randomization

Power calculation

How many data points removed?

  - why

2. Animals

Age

Sex

Genetic background of mutation

Supplier

Weight Range

Behavioral Abnormalities

Any additional comments

3. Environment

a. *Housing*

Diet

Bedding

Cage rack ventilation

Home cage enrichment

Habituation time before experiments (in days)

Handling frequency before testing

Cage cleaning frequency

housed per cage

House experimental/ control groups together or separately

Different species housed in same room

Lights on time

Lights off time

Procedural anesthetic

Post-operative analgesia

  -Analgesic and dose

b. *Testing*

of testers

Experience of tester(s)

Lighting intensity (lux)

Time testing ends

Test environment noise

Recent calibration of testing equipment

Cleaning of test equip. between subjects

  -with

Habituation time before testing (in minutes)

Oestrus stage of females

Number of animals present in testing room

Distance separated

In visual contact

Arousal state

Comments on this form to: Andrew Rice *a.rice@imperial.ac.uk*

Fig. 2. A checklist to improve the reporting transparency for the methods used in research involving animal models of pain (from Rice et al. [86]).

Conclusion

In conclusion, I have discussed several ways in which the predictive validity of animal models of neuropathic pain may be improved. Some of these efforts, such as attempts to develop more clinically relevant models and outcome measures, are already in progress, but it will still take a concerted collaborative effort from industrially and academically based research groups before the validity and reproducibility of such models and outcome measures are fully established. Other strategies, particularly the use of techniques aimed at minimizing experimental bias, could be more readily and rapidly addressed by widespread adoption of simple bias-reduction techniques and transparent reporting standards.

The issues discussed in this chapter are recognized and being actively addressed by many people working in this field. Indeed, a partnership between the European Union and a collective of pharmaceutical companies (EFPIA) recently launched a major program called the "Innovative Medicines Initiative," which will address many of the generic issues discussed in this chapter across a number of disease areas, including pain, by encouraging large-scale collaborative approaches between industry and academic groups (www.imi.europa.eu).

References

[1] Aicher SA, Silverman MB, Winkler CW, Bebo J. Hyperalgesia in an animal model of multiple sclerosis. Pain 2004;110:560–70.

[2] Andersen ML, Tufik S. Sleep patterns over 21-day period in rats with chronic constriction of sciatic nerve. Brain Res 2003;984:84–92.

[3] Attal N, Bouhassira D, Gautron M, Vaillant JN, Mitry E, Lepere C, Rougier P, Guirimand F. Thermal hyperalgesia as a marker of oxaliplatin neurotoxicity: a prospective quantified sensory assessment study. Pain 2009;144:245–52.

[4] Attal N, Fermanian C, Fermanian J, Lanteri-Minet M, Alchaar H, Bouhassira D. Neuropathic pain: are there distinct subtypes depending on the aetiology or anatomical lesion? Pain 2008;138:343–53.

[5] Authier N, Balayssac D, Marchand F, Ling B, Zangarelli A, Descoeur J, Coudore F, Bourinet E, Eschalier A. Animal models of chemotherapy-evoked painful peripheral neuropathies. Neurotherapeutics 2009;6:620–9.

[6] Authier N, Gillet JP, Fialip J, Eschalier A, Coudore F. A new animal model of vincristine-induced nociceptive peripheral neuropathy. Neurotoxicology 2003;24:797–805.

[7] Authier N, Gillet JP, Fialip J, Eschalier A, Coudore F. An animal model of nociceptive peripheral neuropathy following repeated cisplatin injections. Exp Neurol 2003;182:12–20.

[8] Backonja MM, Stacey B. Neuropathic pain symptoms relative to overall pain rating. J Pain 2004;5:491–7.

[9] Barnett SA, Whilshaw IQ, Kolb B. The behaviour of the laboratory rat, Vol. 1. Oxford: Oxford University Press; 2006.

[10] Baron R, Tölle TR, Gockel U, Brosz M, Freynhagen R. A cross-sectional cohort survey in 2100 patients with painful diabetic neuropathy and postherpetic neuralgia: Differences in demographic data and sensory symptoms. Pain 2009;146:34–40.

[11] Bath PM, Gray LJ, Bath AJ, Buchan A, Miyata T, Green AR. Effects of NXY-059 in experimental stroke: an individual animal meta-analysis. Br J Pharmacol 2009;157:1157–71.

[12] Bennett GJ, Xie YK. A peripheral mononeuropathy in rat that produces disorders of pain sensation like those seen in man. Pain 1988;33:87–107.

[13] Bhangoo SK, Ren D, Miller RJ, Chan DM, Ripsch MS, Weiss C, McGinnis C, White FA. CXCR4 chemokine receptor signaling mediates pain hypersensitivity in association with antiretroviral toxic neuropathy. Brain Behav Immun 2007;21:581–91.

[14] Bhangoo SK, Ripsch MS, Buchanan DJ, Miller RJ, White FA. Increased chemokine signaling in a model of HIV1-associated peripheral neuropathy. Mol Pain 2009;5:48.

[15] Blackburn-Munro G. Pain-like behaviours in animals: how human are they? Trends Pharmacol Sci 2004;25:299–305.

[16] Bove G. Mechanical sensory threshold testing using nylon monofilaments: the pain field's "tin standard." Pain 2006;124:13–7.

[17] Boyce S, Hill RG. Discrepant results from preclinical and clinical studies on the potential of substance P-receptor antagonist compounds as analgesics. In: Devor M, Rowbotham MC, Wiesenfeld-Hallin Z, editors. Proceedings of the 9th World Congress on Pain. Seattle: IASP Press, 2000. p. 313–24.

[18] Carroll D, Tramer M, McQuay H, Nye B, Moore A. Randomization is important in studies with pain outcomes: systematic review of transcutaneous electrical nerve stimulation in acute postoperative pain. Br J Anaesth 1996;77:798–803.

[19] Chen X, Levine J. Mechanically-evoked C-fiber activity in painful alcohol and AIDS therapy neuropathy in the rat. Mol Pain 2007;3:5.

[20] Chesler EJ, Wilson SG, Lariviere WR, Rodriguez-Zas SL, Mogil JS. Identification and ranking of genetic and laboratory environment factors influencing a behavioral trait, thermal nociception, via computational analysis of a large data archive. Neurosci Biobehav Rev 2002;26:907–23.

[21] Courteix C, Eschalier A, Lavarenne J. Streptozocin-induced diabetic rats: behavioural evidence for a model of chronic pain. Pain 1993;53:81–8.

[22] Crossley NA, Sena E, Goehler J, Horn J, van der Worp B, Bath PMW, Macleod M, Dirnagl U. Empirical evidence of bias in the design of experimental stroke studies: a metaepidemiologic approach. Stroke 2008;39:929–34.

[23] Cryan JF, Holmes A. The ascent of mouse: advances in modelling human depression and anxiety. Nat Rev Drug Discov 2005;4:775–90.

[24] Daniel HC, Narewska J, Serpell M, Hoggart B, Johnson R, Rice AS. Comparison of psychological and physical function in neuropathic pain and nociceptive pain: implications for cognitive behavioral pain management programs. Eur J Pain 2008;12:731–41.

[25] Day S. Dictionary for clinical trials, Vol. 1. Chichester: John Wiley & Sons; 1999.

[26] De Angelis C, Drazen JM, Frizelle FA, Haug C, Hoey J, Horton R, Kotzin S, Laine C, Marusic A, Overbeke AJ, et al. Clinical trial registration: a statement from the International Committee of Medical Journal Editors. Lancet 2004;364:911–2.

[27] Deacon RMJ. Housing, husbandry and handling of rodents for behavioral experiments. Nat Protocols 2006;1:936–46.

[28] Dirnagl U, Macleod MR. Stroke research at a road block: the streets from adversity should be paved with meta-analysis and good laboratory practice. Br J Pharmacol 2009;157:1154–6.

[29] Dorsey SG, Leitch CC, Renn CL, Lessans S, Smith BA, Wang XM, Dionne RA. Genome-wide screen identifies drug-induced regulation of the gene giant axonal neuropathy (GAN) in a mouse model of antiretroviral-induced painful peripheral neuropathy. Biol Res Nurs 2009;11:7–16.

[30] Doth AH, Hansson PT, Jensen MP, Taylor RS. The burden of neuropathic pain: a systematic review and meta-analysis of health utilities. Pain 2010; Epub Mar 12.

[31] Dworkin RH, O'Connor AB, Backonja M, Farrar JT, Finnerup NB, Jensen TS, Kalso EA, Loeser JD, Miaskowski C, Nurmikko TJ, et al. Pharmacologic management of neuropathic pain: evidence-based recommendations. Pain 2007;132:237–51.

[32] Dworkin RH, Turk DC, McDermott MP, Peirce-Sandner S, Burke LB, Cowan P, Farrar JT, Hertz S, Raja SN, Rappaport BA, et al. Interpreting the clinical importance of group differences in chronic pain clinical trials: IMMPACT recommendations. Pain 2009;146:238–44.

[33] Dworkin RH, Turk DC, Wyrwich KW, Beaton D, Cleeland CS, Farrar JT, Haythornthwaite JA, Jensen MP, Kerns RD, Ader DN, et al. Interpreting the clinical importance of treatment outcomes in chronic pain clinical trials: IMMPACT recommendations. J Pain 2008;9:105–21.

[34] Dworkin RH, Turk DC, Farrar JT, Haythornthwaite JA, Jensen MP, Katz NP, Kerns RD, Stucki G, Allen RR, Bellamy N. Core outcome measures for chronic pain clinical trials: IMMPACT recommendations. Pain 2005;113:9–19.

[35] Dworkin RH, Turk DC, Peirce-Sandner S, Baron R, Bellamy N, Burke LB, Chappell A, Chartier K, Cleeland CS, Costello A, et al. Research design considerations for confirmatory chronic pain clinical trials: IMMPACT recommendations. Pain 2010; Epub Mar 6.

[36] Egger M, Smith GD, Schneider M, Minder C. Bias in meta-analysis detected by a simple, graphical test. BMJ 1997;315:629–34.

[37] Ernst E, White AR. Acupuncture for back pain: a meta-analysis of randomized controlled trials. Arch Intern Med 1998;158:2235–41.

[38] Finnerup NB, Otto M, McQuay HJ, Jensen TS, Sindrup SH. Algorithm for neuropathic pain treatment: an evidence based proposal. Pain 2005;118:289–305.

[39] Flatters SJL, Bennett GJ. Ethosuximide reverses paclitaxel- and vincristine-induced painful peripheral neuropathy. Pain 2004;109:150–61.

[40] Fleetwood-Walker SM, Quinn JP, Wallace C, Blackburn-Munro G, Kelly BG, Fiskerstrand CE, Nash AA, Dalziel RG. Behavioural changes in the rat following infection with varicella zoster virus. J Gen Virol 1999;80:2433–6.

[41] Garry EM, Delaney A, Anderson HA, Sirinathsinghji EC, Clapp RH, Martin WJ, Kinchington PR, Krah DL, Abbadie C, Fleetwood-Walker SM. Varicella zoster virus induces neuropathic changes in rat dorsal root ganglia and behavioral reflex sensitisation that is attenuated by gabapentin or sodium channel blocking drugs. Pain 2005;118:97–111.

[42] Hackam DG. Translating animal research into clinical benefit. BMJ 2007;334:163–4.

[43] Hasnie FS, Breuer J, Parker S, Wallace V, Blackbeard J, Lever I, Kinchington PR, Dickenson AH, Pheby T, Rice ASC. Further characterization of a rat model of varicella zoster virus-associated pain: Relationship between mechanical hypersensitivity and anxiety-related behavior, and the influence of analgesic drugs. Neuroscience 2007;144:1495–1508.

[44] Hasnie FS, Wallace VCJ, Hefner K, Holmes A, Rice ASC. Mechanical and cold hypersensitivity in nerve-injured C57BL/6J mice is not associated with fear-avoidance- and depression-related behaviour. Br J Anaesth 2007;98:816–22.

[45] Hempenstall K, Nurmikko TJ, Johnson RW, A'Hern R, Rice ASC. Analgesic therapy in postherpetic neuralgia: a quantitative systematic review. PLoS Med 2005;2:628–44.

[46] Hill R. NK1 (substance P) receptor antagonists: why are they not analgesic in humans? Trends Pharmacol Sci 2000;21:244–6.

[47] Hu B, Doods H, Treede RD, Ceci A. Depression-like behaviour in rats with mononeuropathy is reduced by the CB2-selective agonist GW405833. Pain 2009;143:206–12.

[48] Jadad AR, Moore RA, Carroll D, Jenkinson C, Reynolds DJ, Gavaghan DJ, McQuay HJ. Assessing the quality of reports of randomized clinical trials: is blinding necessary? Control Clin Trials 1996;17:1–12.

[49] Jensen MP, Chodroff MJ, Dworkin RH. The impact of neuropathic pain on health-related quality of life: review and implications. Neurology 2007;68:1178–82.

[50] Joseph EK, Chen X, Khasar SG, Levine JD. Novel mechanism of enhanced nociception in a model of AIDS therapy-induced painful peripheral neuropathy in the rat. Pain 2004;107:147–58.

[51] Joseph EK, Levine JD. Mitochondrial electron transport in models of neuropathic and inflammatory pain. Pain 2006;121:105–14.

[52] Kim KJ, Yoon YW, Chung JM. Comparison of three rodent neuropathic pain models. Exp Brain Res 1997;113:200–6.

[53] Kim SH, Chung JM. An experimental model for peripheral neuropathy produced by segmental spinal nerve ligation in the rat. Pain 1992;50:355–63.

[54] King T, Vera-Portocarrero L, Gutierrez T, Vanderah TW, Dussor G, Lai J, Fields HL, Porreca F. Unmasking the tonic-aversive state in neuropathic pain. Nat Neurosci 2009;12:1364–6.

[55] Kola I, Landis J. Can the pharmaceutical industry reduce attrition rates? Nat Rev Drug Discov 2004;3:711–5.

[56] Kontinen VK, Meert TF. Predictive validity of neuropathic pain models in pharmacological studies with a behavioral outcome in the rat: a systematic review. In: Dostrovsky JO, Carr DB, Koltzenburg M, editors. Proceedings of the 10th World Congress on Pain. Seattle: IASP Press; 2003. p. 489–98.

[57] LaBuda CJ, Fuchs PN. Morphine and gabapentin decrease the mechanical hyperalgesia and escape/avoidance behavior in a rat model of neuropathic pain. Neurosci Lett 2000;290:137–40.

[58] LaBuda CJ, Fuchs PN. Place avoidance paradigm: a simple method for measuring the aversive quality of inflammatory and neuropathic pain in rats. Exp Neurol 2000;163:490–4.

[59] Lang L. High clinical trials attrition rate is boosting drug development costs. Gastroenterology 2004;127:1026.

[60] Langford DJ, Bailey AL, Chanda ML, Clarke SE, Drummond TE, Echols S, Glick S, Ingrao J, Klassen-Ross T, Lacroix-Fralish ML, et al. Coding of facial expressions of pain in the laboratory mouse. Nat Methods 2010; in press.

[61] Liberati A, Altman DG, Tetzlaff J, Mulrow C, Gotzsche PC, Ioannidis JP, Clarke M, Devereaux PJ, Kleijnen J, Moher D. The PRISMA statement for reporting systematic reviews and meta-analyses of studies that evaluate health care interventions: explanation and elaboration. PLoS Med 2009;6:e1000100.

[62] Ling B, Authier N, Balayssac D, Eschalier A, Coudore F. Behavioral and pharmacological description of oxaliplatin-induced painful neuropathy in rat. Pain 2007;128:225–34.

[63] Lynch III, Wade CL, Zhong CM, Mikusa JP, Honore P. Attenuation of mechanical allodynia by clinically utilized drugs in a rat chemotherapy-induced neuropathic pain model. Pain 2004;110:56–63.

[64] Macleod MM, Fisher M, O'Collins V, Sena ES, Dirnagl U, Bath PMW, Buchan A, van der Worp HB, Traystman R, Minematsu K, Donnan GA, Howells DW. Good laboratory practice. Preventing introduction of bias at the bench. Stroke 2009;40:e50–e52.

[65] Macleod MR, van der Worp HB, Sena ES, Howells DW, Dirnagl U, Donnan GA. Evidence for the efficacy of NXY-059 in experimental focal cerebral ischaemia is confounded by study quality. Stroke 2008;39:2824–9.

[66] Malcangio M, Tomlinson DR. A pharmacologic analysis of mechanical hyperalgesia in streptozocin/diabetic rats. Pain 1998;76:151–7.

[67] Maratou K, Wallace VC, Hasnie FS, Okuse K, Hosseini R, Jina N, Blackbeard J, Pheby T, Orengo C, Dickenson AH, McMahon SB, Rice ASC. Comparison of dorsal root ganglion gene expression in rat models of traumatic and HIV-associated neuropathic pain. Eur J Pain 2009;13:398.

[68] Matsuzawa-Yanagida K, Narita M, Nakajima M, Kuzumaki N, Niikura K, Nozaki H, Takagi T, Tamai E, Hareyama N, Terada M, et al. Usefulness of antidepressants for improving the neuropathic pain-like state and pain-induced anxiety through actions at different brain sites. Neuropsychopharmacology 2007;33:1952–65.

[69] Maurer K, Bostock H, Koltzenburg M. A rat in vitro model for the measurement of multiple excitability properties of cutaneous axons. Clin Neurophysiol 2007;118:2404–12.

[70] Medhurst SJ, Collins SD, Billinton A, Bingham S, Dalziel RG, Brass A, Roberts JC, Medhurst AD, Chessell IP. Novel histamine H3 receptor antagonists GSK189254 and GSK334429 are efficacious in surgically-induced and virally-induced rat models of neuropathic pain. Pain 2008;138:61–9.

[71] Meyer-Rosberg K, Kvarnstrom A, Kinnman E, Gordh T, Nordfors LO, Kristofferson A. Peripheral neuropathic pain: a multidimensional burden for patients. Eur J Pain 2001;5:379–89.

[72] Mignini LE, Khan KS. Methodological quality of systematic reviews of animal studies: a survey of reviews of basic research. BMC Med Res Methodol 2006;6:10.

[73] Mogil JS. The genetic mediation of individual differences in sensitivity to pain and its inhibition. Proc Natl Acad Sci USA 1999;96:7744–51.

[74] Mogil JS, Chanda ML. The case for the inclusion of female subjects in basic science studies of pain. Pain 2005;117:1–5.

[75] Mogil JS. Animal models of pain: progress and challenges. Nat Rev Neurosci 2009;10:283–94.

[76] Mogil JS, Crager SE. What should we be measuring in behavioral studies of chronic pain in animals? Pain 2004;112:12–5.

[77] Monassi CR, Bandler R, Keay KA. A subpopulation of rats show social and sleep-waking changes typical of chronic neuropathic pain following peripheral nerve injury. Eur J Neurosci 2003;17:1907–20.

[78] Moore RA, Derry S, McQuay HJ, Straube S, Aldington D, Wiffen P, Bell RF, Kalso E, Rowbotham MC. Clinical effectiveness: an approach to clinical trial design more relevant to clinical practice, acknowledging the importance of individual differences. Pain 2009; Epub Sep 10.

[79] Olmarker K, Storkson R, Berge OG. Pathogenesis of sciatic pain: a study of spontaneous behavior in rats exposed to experimental disc herniation. Spine 2002;27:1312–7.

[80] Pedersen LH, Blackburn-Munro G. Pharmacological characterisation of place escape/avoidance behaviour in the rat chronic constriction injury model of neuropathic pain. Psychopharmacology (Berl) 2006;185:208–17.

[81] Pedersen LH, Scheel-Kruger J, Blackburn-Munro G. Amygdala GABA-A receptor involvement in mediating sensory-discriminative and affective-motivational pain responses in a rat model of peripheral nerve injury. Pain 2007;127:17–26.

[82] Perel P, Roberts I, Sena E, Wheble P, Briscoe C, Sandercock P, Macleod M, Mignini LE, Jayaram P, Khan KS. Comparison of treatment effects between animal experiments and clinical trials: systematic review. BMJ 2007;334:197.

[83] Pickering G, Jourdan D, Millecamps M, Chapuy E, Alliot J, Eschalier A. Age-related impact of neuropathic pain on animal behaviour. Eur J Pain 2006;10:749–55.

[84] Rice ASC, Lever IJ, Zarnegar R. Cannabinoids and analgesia, with special reference to neuropathic pain. In: McQuay HJ, Kalso E, Moore RA, editors. Systematic reviews and meta-analyses in pain. Seattle: IASP Press; 2008. p. 233–46.

[85] Rice ASC, Maton S; Postherpetic Neuralgia Study Group. Gabapentin in postherpetic neuralgia; a randomised, double-blind, controlled study. Pain 2001;94:215–24.

[86] Rice ASC, Cimino-Brown D, Eisenach JC, Kontinen VK, Lacroix-Fralish ML, Machin I, Mogil JS, Stöhr T. Animal models and the prediction of efficacy in clinical trials of analgesic drugs: a critical appraisal and call for uniform reporting standards. Pain 2008;139:243–7.

[87] Roeska K, Doods H, Hu B, Kremer A, Treede RD, Ceci A. Anxiety-like behaviour is observed in two rat models of mononeuropathy. Eur J Pain 2007;11:71.

[88] Roeska K, Doods H, Arndt K, Treede RD, Ceci A. Anxiety-like behaviour in rats with mononeuropathy is reduced by the analgesic drugs morphine and gabapentin. Pain 2008;139:349–57.

[89] Rolke R, Baron R, Maier C, Tölle TR, Treede RD, Beyer A, Binder A, Birbaumer N, Birklein F, Botefur IC. Quantitative sensory testing in the German Research Network on Neuropathic Pain (DFNS): standardized protocol and reference values. Pain 2006;123:231–43.

[90] Rolke R, Magerl W, Campbell KA, Schalber C, Caspari S, Birklein F, Treede RD. Quantitative sensory testing: a comprehensive protocol for clinical trials. Eur J Pain 2006;10:77–88.

[91] Rowbotham MC. The case for publishing 'negative' clinical trials. Pain 2009;146:225–6.

[92] Scholz J, Mannion RJ, Hord DE, Griffin RS, Rawal B, Zheng H, Scoffings D, Phillips A, Guo J, Laing RJC, et al. A novel tool for the assessment of pain: validation in low back pain. PLoS Med 2009;6:e1000047.

[93] Schulz KF, Altman DG, Moher D, for the CONSORT Group. CONSORT 2010 statement: updated guidelines for reporting parallel group randomised trials. PLoS Med 2010;7:e1000251.

[94] Scott FT, Leedham-Green ME, Barrett-Muir WY, Hawrami K, Gallagher WJ, Johnson R, Breuer J. A study of shingles and the development of postherpetic neuralgia in East London. J Med Virol 2003;70(Suppl 1):S24–S30.

[95] Seltzer Z, Dubner R, Shir Y. A novel behavioral model of neuropathic pain disorders produced in rats by partial sciatic nerve injury. Pain 1990;43:205–18.

[96] Sena E, van der Worp HB, Howells D, Macleod M. How can we improve the pre-clinical development of drugs for stroke? Trends Neurosci 2007;30:433–9.

[97] Sena E, Wheble P, Sandercock P, Macleod M. Systematic review and meta-analysis of the efficacy of tirilazad in experimental stroke. Stroke 2007;38:388–94.

[98] Serra J. Microneurography: an opportunity for translational drug development in neuropathic pain. Neurosci Lett 2010;470:155–7.

[99] Serra J, Bostock H, Navarro X. Microneurography in rats: a minimally invasive method to record single C-fiber action potentials from peripheral nerves in vivo. Neurosci Lett 2010;470:168–74.

[100] Vierck CJ, Acosta-Rua AJ, Johnson RD. Bilateral chronic constriction of the sciatic nerve: a model of long-term cold hyperalgesia. J Pain 2005;6:507–17.

[101] Vierck CJ, Hansson PT, Yezierski RP. Clinical and pre-clinical pain assessment: are we measuring the same thing? Pain 2008;135:7–10.

[102] Vierck CJ, Jr., Kline R, Wiley RG. Comparison of operant escape and innate reflex responses to nociceptive skin temperatures produced by heat and cold stimulation of rats. Behav Neurosci 2004;118:627–35.

[103] Vierck CJ, Acosta-Rua A, Nelligan R, Tester N, Mauderli A. Low dose systemic morphine attenuates operant escape but facilitates innate reflex responses to thermal stimulation. J Pain 2002;3:309–19.

[104] Walf AA, Frye CA. The use of the elevated plus maze as an assay of anxiety-related behavior in rodents. Nat Protocols 2007;2:322–8.

[105] Wallace VC, Segerdahl AR, Blackbeard J, Pheby T, Rice AS. Anxiety-like behaviour is attenuated by gabapentin, morphine and diazepam in a rodent model of HIV anti-retroviral-associated neuropathic pain. Neurosci Lett 2008;448:153–6.

[106] Wallace VCJ, Segerdahl AR, Lambert DM, Vandevoorde S, Blackbeard J, Pheby T, Hasnie F, Rice ASC. The effect of the palmitoylethanolamide analogue, palmitoylallylamide (L-29) on pain behaviour in rodent models of neuropathy. Br J Pharmacol 2007;151:1117–28.

[107] Wallace VCJ, Blackbeard J, Segerdahl A, Hasnie FS, Pheby T, McMahon SB, Rice ASC. Characterisation of rodent models of HIV-gp120 and anti-retroviral associated neuropathic pain. Brain 2007;130:2688–702.

[108] Wallace VCJ, Blackbeard J, Pheby T, Segerdahl AR, Davies M, Hasnie F, Hall S, McMahon SB, Rice ASC. Pharmacological, behavioural and mechanistic analysis of HIV-1 gp120 induced painful neuropathy. Pain 2007;133:47–63.

[109] Wallace VCJ, Norbury TA, Rice ASC. Ultrasound vocalisation by rodents does not correlate with behavioural measures of persistent pain. Eur J Pain 2005;9:445–52.

[110] Whiteside GT, Adedoyin A, Leventhal L. Predictive validity of animal pain models? A comparison of the pharmacokinetic-pharmacodynamic relationship for pain drugs in rats and humans. Neuropharmacology 2008;54:767–75.

[111] Willner P. Animal models of depression: an overview. Pharmacol Ther 1990;45:425–55.

[112] Wilson SG, Smith SB, Chesler EJ, Melton KA, Haas JJ, Mitton B, Strasburg K, Hubert L, Rodriguez-Zas SL, Mogil JS. The heritability of antinociception: common pharmacogenetic mediation of five neurochemically distinct analgesics. J Pharmacol Exp Ther 2003;304:547–59.

Correspondence to: Prof. Andrew S.C. Rice, Department of Anaesthetics, Pain Medicine and Intensive Care, Imperial College London, Chelsea & Westminster Hospital Campus, 369 Fulham Road, London SW10 9NH, United Kingdom. Email: a.rice@imperial.ac.uk.

From "First-in-Human" Trials to Efficacy in Patients: Identifying Tomorrow's Analgesics in a Sea of Failed Optimism

John P. Huggins, PhD

Pfizer Pharmatherapeutics, Sandwich, Kent, United Kingdom

There are few examples from the last century of medically used analgesics that have been discovered and developed from first principles. Opiates and nonsteroidal anti-inflammatory drugs (NSAIDs) obviously predate the modern scientific era, although, arguably, many of the newer agents and formulations have improved dosing frequency and patient acceptability. Gabapentin [5] and duloxetine [69] were originally developed for their antiepileptic properties and antidepressant properties, respectively. Pregabalin [66], ziconotide [54], and selective cyclooxygenase (COX)-2 inhibitors [53] are probably the best examples of the success of the thousands of human-years' effort within academia and industry to deliver novel analgesics to patients in need. (The development of tanezumab, a neutralizing antibody to nerve growth factor, may be the next example [11].) At the same time there has been a quantum increase in molecular and functional science over the last decade or so. What can be learned from this mountain of effort to more effectively apply scientific advances to address the misery caused by pain in patients?

Proof of Concept

"Proof of concept" (PoC) is a widely employed, but often poorly defined, term within the pharmaceutical world; it is a landmark in the development of any novel drug. It is best defined in terms of risk and will be used here (with application to pain) as "the point at which sufficient evidence has been accrued to justify the (enormous) expense associated with large dose-setting, efficacy and safety trials in patients suffering from pain" (formally, Phase 2b and Phase 3 trials). Such an apparently loose definition is ironically helpful, as making decisions on the type of data that is critical for PoC to be "declared" forces an evaluation of what is most likely to fail ("attrition") for any particular novel analgesic. In turn, this evaluation drives the clinical development plan for any particular novel potential analgesic agent. Traditionally, attrition has occurred mainly because of one of three factors: (1) pharmacokinetics that are too poor to be associated with clinically acceptable dosing paradigms; (2) safety issues that have either not been observed from preclinical testing, or were observed, but the safety margin in humans proved smaller than hoped (transient receptor potential V1 [TRPV1] antagonists were an example of potential analgesics falling into this category [38]); or (3) failure to demonstrate efficacy in patients in the manner hypothesized from preclinical models. The history of neurokinin-1 antagonists is a well-publicized example of such a failure, but it may actually be unusual in only one respect: that it has been openly reported [36] (see the chapter in this volume by A.S.C. Rice).

Pain 2010—An Updated Review: Refresher Course Syllabus
edited by Jeffrey S. Mogil
IASP Press, Seattle, © 2010

427

If the novel analgesic being developed acts by a mechanism with clear clinical precedent, then the chances of failure of efficacy are evidently much lower, and if it has a chemotype similar to drugs that have been used with an acceptable safety profile in millions of patients, failure due to safety is evidently a lower hurdle. However, both of these statements have to be balanced by an ever-rising (and arguably unrealistic) societal demand for higher burdens of proof in both of these domains. By contrast, for potential analgesics working through novel mechanisms there is a high probability of attrition when a drug is tested for the first time in patients. Given the low responder rates for existing analgesics (see, e.g., ref. [35]), it seems likely that major leaps in therapeutic benefit for patients in chronic pain are most likely to be achieved from exploiting novel mechanisms and drug targets, and as such, solutions to the Phase 2 attrition problem are urgently required. This subject extends beyond the scope of this chapter, but there are three elements that will be included that help.

First, examination of drugs acting on mechanisms where pharmacology was demonstrated in humans prior to testing in patient efficacy trials shows that these drugs survive more often than those where no pharmacology was demonstrated (see ref. [70]). This may simply be because tolerability concerns have prevented sufficient exposure at the target site and so efficacious doses have not been achieved in patients. One error that has widely been used in this area is the use of drug exposure goals in humans derived from *minimally* effective doses in pain animal models. Such an approach evidently predisposes early clinical trials toward likely failure owing to insufficient exposure of the individual to the drug under examination.

Second, because clinical trials in patients are not normally aimed at achieving regulatory approval, it is financially and ethically beneficial to explore options for novel trial designs in PoC studies. Some examples will be given here, and the material in the chapter by S. Quessy in this volume is also relevant to this discussion.

Third, nonpublication of failed clinical trials on potential analgesics (either due to the effect on investor perception or due to the bias of journal policies) may have driven widespread redundancy of effort in the drive to develop novel analgesics. Worse still, if pharmacology cannot be demonstrated in humans and a clinical trial of a compound working through a novel mechanism fails, it is impossible to

determine whether future intellectual or financial investment in that target is of value. In other words, is the failure of (animal or human) models that predicted success caused by differences in the inability of the drug to affect the target sufficiently or by the target not being sufficiently important in affecting mechanisms underlying pain in patients?

Purpose and Design of Phase 1 Studies

Phase 1 clinical trials are uniformly designed to gradually increase exposure in terms of time, dose, and subject numbers in order to understand more about a potential drug's tolerability and absorption, distribution, metabolism, and excretion prior to dosing to patients. Although in some areas of high medical need, typically in oncology trials, novel agents are dosed directly to patients after preclinical testing, this strategy is often considered ethically unjustified for patients in pain, although it is theoretically possible to imagine a case for it if a drug target were overexpressed in patients compared to healthy volunteers, for example.

As described above, there has been increasing focus on measuring biomarkers in human studies to determine whether exposures that elicit pharmacological effects are achieved in Phase 1 studies [26,70]. According to the Biomarkers Definitions Working Group, initiated by the U.S. National Institutes of Health, a biomarker is defined as "a characteristic that is objectively measured and evaluated as an indicator of normal biological processes, pathogenic processes, or pharmacologic responses to a therapeutic intervention" [7]. As such, it may reflect simply the ability of a novel analgesic to interact with its target; technologies such as positron emission tomography would provide a particular good exemplar for such an approach [20]. Of more value, however, is a demonstration that a novel analgesic has an effect on the pathway that is hypothesized to be important in pain patients in order to demonstrate analgesic efficacy. This leads directly into the field of experimental pain in healthy volunteers.

Experimental Pain Models

A complete description of all the models of experimental models of pain that have been developed in humans is well beyond the scope of this chapter, but recent reviews are recommended as an introduction to the field [4,15,17].

The third molar extraction model employs volunteers with recurrent pericoronitis associated with lower third molars, who have one or both of the offending teeth removed, and pain is monitored as local anesthesia dissipates after administration of either an experimental drug or placebo [12]. The advantages of the model are its acceptability to the U.S. Food and Drug Administration (FDA) and the European Medicines Agency (EMEA) as a clinical model of acute pain, as well as its responsiveness to agents affecting prostaglandin pathways [12]. Its disadvantages are that it does not involve severe pain, it may underreport the effects of analgesics effective in severe pain (such as opiates) relative to NSAIDs [56], and it requires quite large numbers of patients (typically 50 subjects/arm) to observe effects, making it an expensive option unless the final therapeutic goal for registration is acute pain. Interestingly, recent reports suggest that implementation of more careful surgical techniques and sequential removal of each impacted lower third molar enable crossover designs that dramatically reduce variability and hence the number of subjects required for a study (M. Howard, unpublished observations; see also below).

A similar, but more severe, model of acute postoperative pain is the bunionectomy model [21]. Both third molar extraction and bunionectomy models are aiming to directly demonstrate effects on pain in subjects, either as a step toward registration for acute pain, or as a step in reducing the likelihood of failure in patients with acute postinflammatory pain (e.g., osteoarthritis pain) in potential analgesics affecting inflammatory (especially prostaglandin-mediated) pathways.

Laser- or heat-evoked pain responses (and laser-evoked potentials) have similarly been used to demonstrate effects of opiates in healthy volunteers [52,61]. An additional model of relevance here is the cold pressor test [39], in which subjects immerse their hands in water at 4°C for 2 minutes and self-reported pain is measured with a visual analogue scale (VAS); this test is similarly reported to be sensitive to opiates [39].

One of the issues with the aforementioned models is that they attempt to detect and quantify effects of novel analgesics on relatively normal, acute pain pathways and, indeed, producing models in healthy human subjects that reflect chronic pain states without creating chronic pain for the volunteers (a self-evidently unacceptable sequela) has been a major challenge for all investigators working in this area.

Three approaches of note have been employed to try to address this issue:

1) *Establish translationally viable techniques that interrogate specific parts of the pain pathway that are hypothesized to be involved in chronic pain.* An example of this approach is determination of capsaicin-induced hyperemia, measured using a scanning laser Doppler of the volar forearm [75]. (The capsaicin is applied topically in alcohol or as a cream and elicits no or minimal pain.) Effectively, the technique measures C-fiber sensory activation and transmission via an axon reflex to cutaneous blood vessels; mast cell activation may also be involved. This technique is sufficiently reproducible in humans in a crossover setting that effects may be observed with a reasonable number of subjects [75]. It is sensitive to pharmacological challenge—calcitonin gene-related peptide (CGRP) and TRPV1 antagonists both give effects [16,76]—and it can be established in rodents and nonhuman primates so that novel mechanisms can be tested prior to studies in human subjects. As such, this simple model is probably one of the best-performing of all human experimental pain models.

2) *Induce short-term hypersensitivity in human subjects that may mimic some of the characteristics of longer-term hypersensitivity (hyperalgesia and allodynia) in chronic pain patients.* This goal has been a major focus of human experimental pain research for many years. Again, only a few examples will be given here to illustrate the point. The best-known example of induced hypersensitivity is by application of capsaicin, either by intradermal injection (see Table I) or by dermal application, in conjunction with heat application from a thermode [60]. As well as the intense pain caused by intradermal injection, ongoing brush and von Frey hair or pinprick hyperalgesia is created for a period of time in the area around the injection or capsaicin/heat application site. Although this "model" is well known, it suffers from an issue that is somewhat typical of research in the human experimental pain area, which represents both a need and an opportunity for the field to progress. This issue is the wide variability of methodologies used between, and even within, groups (see Table I), making comparative pharmacology difficult to assess from the literature. The differences include different amounts, sources, sites, and vehicle for injected capsaicin; varying times of administration and doses of test drugs post-capsaicin; and varying endpoints and ways of measuring them. The opportunity here is for

Table I
Summary of publications on the intradermal capsaicin model between 1995 and 2004, highlighting methodological variability

Capsaicin Concentration	Injection Site	Drugs Tested	Notes	Ref.
250 µg/25 µL		Alfentanil, ketamine	Both drugs reduce spontaneous pain, punctate hyperalgesia, and dynamic allodynia	59
300 µg/50 µL in polysorbate 80	Volar forearm	Dextromethorphan	No significant effect	40
100 µg/10 µL 20% cyclodextrin	Volar forearm	Lidocaine	Crossover design; large effects on secondary hyperalgesia	79
100 µg/10 µL in polysorbate 80	Volar forearm or lateral calf	Alfentanil, amitriptyline		25
300 µg in 50 µL		Morphine	Von Frey hair area substantially reduced	41
10 µg in 10 µL	Volar forearm	Ondansetron		28
250 µg/25 µL	Volar forearm	Alfentanil, ketamine and combination	No placebos used	68
100 µg/10 µL	Lateral calf	Intrathecal and intravenous clonidine	Only high intrathecal dose affects area of hyperalgesia	23
100 µg/20 µL in polysorbate 80	Volar forearm	Ketamine, lidocaine	Small effect sizes	30
100 µg/20 µL in polysorbate 80	Volar forearm	Lidocaine	Small effect sizes	45
100 µg/10 µL in polysorbate 80	Volar forearm or lateral calf	Clonidine	Large effects on area of hyperalgesia	24
100 µg/20 µL in polysorbate 80	Forearm	Lidocaine, ketamine	Good reproducibility and effect sizes	29
100 µg/10 µL 20% cyclodextrin	Volar forearm	Mexiletine	Effect on punctate allodynia only	1
100 µg/10 µL 20% cyclodextrin	Volar forearm	Alfentanil, ketamine	Large effects	81
100 µg/10 µL 20% cyclodextrin		Alfentanil, ketamine	As Wallace et al. [81], plus effects on spontaneous pain	78
100 µg/10 µL 20% cyclodextrin	Volar forearm	Desipramine	No significant effects of drugs	77
250 µg/25 µL 7.5% polysorbate 80	Volar forearm	None		37
100 µg/10 µL 20% cyclodextrin	Volar forearm	Lamotrigine, 4030W92	Crossover design	80
100 µg/20 µL 20% polysorbate 80 (heated)	Volar forearm	Gabapentin	Von Frey hair area slightly reduced	31

academic and industrial experts to agree and publish model methodology in sufficient detail such that statistical and pharmacological properties of a particular model can be established across sites. The interest in the capsaicin-hyperalgesia models is the belief that the secondary hyperalgesia produced by capsaicin involves central sensitization [44], although this view is not unchallenged [67].

At informal precompetitive gatherings of industry experts in the United Kingdom in 2008 and 2009, involving representatives from most pharmaceutical companies active in pain research (including some that are no longer), wide agreement was expressed on

simple criteria for a successful human experimental pain model to make it of value in drug development for chronic pain. The model needs to:

• Be sufficiently reproducible to demonstrate effects in "small" numbers of subjects (certainly no more than 24 volunteers in a crossover design);

• Be sufficiently well described that it can be repeated at different sites across the world (many models fail at this hurdle);

• Show reproducible and comprehensible modulation by pharmacological agents in an exposure-dependent manner (comprehensible does necessarily not mean "the same as in a particular type of patient," but understandably representing a pathway in a manner that can be understood from a mechanistic viewpoint);

• Be mimicked in preclinical models (preferably) and so be translatable in this sense;

• Act via a mechanism known to be affected in chronic pain patients.

There are no human experimental pain models that pass all of these criteria. However, two additional models have been identified in this category that may be of particular potential for drug development. The first model is that of electrically induced hyperalgesia (see Table II), which, although being more technically demanding, appears to offer more predictable pharmacology and reliability. Again, there is evidence from elegant experiments using local anesthetics that the hyperalgesia evoked by this model has a central origin [42]. The second model is that of ultraviolet (UV) light-induced burn and hyperalgesia (essentially experimentally induced sunburn). There is controversy over the ability to detect secondary hyperalgesia in this model [8,32,34], and the effect size may not be large enough to demonstrate exposure-dependent effects, but the model nevertheless looks promising [8,71]. The TRPV1 antagonist, SB-705498, was shown to increase heat pain tolerance at the site of UV inflammation [16].

3) *Focus on mechanism in patients.* This approach has obvious advantages, but it clearly requires accessibility to patients. Three approaches here are noteworthy. The first is the magnificent efforts of the German Neuropathic Pain Network to establish quantitative sensory testing techniques in a reproducible manner to understand and measure specific pain phenotypes in patients with neuropathic pain [62]. However, to my knowledge, such an approach has not been used to date in the development of any novel analgesic, and it poses a strong challenge to regulatory authorities and to medical practice. To wit, if an agent were found that affected some pain phenotypes but not others, how would this be viewed by these two parties, and is the pain community (industrial and academic) sufficiently flexible to develop such an agent to provide value for patients? The second approach is direct recordings of individual axonal activity by raster analysis via microneurography recordings from the vicinity of peripheral nerves in patients [57]. While the advantages of this technique are obvious from a transitional perspective (the human equivalent of electrophysiology in animal species), there are practical issues with this approach, namely that there are very few trained or sufficiently

patient microneurography experts in the world, and analysis of recordings is time-consuming. Nevertheless the Pain Consortium within the European Union's Innovative Medicines Initiative is investing in this area to determine whether patient recordings of ectopia provide insights into disease mechanisms. The third approach is neuroimaging, especially fMRI, which is discussed in more detail below.

Approaches to Efficient Proof-of-Concept Clinical Trials in Patients

Some time ago, PoC trials were sometimes referred to as "pilot studies" and were effectively small, underpowered clinical trials from which researchers would attempt to guess whether or not novel agents were likely to be effective in properly designed clinical trials. Human optimism ensured that slight signals, often in secondary endpoints, were overinterpreted, which in turn fueled a flurry of eventually pointless activity.

As also discussed in the accompanying chapter by S. Quessy, the appropriate statistical and clinical design of genuine PoC studies for novel potential analgesics requires several factors to coincide: appropriate dose selection, a balance between "ideal" patients and those who can realistically be recruited, careful analysis of historical data to determine variability and effect sizes, interim analyses to stop or resize the study if (for example) the drug performs better or worse than expected, and predetermined decision-making criteria to ensure that the efficacy achieved can be interpreted without undue influence from unfounded optimism, given that so much effort and funds have been invested to progress a novel molecule to this point.

The greatest reason for attrition in the pharmaceutical pipeline at this time is failure of compounds to demonstrate efficacy when first tested in patients [43]. For those compounds, where good pharmacokinetic and toleration profiles have enabled patient exposures that elicit pharmacology, and yet efficacy is still not observed, this attrition represents a real failure in the science of pain. In many cases, the target affected by the compound will have been selected based on an apparently sound mechanistic basis, bearing in mind results from pharmacological or genetic manipulation in so-called animal models of disease, and it is essential that results of such studies are published and that the pain community is able to reflect and improve scientific understanding to learn from these failures. One way of improving target selection to reduce attrition in PoC clinical trials is to select targets based on knowledge of the biology of patients, rather than the biology of animals. Such information is gleaned from prior precedence with analgesics, genetics, and functional information from physiological studies all in patients themselves.

Two consequences of high attrition at PoC are: (a) that PoC studies should be as simple (i.e., inexpensive) as possible whilst allowing statistically valid decision-making and (b) that the decision-making must be quantitatively sound so that failing compounds are not endlessly tested in different patient populations, with a hope that they "might work somewhere."

The need for simple studies has prompted a number of generally held (but nevertheless controversial in some cases) principles for PoC studies:

1) Given the first principles of clinical trials and the well-described placebo effects [19] in pain trials, all trials should be placebo controlled (as well as fully randomized and blinded, of course); efforts to reduce the placebo effect (an example is given below) should be included in these trials, even if not viable for later-stage trials.

Table II
Pharmacological responses reported in the electrically induced hyperalgesia model

Drug Tested	Pain Rating (NRS)	Area of Hyperalgesia	Area of Dynamic (Brush) Allodynia	Flare Area
Alfentanil i.v. [47]	↓↓↓	↓↓	↓↓	↓
S-ketamine i.v. [47][a]	↓↓↓	↓↓↓	↓↓↓	↓
Lidocaine i.v. [47]	↓	↓↓	↓↓	↓↓
Lidocaine i.d. (microdialysis) [42]	No data	→	→	↓↓↓
Remifentanil i.v. or Naloxone i.v.[b] [33]	↓↓[c] →	↓↓ →	↓↓ →	Not done
Remifentanil i.v. or S-ketamine i.v. Remifentanil + S-ketamine i.v. or Remifentanil + clonidine i.v. [50]	↓↓↓ ↓↓ ↓↓↓ ↓↓↓[d]	↓↓ ↓ ↓↓↓[d] ↓[d]	↓↓ ↓ ↓↓↓[d] ↓↓↓[d]	Not done
S-ketamine i.v. or Placebo i.v. + S-ketamine i.v. or Placebo/remifentanil i.v. + S-ketamine i.v. [46]	Not done	↓↓ ↓↓ ↓↓↓[d]	Not done	Not done
Naloxone i.v. [48][e]	↓	→	→	Not done
Parecoxib i.v. [51]	→	↓↓	↓↓	↓
Paracetamol i.v. [51]	→	↓↓	↓↓	↓
Adenosine i.v. [13]	→	↓↓[f]	↓	→
Buprenorphine i.v. [49]	↓↓	↓↓↓	Not done	Not done
Buprenorphine s.l. [49]	↓	↓↓	Not done	Not done
Pregabalin oral 1 wk [14]	(↓)	↓↓	↓↓	Not done
Aprepitant oral 6 days [14]	(↓)	→	↓	Not done
Parecoxib i.v. plus pregabalin oral 1 wk or Aprepitant oral 6 days [14]	Effect of parecoxib not separated in analysis			Not done
Remifentanil i.v. or Remifentanil + parecoxib (predosed or during electrical stimulation)[g] [2,74]	↓	↓↓	Not done	Not done
Morphine i.v. or Alfentanil i.v. [63]	↓↓↓[c] ↓↓↓	↓[c] ↓	Not done	Not done
Gabapentin oral, single/multiple dose (1 day)[h] [65]	Not done	↓	Not done	Not done

Abbreviations: i.d.: intradermal; i.v.: intravenous; NRS: pain assessed using a numerical rating scale.

[a] May have been functionally unblinded from adverse events (e.g., 12/12 hypacusis).

[b] Hyperalgesia in area of pain and hyperalgesia after stopping infusion of either drug.

[c] Dose-dependent.

[d] Rebound hyperalgesia post-remifentanil blocked by ketamine [2,50] and clonidine [50].

[e] Naloxone reduced intraperiod rundown of NRS and hyperalgesic area, viewed as reducing descending inhibition; interperiod rundown was not affected (but naloxone was not given between periods).

[f] Smaller effect on second period.

[g] Pretreatment with parecoxib prevented rebound hyperalgesia.

[h] Current titration performed after dosing suggests possible flaw in design.

2) Comparators should not be included in PoC trials. Rather, decision rules should be built on historical effect sizes where available and possible. Non-inferiority designs should be avoided (they are "expensive" on patients and require difficult judgements about acceptable margins of inferiority). Active controls may be of value, just to ensure that the study design has yielded a useable result, but any conclusions made from such controls should be absorbed into the effect size used for comparative purposes, such as with a Bayesian approach.

3) Statistical approaches such as Bayesian statistics should be considered with an open mind for PoC trials, even when they are rarely adopted in later-phase clinical trials because of non-acceptance by regulatory authorities. Similarly, novel designs that use, for example, much shorter durations of exposure than later-stage trials should be carefully employed. The guiding principle in trial design should be a "no-regrets" policy. In other words, if the novel compound proves inefficacious in the PoC trial, post hoc arguments cannot be used to argue that this result was because of issues in trial design. (This statement should be used to drive not conservatism, but innovation.)

4) The number of dosing arms used in PoC trials should be minimized. Even the use of a model-based approach to determining significance in a multi-dose trial will have less significance at any one particular dose than if all patients were randomized to just placebo or one dose of active treatment. There may, however, be good reasons for including more than one dose of "active" in a PoC trial, for example if there are issues around expected toleration or compliance at the highest dose.

5) The number of endpoints should be carefully controlled in such studies. There is value in working with fewer study centers to include endpoints that could never be entertained in huge multi-continent later-phase trials, yet practical experience continually teaches us that trials with too many trial endpoints fail (for example, because patients refuse to answer all the questions in an "encyclopedia" of patient-reported outcomes), that some endpoints of great potential value in later stage trials have insufficient power for their inclusion to be of value (many patient-reported outcome questionnaires and most health-economic measures fall into this category), and that we are continually confused by trial outcomes where the primary outcome fails but secondary outcomes succeed (for example, is this outcome the result of not correcting for endpoint multiplicity?).

6) Tolerability compared to "standard of care" can rarely be quantitatively assessed from adverse event frequencies in PoC trials, because patient numbers needed for even fairly frequent adverse events are much larger than can usually be afforded for such trials. Therefore, if tolerability is the area that is likely to result in differentiation of a new agent from an existing medication, more specialized "niche" studies and techniques are called for, such as cognitive testing batteries [18].

The above rules are all open to interpretation for any particular study and will not apply for all drugs in development. If a company is developing a novel opiate formulation, for example, then sufficient pharmacokinetics and results in experimental pain models may well justify direct progression to large multidose clinical trials, or at least a seamless trial design where a positive PoC result immediately triggers an expansion of patients numbers into such a Phase 2b design.

One example of the valuable use of "nonstandard" clinical designs for PoC trials that has proven beneficial is the use of crossover rather than parallel-group designs [27]. Because intrasubject variability in pain score assessment is smaller than intersubject assessment, greater power can be achieved in such studies than from more traditional parallel group designs; evidence to date suggests that period effects are sufficiently reliable that they can be corrected for, and carryover does not prove to be a problem. Whether such designs can be generalized to all patient groups remains to be seen. Obviously, a crossover design is only applicable for a drug with a reasonably short pharmacokinetic and pharmacodynamic washout period; biologics, for example, cannot normally be tested using this method. Another example is that subjects can be administered placebo prior to and after the treatment period, and blinded not only to their randomization within the treatment period but also to when they are switched to active drug. Such an approach has given a remarkable reduction of the placebo effect (presumably because of inability to anticipate analgesia) in some cases (F. Hackman, Z. Ali, private communications).

Novel Approaches for Tomorrow's Analgesics

A chapter of this kind would not be complete without reference to neuroimaging of the brain, in particular functional magnetic resonance imaging (fMRI; spinal cord fMRI is still challenging due to resolution and movement artefacts). So-called blood oxygenation level-dependent (BOLD) fMRI has been used for some time to demonstrate the existence of a number of brain regions that are activated in painful conditions [3]. Because of the signal : noise ratio in BOLD fMRI, and the fact that the output is relative, not absolute, this technology is best at quantitating responses to repeated painful stimuli, although Apkarian has used an ingenious variant of the technique to detect natural variability in ongoing pain [6]. Of great interest, however, is an emerging technology known as arterial spin-labeling (ASL), which directly measures blood flow responses throughout the brain in absolute terms and so has the potential to be a physiological measure of ongoing pain [58,73]. To date, however, the vast majority of fMRI studies have been performed in healthy volunteers in whom pain is elicited intermittently as described above. In those studies examining pain in patients, differences in brain activation associated with pain in these patients compared to healthy volunteers have been spatially quite subtle (see, e.g., refs. [22] and [64]).

Interest in this field for drug development is driven by three main factors. First, fMRI has the potential to be used as a functional biomarker of central activity for a drug whose putative action is in the brain; second, it could be used as an efficacy readout that may determine likely efficacy from studies involving small numbers of patients; and third, it could be used to better understand pain pathways that should be targeted to yield better analgesics in the future (see refs. [9,72]). However, many challenges remain, not least how to derive straightforward decisions ("Should drug X be continued to the next stage of development or not?") from the complexity of data that emerges from whole-brain voxelwise analysis. Even simple questions such as "What is the best way to summarize brain activation in a particular region of interest?" are remarkably complex, and further work is needed in terms of improved functional understanding and mathematical analysis to evolve decision-making algorithms for drug development [55]. Despite these unanswered questions, it seems intuitively obvious to many in the field that a physiological measure of pain that is less reliant on other factors of how a patient completes a pain questionnaire would be a quantum step forward.

Conclusions

The early development of potential new analgesics is an area that requires innovation to ensure that in the future such work unequivocally establishes at least pharmacology, and preferably functional activity, in human subjects prior to initiation of PoC studies. Also, PoC studies must be designed innovatively and wisely, both to maximize the chances of identifying novel analgesics and to stop work on those that are doomed to fail. Notwithstanding the reasonable bounds of commercial secrecy, there is a need for openness and collaboration to understand and standardize human experimental pain models, and to much better understand the pathways and their molecular attributes to steer us all toward targets that will yield less attrition than has hitherto been observed. Most of all, there is a strong need for a better understanding of patient pathophysiology to select targets and drugs more likely to succeed, and all parties involved need to commit to full publication of results of both negative and positive early clinical trials, in order that as a pain community we may serve the patients in our corporate care better in the future than they have been in the past [10].

References

[1]   Ando K, Wallace MS, Braun J, Schulteis G. Effect of oral mexiletine on capsaicin-induced allodynia and hyperalgesia: a double-blind, placebo-controlled, crossover study. Reg Anaesth Pain Med 2000;25:468–74.

[2]   Angst MS, Koppert W, Pahl I, Clark DJ, Schmelz M. Short-term infusion of the μ-opioid agonist remifentanil in humans causes hyperalgesia during withdrawal. Pain 2003;106:49–57.

[3]   Apkarian AV, Bushnell MC, Treede RD, Zubieta JK. Human brain mechanisms of pain perception and regulation in health and disease. Eur J Pain 2005;9:463–84.

[4]   Arendt-Nielsen L, Curatolo M, Drewes A. Human experimental pain models in drug development: translational pain research. Curr Opin Investig Drugs 2007;8:41–53.

[5]   Backonja M, Glanzman RL. Gabapentin dosing for neuropathic pain: evidence from randomized, placebo-controlled clinical trials. Clin Ther 2003;25:81–104.

[6]   Baliki MN, Geha PY, Jabakhanji R, Harden N, Schnitzer TJ, Apkarian AV. A preliminary fMRI study of analgesic treatment in chronic back pain and knee osteoarthritis. Mol Pain 2008;4:47.

[7]   Biomarkers Definitions Working Group. Biomarkers and surrogate endpoints: preferred definitions and conceptual framework. Clin Pharmacol Ther 2001;69:89–95.

[8]   Bishop T, Ballard A, Holmes H, Young AR, McMahon SB. Ultraviolet-B induced inflammation of human skin: Characterisation and comparison with traditional models of hyperalgesia. Eur J Pain 2009;13:524–32.

[9]   Borsook D, Ploghaus A, Becerra L. Utilizing brain imaging for analgesic drug development. Curr Opin Invest Drugs 2002;3:1342–7.

[10]   Breivik H, Collett B, Ventafridda V, Cohen R, Gallacher D. Survey of chronic pain in Europe: prevalence, impact on daily life, and treatment. Eur J Pain 2006;10:287–333.

[11]   Cattaneo A. Tanezumab, a recombinant humanized mAb against nerve growth factor for the treatment of acute and chronic pain. Curr Opin Mol Ther 2010;12:94–106.

[12]   Chen LC, Elliott RA, Ashcroft DM. Systematic review of the analgesic efficacy and tolerability of COX-2 inhibitors in post-operative pain control. J Clin Pharm Ther 2004;29:215–29.

[13] Chizh BA, Dusch M, Puthawala M, Schmelz M, Cookson LM, Martina R, Brown J, Koppert W. The effect of intravenous infusion of adenosine on electrically evoked hyperalgesia in a healthy volunteer model of central sensitisation. Anesth Analg 2004;99:816–22.

[14] Chizh BA, Gohring M, Troster A, Quartey GK, Schmelz M, Koppert W. Effects of oral pregabalin and aprepitant on pain and central sensitization in the electrical hyperalgesia model in human volunteers. Br J Anaesth 2007;98:246–54.

[15] Chizh BA, Hobson AR. Using objective markers and imaging in the development of novel treatment of chronic pain. Expert Rev Neurother 2007;7:443–7.

[16] Chizh BA, O'Donnell MB, Napolitano A, Wang J, Brooke AC, Aylott MC, Bullman JN, Gray EJ, Lai RY, Williams PM, Appleby JM. The effects of the TRPV1 antagonist SB-705498 on TRPV1 receptor-mediated activity and inflammatory hyperalgesia in humans. Pain 2007;132:132–41.

[17] Chizh BA, Priestley T, Rowbotham M, Schaffler K. Predicting therapeutic efficacy: experimental pain in human subjects. Brain Res Rev 2009;60:243–54.

[18] Collie A, Darekar A, Weissgerber G, Toh MK, Snyder PJ, Maruff P, Huggins JP. Cognitive testing in early-phase clinical trials: development of a rapid computerized test battery and application in a simulated Phase I study. Contemp Clin Trials 2007;28:391–400.

[19] Colloca L, Benedetti F. Placebos and painkillers: is mind as real as matter? Nat Rev Neurosci 2005;6:545–52.

[20] Comar D. PET for drug development and education. Dordrecht: Kluwer Academic; 1995.

[21] Desjardins PJ, Shu VS, Recker DP, Verburg KM, Woolf CJ. A single preoperative oral dose of valdecoxib, a new cyclooxygenase-2 specific inhibitor, relieves post-oral surgery or bunionectomy pain. Anesthesiology 2002;97:565–73.

[22] Dunkley P, Wise RG, Fairhurst M, Hobden P, Aziz Q, Chang L, Tracey I. A comparison of visceral and somatic pain processing in the human brainstem using functional magnetic resonance imaging. J Neurosci 2005;25:7333–41.

[23] Eisenach JC, Hood DD, Curry R. Intrathecal, but not intravenous, clonidine reduces experimental thermal or capsaicin-induced pain and hyperalgesia in normal volunteers. Anesth Analg 1998;87:591–6.

[24] Eisenach JC, Hood DD, Curry R. Relative potency of epidural to intrathecal clonidine differs between acute thermal pain and capsaicin-induced allodynia. Pain 2000;84:57–64.

[25] Eisenach JC, Hood DD, Curry R, Tong C. Alfentanil, but not amitriptyline, reduces pain, hyperalgesia, and allodynia from intradermal injection of capsaicin in humans. Anesthesiology 1997;86:1279–87.

[26] Frank R, Hargreaves R. Clinical biomarkers and drug discovery and development. Nat Drug Discov 2003;2:566–80.

[27] Gilron I, Bailey JM, Tu D, Holden RH, Weaver DF, Houlden RL. Morphine, gabapentin, or their combination for neuropathic pain. N Engl J Med 2005;352:1324–34.

[28] Giordano J, Daleo C, Sacks SM. Topical ondansetron attenuates nociceptive and inflammatory effects of intradermal capsaicin in humans. Eur J Pharmacol 1998;354:R13–4.

[29] Gottrup H, Bach FW, Arendt-Nielsen L, Jensen TS. Peripheral lidocaine but not ketamine inhibits capsaicin-induced hyperalgesia in humans. Br J Anaesth 2000;85:520–8.

[30] Gottrup H, Hansen PO, Arendt-Nielsen L, Jensen TS. Differential effects of systemically administered ketamine and lidocaine on dynamic and static hyperalgesia induced by intradermal capsaicin in humans. Br J Anaesth 2000;84:155–62.

[31] Gottrup H, Juhl G, Kristensen AD, Lai R, Chizh BA, Brown J, Bach FW, Jensen TS. Chronic oral gabapentin reduces elements of central sensitization in human experimental hyperalgesia. Anesthesiology 2004;101:1400–8.

[32] Gustorff B, Anzenhofer S, Sycha T, Lehr S, Kress HG. The sunburn pain model: the stability of primary and secondary hyperalgesia over 10 hours in a crossover setting. Anesth Analg 2004;98:173–7.

[33] Gustorff B, Hoechtl K, Sycha T, Felouzis E, Lehr S, Kress HG. The effects of remifentanil and gabapentin on hyperalgesia in a new extended inflammatory skin pain model in healthy volunteers. Anesth Analg 2003;98:401–7.

[34] Hamilton SG, Warburton J, Bhattacharjee A, Ward J, McMahon SB. ATP in human skin elicits a dose-related pain response which is potentiated under conditions of hyperalgesia. Brain 2000;123:1238–46.

[35] Hempenstall K, Nurmikko TJ, Johnson RW, A'Hern RP, Rice ASC. Analgesic therapy in postherpetic neuralgia: a quantitative systematic review. PLoS Med 2005;2:e164.

[36] Hill R. NK1 (substance P) receptor antagonists: why are they not analgesic in humans? Trends Pharmacol Sci 2000;21:244–6.

[37] Hughes A, Macleod A, Growcott J, Thomas I. Assessment of the reproducibility of intradermal administration of capsaicin as a model for inducing human pain. Pain 2002;99:323–31.

[38] Immke DC, Gavva NR. The TRPV1 receptor and nociception. Semin Cell Dev Biol 2006;17:582–91.

[39] Jones SF, McQuay HJ, Moore RA, Hand CW. Morphine and ibuprofen compared using the cold pressor test. Pain 1988;34:117–22.

[40] Kinnman E, Nygårds EB, Hansson-P. Effects of dextromethorphan in clinical doses on capsaicin-induced ongoing pain and mechanical hypersensitivity. J Pain Symptom Manage 1997;14:195–201.

[41] Kinnman E, Nygårds EB, Hansson P. Peripherally administered morphine attenuates capsaicin-induced mechanical hypersensitivity in humans. Anesth Analg 1997;84:595–9.

[42] Klede M, Handwerker HO, Schmelz M. Central origin of secondary mechanical hyperalgesia. J Neurophysiol 2002;90:353–9.

[43] Kola I, Landis J. Can the pharmaceutical industry reduce attrition rates? Nat Rev 2004;3:711–5.

[44] Koltzenburg M, Lundberg LE, Torebjork HE. Dynamic and static components of mechanical hyperalgesia in human hairy skin. Pain 1992;51:207–19.

[45] Koppert W, Ostermeier N, Sittl R, Weidner C, Schmelz M. Low-dose lidocaine reduces secondary hyperalgesia by a central mode of action. Pain 2000;85:217–24.

[46] Koppert W, Angst M, Alsheimer M, Sittl R, Albrecht S, Schuttler J, Schmelz M. Naloxone provokes similar pain facilitation as observed after short-term infusion of remifentanil in humans. Pain 2003;106:91–9.

[47] Koppert W, Dern SK, Sittl R, Albrecht S, Schuttler J, Schmelz M. A new model of electrically evoked pain and hyperalgesia in human skin, Anesthesiology 2001;95:395–402.

[48] Koppert W, Filitz J, Tröster, A, Ihmsen A, Angst M, Flor H, Schüttler J, Schmelz M. Activation of naloxone-sensitive and insensitive inhibitory systems in a human pain model. J Pain 2005;6:757–64.

[49] Koppert W, Ihmsen H, Korber N, Wehrfritz A, Sittl R, Schmelz M, Schuttler J. Different profiles of buprenorphine-induced analgesia and antihyperalgesia in a human pain model, Pain 2005;118:15–22.

[50] Koppert W, Sittl R, Scheuber K, Alsheimer M, Schmelz M, Schüttler J. Differential modulation of remifentanil-induced analgesia and postinfusion hyperalgesia by s-ketamine and clonidine in humans. Anesthesiology 2003;99:152–9.

[51] Koppert W, Wehrfritz A, Korber N, Sittl R, Albrecht S, Ihmsen H, Schuttler J, Schmelz M. The cyclooxygenase isozyme inhibitors parecoxib and paracetamol reduce central hyperalgesia in humans. Pain 2004;108:148–53.

[52] Lorenz J, Beck H, Bromm B. Differential changes of laser evoked potentials, late auditory evoked potentials and P300 under morphine in chronic pain patients. Electroencephalogr Clin Neurophysiol 1997;104:514–21.

[53] Marnett LJ. The COXIB experience: a look in the rearview mirror. Annu Rev Pharmacol Toxicol 2009;49:265–90.

[54] McGivern JG. Ziconotide: a review of its pharmacology and use in the treatment of pain. Neuropsychiatr Dis Treat 2007;3:69–85.

[55] Mitsis GD, Iannetti GD, Smart TS, Tracey I, Wise RG. Regions of interest analysis in pharmacological fMRI: How do the definition criteria influence the inferred result? Neuroimage 2008;40:121–32.

[56] Moore RA, McQuay HJ. Single-patient data meta-analysis of 3453 postoperative patients: oral tramadol versus placebo, codeine and combination analgesics. Pain 1997;69:287–94.

[57] Ørstavik K, Namer B, Schmidt R, Schmelz M, Hilliges M, Weidner C, Carr RW, Handwerker H, Jørum E, Torebjo HE. Abnormal function of C-fibers in patients with diabetic neuropathy. J Neurosci 2006;26:11287–94.

[58] Owen DG, Bureau Y, Thomas AW, Prato FS, St. Lawrence KS. Quantification of pain-induced changes in cerebral blood flow by perfusion MRI. Pain 2008;136:85–96.

[59] Park KM, Max MB, Robinovitz E, Gracely RH, Bennett GJ. Effects of intravenous ketamine, alfentanil, or placebo on pain, pinprick hyperalgesia, and allodynia produced by intradermal capsaicin in human subjects. Pain 1995;63:163–72.

[60] Petersen KL, Rowbotham MC: A new human experimental pain model: the heat/capsaicin sensitization model. Neuroreport 1999;10:1511–6.

[61] Plaghki L, Mouraux A. EEG and laser stimulation as tools for pain research. Curr Opin Investig Drugs 2005;6:58–64.

[62] Rolke R, Magerl W, Campbell KA, Schalber C, Caspari S, Birklein F, Treede R-D. Quantitative sensory testing: a comprehensive protocol for clinical trials. Eur J Pain 2006;10:77–88.

[63] Schulte H, Sollevi A, Segerdahl M. Dose-dependent effects of morphine on experimentally induced cutaneous pain in healthy volunteers. Pain 2005;116:366–74.

[64] Schweinhardt P, Glynn C, Brooks J, McQuay H, Jack T, Chessell I, Bountra C, Tracey I. An fMRI study of cerebral processing of brush-evoked allodynia in neuropathic pain patients. Neuroimage 2006;32:256–65.

[65] Segerdahl M. Multiple dose gabapentin attenuates cutaneous pain and central sensitisation but not muscle pain in healthy volunteers. Pain 2006;125:158–64.

[66] Selak I. Pregabalin (Pfizer). Curr Opin Investig Drugs 2001;2:828–34.

[67] Serra J, Campero M, Bostock H, Ochoa J. Two types of C nociceptors in human skin and their behavior in areas of capsaicin-induced secondary hyperalgesia. J Neurophysiol 2004;91:2770–81.

[68] Sethna NF, Liu M, Gracely R, Bennett GJ, Max MB. Analgesic and cognitive effects of intravenous ketamine-alfentanil combinations versus either drug alone after intradermal capsaicin in normal subjects. Anesth Analg 1998;86:1250–6.

[69] Sultan A, Gaskell H, Derry S, Moore RA. Duloxetine for painful diabetic neuropathy and fibromyalgia pain: systematic review of randomised trials. BMC Neurol 2008;8:29.

[70] Sultana SR, Roblin D, O'Connell D. Translational research in the pharmaceutical industry: from theory to reality. Drug Discov Today 2007;12:419–25.

[71] Sycha T, Gustorff B, Lehr S, Tanew A, Eichler HG, Schmetterer L. A simple pain model for the evaluation of analgesic effects of NSAIDs in healthy subjects. Br J Clin Pharmacol 2003;56:165–72.

[72] Tracey I. Nociceptive processing in the human brain. Curr Opin Neurobiol 2005;15:478–87.

[73] Tracey I, Johns E. The pain matrix: Reloaded or reborn as we image tonic pain using arterial spin labelling. Pain 2010;148:359–60.

[74] Troster A, Sittl R, Singler B, Schmelz M, Schuttler J, Koppert W. Modulation of remifentanil-induced analgesia and postinfusion hyperalgesia by parecoxib in humans, Anesthesiology 2006;105:1016–23.

[75] Van der Schueren BJ, de Hoon JN, Vanmolkot FH, Van Hecken A, Depré M, Kane SA, De Lepeleire I, Sinclair SR. Reproducibility of the capsaicin-induced dermal blood flow response as assessed by laser Doppler perfusion imaging. Br J Clin Pharmacol 2007;64:580–90.

[76] Van der Schueren BJ, Rogiers A, Vanmolkot FH, Van Hecken A, Depré M, Kane SA, De Lepeleire I, Sinclair SR, de Hoon JN. Calcitonin gene-related peptide$_{8-37}$ antagonizes capsaicin-induced vasodilation in the skin: evaluation of a human in vivo pharmacodynamic model. J Pharmacol Exp Ther 2008;325:248–55.

[77] Wallace MS, Barger D, Schulteis G. The effect of chronic oral desipramine on capsaicin-induced allodynia and hyperalgesia: a double-blinded, placebo-controlled, crossover study. Anesth Analg 2002;95:973–8.

[78] Wallace MS, Braun J, Schulteis G. Postdelivery of alfentanil and ketamine has no effect on intradermal capsaicin-induced pain and hyperalgesia. Clin J Pain 2002;18:373–9.

[79] Wallace MS, Laitin S, Licht D, Yaksh TL. Concentration-effect relations for intravenous lidocaine infusions in human volunteers: effects on acute sensory thresholds and capsaicin-evoked hyperpathia. Anesthesiology 1997;86:1262–72.

[80] Wallace MS, Quessy S, Schulteis G. Lack of effect of two oral sodium channel antagonists, lamotrigine and 4030W92, on intradermal capsaicin-induced hyperalgesia model. Pharm Biochem Behav 2004;78:349–55.

[81] Wallace MS, Ridgeway B 3rd, Leung A, Schulteis G, Yaksh TL. Concentration-effect relationships for intravenous alfentanil and ketamine infusions in human volunteers: effects on acute thresholds and capsaicin-evoked hyperpathia. J Clin Pharm 2002;42:70–80.

Correspondence to: John P. Huggins, PhD, Lead Clinician and Senior Director, Pfizer Pharmatherapeutics, Sandwich, Kent, CT13 9NJ, United Kingdom. Email: john.p.huggins@pfizer.com.

Issues Relating to the Clinical Development Process of New Analgesics

Steve Quessy, PhD

qd consulting, LLC, Durham, North Carolina, USA

Background

Despite a rich expansion in biological targets for pain over the past 10 years, there have been many translational failures from animal models to humans [43,45]. These new targets represent mechanisms of action that are unprecedented, meaning there is little or no body of clinical experience to guide a development pathway. Many, if not all, have plausible potential for a variety of indications including inflammatory pain, neuropathic pain, migraine, gastrointestinal disorders, and many nonpain conditions. A drug mechanism that represents a common target for multiple disorders has efficiency at the drug discovery level, as there is a higher chance of development in at least one potential indication. The challenge of prioritizing the target population for initial testing of a new drug for a "proof-of-concept" study is a real-life occurrence in analgesic drug development. Some issues affecting analgesic drug development that were identified in a joint workshop of the U.S. National Institutes of Health (NIH) and the U.S. Food and Drug Administration (FDA) in 2002 are shown in Table I.

It is estimated that 35–50 million people in the United States have some type of chronic pain. The economic cost in quality of life is estimated at over US$100 billion in the United States and at US$1 trillion across developed countries, yet access to safe and effective pain treatments remains an issue. It is estimated that clinically meaningful pain relief is only effected in 30% of patients suffering pain [21,46], and the majority of analgesics in the armamentarium have significant safety issues [80]. Nonmedical use of opioids is increasing, and misuse, abuse, accidental exposure or serious adverse complication related to products containing opioids, nonsteroidal anti-inflammatory drugs (NSAIDs), and acetaminophen (paracetamol) is a major cause of emergency room visits, with over 250,000 visits in the United States in 2006 [80]. More effective drugs with easier-to-manage risks are clearly needed.

This chapter is organized into three main sections. First, I discuss a number of challenges that are particularly pertinent to Phase 2 development of a new analgesic, although many of the same challenges are relevant throughout later phases of development. Second, I discuss challenges confronting meeting the need to gain regulatory approval for one or more pain indication. Third, I discuss the challenge of viability post-approval.

The Phase 2 or "Proof-of-Concept" Challenge

Most companies would like to do a single "killer" experiment; that is, to make a rational "go or no-go" decision based on one, or maybe two, relatively small and short-duration studies. No one entity has the resources to

Pain 2010—An Updated Review: Refresher Course Syllabus
edited by Jeffrey S. Mogil
IASP Press, Seattle, © 2010

Table I
Issues affecting analgesic drug development identified at the
2002 NIH-FDA analgesic drug development workshop

Animal models of pain are not predictive of the clinical situation.
Clinical models of pain not representative of the heterogeneous population (inclusion criteria are too restrictive for generalization).
No consensus on a pain measure that is applicable across all pain conditions (impedes meta-analyses).
Development is focused on monotherapy, whereas in clinical practice chronic pain is treated by combination therapy.
Novel drugs should address mechanisms contributing to the pain condition.
FDA guidelines are deficient, especially for chronic pain.

Source: Adapted from Dionne and Witter [11].

run multiple, large, independent studies to make such a decision, and even in large companies with huge resources, an early poor result will have to compete for resources against other potential products in the portfolio. Standard study designs do not readily allow testing more than one hypothesis at a time, nor are they amenable to testing multiple sets of conditions. With so many choices for selecting the right study (i.e., an optimum trial to answer the basic go or no-go question), one must prioritize which patient population to test initially amongst the many plausible conditions. (We will put aside the issue of choosing among various plausible diseases as outside the scope of this chapter, and assume that a pain population trial is one of the priorities). In practice, this process may be influenced by the perceived size of the indication, regulatory precedent for the indication, competitive landscape, and development economics. However, this choice has consequences, as even a truly effective drug could fail at the early stages of development due to inappropriate choice of population or its characteristics, dose, duration of trial, and so on.

The key questions to be addressed in the early stages of a novel analgesic are:

1) Does it have activity? (i.e., is this drug worth further investment?)

2) Under what conditions does it work or fail to work? (i.e., what types of medical need does it address?)

3) What is a dose range is of interest? (i.e., what is the balance of efficacy and tolerability?)

The early-stage development plan should provide actionable information on these issues. For some additional insights, please refer to the background materials from the IMMPACT IX meeting, available at www.immpact.org/meetings/Immpact9/background (accessed February 21, 2010).

The Challenge in Choosing What Compounds to Select for Study

The pool of available analgesic candidates depends on the status of basic research knowledge, and the strategic decisions and priorities made by research institutions on which targets to pursue (and just as importantly those not pursued). Analgesic drug candidates are advanced based on fulfilling a variety of development characteristics, but predictions made from animal pain behavioral models remain a key factor in drug selection. However, it has become clear that the current models of experimental pain in rodents are poorly predictive in terms of patient populations likely to respond [11,43,45,48,53]. There have been many failures of promising drug candidates with novel mechanisms of action [9,33,43,45,48,53]. The extent to which these results reflect failure of predictive validity from animal models, clinical trial design flaws, or inappropriate selection of the study population characteristics is not known [9,33,43,48,50,53,72] (also refer to the chapter in this volume by A.S.C. Rice). Despite the failure of neurokinin-1 antagonists in acute pain, migraine, osteoarthritis, and neuropathic pain, there was evidence of on-target activity such as antidepressant and antiemetic effects [30]. In other examples failure of the mechanism itself is less clear, although in several cases the sensory responses in rodent models upon which the drugs were selected were not translated to humans [24,77,78]. Therefore, for new analgesics with an unprecedented mechanism of action (i.e., without existing clinical experience), the development risk remains high.

The Challenge of What "Indication" to Target

Target indications and study populations are influenced by medical need and practice, but they are also heavily influenced by commercial factors and regulatory agency philosophy. The current process by which labeled indications are structured and approved by regulatory agencies remains a challenge because it channels clinical development pathways toward indications (usually narrowly defined) with regulatory precedent, constrains alternative development pathways due to perceived higher risks, and imposes barriers to seamless expansion or broadening indications. For example, to date the U.S. FDA has limited approved indications to the actual population studied (usually requiring two trials in each type). Although there appears to be some flexibility to allow a more general chronic pain indication, as of 2009 no drug had gained approval for a chronic pain indication. In Europe there has been more flexibility in the structure of indications for neuropathic pain (for example more general indications for peripheral and central neuropathic pains). Establishing the regulatory process for new indications can be lengthy, iterative, and full of uncertainties, often to the disadvantage of the innovator. It took a long time to obtain drug approvals in fibromyalgia syndrome (FMS). Three products have been approved for FMS in the United States but so far none in Europe. As of 2009, no drug had been approved for chronic low back pain (CLBP). There is no template for targeting indications in orofacial pain disorders and visceral pain. Downstream, labeled indications matter because the label (the package insert or summary of product characteristics) has an impact on medical practice and reimbursement and strictly controls what a manufacturer may communicate about a product. Because pain is a major symptom in such a wide variety of diseases, the interplay of development decisions and requirements for approval of pain indications presents a greater challenge in the development of analgesics than perhaps applies in most other areas.

The Challenge of Who We Choose to Study

There are many types of neuropathic and inflammatory pain conditions, necessitating choices dependent on accepted disease definitions and diagnostic criteria or on definition of specific patient characteristics. Furthermore, the incidences of the various pain conditions cover a wide range (e.g., from less than 0.3% for trigeminal neuralgia to 10–15% for osteoarthritis), and in some cases they are poorly characterized. Treatment usage ranges from a high-volume but short treatment course (postoperative pain) to a low-volume but lifetime treatment course (chronic pains). These factors combined not only affect what patient populations are available for clinical trials, but also influence commercial attractiveness, selection of dose forms, and range of dose strength.

Issues in Selecting the Pain Population

Choosing an efficient clinical development plan is a lot easier if there is already clinical and regulatory precedent to guide the pathway. Selective cyclooxygenase-2 (COX-2) inhibitors (coxibs) were able to follow the well-established clinical models successful for earlier classes of NSAIDs, namely third molar tooth extraction and osteoarthritis studies. Confirmation of this pathway for the first COX-2 inhibitors, celecoxib and rofecoxib, was enabling for subsequent coxibs (e.g., valdecoxib, etoricoxib, and lumiracoxib). The development of pregabalin relied heavily on the known clinical profile of gabapentin [29,40], which was first introduced for epilepsy and was subsequently found to be effective in neuropathic pain, such as postherpetic neuralgia (PHN) and painful diabetic neuropathy (PDN) [1,56]. Thus, initially testing pregabalin in PHN and PDN was a relatively straightforward decision [42,54,60]. Duloxetine was initially targeted as an antidepressant, but early on it was explored in neuropathic pain indications in line with the wealth of clinical knowledge about tricyclic antidepressants [21], as well as a number of pain trials on venlafaxine [58]. This pathway was enabling for a number of other monamine reuptake inhibitors that entered development during this time. The development of tapentadol adopted the body of knowledge on tramadol as well as opioid analgesics. Initial studies of tramadol were in acute postoperative pain [71] and subsequently in osteoarthritis and PDN [7,28]. A similar path was used for tapentadol.

Although these established models have served well for the above examples, this may not hold true for new drugs with little or no clinical precedent. The question becomes: How does one decide the right population for proof-of-concept in the absence of clinical precedent? The question is more complex if there is no evidence yet for a desired biological effect in any other potential population.

Issues in Defining Patient Characteristics

Having selected a population (disease etiology), the issue becomes defining inclusion/exclusion criteria to maximize the chance of detecting a signal. The tendency has been to select a single homogeneous population, to reduce unwanted noise from the experiment, and, for consistency with regulatory notions, to determine a rigorously defined target population. However, choices made in the selection criteria affect not only inference to the wider real-world population (which can affect a drug's degree of success post-approval) but also the success of the study if the wrong population characteristics are selected.

Most trials have attempted to exclude subjects who may be unlikely to be responsive. This can mean excluding prior nonresponders to similar therapy (for example, early trials of pregabalin excluded subjects who did not respond to or tolerate gabapentin) [70], excluding subjects who have failed multiple prior therapies (and are assumed to be treatment refractory) [23,68], and including only those who have shown response to or who tolerate a similar therapy (for example, many opioid trials recruited subjects already stabilized on and benefiting from an established opioid regimen) [44,49]. NSAID/coxib and opioid trials commonly required a worsening (or flare-up) of symptoms on washout of prior NSAID or opioid therapy [37,61]. This practice enriched for subjects likely to be responders to the test NSAID/coxib or opioid. Alternative approaches include the use of pharmacological probes such as enrichment based on test responses to intravenous lidocaine, fentanyl, or capsaicin challenge [9].

In animal models the common efficacy measures are mechanical and thermal hyperalgesia or allodynia. One could argue that selecting patients with evidence of these symptoms might be an attractive approach to proof-of-concept or proof-of-mechanism. However, two proof-of-concept trials in which patients were specifically selected to have well-defined allodynia symptoms did not reproduce in humans the corresponding sensory testing results on which the compounds were selected in animal studies [77,78]. A more recent study of topical ketamine in patients with complex regional pain syndrome (CRPS) and well-defined allodynia was more successful [20]. Phenotyping patients on specific signs and symptoms rather than on disease etiology may be a more promising approach to defining patient populations for study. The work of the German Research Network on Neuropathic Pain in sensory mapping of various pain syndromes holds promise to be enabling for such trials [2,55].

How We Design Trials

In the early phase of clinical development there is a need for trial designs that are efficient with regard to patient sample size; this requirement is for reasons of economics and time-to-decision as well as for reasons of ethics (to ensure minimum exposure to ineffective or potentially harmful test analgesics). The advantages and disadvantages of various trial designs have been discussed previously [14,33,44,49,57,63]. Crossover designs in general provide a high level of efficiency when limited sample size is the goal, and these designs have been employed for proof-of-concept trials, with varying degrees of success [20,38,39,49,77,78]. In general,

a condition with expectation of a relatively stable pain for the duration of the trial is necessary in crossover designs, but episodic pain is also suitable, and many trials in migraine or cancer breakthrough pain have employed multi-crossover arms with interspersed placebo and active treatment sessions [49]. Crossover designs become less practical compared to parallel group designs when there are more than two treatment arms. Trials aimed at drug approval tend to employ randomized parallel group designs—usually with fixed dose assignments—because this is the accepted evidentiary design standard [16,33]. The expectation by regulatory agencies (e.g., FDA, EMEA) for analgesic trials is for exposure to fixed doses (covering the proposed label dose range) for a period of 8 to 24 weeks, depending on the indicated population.

The two greatest challenges in studies with this design are: (1) the impact of a high placebo response in many pain populations on the ability to demonstrate a clinically meaningful drug response [33,50,81], and (2) the data analysis issue for those subjects who do not complete the trial. Imputation of missing data is a controversial issue that will not be discussed here; suffice it say that for drugs requiring a lengthy titration to assigned dose for safety or tolerability reasons (e.g., opioids and many anticonvulsant drugs), the impact of missing data is even greater. Therefore, strategies to minimize dropout from the trial are important, and the FDA in particular appears to be becoming more flexible with respect to this problem. However, there is still a need for new approaches to exploratory trial designs [31,49,57].

Issues Relating to Dose and Dose Regimen

A range of doses for early trials is usually established from the safety and tolerability profile in human Phase 1 trials and from allometric scaling from pharmacokinetic/pharmacodynamic modeling in animal models. The number of dose levels that are tested directly affects the size, cost, complexity, and time to completion of a trial. Selecting the highest well-tolerated dose has been a popular option if no titration is required [77,78], but it leads to problems if too many subjects do not tolerate the drug for the full trial duration, or if this dose is suboptimal for patients who might have tolerated a higher dose. Flexible dosing options have been used to overcome this issue—in essence patients are titrated individually to their highest well-tolerated dose [1,52,56,62,76]. This strategy is attractive, but it confounds time with dose such that the effective dose may be overestimated if onset is slow. Strategies for minimizing dropouts for intolerable adverse events within the randomized, assigned dose design include: allowing one-step dose reduction if the assigned dose is not tolerated [26,52,72], allowing for at least one arm to be fixed/flexible dosing (a minimum dose with progression to the maximum level only if the minimum dose is tolerated) [67], and randomized reassignment of the active arm to the same dose or a higher dose during the trial [8]. An alternative design is to select and randomize only those subjects who tolerate the test drug. Examples of this approach include the enriched-enrollment randomized withdrawal design [44] and related enrichment designs [49]. Because the randomization point occurs after selection of those who tolerate the test drug (and usually also those who respond to it), this design has the advantage of minimizing post-randomization dropouts and the consequent impact of imputing missing data. The endpoint of interest in these designs becomes loss of effect rather than improvement. Enrichment designs have many of the same drawbacks as crossover designs, particularly carry-over effects and issues of unblinding due to prior exposure of the test drug, and they have been criticized [69], but they may offer a number of powerful advantages for early proof-of-concept trials [49].

More recent proposals for improving the efficiency of clinical trials (especially multi-arm dose-response trials) involve the use of adaptive designs [13,25]. An adaptive design involves a multistep process that utilizes accumulating data within the study to modify (adapt) design elements such as sample size, treatment allocation, or termination according to pre-defined decision rules. To date, the focus has been on adaptive allocation of dose (for efficiency in optimum dose selection) and on staged interim analyses with predefined decision rules to allow adaptive modification of dose (dropping of doses or adding new doses), adjustment of the final sample size, or termination of the study. There have been few attempts to explore the power of adaptive type designs in analgesic studies, although the approach has been reported in migraine [27,41,66] and anesthesia [12] trials.

Issues in Defining Background Therapy

Most pain trials have been conducted as monotherapy, with all prior analgesics discontinued during a baseline phase prior to randomization [33,35]. One reason for this methodology is to avoid confounding, but the perception that resultant labeling would limit the product to second-line therapy is a commercial consideration. Uncritical application of this decision path may preclude understanding the best way to use a drug. If a trial fails in a monotherapy design, would it have been successful as add-on therapy? Because the underlying mechanisms driving pain are not unitary, the expectation that a single drug would be sufficient to overcome significant pain in a chronic pain trial may be unrealistic [51]. There is no clear rationale for whether monotherapy or add-on therapy design is the best initial approach. There is some advocacy for allowing concomitant background therapy in partial responders whose pain intensity is above a pre-specified threshold [16].

Issues on Active Control

The purpose of an active control is usually assay sensitivity. Many postoperative pain (acute pain) trials have included both placebo and active control arms [4,19,59,74]. Many trials of coxibs in osteoarthritis have also included placebo and active control (e.g., NSAID) [10,22]. This method allows scientific interpretation of the result (e.g., if the test drug fails but the positive control works) as well as allowing a level of benchmarking for relative effect (e.g., peak effect or duration). Few trials in neuropathic pain have included a positive control arm. Some reasons include lack of confidence in the test drug, impact on total sample size, and cost/time. The disadvantage is that many unexpectedly negative trials are hard to interpret.

How We Measure Pain: Issues Relating to Endpoints

Choosing the right endpoint is important. Most studies use a primary endpoint of change in pain intensity score—on a visual analogue scale (VAS) or numerical rating scale (NRS)—from baseline to the average over the last week of the trial. This approach is the one recommended by the IMMPACT consortium [15,73]. However, it is common for trials to incorporate many pain-scoring endpoints such as those contained in the Brief Pain Inventory (BPI), the McGill Pain Questionnaire, the Neuropathic Pain Scale, the Western Ontario and McMasters (WOMAC) index for osteoarthritis, or the Gracely Scale [8,65,75,79]. It is recognized, but not well documented in the literature, that individual pain scores vary widely on a day-to-day basis, and that individual pain scores reported in the primary VAS/NRS measures can differ widely from values reported by the same subject in other instruments assessing pain, even though there is tendency for correlation of mean values across instruments [72]. Pain scores also fluctuate depending on whether pain is assessed in the morning or evening. The fact that individuals may report inconsistent responses to the different assessment instruments at the same time, together with the very strong placebo response in many pain trials, suggests that there is still room to explore whether analgesic trials are using too many instruments to assess pain, whether the patient's interpretation of what is being reported is the intended one, and whether there is a best set of instruments or question construction that can distinguish signal from noise.

Challenges Beyond Phase 2: Meeting Standards for Regulatory Approval

Generalizing outcome (either positive or negative) from one population to another is not a straightforward process, or even possible at the current level of understanding. For example, efficacy in osteoarthritis pain does not inform on the likelihood of efficacy in PDN, and vice versa. To add to the problem, efficacy in PDN does not inform on efficacy in other types of neuropathic pain, and efficacy in osteoarthritis of the knee may not be accepted as predictive of osteoarthritis in other locations. Many drugs have reached Phase 3 development based on efficacy in one population, only to fail in new populations. In some cases this outcome may have been due to a failure to conduct careful Phase 2 trials before launching into large Phase 3 trials, and in other cases it may have been lack of correspondence in efficacy between pain conditions. One example is lamotrigine, a drug established as an anticonvulsant, which appeared to be effective in a number of small trials in neuropathic pain (including diabetic neuropathy and HIV-associated neuropathy), but in two large Phase 3 diabetic neuropathy trials [75] and one large Phase 3 HIV-associated neuropathy trial [64], lamotrigine failed to separate from placebo. Topiramate, another established anticonvulsant, also failed in three large Phase 3 trials in diabetic neuropathy [72]. Pregabalin, which was originally approved as an anticonvulsant and for PHN and PDN, has subsequently shown mixed results in other types of neuropathic pain or chronic pain [47,65,76]. Bupropion, an established antidepressant with evidence of efficacy in a small mixed neuropathic pain trial, failed in a CLBP trial [34].

There are many potential reasons for attrition in Phase 3, and while most are not unique to analgesics, the rate of attrition for analgesics does seem to be above average. By far the greatest challenge in Phase 3 analgesic trials is the placebo effect in long-term trials [33,50]. The combined interactions of a placebo response and analytic methods for handling missing data for dropouts is making it difficult to achieve positive results that meet regulatory evidentiary requirements using standard designs. The problem is compounded for drugs that are poorly tolerated initially, or that require a titration to effective dose [49]. Despite many attempts at analyzing factors that influence positive or negative outcomes in pain trials [9,14,16,24,32,33,35,36,44,49,50,57,72,81], there is no clear convergence on the "best" way to design and conduct a trial to maximize success. A summary of identified issues thought to affect trial success is given in Table II.

Table II
Factors associated with study failure or high placebo response

Study Factor	Ref.
Baseline pain scores too low (sensitivity)	33
Too many treatment groups (anticipation)	
Forced fixed dose levels (flexible dosing regimen reduces dropouts)	
Unrealistic patient expectations (motivations)	
Influences/communications by site personnel	
Inability to identify and select out placebo responders (noise)	
Selection of pain instrument different from primary endpoint instrument (sensitivity loss on primary endpoint)	72
Pain questionnaire is not specific to painful location (sensitivity)	
Analgesic use allowed during washout period (confounded baseline)	
Analgesic washout period prior to randomization too short (unstable baseline)	
Long-term placebo response (sensitivity)	
Impact of early dropouts during titration period (i.e., before achieving assigned target dose)	75
Long-term placebo response (sensitivity)	
Centers with rapid recruitment associated with greater placebo response	32

Source: Compilations from sources shown.

As development progresses to trial exposures of longer duration and in a broader range of populations, some of the following issues may arise that affect the probability of success or the timing of potential approval.

• Tachyphylaxis may occur (a loss of effect over time) (this issue applies to opioids).

- There may be an unacceptable safety profile or poor toleration at doses anticipated for effectiveness (which applies to many anticonvulsant type drugs used as analgesics).

- There may be unanticipated serious toxicity on long-term exposure or rare events that are difficult to predict (examples include liver toxicity associated with lumiracoxib or duloxetine and thromboembolic events with rofecoxib and other coxibs).

- New safety findings can cause delays in the development process (e.g., pregabalin had a development hiatus for more than a year due to a mouse hemangiosarcoma finding during animal safety studies).

- Regulatory agency review issues may delay approval, usually reflecting an evolution of regulatory expectations in the dossier while the review is ongoing. For example, the duloxetine chronic pain indication dossier was withdrawn and resubmitted; a topical fentanyl product approval was delayed while criteria for a risk evaluation and mitigation strategy [REMS] were defined; and the acute pain indication for celecoxib was delayed, although other indications were approved.

- New safety findings with related drugs can have a global impact on pending reviews and development plan requirements for similar classes of drugs. The classic example is the thromboembolic findings in a rofecoxib outcome trial aimed at establishing a reduced risk of gastrointestinal toxicity [3]. The resulting debate had a profound impact on the pending FDA reviews of etoricoxib and lumiracoxib, which resulted in neither drug gaining approval in the United States despite controlled, randomized outcome trials in over 20,000 patients in each submission [5,6,17,18]. There were several other coxibs in late-stage development at that time, and those programs shut down shortly after.

Challenges Beyond Approval: Market Viability

Clinical development and accumulation of risk-benefit information do not cease with approval, nor with patent expiration. New or more appropriate uses of older drugs as analgesics have been developed, along with advances in basic science and clinical experience (e.g., the use of tricyclic antidepressants as analgesics to treat neuropathic pain; the use of propranolol for migraine; and epidural, topical, and transdermal drug delivery). Expansion of indications is often cost-effective after initial approval (e.g., clinical development plans

for various coxib drugs were exploring CLBP, gouty arthritis, and ankylosing spondylitis before their withdrawal from the market; various other types of neuropathic pain were explored with pregabalin; duloxetine is being explored in osteoarthritis and CLBP).

Safety signals identified post-launch may lead to a need for additional studies, revised labeling, or stricter warnings and in extreme cases withdrawal from the market. In the past 50 years, at least 15 analgesic drugs have been removed from the marketplace in Europe and North America for safety issues, including five in the 10-year period from 1998 to 2007: bromfenac (hepatotoxicity), rofecoxib and valdecoxib (cardiovascular safety), lumiracoxib (hepatotoxicity), and propoxyphene (abuse/risk-benefit). In addition, potent opioids such as fentanyl-containing products and extended-release morphine- and oxycodone-containing products have come under increasing scrutiny, restrictions, and label warnings regarding potential for abuse and diversion. In fact, during the past 10 years or so, almost all analgesic products (both prescription and over-the-counter) have undergone renewed scrutiny for issues relating to abuse, addiction, serious adverse events, and death (accidental or suicidal) [80]. The safety of acetaminophen and acetaminophen-containing products was the subject of an FDA review in June, 2009. The safety of all NSAIDs was the subject of FDA and European Medicines Agency (EMEA) review in mid-2005 following worldwide withdrawal of rofecoxib from the market, which led to significant strengthening of warnings and recommendations for use. In February, 2009, the FDA required all manufacturers of potent opioid products to institute a REMS program to address abuse and misuse of these products. Anticonvulsant drugs and antidepressant drugs with analgesic indications (e.g., pregabalin and duloxetine) have new class warnings around the need for tapering dose or for suicidal ideation. Hepatoxicity warnings were strengthened in the labeling of duloxetine in October, 2005.

These issues that accumulate with ongoing clinical experience with drugs also feed back into the challenges in developing new analgesics by raising the bar on the number and type of clinical data that need to be generated. They also affect the expectations for commitments in the peri-post-approval period. As a result, the size and cost of preapproval clinical programs are inflated. The impact is particularly challenging for analgesic drugs, not just because of their safety history and drug abuse issues, but also because of the wide variation in populations in whom safety needs to be demonstrated.

References

[1] Backonja M, Beydoun A, Edwards KR, Schwartz SL, Fonseca V, Hes M, Lamoreaux L, Garofalo E. Gabapentin for the symptomatic treatment of painful neuropathy in patients with diabetes mellitus: a randomized controlled trial. JAMA 1998;280:1831–6.

[2] Baron R, Tolle TR, Gockel U, Brosz M, Freynhagen R. A cross-sectional cohort survey in 2100 patients with painful diabetic neuropathy and postherpetic neuralgia: differences in demographic data and sensory symptoms. Pain 2009;146:34–40.

[3] Bombardier C, Laine L, Reicin A, Shapiro D, Burgos-Vargas R, Davis B, Day R, Ferraz MB, Hawkey CJ, Hochberg MC, et al. Comparison of upper gastrointestinal toxicity of rofecoxib and naproxen in patients with rheumatoid arthritis. VIGOR Study Group. N Engl J Med 2000;343:1520–8.

[4] Bulley S, Derry S, Moore RA, McQuay HJ. Single dose oral rofecoxib for acute postoperative pain in adults. Cochrane Database Syst Rev 2009;CD004604.

[5] Cannon CP, Curtis SP, Bolognese JA, Laine L. Clinical trial design and patient demographics of the Multinational Etoricoxib and Diclofenac Arthritis Long-term (MEDAL) study program: cardiovascular outcomes with etoricoxib versus diclofenac in patients with osteoarthritis and rheumatoid arthritis. Am Heart J 2006;152:237–45.

[6] Cannon CP, Curtis SP, FitzGerald GA, Krum H, Kaur A, Bolognese JA, Reicin AS, Bombardier C, Weinblatt ME, van der HD, et al. Cardiovascular outcomes with etoricoxib and diclofenac in patients with osteoarthritis and rheumatoid arthritis in the Multinational Etoricoxib and Diclofenac Arthritis Long-term (MEDAL) programme: a randomised comparison. Lancet 2006;368:1771–81.

[7] Cepeda MS, Camargo F, Zea C, Valencia L. Tramadol for osteoarthritis: a systematic review and metaanalysis. J Rheumatol 2007;34:543–55.

[8] Chappell AS, Ossanna MJ, Liu-Seifert H, Iyengar S, Skljarevski V, Li LC, Bennett RM, Collins H. Duloxetine, a centrally acting analgesic, in the treatment of patients with osteoarthritis knee pain: a 13-week, randomized, placebo-controlled trial. Pain 2009;146:253–60.

[9] Chizh BA, Priestley T, Rowbotham M, Schaffler K. Predicting therapeutic efficacy: experimental pain in human subjects. Brain Res Rev 2009;60:243–54.

[10] Clemett D, Goa KL. Celecoxib: a review of its use in osteoarthritis, rheumatoid arthritis and acute pain. Drugs 2000;59:957–80.

[11] Dionne RA, Witter J. NIH-FDA Analgesic Drug Development Workshop: translating scientific advances into improved pain relief. Clin J Pain 2003;19:139–47.

[12] Dougherty TB, Porche VH, Thall PF. Maximum tolerated dose of nalmefene in patients receiving epidural fentanyl and dilute bupivacaine for postoperative analgesia. Anesthesiology 2000;92:1010–6.

[13] Dragalin V. Adaptive designs: terminology and classification. Drug Inf J 2006;40:425–35.

[14] Dworkin RH, Katz J, Gitlin MJ. Placebo response in clinical trials of depression and its implications for research on chronic neuropathic pain. Neurology 2005;65:S7–19.

[15] Dworkin RH, Turk DC, Farrar JT, Haythornthwaite JA, Jensen MP, Katz NP, Kerns RD, Stucki G, Allen RR, Bellamy N, et al. Core outcome measures for chronic pain clinical trials: IMMPACT recommendations. Pain 2005;113:9–19.

[16] Dworkin R, Turk D, Peirce-Sandner S, Baron R, Bellamy N, Burke L, Chappell A, Chartier K, Cleeland C, Costello A, et al. Research design considerations for confirmatory chronic pain clinical trials: IMMPACT recommendations. Pain 2010;149;177–93.

[17] Farkouh ME, Greenberg JD, Jeger RV, Ramanathan K, Verheugt FW, Chesebro JH, Kirshner H, Hochman JS, Lay CL, Ruland S, et al. Cardiovascular outcomes in high risk patients with osteoarthritis treated with ibuprofen, naproxen or lumiracoxib. Ann Rheum Dis 2007;66:764–70.

[18] Farkouh ME, Kirshner H, Harrington RA, Ruland S, Verheugt FW, Schnitzer TJ, Burmester GR, Mysler E, Hochberg MC, Doherty M, et al. Comparison of lumiracoxib with naproxen and ibuprofen in the Therapeutic Arthritis Research and Gastrointestinal Event Trial (TARGET), cardiovascular outcomes: randomised controlled trial. Lancet 2004;364:675–84.

[19] Fenton C, Keating GM, Wagstaff AJ. Valdecoxib: a review of its use in the management of osteoarthritis, rheumatoid arthritis, dysmenorrhoea and acute pain. Drugs 2004;64:1231–61.

[20] Finch PM, Knudsen L, Drummond PD. Reduction of allodynia in patients with complex regional pain syndrome: A double-blind placebo-controlled trial of topical ketamine. Pain 2009;146:18–25.

[21] Finnerup NB, Otto M, McQuay HJ, Jensen TS, Sindrup SH. Algorithm for neuropathic pain treatment: an evidence-based proposal. Pain 2005;118:289–305.

[22] Frampton JE, Keating GM. Celecoxib: a review of its use in the management of arthritis and acute pain. Drugs 2007;67:2433–72.

[23] Freynhagen R, Grond S, Schupfer G, Hagebeuker A, Schmelz M, Ziegler D, Von Giesen HJ, Junker U, Wagner KJ, Konrad C. Efficacy and safety of pregabalin in treatment refractory patients with various neuropathic pain entities in clinical routine. Int J Clin Pract 2007;61:1989–96.

[24] Galer BS, Lee D, Ma T, Nagle B, Schlagheck TG. MorphiDex (morphine sulfate/dextromethorphan hydrobromide combination) in the treatment of chronic pain: three multicenter, randomized, double-blind, controlled clinical trials fail to demonstrate enhanced opioid analgesia or reduction in tolerance. Pain 2005;115:284–95.

[25] Gallo P, Chuang-Stein C, Dragalin V, Gaydos B, Krams M, Pinheiro J. Adaptive designs in clinical drug development: an Executive Summary of the PhRMA Working Group. J Biopharm Stat 2006;16:275–83.

[26] Gimbel JS, Richards P, Portenoy RK. Controlled-release oxycodone for pain in diabetic neuropathy: a randomized controlled trial. Neurology 2003;60:927–34.

[27] Hall DB, Meier U, Diener HC. A group sequential adaptive treatment assignment design for proof of concept and dose selection in headache trials. Contemp Clin Trials 2005;26:349–64.

[28] Harati Y, Gooch C, Swenson M, Edelman S, Greene D, Raskin P, Donofrio P, Cornblath D, Sachdeo R, Siu CO, Kamin M. Double-blind randomized trial of tramadol for the treatment of the pain of diabetic neuropathy. Neurology 1998;50:1842–6.

[29] Harden RN. Gabapentin: a new tool in the treatment of neuropathic pain. Acta Neurol Scand Suppl 1999;173:43–7.

[30] Hill R. NK1 (substance P) receptor antagonists: why are they not analgesic in humans? Trends Pharmacol Sci 2000;21:244–6.

[31] Ho TW, Backonja M, Ma J, Leibensperger H, Froman S, Polydefkis M. Efficient assessment of neuropathic pain drugs in patients with small fiber sensory neuropathies. Pain 2009;141:19–24.

[32] Irizarry MC, Webb DJ, Ali Z, Chizh BA, Gold M, Kinrade FJ, Meisner PD, Blum D, Silver MT, Weil JG. Predictors of placebo response in pooled lamotrigine neuropathic pain clinical trials. Clin J Pain 2009;25:469–76.

[33] Katz J, Finnerup NB, Dworkin RH. Clinical trial outcome in neuropathic pain: relationship to study characteristics. Neurology 2008;70:263–72.

[34] Katz J, Pennella-Vaughan J, Hetzel RD, Kanazi GE, Dworkin RH. A randomized, placebo-controlled trial of bupropion sustained release in chronic low back pain. J Pain 2005;6:656–61.

[35] Katz N. Methodological issues in clinical trials of opioids for chronic pain. Neurology 2005;65:S32–49.

[36] Katz N. Enriched enrollment randomized withdrawal trial designs of analgesics: focus on methodology. Clin J Pain 2009;25:797–807.

[37] Katz N, Ju WD, Krupa DA, Sperling RS, Bozalis RD, Gertz BJ, Gimbel J, Coleman S, Fisher C, Nabizadeh S, Borenstein D. Efficacy and safety of rofecoxib in patients with chronic low back pain: results from two 4-week, randomized, placebo-controlled, parallel-group, double-blind trials. Spine (Phila Pa 1976) 2003;28:851–8.

[38] Khoromi S, Cui L, Nackers L, Max MB. Morphine, nortriptyline and their combination vs. placebo in patients with chronic lumbar root pain. Pain 2007;130:66–75.

[39] Khoromi S, Patsalides A, Parada S, Salehi V, Meegan JM, Max MB. Topiramate in chronic lumbar radicular pain. J Pain 2005;6:829–36.

[40] Laird MA, Gidal BE. Use of gabapentin in the treatment of neuropathic pain. Ann Pharmacother 2000;34:802–7.

[41] Lemmens HJ, Wada DR, Munera C, Eltahtawy A, Stanski DR. Enriched analgesic efficacy studies: an assessment by clinical trial simulation. Contemp Clin Trials 2006;27:165–73.

[42] Lesser H, Sharma U, Lamoreaux L, Poole RM. Pregabalin relieves symptoms of painful diabetic neuropathy: a randomized controlled trial. Neurology 2004;63:2104–10.

[43] Mao J. Translational pain research: achievements and challenges. J Pain 2009;10:1001–11.

[44] McQuay HJ, Derry S, Moore RA, Poulain P, Legout V. Enriched enrolment with randomised withdrawal (EERW): time for a new look at clinical trial design in chronic pain. Pain 2008;135:217–20.

[45] Mogil JS. Animal models of pain: progress and challenges. Nat Rev Neurosci 2009;10:283–94.

[46] Moore RA, Moore OA, Derry S, McQuay HJ. Numbers needed to treat calculated from responder rates give a better indication of efficacy in osteoarthritis trials than mean pain scores. Arthritis Res Ther 2008;10:R39.

[47] Pfizer Inc. A randomized placebo-controlled trial of the efficacy and safety of pregabalin in the treatment of subjects with neuropathic pain associated with lumbo-sacral radiculopathy. Protocol No. A0081007. Available at: www.clinicalstudyresults.org.

[48] Quessy SN. Comment on: Animal models and the prediction of efficacy in clinical trials of analgesic drugs: a critical appraisal and a call for uniform reporting standards. Pain 2009;142:284–5.

[49] Quessy SN. Two-stage enriched enrolment pain trials: a brief review of designs and opportunities for broader application. Pain 2010;148:8–13.

[50] Quessy SN, Rowbotham MC. Placebo response in neuropathic pain trials. Pain 2008;138:479–83.

[51] Raja SN, Haythornthwaite JA. Combination therapy for neuropathic pain: which drugs, which combination, which patients? N Engl J Med 2005;352:1373–5.

[52] Rauck RL, Shaibani A, Biton V, Simpson J, Koch B. Lacosamide in painful diabetic peripheral neuropathy: a phase 2 double-blind placebo-controlled study. Clin J Pain 2007;23:150–8.

[53] Rice AS, Cimino-Brown D, Eisenach JC, Kontinen VK, Lacroix-Fralish ML, Machin I, Mogil JS, Stohr T. Animal models and the prediction of efficacy in clinical trials of analgesic drugs: a critical appraisal and call for uniform reporting standards. Pain 2008;139:243–7.

[54] Richter RW, Portenoy R, Sharma U, Lamoreaux L, Bockbrader H, Knapp LE. Relief of painful diabetic peripheral neuropathy with pregabalin: a randomized, placebo-controlled trial. J Pain 2005;6:253–60.

[55] Rolke R, Baron R, Maier C, Tolle TR, Treede RD, Beyer A, Binder A, Birbaumer N, Birklein F, Botefur IC, et al. Quantitative sensory testing in the German Research Network on Neuropathic Pain (DFNS): standardized protocol and reference values. Pain 2006;123:231–43.

[56] Rowbotham M, Harden N, Stacey B, Bernstein P, Magnus-Miller L. Gabapentin for the treatment of postherpetic neuralgia: a randomized controlled trial. JAMA 1998;280:1837–42.

[57] Rowbotham MC. Mechanisms of neuropathic pain and their implications for the design of clinical trials. Neurology 2005;65:S66–73.

[58] Rowbotham MC, Goli V, Kunz NR, Lei D. Venlafaxine extended release in the treatment of painful diabetic neuropathy: a double-blind, placebo-controlled study. Pain 2004;110:697–706.

[59] Roy YM, Derry S, Moore RA. Single dose oral lumiracoxib for postoperative pain. Cochrane Database Syst Rev 2007;CD006865.

[60] Sabatowski R, Galvez R, Cherry DA, Jacquot F, Vincent E, Maisonobe P, Versavel M. Pregabalin reduces pain and improves sleep and mood disturbances in patients with post-herpetic neuralgia: results of a randomised, placebo-controlled clinical trial. Pain 2004;109:26–35.

[61] Scott-Lennox JA, McLaughlin-Miley C, Lennox RD, Bohlig AM, Cutler BL, Yan C, Jaffe M. Stratification of flare intensity identifies placebo responders in a treatment efficacy trial of patients with osteoarthritis. Arthritis Rheum 2001;44:1599–607.

[62] Serpell MG. Gabapentin in neuropathic pain syndromes: a randomised, double-blind, placebo-controlled trial. Pain 2002;99:557–66.

[63] Sheiner LB, Beal SL, Sambol NC. Study designs for dose-ranging. Clin Pharmacol Ther 1989;46:63–77.

[64] Simpson DM, McArthur JC, Olney R, Clifford D, So Y, Ross D, Baird BJ, Barrett P, Hammer AE. Lamotrigine for HIV-associated painful sensory neuropathies: a placebo-controlled trial. Neurology 2003;60:1508–14.

[65] Simpson DM, Schifitto G, Clifford DB, Murphy TK, Durso-De CE, Glue P, Whalen E, Emir B, Scott GN, Freeman R. Pregabalin for painful HIV neuropathy: a randomized, double-blind, placebo-controlled trial. Neurology 2010;74:413–20.

[66] Smith MK, Jones I, Morris MF, Grieve AP, Tan K. Implementation of a Bayesian adaptive design in a proof of concept study. Pharm Stat 2006;5:39–50.

[67] Stacey BR, Barrett JA, Whalen E, Phillips KF, Rowbotham MC. Pregabalin for postherpetic neuralgia: placebo-controlled trial of fixed and flexible dosing regimens on allodynia and time to onset of pain relief. J Pain 2008;9:1006–17.

[68] Stacey BR, Dworkin RH, Murphy K, Sharma U, Emir B, Griesing T. Pregabalin in the treatment of refractory neuropathic pain: results of a 15-month open-label trial. Pain Med 2008;9:1202–8.

[69] Staud R, Price DD. Long-term trials of pregabalin and duloxetine for fibromyalgia symptoms: how study designs can affect placebo factors. Pain 2008;136:232–4.

[70] Straube S, Derry S, McQuay HJ, Moore RA. Enriched enrollment: definition and effects of enrichment and dose in trials of pregabalin and gabapentin in neuropathic pain: a systematic review. Br J Clin Pharmacol 2008;66:266–75.

[71] Sunshine A. New clinical experience with tramadol. Drugs 1994;47(Suppl 1):8–18.

[72] Thienel U, Neto W, Schwabe SK, Vijapurkar U. Topiramate in painful diabetic polyneuropathy: findings from three double-blind placebo-controlled trials. Acta Neurol Scand 2004;110:221–31.

[73] Turk DC, Dworkin RH, Allen RR, Bellamy N, Brandenburg N, Carr DB, Cleeland C, Dionne R, Farrar JT, Galer BS, et al. Core outcome domains for chronic pain clinical trials: IMMPACT recommendations. Pain 2003;106:337–45.

[74] Varner J, Lomax M, Blum D, Quessy S. A randomized, controlled, dose-ranging study investigating single doses of GW406381, naproxen sodium, or placebo in patients with acute pain after third molar tooth extraction. Clin J Pain 2009;25:577–83.

[75] Vinik AI, Tuchman M, Safirstein B, Corder C, Kirby L, Wilks K, Quessy S, Blum D, Grainger J, White J, Silver M. Lamotrigine for treatment of pain associated with diabetic neuropathy: results of two randomized, double-blind, placebo-controlled studies. Pain 2007;128:169–79.

[76] Vranken JH, Dijkgraaf MG, Kruis MR, van der Vegt MH, Hollmann MW, Heesen M. Pregabalin in patients with central neuropathic pain: a randomized, double-blind, placebo-controlled trial of a flexible-dose regimen. Pain 2008;136:150–7.

[77] Wallace MS, Rowbotham M, Bennett GJ, Jensen TS, Pladna R, Quessy S. A multicenter, double-blind, randomized, placebo-controlled crossover evaluation of a short course of 4030W92 in patients with chronic neuropathic pain. J Pain 2002;3:227–33.

[78] Wallace MS, Rowbotham MC, Katz NP, Dworkin RH, Dotson RM, Galer BS, Rauck RL, Backonja MM, Quessy SN, Meisner PD. A randomized, double-blind, placebo-controlled trial of a glycine antagonist in neuropathic pain. Neurology 2002;59:1694–700.

[79] Wernicke JF, Pritchett YL, D'Souza DN, Waninger A, Tran P, Iyengar S, Raskin J. A randomized controlled trial of duloxetine in diabetic peripheral neuropathic pain. Neurology 2006;67:1411–20.

[80] Woodcock J. A difficult balance: pain management, drug safety, and the FDA. N Engl J Med 2009;361:2105–7.

[81] Zhang W, Robertson J, Jones AC, Dieppe PA, Doherty M. The placebo effect and its determinants in osteoarthritis: meta-analysis of randomised controlled trials. Ann Rheum Dis 2008;67:1716–23.

Correspondence to: Steve Quessy, PhD, 20 Wythebrook Lane, Durham, NC 27713, USA. Email: quessy@qd-consulting.com.

Index

Page numbers followed by f refer to figures; page numbers followed by t refer to tables.